I0044596

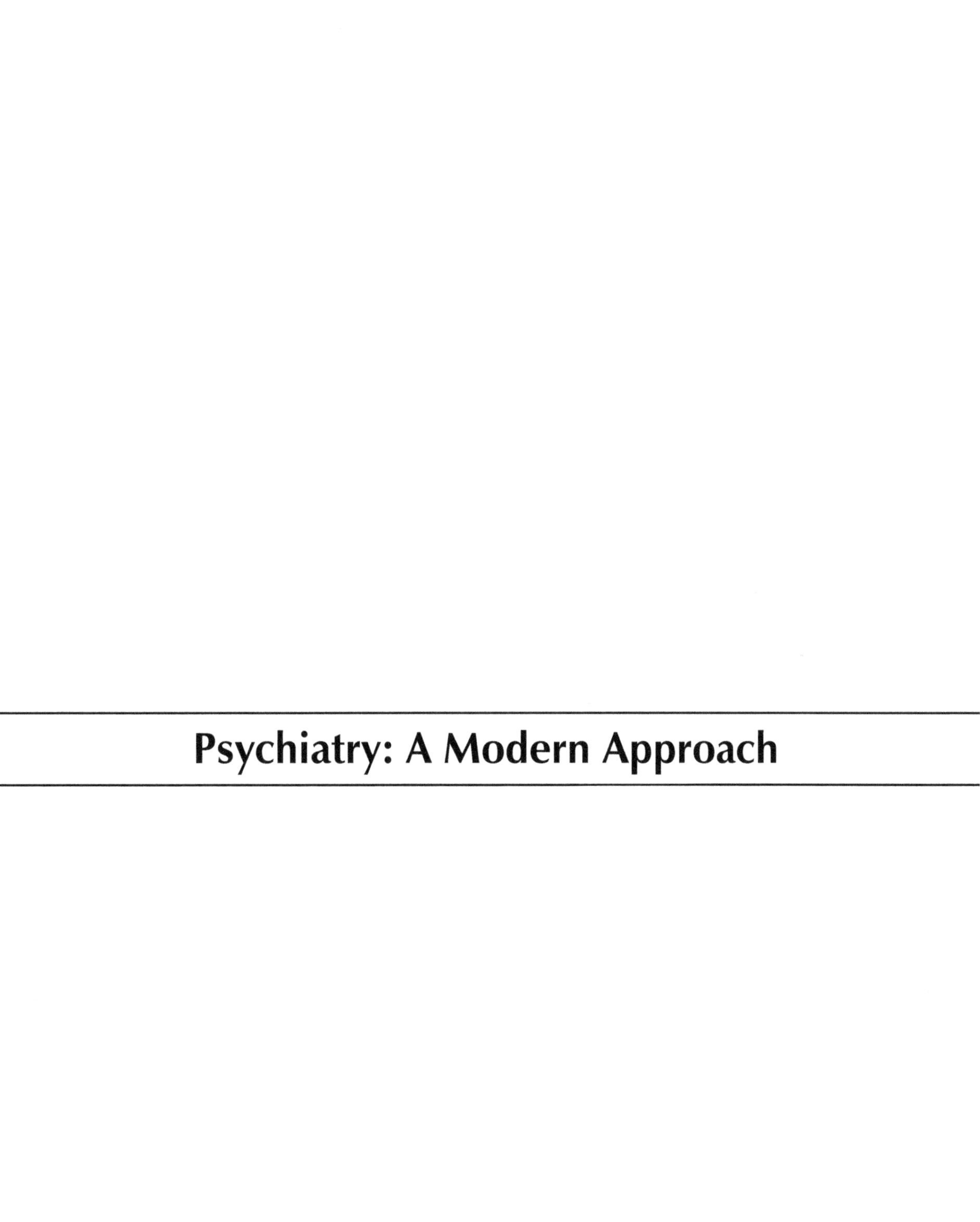

Psychiatry: A Modern Approach

Psychiatry: A Modern Approach

Editor: Chase Harris

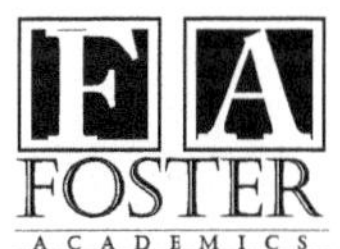

www.fosteracademics.com

www.fosteracademics.com

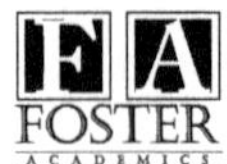

Cataloging-in-Publication Data

Psychiatry : a modern approach / edited by Chase Harris.
p. cm.
Includes bibliographical references and index.
ISBN 978-1-63242-786-1
1. Psychiatry. 2. Psychology, Pathological. 3. Mental health.
4. Medicine and psychology. I. Harris, Chase.
RC454 .P79 2019
616.89--dc23

© Foster Academics, 2019

Foster Academics,
118-35 Queens Blvd., Suite 400,
Forest Hills, NY 11375, USA

ISBN 978-1-63242-786-1 (Hardback)

This book contains information obtained from authentic and highly regarded sources. Copyright for all individual chapters remain with the respective authors as indicated. All chapters are published with permission under the Creative Commons Attribution License or equivalent. A wide variety of references are listed. Permission and sources are indicated; for detailed attributions, please refer to the permissions page and list of contributors. Reasonable efforts have been made to publish reliable data and information, but the authors, editors and publisher cannot assume any responsibility for the validity of all materials or the consequences of their use.

Trademark Notice: Registered trademark of products or corporate names are used only for explanation and identification without intent to infringe.

Contents

Preface

A medical specialty that studies the diagnosis, prevention and treatment of mental disorders is known as psychiatry. Neurology and psychology are the fields which are closely related to psychiatry. The mental disorders which fall under psychiatry include disorders related to mood, perception, behavior and cognition. To assess the initial psychiatric condition of a person, the process begins with a case history and mental status examination. Physical examinations, psychological tests, neuroimaging and neurophysiological techniques are used to assess the mental status of a person. Psychotherapy, psychiatric medication, assertive community treatment (ACT) and community reinforcement approach and family training (CRAFT) are some of the common psychiatric treatments. This book provides comprehensive insights into the field of psychiatry. It is a compilation of chapters that discuss the most vital concepts and emerging trends in this field. Those with an interest in psychiatry would find this book helpful.

Various studies have approached the subject by analyzing it with a single perspective, but the present book provides diverse methodologies and techniques to address this field. This book contains theories and applications needed for understanding the subject from different perspectives. The aim is to keep the readers informed about the progresses in the field; therefore, the contributions were carefully examined to compile novel researches by specialists from across the globe.

Indeed, the job of the editor is the most crucial and challenging in compiling all chapters into a single book. In the end, I would extend my sincere thanks to the chapter authors for their profound work. I am also thankful for the support provided by my family and colleagues during the compilation of this book.

Editor

1

Personality traits, gender roles and sexual behaviours of young adult males

Jacek Kurpisz[1*], Monika Mak[1], Michał Lew-Starowicz[2], Krzysztof Nowosielski[3,4], Przemysław Bieńkowski[5], Robert Kowalczyk[6], Błażej Misiak[7], Dorota Frydecka[8] and Jerzy Samochowiec[1]

Abstract

Background: Previous studies have shown that personality characteristics affect sexual functioning. The aim of this exploratory study was to assess and describe the relationship between global personality traits and the stereotypical femininity and masculinity levels with the broad aspects of sexual behaviours and attitudes in the group of 97 heterosexual young adult men aged 19–39 and living in Poland.

Methods: The 'Big Five' personality traits were measured with the NEO-FFI questionnaire; stereotypical femininity and masculinity with the Bem sex role inventory (BSRI); sexual disorders with the International index of erectile function (IIEF); socio-epidemiological data, sexual behaviours and attitudes towards sexuality with a self-constructed questionnaire.

Results: We identified weak to moderate associations with particular sexual behaviours and attitudes. Neuroticism correlated positively with lower sexual satisfaction, self-acceptance and more negative attitudes towards sexuality; extraversion with higher desire, frequency of sexual intercourses, their diversity, sexual satisfaction, masculinity level and lower report of erectile problems; openness to experience with better quality of partnership, more positive attitudes towards sexual activity and masculinity level; conscientiousness with later sexual initiation age, more frequent and diverse sexual behaviours (but lower interest in masturbation and coitus interruptus), overall sexual satisfaction, satisfaction with one's body and femininity level; agreeableness with a better quality of relationship with a partner, satisfaction from body, lower number of previous partners and more frequent sexual encounters (but less masturbation). Stereotypical masculinity, more so than femininity, was related to a wide range of positive aspects of sexuality.

Conclusions: The Big Five personality traits and stereotypical femininity/masculinity dimensions were found to have a noticeable, but weak to moderate influence on sexual behaviour in young adult males.

Keywords: Sexual behaviour, Big Five personality traits, Gender roles

Background

There is a paucity of studies on relationships between personality structure and sexual functions, as well as expression of sexuality in the period of early adulthood [1, 2]. The quest for exploring the relationship between traits that describe human personality and sexual expression was initiated by Eysenck [3]. He used his 3-factor model (EPQ) to examine extraversion, neuroticism and psychoticism and describe patterns of sexual activity. He proposed to use 'libido' and 'satisfaction' scales to measure a number of continuums comprising various aspects of human sexual experience [4]. Other researchers suggested different theories and psychometric tools for measuring sexual-related traits as a separate entity, e.g. erotophobia-erotophilia scale [5] and self-monitoring scale [6]. Some researchers followed the idea of sexual-related traits in their studies, while others were still using the recognised personality taxonomies to investigate the field of sexuality [7]. In the latter group, the initial studies were based on Eysenck's concept [3, 8], while the later ones shifted to exploit 'The Big Five Model' [3]. Discussion concerning a potential overlap and other relations to

*Correspondence: jacek.kurpisz@gmail.com
[1] Department of Psychiatry, Pomeranian Medical University, Szczecin, Poland
Full list of author information is available at the end of the article

the Eysenck's model can be found elsewhere [3, 9, 10]. In this study, we followed the 'Big Five' way of exploration.

According to Buss [11], the Big Five may capture some important features that represent individual differences in evolutionary strategies, which could be significantly related to engaging in specific sexual behaviours.

Previous studies, although limited in number, proved that existing personality taxonomies are indeed useful for explanation of some sexual attitudes and behaviours [3]. Shafer [4] states that global personality traits, such as the 'Big Five', have been shown to be moderate predictors of individual differences within sexuality.

We decided to verify that assumption, but in our study the main objective was to check if the 'Big Five' personality traits are related to engagement in particular sexual behaviours, occurrence of sexual problems and selected attitudes towards sexual expression.

Besides global personality traits, we hypothesised that in young adult men their perception of gender role may correlate with engagement in particular sexual activities and sexual expression. In brief, gender role is a social construct containing rules and characteristics (physical, emotional, intellectual) of stereotypically perceived femininity and masculinity [12, 13]. Under the pressure of social expectations, all members of society have to develop their personal gender role, as a part of their personality in the process of enculturation. S. L. Bem distinguished four gender role types, depending on the relationship of stereotypically masculine and feminine traits: masculine (high level of masculine and low of feminine traits), feminine (low level of masculine and high of feminine traits), androgynous (high levels of both masculine and feminine traits), or undifferentiated (low levels of both masculine and feminine traits; such individuals describe themselves differently than by using gender-related characteristics). Identification with a particular type affects the way that individuals construct their cognitions about the world and others.

In our study we decided to provide the answer to the following questions:

(1) What is the relationship between the 'Big Five' characteristics, femininity and masculinity levels and tendency to engage in sexual behaviours like: penile-vaginal encounter, sexual activities without penetration, oral sex, anal sex, masturbation and mutual masturbation with partner, orgasm frequency and contraception usage?
(2) What is the relationship between the 'Big Five' characteristics, femininity and masculinity levels and erectile functions?
(3) What is the relationship between the 'Big Five' characteristics, femininity and masculinity levels and positive/negative attitudes towards sexual activity, satisfaction with sexual life, one's body and self?
(4) What is the relationship between the 'Big Five' characteristics, femininity and masculinity levels and relationship with a partner?
(5) What is the relationship between the 'Big Five' characteristics, femininity and masculinity levels and sexual disorders report?

Methods

Participants

The 97 respondents were aged between 19 and 39 years (M = 29.28, SD = 5.83). The sample was composed of male students and workers of Pomeranian Medical University, patients of the occupational medicine centre, workers from a local building company, state office workers, public hospital staff and other volunteers who agreed to take part in the study. Participants were recruited between January 2014 and May 2015 in the city of Szczecin. Out of the total sample, 89 % were city dwellers and 11 % were rural residents. The majority of the sample had secondary (50 %) and college (39 %) education, which is quite a typical phenomenon in sexological studies [14]. About 75 % of the studied subjects were in a relationship. In regard to religion, 66 % identified themselves as Catholics, 29 % as non-believers and 3 % as 'other'. Socio-demographic characteristics of the sample are presented in Table 1.

Procedure

The participants were selected according to age, to gather a relatively representative group for Polish young adults (basing on national census from 2012 [15]). Because of the expected problems which commonly follow sexological studies during the development of the study design, we decided not to use any additional criterion for the recruitment process. We have made such decision with awareness of its limitation to avoid the influence of taboo concerning information about sexual life in the Polish society, which could result in a great decrease in response rate.

In this paper, we decided to apply the quota sampling method. The respondents were qualified to sub-groups by age: 19–24 years (27 % of the sample), 25–29 years (25 % of the sample), 30–34 years (25 % of the sample) and 35–39 years (23 % of the sample). After giving their consent to take part in the study, the participants were given a paper-and-pencil version of the questionnaires to fill in at home and send back anonymously in the provided envelope with a stamp and address. They were provided with all the necessary instructions about the study, as well as the study procedure. Recruitment to the study was continued until a representative group of 100 respondents was gathered. The response rate was 36.7 %.

Table 1 Socio-demographic characteristics of the sample ($n = 97$)

	n	%
Education		
Elementary	10	10
Secondary	48	50
College	38	39
No answer	1	1
Residency		
City	86	86
Country	10	10
No answer	4	4
Relationship		
Single	20	21
In relationship	74	76
No answer	3	3
Religion		
Catholic	64	66
Other	3	3
Non-believer	28	29
No answer	2	2

Men who reported being treated for sexual dysfunction at the time of the study or suffered from a serious somatic illness, mental illness or disabilities were excluded from the study. We decided to apply such criteria to exclude the possibility of sexual expression being in any way affected by such external causes. Our intention was to assess the exclusive impact of personality and gender characteristics on sexual behaviour and attitudes.

During the data analysis phase, we decided to exclude three non-heterosexual persons from the sample to make it more homogenous in relation to sexual orientation.

Measures

Personality traits were assessed by the Polish version of NEO-FFI, a 60-item Big Five inventory. The Cronbach's alpha reliability coefficients were as follows: 0.80 for neuroticism, 0.77 for extraversion, 0.82 for conscientiousness, 0.68 for agreeableness and 0.68 for openness to experience [16].

Masculinity-Femininity and gender roles were evaluated with the Polish version of the Bem sex role inventory (BSRI) [12, 17]. In this 35-item questionnaire the respondents were asked to assess on a scale from 1 (I strongly disagree) to 5 (I strongly agree) the extent to which given adjectives relating to stereotypical femininity and masculinity described them personally. The Cronbach's alpha reliability coefficients were 0.78 for masculinity scale and 0.79 for femininity scale.

Sexual function was evaluated using a 15-question standardised and validated Polish version of the international index of erectile function (IIEF) questionnaire, which measures five domains of sexual functions in men: erectile and orgasmic functions, sexual desire, intercourse satisfaction, and overall satisfaction. Individuals who scored 26 or more points in the erectile function scale (EF) were considered as having normal erectile function. Mild dysfunction was diagnosed in patients with 22–25 point score, mild to moderate, 17–21, moderate, 11–16, and severe, 10 or less. Orgasmic function (OF), sexual desire (SD) and overall satisfaction (OS) were considered normal in patients with a score of 9 or more, whereas intercourse satisfaction (IS) was considered decreased in those with a score of 12 or less [18, 19]. Cronbach's alpha range for the IIEF scales was from 0.73 to 0.99.

For socio-epidemiological data assessment we used a self-constructed questionnaire. It included questions concerning frequency of sexual behaviours such as condom usage, coitus interruptus on scales from 1-never to 5-always. Other questions measured the respondent's and their partner's perceived attitudes towards sexuality, quality of the relationship with a current sexual partner, satisfaction with sex life, satisfaction with one's body, with self as a man, and self-esteem (on Likert's scales from 1-very low level/bad to 5-very high level/very good). Religiosity type was assessed through a question asking for self-identification (catholic/other/non-believer) and religiosity level was measured on a scale based on a single question, ranging from 1-totally not religious to 5-very religious.

Sexual activity was defined as any of the following: caressing, foreplay, masturbation, vaginal or anal intercourse, or oral sex (declared mean number per month). There were also yes/no questions about pornography usage and staying in a relationship.

Frequency of sexual problems, such as erectile dysfunction, premature ejaculation, and delayed ejaculation were measured on scales from 1 (never) to 4 (almost always). All questions concerning sexual problems considered the period of the last 3 months.

Statistical methods

For a statistical evaluation, we have chosen correlation and quasi-experimental plans. We used Pearson's r and Spearman's rho for the particular correlation analysis. For group comparisons we utilised the Kruskal–Wallis and Mann–Whitney tests because of their inequality. Additionally, we used the Bonferroni correction to highlight the strongest relationships, although we decided to set p value on a 0.05 level to avoid type II error. We checked the normality of variable distribution with the Shapiro–Wilk test.

Before we started the statistical analysis, the variables assessing frequency of particular sexual behaviours (sexual activity per month) were modified from continuous to discrete form of 10 equal groups, according to the percentile distribution observed in our sample. Such procedure was applied to avoid any possible bias related to the continuous form of the primary variables.

Results

Table 2 shows statistical characteristics of the sexual behaviours in the sample. It proves that the studied sample presented a great individual diversity of these measures.

Table 3 depicts statistical characteristics of the 'Big Five' traits in the investigated group. None of the measured traits in the sample has met close to normal distribution in the Shapiro–Wilk test.

Table 4 shows description of the gender role measures. In the Shapiro–Wilk test, masculinity scores did not reach close to normal distribution, while femininity did [$W(95) = 0.98, p > 0.05$]. The dominating gender role type was stereotypically masculine, then androgynous, undifferentiated, with the feminine being the rarest.

Description of the sexual functioning (IIEF scores) is shown in Table 5, while prevalence of sexual problems is presented in Table 6. As expected, the studied sample was relatively sexually healthy.

In relation to age in the studied sample of males, we indicated significant correlations with masculinity level ($r = -0.26$; $p < 0.05$), number of previous partners ($r = 0.24$; $p < 0.05$), education level ($r_s = 0.35$; $p < 0.001$), condom usage ($r_s = -0.25$; $p < 0.05$), frequency of sexual encounters without penetration ($r_s = -0.40$; $p < 0.001$), anal sex ($r_s = 0.29$; $p < 0.01$), oral sex ($r_s = -0.28$; $p < 0.01$), and masturbation ($r_s = -0.35$; $p < 0.01$). The studied age sub-group comparison has revealed statistically significant differences in frequency of sexual activities without penetration, anal sex, oral sex and masturbation per month. There were also differences in satisfaction with one's body. These findings are presented in Table 7.

With reference to the 'Big Five' traits, Neuroticism was significantly negatively correlated with conscientiousness ($r = -0.59$; $p < 0.001$) and agreeableness ($r = -0.25$; $p < 0.01$). In the IIEF scales, it was correlated only with OS

Table 2 Characteristics of the sexual behaviour in the sample (n = 97)

	Mean score	SE	SD
Sexual initiation (age)	17.79	0.26	2.47
Number of previous sexual partners	5.97	0.53	5.16
No. of sexual encounters per month (penile-vaginal)	11.90	0.88	8.52
No. of sexual activities without penetration per month	6.33	0.90	8.76
No. of anal sex per month	2.73	0.64	6.14
No. of oral sex per month	5.25	0.69	6.57
No. of mutual masturbation with partner per month	4.91	0.73	7.15
No. of masturbation per month	5.26	0.74	7.11
No. of orgasms per month	15.44	1.01	9.81
No. of any sexual activity per month	14.73	0.96	9.24
No. of satisfying sexual activities per month	12.60	0.98	9.22
Mean time of ejaculation latency	19.40	1.43	13.66

Variables are shown in a primary form, as continuous ones

Table 3 The 'Big Five' statistical description (n = 97)

	Min	max	Mean score	SE	SD
N	1	8	4.41	0.21	2.11
E	1	10	5.88	0.21	2.05
O	1	10	4.86	0.21	2.03
C	1	10	6.74	0.22	2.17
A	1	10	5.81	0.20	1.99

Table 4 Femininity, masculinity and gender roles prevalence in the sample (n = 95)

	Mean score	SE	SD
F	51.85	0.79	7.70
M	52.71	0.85	8.32
Gender role type prevalence			
Masculine (%)	**Feminine (%)**	**Androgynous (%)**	**Undifferentiated (%)**
43	4	32	20

F stereotypical femininity, *M* stereotypical masculinity. Gender role types: Masculine low F, high M; Feminine high F, low M; Androgynous high both F and M; Undifferentiated low both F and M

Table 5 IIEF scores—statistical description

	Mean score	SE	SD
EF ($n = 88$)	27.20	0.37	3.43
OF ($n = 88$)	9.11	0.16	1.45
SD ($n = 96$)	7.74	0.16	1.56
IS ($n = 88$)	12.39	0.21	1.93
OS ($n = 88$)	9.10	0.14	1.28

Eight subjects were not sexually active in the past 4 weeks so only SD was measured for them. 1 response was lacking

EF erectile function, *OF* orgasmic function, *SD* sexual desire, *IS* intercourse satisfaction, *OS* overall satisfaction

Table 6 Sexual problems frequency report ($n = 97$)

	Never (%)	Sometimes (%)	Less than in a half of sexual encounters (%)	Almost always (%)
Erectile dysfunction	74	26	0	0
Premature ejaculation	59	34	4	3
Delayed ejaculation	74	25	0	1

Table 7 The age sub-groups (19–24, 25–29, 30–34, 35–39) comparison for measured variables

	Df	Chi^2	*p* value	
Masculinity	3	12.07	<0.01	19–24 > 25–29 > 30–34 > 35-39
Education	3	16.72	<0.001[a]	19–24 < 25–29, 35–39 < 30–34
No. of sexual activities without penetration per month	3	15.16	<0.01	19–24 > 25–29 > 30–34 > 35–39
No. of anal sex per month	3	8.82	<0.05	19–24 < 25–29 < 30–34 < 35–39
No. of oral sex per month	3	11.51	<0.01	19–24 > 30–34 > 25–29 > 35–39
No. of masturbation per month	3	12.45	<0.01	19–24 > 25–29 > 30–34 > 35–39
Satisfaction with one's body	3	8.01	<0.05	19–24 < 25–29 < 30–34 < 35–39

There are presented only these variables which had $p < 0.05$ in the Kruskal–Wallis test (all the variables measured in the study were tested). The last column shows relations of the variable levels between groups

[a] Means passing requirements of the Bonferroni correction ($p < 0.0013158$)

($r = -0.23$; $p < 0.05$). There was no significant correlation with BSRI femininity or masculinity, nor with any sexual disorders. Among sexual behaviours, Neuroticism was negatively associated with anal sex ($r_s = -0.39$; $p < 0.001$) and positively with condom usage ($r_s = 0.23$; $p < 0.05$), as well as coitus interruptus ($r_s = 0.26$; $p < 0.05$). Regarding the attitudes, neuroticism was negatively correlated with satisfaction with one's body ($r_s = -0.52$; $p < 0.001$), satisfaction with self as a man ($r_s = -0.26$; $p < 0.01$), satisfaction with sex life ($r_s = -0.22$; $p < 0.05$), one's attitude toward sexual activity ($r_s = -0.24$; $p < 0.05$), partner's attitude towards sexual activity ($r_s = -0.22$; $p < 0.05$), and quality of relationship with a partner ($r_s = -0.23$; $p < 0.05$).

Extraversion was found to be correlated with openness to experience ($r = 0.30$; $p < 0.01$). Among IIEF facets, extraversion was associated only with SD ($r = 0.21$; $p < 0.05$). In the field of sexual problems, there was a negative correlation with erectile dysfunction ($r_s = -0.23$; $p < 0.05$). Notably, there was a medium correlation with the BSRI dimension of masculinity ($r = 0.39$; $p < 0.001$). In the area of sexual behaviours, extraversion was correlated with sex per month ($r_s = 0.34$; $p < 0.01$), oral sex per month ($r_s = 0.31$; $p < 0.01$), orgasms per month ($r_s = 0.26$; $p < 0.05$), any sexual activity per month ($r_s = 0.24$; $p < 0.05$), and satisfying intercourses per month ($r_s = 0.43$; $p < 0.001$). Extraversion was also correlated with satisfaction with sex life ($r_s = 0.22$; $p < 0.05$). There was no significant correlation with personal attitudes, demographic features or other sexual characteristics.

Openness to experience was positively associated with extraversion and negatively with conscientiousness ($r = -0.22$; $p < 0.05$). There was no correlation with IIEF facets. Among the BSRI dimensions, Openness to experience was connected with masculinity ($r = 0.21$; $p < 0.05$). Surprisingly, neither the investigated sexual behaviours per month or demographic characteristics, nor personal attitudes were associated with this personality feature. However, Openness to experience correlated with the positive quality of relationship with a partner ($r_s = 0.28$; $p < 0.01$), partner's positive attitude toward sexual activity ($r_s = 0.34$; $p < 0.01$) and satisfaction with sexual life ($r_s = 0.32$; $p < 0.01$).

Conscientiousness, apart from inverse correlations with Neuroticism ($r = -0.59$; $p < 0.001$) and openness to experience ($r = -0.22$; $p < 0.05$), was also positively associated with agreeableness ($r = 0.45$; $p < 0.001$). It correlated with OS ($r = 0.28$; $p < 0.01$) and BSRI femininity ($r = 0.26$; $p < 0.01$). Conscientiousness was on the one hand associated with later sexual initiation age ($r = 0.24$; $p < 0.05$), but on the other with more frequent sexual intercourse per month ($r_s = 0.27$; $p < 0.01$), anal sex per month ($r_s = 0.28$; $p < 0.01$), satisfying intercourses per month ($r_s = 0.31$; $p < 0.01$) and negatively with masturbation per month ($r_s = -0.30$; $p < 0.01$). None of the investigated demographic characteristics were associated with this personality feature. Conscientiousness was correlated with less frequent engaging in coitus interruptus ($r_s = -0.36$; $p < 0.001$) and premature ejaculation

($r_{s=}$−0.22; $p < 0.05$). Regarding personal attitudes, there were correlations with satisfaction with one's body ($r_s = 0.43$; $p < 0.001$).

Agreeableness, as previously mentioned, was inversely associated with neuroticism and conscientiousness. It was not connected with any of the IIEF facets. In reference to BSRI dimensions, Agreeableness positively correlated with femininity ($r = 0.25$; $p < 0.05$) but negatively with masculinity ($r = -0.22$; $p < 0.05$). It was also negatively associated with the number of previous sexual partners ($r = -0.28$; $p < 0.01$). As regards sexual behaviours, agreeableness was connected with engaging in sexual intercourse per month ($r_s = 0.25$; $p < 0.05$), mutual masturbation with partner per month ($r_s = 0.21$; $p < 0.05$) and negatively with masturbation ($r_s = -0.25$; $p < 0.05$). None of the investigated demographic characteristics were associated with this personality feature. Agreeableness correlated with satisfaction with one's body ($r_s = 0.25$; $p < 0.01$), self-acceptance ($r_s = 0.20$; $p < 0.05$), good relationship with a sexual partner ($r_s = 0.26$; $p < 0.05$) and negatively with frequency of premature ejaculation ($r_s = -0.24$; $p < 0.05$).

All the findings concerning associations between the 'Big Five' traits and the other investigated variables are presented in Table 8.

In our study, BSRI stereotypical femininity dimension correlated with EF ($r = 0.27$; $p < 0.05$) and OF ($r = 0.22$; $p < 0.05$), time needed to ejaculate in minutes ($r = 0.33$; $p < 0.01$), anal sex per month ($r = 0.28$; $p < 0.01$) and, surprisingly, with masculinity ($r = 0.31$; $p < 0.01$).

Stereotypical masculinity additionally correlated with EF ($r = 0.30$; $p < 0.01$), SD ($r = 0.29$; $p < 0.01$), age ($r = -0.26$; $p < 0.01$), number of previous sexual partners ($r = 0.21$; $p < 0.05$), sex without penetration per month ($r_s = 0.35$; $p < 0.001$), orgasms per month ($r_s = 0.32$; $p < 0.01$), any sexual activity per month ($r_s = 0.31$; $p < 0.01$), satisfying sexual intercourses per month ($r_s = 0.25$; $p < 0.05$), satisfaction with sex life ($r_s = 0.30$; $p < 0.01$) lower erectile dysfunction frequency ($r_s = -0.31$; $p < 0.01$), one's better attitude toward sexual activity ($r_s = 0.30$; $p < 0.05$), partner's attitude toward sexual activity ($r_s = 0.21$; $p < 0.05$), satisfaction with sexual life ($r_s = 0.30$; $p < 0.05$), partner's attitude toward sexual activity ($r_s = 0.25$; $p < 0.05$) and femininity.

All the investigated associations between BSRI dimensions and other variables are depicted in Table 9.

The particular gender role types (stereotypical masculine, feminine, androgynous, undifferentiated) did not differentiate our sample in any of the measured variables in the Kruskal–Wallis test (all p values >0.05), except for extraversion level ($H = 10.16$; $p < 0.05$), which was the highest for the androgynous and lowest for undifferentiated type.

There was no significant difference between pornography users (79 % of the whole group) and non-users (22 %) in the Mann–Whitney test (ps > 0.05) regarding the Big Five trait levels, masculinity, femininity and erectile functions. Differences between these groups were observed for religiosity level, sexual initiation age, number of previous sexual partners and frequency of masturbation. The statistically relevant findings are shown in Table 10.

Those men who reported being in a romantic relationship did not differ from the singles in the Big Five features in Mann–Whitney test, or the levels of stereotypical femininity and masculinity (all ps > 0.05). The significant differences were observed for age, EF, IS, OS, relationship quality, condom usage frequency, one's and partner's attitudes toward sexuality, satisfaction with sexual life, self-acceptance, sexual encounters, any sexual activity, orgasms and satisfying sexual contacts per month. The findings are shown in Table 11.

The religiosity level did not correlate with any of the investigated variables (measured with Spearman's rho, all ps > 0.05). The comparison of groups consisted of catholics and non-believers ('other' type group was omitted because of low prevalence) has not revealed any significant differences in any of the measured variables (ps > 0.05), except for religiosity level ($Z = -7.34$, $p < 0.05$).

Education level correlated positively with age ($r_s = 0.35$; $p < 0.001$), EF ($r_s = 0.24$; $p < 0.05$), OF ($r_s = 0.29$; $p < 0.01$), IS ($r_s = 0.32$; $p < 0.01$), delayed ejaculation ($r_s = 0.22$; $p < 0.05$), while negatively with frequency of sexual contacts without penetration ($r_s = -0.21$; $p < 0.05$),

Concerning condom usage frequency, besides the observed relationship with Neuroticism, it also negatively correlated with age ($r_s = -0.25$; $p < 0.05$) and relationship quality ($r_s = -0.30$; $p < 0.01$). Coitus interruptus frequency was also negatively related to frequency of anal sexual contacts ($r_s = -0.22$; $p < 0.05$), as well as one's ($r_s = -0.30$; $p < 0.01$) and partner's ($r_s = 0.29$; $p < 0.01$) more negative overall attitude toward sexual activity.

Among the additional findings, it is noteworthy that there seems to be a high compatibility between the participants' and their partners' attitude toward sexual activity ($r_s = 0.79$; $p < 0.001$), partners' attitude toward sexual activity and investigated men's satisfaction with sex life ($r_s = 0.76$; $p < 0.001$), investigated men's attitude toward sexual activity and the perceived quality of relationship with a partner ($r_s = 0.51$; $p < 0.001$), partners' attitude toward sexual activity and relationship with a partner ($r_s = 0.55$; $p < 0.001$), relationship with a partner and investigated men's satisfaction with sex life ($r_s = 0.69$; $p < 0.001$).

Table 8 Correlations between the Big Five traits and other variables

Big Five domain	Neuroticism		Extraversion		Openness to experience		Conscientiousness		Agreeableness	
	r	p	r	p	r	p	r	p	r	p
EF ($n = 88$)	−0.17	NS	0.18	NS	−0.12	NS	0.05	NS	−0.13	NS
OF ($n = 88$)	−0.08	NS	0.01	NS	0.11	NS	−0.07	NS	−0.13	NS
SD ($n = 96$)	0.07	NS	0.21*	<0.05	0.16	NS	−0.10	NS	−0.14	NS
IS ($n = 88$)	−0.02	NS	0.09	NS	−0.03	NS	0.05	NS	−0.14	NS
OS ($n = 88$)	−0.23*	<0.05	0.03	NS	0.03	NS	0.28**	<0.01	0.04	NS
Femininity ($n = 97$)	−0.13	NS	0.09	NS	0.01	NS	0.26**	<0.01	0.25*	<0.05
Masculinity ($n = 97$)	−0.19	NS	0.39***[a]	<0.001	0.21*	<0.05	0.18	NS	−0.22*	<0.05
Sexual initiation (age) ($n = 92$)	−0.15	NS	−0.05	NS	−0.12	NS	0.24*	<0.05	0.19	NS
Time needed to ejaculate (min) ($n = 91$)	−0.11	NS	0.01	NS	0.02	NS	0.08	NS	−0.12	NS
Number of previous sexual partners ($n = 96$)	0.11	NS	0.18	NS	0.10	NS	−0.17	NS	−0.28**	<0.01
No. of sexual encounters per month ($n = 82$)	−0.11	NS	0.34**	<0.01	0.12	NS	0.27*	<0.05	0.25*	<0.05
No. of sexual activities without penetration per month ($n = 95$)	0.26	<0.05	0.19	NS	0.18	NS	−0.22*	<0.05	−0.15	NS
No. of anal sex per month ($n = 93$)	−0.39***[a]	<0.001	−0.07	NS	−0.05	NS	0.28**	<0.01	0.19	NS
No. of oral sex per month ($n = 92$)	0.10	NS	0.31**	<0.01	0.17	NS	−0.01	NS	−0.05	NS
No. of mutual masturbation with partner per month ($n = 95$)	−0.10	NS	0.10	NS	−0.04	NS	0.12	NS	0.21*	<0.05
No. of masturbation per month ($n = 93$)	0.04	NS	−0.05	NS	0.07	NS	−0.30**	<0.01	−0.25*	<0.05
No. of orgasms per month ($n = 94$)	−0.07	NS	0.26*	<0.05	0.17	NS	0.10	NS	0.02	NS
No. of any sexual activity per month ($n = 93$)	−0.17	NS	0.24*	<0.05	0.10	NS	0.24*	<0.05	0.14	NS
No. of satisfying sexual activities per month ($n = 89$)	−0.20	NS	0.43***[a]	<0.001	0.09	NS	0.31**	<0.01	0.19	NS
Condom usage frequency ($n = 94$)	0.23*	<0.05	−0.02	NS	−0.08	NS	−0.03	NS	−0.09	NS
Coitus interruptus frequency ($n = 94$)	0.26*	<0.05	0.18	NS	0.08	NS	−0.36***	<0.001	−0.20	NS
Satisfaction with one's body ($n = 96$)	−0.52***[a]	<0.001	0.08	NS	−0.01	NS	0.43***[a]	<0.001	0.26**	<0.01
Satisfaction with self as a man ($n = 97$)	−0.26**	<0.01	0.18	NS	0.05	NS	0.13	NS	0.05	NS
Satisfaction with sexual life ($n = 95$)	−0.22*	<0.05	0.23*	<0.05	0.32**	<0.01	0.15	NS	0.12	NS
Self-acceptance ($n = 97$)	−0.08	NS	0.01	NS	0.12	NS	0.17	NS	0.20*	<0.05
Quality of relationship with a partner ($n = 92$)	−0.23*	<0.05	0.15	NS	0.28**	<0.01	0.19	NS	0.26*	<0.05
One's attitude toward sexual activity ($n = 97$)	−0.22*	<0.05	0.14	NS	0.20	<0.05	0.17	NS	0.06	NS
Partner's attitude toward sexual activity sex ($n = 91$)	−0.25*	<0.05	0.10	NS	0.34**	<0.01	0.19	NS	0.09	NS
Erectile dysfunction ($n = 95$)	0.03	NS	−0.23*	<0.05	−0.02	NS	−0.19	NS	−0.02	NS
Premature ejaculation ($n = 95$)	0.06	NS	−0.07	NS	−0.04	NS	−0.22*	<0.05	−0.25*	<0.05
Delayed ejaculation ($n = 95$)	−0.06	NS	0.08	NS	0.01	NS	−0.15	NS	−0.08	NS

The table shows correlations with the IIEF scales, stereotypical femininity and masculinity from the BSRI, frequency of sexual behaviours, measured attitudes and declared sexual problems. Different numbers of n for particular comparisons mean lack of given answer. Pearson's *r* was used for: the IIEF and BSRI scales, sexual initiation age and time needed to ejaculate. Spearman's rho was used for: frequency of sexual behaviours, attitudes and declared sexual problems

IIEF abbreviations: *EF* erectile function, *OF* orgasmic function, *SD* sexual desire, *IS* intercourse satisfaction, *OS* overall satisfaction

* $p < 0.06$, ** $p < 0.01$, *** $p < 0.001$

[a] Means passing requirements of the Bonferroni correction ($p < 0.0003226$). In the IIEF eight subjects submitted that they were not sexually active in the past 4 weeks, so only SD was measured for them

Table 9 Correlations between the BSRI femininity, masculinity and other variables

BSRI	Femininity		Masculinity	
	r	*p*	*r*	*p*
EF ($n = 86$)	0.30*	<0.05	0.29**	<0.01
OF ($n = 86$)	0.22*	<0.05	0.07	NS
SD ($n = 94$)	0.04	NS	0.28**	<0.01
IS ($n = 85$)	0.18	NS	0.18	NS
OS ($n = 86$)	0.12	NS	0.19	NS
Sexual initiation (age) ($n = 90$)	−0.08	NS	−0.21	NS
Time needed to ejaculate (min) ($n = 89$)	0.33**	<0.01	0.15	NS
Number of previous sexual partners ($n = 94$)	0.06	NS	0.21*	<0.05
No of Sexual encounters per month ($n = 81$)	−0.04	NS	0.16	NS
No of sexual activities without penetration per month ($n = 81$)	−0.10	NS	0.35***	<0.001
No of anal sex per month ($n = 91$)	0.28**	<0.01	−0.13	NS
No of oral sex per month ($n = 90$)	−0.19	NS	0.13	NS
No of mutual masturbation with partner per month ($n = 93$)	0.17	NS	−0.12	NS
No of masturbation per month ($n = 91$)	−0.12	NS	0.15	NS
No of orgasms per month ($n = 92$)	0.02	NS	0.32**	<0.01
No of any sexual activity per month ($n = 91$)	0.09	NS	0.31**	<0.01
No of satisfying sexual activities per month ($n = 87$)	0.02	NS	0.25*	<0.05
Condom usage frequency ($n = 92$)	−0.07	NS	0.12	NS
Coitus interruptus frequency ($n = 92$)	−0.06	NS	−0.10	NS
Satisfaction with one's body ($n = 94$)	0.13	NS	0.16	NS
Satisfaction with self as a man ($n = 95$)	0.10	NS	0.13	NS
Satisfaction with sex life ($n = 93$)	0.03	NS	0.30**	<0.01
Self-acceptance ($n = 95$)	0.05	NS	−0.18	NS
Quality of relationship with a partner ($n = 90$)	−0.04	NS	0.20	NS
One's attitude toward sexual activity ($n = 95$)	0.04	NS	0.30**	<0.01
Partner's attitude toward sexual activity ($n = 89$)	−0.07	NS	0.25*	<0.05
Erectile dysfunction ($n = 95$)	−0.16	NS	−0.31**	<0.01
Premature ejaculation ($n = 95$)	0.05	NS	0.05	NS
Delayed ejaculation ($n = 95$)	−0.01	NS	0.14	NS

The table shows correlations with IIEF scales, frequency of sexual behaviours, measured attitudes and declared sexual problems. Different numbers of n for particular comparisons mean lack of given answer. Pearson's *r* was used for: IIEF scales, sexual initiation age and time needed to ejaculate. Spearman's rho was used for: frequency of sexual behaviours, attitudes and declared sexual problems. * $p < 0.06$, ** $p < 0.01$, *** $p < 0.001$. None of the correlations passed requirements of Bonferroni correction. In IIEF eight subjects submitted, that they were not sexually active in the past 4 weeks, so only SD was measured for them

IIEF abbreviations: *EF* erectile function, *OF* orgasmic function, *SD* sexual desire, *IS* intercourse satisfaction, *OS* overall satisfaction

Table 10 The Mann–Whitney test for pornography users and non-users

	Z	*p* value	
Religiosity level	−2.64	<0.01	Non-users < users
Sexual initiation age	−2.18	<0.05	Non-users > users
Number of previous sexual partners	−2.02	<0.05	Non-users < users
Frequency of masturbation	−2.36	<0.05	Non-users < users

All the variables measured in the study were tested. Only significant group differences for $p < 0.05$ were listed. The last column shows relationships of the variable levels between groups. None of the findings passed requirements of the Bonferroni correction

Discussion

Before the discussion of our findings relating the Big Five and gender roles we briefly present conclusions from earlier studies. All the data cited from these studies were gathered from age groups comparable to our sample.

Hitherto findings revealed that Neuroticism was associated with higher sexual excitement, sexual curiosity, sexual guilt [3], higher sexual anxiety, sexual depression, sexual self-monitoring (a tendency to be aware of the public impression of one's sexuality), lower sexual esteem and sexual assertiveness [4], lower sexual satisfaction [7], higher chance of infidelity in relationship [20], marital

Table 11 The Mann–Whitney test comparing participants who reported being single or in a relationship

	Z	*p* value	
Age	−2.39	<0.05	In relationship > single
EF	−1.98	<0.05	In relationship > single
IS	−2.83	<0.05	In relationship > single
OS	−2.76	<0.05	In relationship > single
Relationship quality	−3.81	<0.001[a]	In relationship > single
Condom usage frequency	−2.00	<0.05	In relationship < single
Attitude toward sexuality	−2.88	<0.01	In relationship > single
Partners attitude toward sexuality	−2.78	<0.01	In relationship > single
Satisfaction from sexual life	−3.58	<0.001[a]	In relationship > single
Self-acceptance	−2.72	<0.01	In relationship > single
Sexual encounters per month	−3.74	<0.001[a]	In relationship > single
Any sexual activity per month	−3.22	<0.001[a]	In relationship > single
Orgasms per month	−2.45	<0.05	In relationship > single
Satisfying sexual contacts per month	−3.95	<0.001[a]	In relationship > single

All the variables measured in the study were tested. Only significant group differences for $p < 0.05$ were listed. The last column shows relations of the variables levels between groups

[a] Means passing requirements of the Bonferroni correction ($p < 0.0012500$)

dissolution and dissatisfaction [21]. Eysenck [3] demonstrated that higher scores on this trait are associated with being more nervous about sexual performance, reporting lower levels of sexual satisfaction, becoming sexually excited quicker but also reacting more intensely with sexual inhibition.

The results of our study showed that Neuroticism was slightly negatively correlated with overall sexual satisfaction (OS) but not related to other erectile functions, or sexual disorder report. The first finding was expected and it remains in accordance with the previous studies [3, 7]. Lack of association with other erectile functions was a bit surprising. On the one hand, generally higher level of emotional instability, anxiety and tendency to experience negative emotions seems to be disruptive to sexual response. This concerns stress reaction, which has an inhibiting impact on sexual expression in various psychological and biological aspects [1]. On the other hand, more neurotic males are generally more emotionally aroused. Thus, some of them may cognitively interpret such arousal in terms of sexual desire, as described in the excitation-transfer theory [22]. Such tendency was presented in previous studies [1] and was found to be stronger amongst younger men. Our findings do not support the notion concerning negative impact of Neuroticism on sexual functioning in young adult males, nor do they directly allow to draw any conclusions of Excitation-Transfer influence on sexual expression. We are more willing to admit that neuroticism has a very individual impact on sexuality of young males. A careful case study analysis could be a useful method to have a closer look on that problem.

Nevertheless, men scoring higher on neuroticism scale in our study were moderately less satisfied with their bodies and slightly less satisfied with themselves as men. These findings show that to some extent neuroticism is linked to the problems with broad aspects of self-acceptance. These aspects are also strictly associated with self-esteem and feeling of being sexually attractive to others. Negative emotionality also affects sex life in a partnership. More neurotic men were slightly less satisfied with the quality of their intimate relationships, they expressed a bit more negative attitude toward sexual activity, and so did their partners. Men scoring higher on neuroticism may have greater difficulties with emotional openness, which is crucial in an erotic situation. This may also affect sexual communication abilities. Problems arising in a relationship may also manifest themselves as sexual problems. However, such concerns are weakly proven by the gathered data. It can be concluded that a higher score on Neuroticism is a risk factor for sexual dissatisfaction but it cannot be construed as definitely destructive per se.

Neuroticism did not correlate with any of the investigated sexual problems. It seems that despite a less positive attitude toward sexual activity, the capability for physiological response like erection and ejaculation remains intact in men, regardless their level of neuroticism [23]. Because we examined a group of 19–39-year-old men, their age may be an important biological factor protecting them from such problems.

While analysing frequency of engagement in particular sexual behaviours, we found that higher scores on neuroticism were related to moderately reduced chance of having anal sex. Apart from consciousness, the impact of which on anal sex was slightly positive, neuroticism was the only Big Five trait that had a decreasing impact on the tendency to get involved in this particular behaviour. We suppose that males scoring higher on Neuroticism scale may interpret the possibility of engagement in anal intercourse as 'not masculine' or even 'homosexual' behaviour, which may be threatening to their own personal concept of masculinity. As rooted in anxiety, the idea of crossing gender-related borders for accepted, 'proper' sexual scripts may result in avoidance of anal sex. Noteworthy is the fact that stereotypical femininity level positively correlated with engaging in anal sex.

It is interesting that we did not observe any association between Neuroticism and stereotypical masculinity and femininity dimensions. We expected a positive correlation with femininity and at least slightly negative one with masculinity. Probably among Polish young adult men a tendency to experience and express negative emotions and emotional instability are perceived as not much related to any gender.

Neuroticism found its reflection in a somewhat increased condom usage but also, comparably, in higher frequency of coitus interruptus. Thus, males with greater tendency to experience anxiety are also more afraid of unwanted pregnancy and, probably, sexually transmitted infections. As the tendency to use condoms should be judged as a positive factor for sexual health, the preference of coitus interruptus is worrisome. This brings a conclusion that more neurotic young men should be given better education about efficient contraception methods.

Generally, the relationships between sexual response, satisfaction and negative (but non-clinical) emotionality (especially anxiety) are complex and ambiguous [1]. In future studies they should be considered in a much broader context. Nevertheless, our findings partially support Eysenck's hypothesis concerning the role of neuroticism in sexual response [3].

Concerning extraversion, the analysis of previous studies revealed relationships with higher levels of sexual satisfaction [7, 8], sexual permissiveness [24], sexual motivation, but also sexual preoccupation [7], number of sexual partners by age 20, psychoactive substance abuse before or during sexual encounter and an earlier sexual initiation age [25]. One study pointed out lower level of sexual preoccupation and sexual consciousness in more extrovert men [4]. According to Eysenck [3], extroverts, because of their hunger for stimuli, are more likely to experiment with sexual activities, have more sexual partners, or engage in sex more often.

In our study, extraversion was found to be associated with multiple positive aspects of sexual expression. First, it was slightly related to a higher sexual desire and lower rate of erectile dysfunction. This supports findings from previous studies [7, 8]. Extraversion was not associated with any other sexual problems. A modest association with experiencing satisfying intercourses was observed. Mild positive correlations were found with engagement in sexual intercourse, oral sex, orgasm frequency and general frequency of different types of sexual activity per month. These results can be explained similar to the ones from the past studies. Persons scoring higher on extraversion scale are more prone to sensation-seeking activities [3]. Sexual activity of various types gives a possibility to enhance stimulation level by increasing desire, sexual thoughts and behaviours. More extrovert individuals are also more sociable. This is a very helpful characteristic in finding a potential sexual partner. Nevertheless, we did not find a significant relationship with a number of previous sexual partners, as Eysenck suspected [3]. Probably the association of higher extraversion level with a greater number of sexual partners occurs in earlier developmental stage of adolescence [25]. Quite surprising was a lack of any relationship with age of sexual initiation.

More extrovert men seem to be more open to a variety of sexual behaviours, except anal sex. Higher extraversion was found to be moderately correlated with the number of satisfying intercourses and slightly with satisfaction with sex life. Such tendency was also described in previous studies [7, 8]. Although individuals scoring higher on extraversion scale have an increased need for stimulation, there was no association with masturbation rate.

As expected, extraversion correlated with a stereotypical masculinity dimension at a moderate level. Hence, higher extraversion was proven to be an element of masculine gender stereotype.

The subsequent trait was openness to experience. The analysis of the previous findings revealed that its higher levels were correlated with lower scores on sexual nervousness [3], lower sexual anxiety and fear of sex [26], but also greater sexual motivation, sexual monitoring, sexual preoccupation [7], permissiveness [24], higher satisfaction and commitment to intimate relationships [27]. Botwin et al. [28] pointed out that intellectual conversation in a couple seems to be linked to greater love and affection. Being traditional and more conservative (low Openness) was also related to having unprotected sex, having sex and pregnancy (for women) at an early age [25].

In relation to our findings, we observed a positive but moderately low correlation between Openness to experience and the quality of relationship with a sexual partner, partner's positive attitude toward sexual activity and general satisfaction with sexual life. This result can be accounted by the fact that Openness to experience understood as a preference of novel stimuli is also a tendency to entertain such 'novel ideas' [29].

In relation to some usefulness of higher levels of Openness to experience for satisfaction and commitment to intimate relationships [27, 28], this trait may support development of adequate communication skills, which results in keeping accurate level of mutual desire between partners, improves partner's attitude to sex and the overall quality of the relationship. It may also be linked with lower sexual anxiety and fear of sex [26]. As we found in our study, quality of the relationship with a sexual partner was an important factor of sexual satisfaction ($r_s = 0.69$; $p < 0.001$) and higher scores on openness to experience seem to be slightly helpful in gaining higher scores on both of those scales.

It is interesting that none of the sexual behaviours frequency listed in our study correlated with this trait. Engagement in these behaviours and curiosity to experience 'non-classical' sexual activity was found to be more closely linked to extraversion (and openness to experience was mildly positively connected with this trait). Likewise, we did not observe any association with erectile functions and sexual problems report.

Earlier studies reveal that low Openness to experience is associated with having unprotected sex [25]. We did not find any relation of this personality trait with condom usage or frequency of coitus interruptus. Neither do our findings support the opinion of higher sexual permissiveness in men who are more open to experience, as it was stated elsewhere [24]. It was not linked to earlier sexual initiation age either.

As expected, openness to experience was mildly associated with stereotypical masculinity, so to some limited extent higher levels of this trait seem to be a part of that gender stereotype.

In other studies, another 'Big Five' trait, conscientiousness, was found to be negatively correlated with sexual preoccupation [7, 26], and positively with marital and dating satisfaction [30]. Individuals who scored low on conscientiousness were more likely to have sexual affairs [31], while more conscientious men were found to be more disciplined in delaying potential sexual gratification and avoiding risky sexual behaviours [25].

In our study, conscientiousness was found to be slightly associated with later sexual initiation age. Persons with high levels on this trait describe themselves as well-organised and responsible. Probably, they also postpone moment of starting sexual life with a partner and tend to wait for more 'proper circumstances'. However, according to our findings, being more conscientious affected having a bit more frequent sexual intercourses, even anal sex and 'any sexual activity' with their partner. It is quite interesting that more conscientious males, who were found to be more able to delay potential sexual gratification [25], generally have more sexual intercourses than those with lower levels of consciousness. It is noteworthy that males scoring higher on consciousness scale were mildly less willing to engage in sexual activities without penetration.

More conscious males also declared more satisfying sexual activities per month and better overall sexual satisfaction. This finding remains in accordance with previous reports [30]. In our sample conscientiousness did not affect any of the direct aspects of a relationship with partner.

A moderate association of conscientiousness with satisfaction with one's body was also indicated. This tendency seems to have a good influence on general sexual expression.

In our study higher levels of conscientiousness moderately decreased the number of masturbation acts. People with this characteristic may hypothetically perceive masturbation as inappropriate, especially if they are concurrently involved in a relationship with a sexual partner. For more conscientious men, following norms is crucial, while for many Polish men masturbation is perceived as morally inappropriate [14]. Although there was no correlation between conscientiousness and condom usage frequency, there is a noticeably decreased tendency to engage in coitus interruptus. This may partly confirm previous findings [25] that men scoring higher on conscientiousness are also more responsible in sexual activities they take part in.

In our sample, higher conscientiousness was surprisingly a slightly protective factor in case of premature ejaculation problems. We expected that an increased tendency to control one's behaviour causes the opposite effects.

Conscientiousness was found to be moderately correlated with the stereotypical femininity. This can be explained as a culture-induced expectation for women to be more self-controlling and restrained in sexual activity [13]. What is surprising, in our sample of young adult males such 'femininity' was slightly associated with better erectile function and orgasm.

The last of the Big Five traits, agreeableness, in previous studies was found to be negatively correlated with sexual motivation and sexual preoccupation [7, 26], positively with marital and dating satisfaction [28, 30]. Partners who scored lower on agreeableness were more likely to have sexual affairs [31]. Low agreeableness was also related to greater number of sexual partners, engaging in risky sexual behaviour and earlier sexual initiation age [25].

We have observed that agreeableness also correlated with various sexual behaviours. There was a weak, negative association with the number of previous sexual partners. Hypothetically, more agreeable men have better partner retention skills, which results in staying in one relationship for a longer time. On the other hand, such men may have a lower interest or lack of skills to engage in short romances or one night stands.

We found that Agreeableness was positively, but mildly associated with having more frequent sexual intercourses and mutual masturbation acts with their partners. Therefore, this personality trait may be helpful in negotiation and gaining partner's acceptance to initiate sexual activity. Because agreeableness showed a slight negative correlation with frequency of masturbation, it may be a useful trait that helps in reaching a 'sexual consensus' with a partner and thus helps to fulfil one's sexual needs.

It is interesting that we also found a correlation between agreeableness and satisfaction with one's body. Presumably, men with high levels of agreeableness accept any imperfections of their bodies more easily, or a good relationship with a sexual partner provides a positive feedback about feeling physically and sexually attractive.

Among sexual attitudes, we reported a weak positive association of level of Agreeableness with the quality of relationship with a partner. Such observation is comparable with previous findings [31].

We did not notice any significant association between the level of Agreeableness and erectile functions. In relation to sexual problems, similarly to Conscientiousness, higher scores on Agreeableness were found to be a bit protective against premature ejaculation.

Agreeableness was weakly positively associated with stereotypical femininity and similarly, but negatively with masculinity. The tendency to be cooperative, trustful, moral, altruistic, modest and sympathetic seems to be perceived as more typically displayed by women than men. Such a feminine attitude seems to be useful in dealing with relationship problems and improving a couple's sex life.

Besides the Big Five traits, we also focused on gender roles' impact on sexual expression. Some authors [13] state that particular elements of the internalised gender stereotypes should affect sexual expression. As regards the concept of masculinity, it contains a tendency for dominance, aggressiveness, autonomy, self-confidence, staying focused on personal satisfaction or negatively overinterpreting sexual problems. For the femininity stereotype it covers being delicate, sensitive, neat, passive in sex, not very interested in having sexual contacts.

The analysis of data from previous studies has revealed that higher level of masculinity was found to be related to sexual pleasure [32], while other studies suggest that femininity was associated with satisfaction from the current intimate relationship [33] and marriage [34]. Intensity of masculinity was also related to the earlier age of sexual initiation and greater number of previous sexual partners [35]. Among gender role types, androgynous and stereotypically masculine men declared higher levels of sexual satisfaction [32]. Androgyny was also linked to more erotophilic attitude [1, 36].

Extreme levels of internalised masculinity were indicated to be associated with sexual aggression towards women [37]. Nevertheless, in a meta-analysis masculinity measure based on Bem's gender schema Theory has shown small effect size with sexual aggression. It seems that general gender-role traits do not strongly predict sexual violence [37].

According to our findings, there are mild, positive correlations between higher levels of both masculinity and femininity and aspects of better sexual functioning, but with prevalence of positive masculine impact.

Almost one third of the participants were identified as an androgynous type, which could explain a medium correlation between dimensions of masculinity and femininity.

Masculinity was weakly to modestly associated with a better erectile function and higher sexual desire, while femininity with orgasmic function. According to this data, we could speculate that both, masculine and feminine dimensions, are somewhat necessary and helpful in different aspects of male sexual functioning. Nevertheless, masculinity was associated with greater number of sexually-favourable aspects, such as: satisfying sexual intercourses, orgasms, sexual activities without penetration, any sexual activity per month, one's and partner's positive attitude towards sexual activity, satisfaction with sexual life, lower tendency to experience erectile dysfunction. More masculine men also declared a bit higher number of previous sexual partners. All gathered data support previous findings concerning number of partners [35], and sexual pleasure and satisfaction [32]. Unfortunately, analysing our findings, we were not able to say anything about sexual aggressiveness towards women in stereotypically more masculine men. We can only suspect that extremely masculine men [37] build their relationships with partners basing on domination and submission. This problem should be investigated in future studies.

Masculinity was slightly negatively correlated with age. Some interesting findings about personality development, which could be related to the masculinity intensification change, were reported elsewhere [38, 39]. In brief, such change within masculinity-related traits may be the result of social adaptation, becoming emotionally less volatile and more attuned to social demands. Although we studied a group of men in the same developmental stage, we can expect that there is a difference between 19 and 39-year-old men in their psychological profile. Perhaps, for some men getting older also means becoming more balanced in relation to the stereotypical masculine traits. However, for now it is only a hypothesis, which should be verified in further studies.

Higher scores on femininity scale were mildly correlated with erectile and orgasmic functions, longer ejaculation latency and higher frequency of anal sex. We did not find any associations with satisfaction with the intimate relationship, as it was observed in earlier studies [33], nor any other attitude towards sexual expression.

Neither did we observe any relationship between the level of internalised femininity and masculinity gender stereotypes and sexual problems, condom usage or frequency of coitus interruptus.

In the group comparison of gender role types, we did not notice any significant differences in frequency of sexual behaviour, erectile functions or attitudes toward sexuality. Previous findings of higher sexual satisfaction and pleasure [32, 33] were not confirmed in our sample.

The age of participants in our sample was related to a few sexual characteristics. More mature men were slightly less willing to engage in masturbation, sexual contacts without penetration, use of condoms or oral sex. On the other hand, they declared a bit higher number of previous sexual partners, more frequent anal intercourses and, quite surprisingly, were more satisfied with their bodies. Most of these findings could be explained by a greater chance of having a stable intimate relationship for older males in comparison to younger ones. A tendency to prefer anal over oral sexual activity with age is hard to interpret. What is noteworthy is a lower willingness to use condoms by older males and those in an intimate relationship.

As we reported, there was no relationship between religiosity level and any of the measured aspects of male sexual expression. It seems that religiosity had a very limited influence on young males' forms of sexual expression. It was thus close to the earlier reports [40], according to which religious attitudes and practices do not fully determine sexual behaviour. Such tendency was found to be more characteristic of men, as opposed to women [14]. For males, religiosity was only related to later sexual initiation and less common sexual contacts outside of marriage [41].

Our study is mostly exploratory. However, it gives an interesting overview of the relationship between personality traits, gender stereotypes and various aspects of sexual expression. We suggest further, more detailed verification of the observed tendencies in the future studies on bigger groups.

Limitations of the study

First, the study sample is homogeneous and relatively too small to draw any definite conclusions. In our sample, we did not report a normal distribution of the Big Five traits ($p < 0.05$ for all traits in the Shapiro–Wilk test). The group was characterized by an increased level of conscientiousness and lower level of neuroticism and openness to experience than expected in the general population.

Some labels were used in the study to assess sexual behaviours may be hard for interpretation. This concerns, i.e. anal sex or mutual masturbation, which could cover a wide range of different behaviours. If we took under consideration methodological assumption of our study, it would be hard to investigate very specific forms of such behaviours. That is why we decided to construct questionnaire items in a more general form.

Another difficulty was to adequately operationalize sexual behaviours and their measures. We are aware that asking about giving 'mean score' of engagement in particular sexual behaviour per month or 'mean time to ejaculate' is a big, but necessary simplification. These are quite common problems of such studies [1, 14]. Nevertheless, our findings seem to be helpful in revealing the image of sexual expression among Polish young adults.

It is important to highlight the fact that the issue of sexual expression, attitudes and its scientific exploration is still a taboo for a substantial part of Polish population. That explains the low response rate. Nevertheless, it is similar to other studies based on the questionnaire methods. To make our study as representative for the general population of young adult men as possible we reflected the age structure for this group in our sample. Anyhow, we have to take notice that in relation to general population our results are somewhat limited. Future research should make these issues a priority.

Retrospective character of the study may not reflect the actual sexual behaviours in a longer period of time. However, it describes a dynamic construct of sexuality that may change in time. We used only the IIEF for assessing sexual function. Other scales could also be applied. However, the 15-item IIEF meets the standards in satisfying evaluation of sexual function in men.

Last but not least, the present study was exploratory in nature and its basic conclusions need further support from multicenter studies recruiting larger groups of Polish men and women with different socio-demographic characteristics.

Conclusion

Big Five personality traits have noticeable, but weak to moderate, influence on sexual behaviour in young adult males. Stereotypical femininity and masculinity dimensions have the same effect. Psychological profile is built by multiple personality traits that jointly affect one's overall functioning. Similarly, sexual expression is also a result of the interrelation of these traits, not only its separated features.

Abbreviations

'Big Five' personality traits

N: neuroticism; E: extraversion; O: openness to experience; C: conscientiousness; A: agreeableness.

Bem sex role inventory (BSRI)

F: stereotypical femininity; M: stereotypical masculinity.

Index of erectile function (IIEF)

EF: erectile function; OF: orgasmic function; SD: sexual desire; IS: intercourse satisfaction; OS: overall satisfaction.

Authors' contributions

JK: study concept and design, analysis and interpretation, study supervision, critical revision of the manuscript for important intellectual content. MM: analysis and interpretation, critical revision of the manuscript for important intellectual content. MLS: study concept and design, analysis and interpretation, study supervision, critical revision of the manuscript for important intellectual content. KN: study concept and design, analysis and interpretation, study supervision, critical revision of the manuscript for important intellectual content. PB: analysis and interpretation, critical revision of the manuscript for important intellectual content. RK: analysis and interpretation, critical revision of the manuscript for important intellectual content. BM: analysis and interpretation, critical revision of the manuscript for important intellectual content. DF: analysis and interpretation, critical revision of the manuscript for important intellectual content. JS: study concept and design, study supervision, critical revision of the manuscript for important intellectual content. All authors read and approved the final manuscript.

Author details

[1] Department of Psychiatry, Pomeranian Medical University, Szczecin, Poland. [2] Institute of Psychiatry and Neurology, 3rd Psychiatric Clinic, Warsaw, Poland. [3] Department of Sexology and Family Planning, Medical College in Sosnowiec, Sosnowiec, Poland. [4] Department of Obstetrics and Gynaecology, Specialistic Teaching Hospital, Tychy, Poland. [5] Institute of Psychiatry and Neurology, Warsaw, Poland. [6] Department of Sexology, Andrzej Frycz Modrzewski Cracow University, Kraków, Poland. [7] Department of Genetics, Wroclaw Medical University, Wrocław, Poland. [8] Department of Psychiatry, Wroclaw Medical University, Wrocław, Poland.

Acknowledgements

None.

Competing interests

The authors declare that they have no competing interests.

Funding

The study was founded from Pomeranian Medical University FSN-312-07/13. These funds were used for collection, analysis, and interpretation of data.

References

1. Bancroft J. Human sexuality and its problems. 3rd ed. Wrocław: Elsevier; 2011.
2. Boyd DR, Bee HL, Johnson PA. Lifespan development. Boston: Pearson; 2006. p. 333–88.
3. Heaven PCL, Fitzpatrick J, Craig FL, Kelly P, Sebar G. Five personality factors and sex: preliminary findings. Pers Individ Differ. 2000;28:1133–41.
4. Shafer AB. The Big Five and sexuality trait terms as predictors of relationships and sex. J Res Pers. 2001;35:313–38.
5. Fisher W, Byrne D, White L, Kelley K. Erotophobia–erotophilia as a dimension of personality. J Sex Res. 1988;25:123–51.
6. Snyder M, Simpson J, Gangestad S. Personality and sexual relations. J Pers Soc Psychol. 1986;51:181–90.
7. Heaven PCL, Crocker D, Edwards B, Preston N, Ward R, Woodbridge N. Personality and sex. Pers Individ Differ. 2003;35:411–9.
8. Barnes G, Malamuth N, Check J. Personality and sexuality. Pers Individ Differ. 1984;5:159–72.
9. Costa PT Jr, McCrae RR. Revised NEO personality inventory NEO-PI-R and NEO Five-factor inventory (NEO-FFI) professional manual. Odessa: Psychological Assessment Resources; 1992.
10. Eysenck HJ, Eysenck M. Personality and individual differences: a natural science approach. 1st ed. London: Plenum Press; 1985.
11. Buss DM. Social adaptation and five major factors of personality. In: Wiggins JS, editor. Theoretical perspectives for the Five Factor Model. New York: Gulilford; 1996. p. 180–207.
12. Bem SL. Gender schema theory: a cognitive account of sex-typing. Psychol Rev. 1981;88:354–64.
13. Brannon L. Gender: psychological perspectives. 1st ed. Gdańsk: GWP; 2002. p. 196–210.
14. Izdebski Z. Seksualność Polaków na początku XXI wieku. Studium badawcze. 1st ed. Kraków: Wydawnictwo Uniwersytetu Jagiellońskiego; 2012.
15. Central Statistical office. Concise statistical book of Poland. Warszawa: Zakład wydawnictw statystycznych; 2015. p. 119.
16. Zawadzki B. Inwentarz osobowości NEO-FFI Costy i McCrae: adaptacja polska: podręcznik. Warszawa: Pracownia Testów Psychologicznych Polskiego Towarzystwa Psychologicznego; 1998.
17. Kuczyńska A. Inwentarz do oceny płci psychologicznej: podręcznik. Warszawa: Pracownia Testów Psychologicznych Polskiego Towarzystwa Psychologicznego; 1992.
18. Rosen RC, Riley A, Wagner G, Osterloh IH, Kirkpatrick J, Mishra A. The international index of erectile function (IIEF) a multidimensional scale for assessment of erectile dysfunction. Urology. 1997;49(6):822–30.
19. Puchalski B, Szymański FM, Kowalik R, Filipiak KJ. Ocena zachowań seksualnych mężczyzn w ciągu pierwszych 9 miesięcy po zawale serca. Pol Sexol. 2013;11(1):24–8.
20. Judge TA, Higgins CA, Thoresen CJ, Barrick MR. The Big Five personality traits, general mental ability and career success across the life span. Pers Psychol. 1999;52:621–52.
21. Kurdek L. Predicting marital dissolution: a 5-year prospective longitudinal study of newlywed couples. J Pers Soc Psychol. 1993;64:221–42.
22. Zillman D. Transfer of excitation in emotional behavior. In: Cacioppo JT, Petty RE, editors. Social Psychophysiology: a sourcebook. New York: Guilford Press; 1983. p. 215–40.
23. Janssen E. Sexual arousal In men: a review and conceptual analysis. Horm Behav. 2011;50:708–16.
24. Hendrick S, Hendrick C. Multidimensionality of sexual attitudes. J Sex Res. 1987;23:502–26.
25. Miller JD, Lynam D, Zimmerman RS, Logan TK, Leukefeld C, Clayton R. The utility of the Five Factor Model in understanding risky sexual behavior. Pers Individ Differ. 2004;36:1611–26.
26. Snell W, Fisher T, Walters A. The multidimensional sexuality questionnaire. An objective self report measure of psychological tendencies associated with human sexuality. Ann Sex Res. 1993;6:27–55.
27. Shaver PR, Brennan KA. Attachment styles and the Big Five personality traits: their connections with each other and with romantic relationship outcomes. Pers Soc Psychol Bull. 1992;18:536–45.
28. Botwin MD, Buss DM, Shackelford TK. Personality and mate preferences: five factors in mate selection and marital satisfaction. J Pers. 1997;65:107–36.
29. Costa PT Jr, McCrae RR. Manual of the NEO personality inventory: form S and FORM R. Odessa: Psychological Assessment Resources; 1985.
30. Watson D, Hubbard B, Wiese D. General traits of personality and affectivity as predictors of satisfaction in intimate relationships: evidence from self- and partner-ratings. J Pers. 2000;68(3):413–49.
31. Buss DM, Shackelford TK. Susceptibility to infidelity in the first year of marriage. J Res Pers. 1997;31:193–221.
32. Grabowska M. Seksualność we wczesnej, średniej i późnej dorosłości. Wybrane uwarunkowania. Bydgoszcz: Uniwersytet Kazimierza Wielkiego w Bydgoszczy; 2011.
33. Pei-Hui RA, Ward C. A cross-cultural perspective on models of psychological androgyny. J Soc Psychol. 1994;134(3):391–3.
34. Kuczyńska A. Płeć psychologiczna idealnego i rzeczywistego partnera życiowego oraz jej wpływ na jakość realnie utworzonych związków. Przegląd Psychologiczny. 2002;45(4):385–99.
35. Fink B, Brewer G, Fehl K, Neave N. Instrumentality and lifetime number of partners. Pers Individ Differ. 2007;43:747–56.
36. Walfish S, Myerson M. Sex role identity and attitudes toward sexuality. Arch Sex Behav. 1980;9:199–203.
37. Murnen SK, Wright C, Kaluzny G. If, "Boys Will Be Boys", Then Girls Will Be Victims? A meta-analytic review of the research that relates masculine ideology to sexual aggression. Sex Roles. 2002;46(11):359–75.
38. Staudinger UM, Kunzmann U. Positive adult personality development: adjustment and/or growth? Eur Psychol. 2005;10:320–9.
39. McCrae RR, Costa PT, Ostendorf F, Angleitner A, Hrebickova M, Avia MD, Sanz J, Sánchez-Bernardos ML, Kusdil ME, Woodfield R, et al. Nature over nurture: temperament, personality, and life span development. J Pers Soc Psychol. 2000;78:173–86.
40. Lefkowitz ES, Gillen MM, Shearer CL. Religiosity, sexual behaviors and sexual attitudes during emerging adulthood. J Sex Res. 2004;41:150–9.
41. Mark KP, Janssen E, Milhausen RR. Infidelity in heterosexual couples: demographic, Interpersonal, and personality-related predictors of extradyadic sex. Arch Sex Behav. 2011;40:971–82.

2

Analysis of EEG entropy during visual evocation of emotion in schizophrenia

Wen-Lin Chu[1], Min-Wei Huang[1,2], Bo-Lin Jian[3] and Kuo-Sheng Cheng[1*]

Abstract

Background: In this study, the international affective picture system was used to evoke emotion, and then the corresponding signals were collected. The features from different points of brainwaves, frequency, and entropy were used to identify normal, moderately, and markedly ill schizophrenic patients.

Methods: The signals were collected and preprocessed. Then, the signals were separated according to three types of emotions and five frequency bands. Finally, the features were calculated using three different methods of entropy. For classification, the features were divided into different sections and classification using support vector machine (principal components analysis on 95%). Finally, simple regression and correlation analysis between the total scores of positive and negative syndrome scale and features were used.

Results: At first, we observed that to classify normal and markedly ill schizophrenic patients, the identification result was as high as 81.5%, and therefore, we further explored moderately and markedly ill schizophrenic patients. Second, the identification rate in both moderately and markedly ill schizophrenic patient was as high as 79.5%, which at the Fz point signal in high valence low arousal fragments was calculated using the ApEn methods. Finally, the total scores of positive and negative syndrome scale were used to analyze the correlation with the features that were the five frequency bands at the Fz point signal. The results show that the *p* value was less than .001 at the beta wave in the 15–18 Hz frequency range.

Keywords: Electroencephalography, Emotion, Entropy, Schizophrenia, Support vector machine

Background

Schizophrenia typically occurs during young adulthood, leading to social deficits in areas such as interpersonal relationships, employment situations, and self-care in patients. The condition requires long-term medication for treatment, which places a significant expenditure burden on families and the health care system [1, 2]. Up to now, many studies have been conducted in the prognosis of schizophrenia [3], which understandably involves a wide range of aspects. However, the results of these studies vary greatly. Although the reliability and comparability of these studies have been increased due to the use of standardized diagnostic interview and symptom evaluation tools, many problems still remain, including the selection of suitable methodologies, patient definition, consistency in description and evaluation tools, sampling, and research design.

The analysis of EEG signals is a noninvasive and non-radioactive tool that can be used for long-term measurements, and therefore plays a very important role in clinical diagnosis. The analysis of EEG signals is used during functional neurological examinations to assist in the diagnosis of brain dysfunctions caused by nonstructural lesions of the brain such as epilepsy [4], dementia [5], and intellectual developmental disorders [6, 7], as well as in research into schizophrenia and other mental disorders [8]. To further understand the response of schizophrenic patients to various types of stimuli, many studies use visual [9, 10] or auditory [8, 11, 12] stimuli to evoke various emotions in schizophrenic patients, and then capture and analyze their EEG signals to determine whether the signals are associated with physiological mechanisms or

*Correspondence: kscheng@mail.ncku.edu.tw
[1] Department of Biomedical Engineering, National Cheng Kung University, Tainan 701, Taiwan
Full list of author information is available at the end of the article

representative of schizophrenia symptoms. In this study, visual stimulation was used to evoke emotions in normal, moderately, and markedly ill schizophrenic patients, then the corresponding changes in EEG signals were explored to extend the existing body of knowledge in this field of research.

Emotions result from the complex interaction of psychological and physiological phenomena, and the cortex reacts differently according to the type of emotions [13]. Therefore, studies on the elicitation of emotions often use a variety of different methods to induce emotional responses. Gross and Livenson used stimulating fragments from films for emotion induction [14]. Lang et al. recorded the susceptibility of subjects to picture stimulation and objectively developed the scoring criteria for visual complexity and emotional reactions [15]. Palomb et al. induced emotional reactions in subjects using films containing threatening surgery procedures [16]. Kim et al. used colored light, music, and other environmental factors to create different emotional environments [17]. Although subsequent research involved new methods, there is a lack of objective standards of stimulation strength and diversity. The emotion stimulation database built by Lang et al., called the International Affective Picture System (IAPS), contains more than 1000 color images and is currently the most clear content and test–retest reliability database [15]. The use of the IAPS in studies to evoke emotional responses from subjects has received positive evaluations [18, 19]. Therefore, IAPS images were used in this study to induce different emotions in subjects.

In this study, we try to analyze five frequency bands of brain signals by calculating the value of entropy. Entropy is often used to analyze EEG signals [20, 21], and nonlinear statistical analysis methods are used to approximate entropy [22]. The approximate entropy (ApEn) method is often used as the standard method for assessing EEG signals at various frequency bands because it is robust and can quantify EEG signal complexity. With regard to long-term dynamic analysis of EEG signals, the ApEn algorithm can help characterize the dynamics of EEG signals [23]. In addition, permutation entropy (PE) can be also used to eliminate noise, and it has excellent performance in quantifying EEG signal complexity [24, 25]. Azami and Escudero proposed amplitude-aware PE (AAPE), which is more suitable for calculating the EEG signal. It can improve PE and does not consider either the average of the amplitude values or equal amplitude values [26]. Based on the abovementioned discussion of entropy, the ApEn, PE, and AAPE calculation methods were used in this study to evaluate the entropy of different frequencies in EEG signals. Additionally, the analysis of entropy via statistical methods was explored, and the entropy was used as a feature to divide patients into moderately and markedly schizophrenic phases. An identification algorithm was adopted for the training and classification of the feature results. Currently, the well-known identification algorithms include the neural network (NN), support vector machine (SVM), learning vector quantization (LVQ), and other intelligent classifiers. To solve multi-type identification problems, to rapidly establish the available identifier architecture, and to validate the feasibility of the process, the "Classification Learner" application included in MATLAB R2015b (MathWorks, USA) was used for training and classification of the SVM. Currently, this tool is also used in solving EEG signal identification problems [27].

Methods

Participants

We classify the participants into three groups: control, moderately, and markedly ill schizophrenic patients. The control (mean age: 41.7 ± 6.31 years; 4 males 6 females), moderately ill, and markedly ill groups were created according to the total scores of PANSS (positive scale, negative scale, and general psychopathology scale). Leucht et al. [28] proposed an accurate definition of the PANSS score (for patients who have a moderately ill patients with baseline PANSS total score of 75, and for the markedly ill patients with a baseline PANSS total score of 95). The scores for moderately ill [mean score of the total PANSS: 70.06 ± 4.25; mean age: 42.18 ± 7.07 years; age of illness onset: 27 ± 8.75 years old; illness duration: 17.53 ± 6.86 years; 8 male 9 female, medication (e.g., chlorpromazine equivalent, mg): 190.59 ± 101.76 mg)] and markedly ill [mean score of the total PANSS: 95.88 ± 10.53; mean age: 42.47 ± 6.98 years; age of illness onset: 23.82 ± 5.74 years old; illness duration: 19.65 ± 6.72 years; 9 male 8 female, medication (e.g., chlorpromazine equivalent, mg): 232.94 ± 91.09 mg)] patients are shown in Table 1.

The participants were recruited from the outpatient clinic at the Department of Psychiatry, Chiayi and Wanqiao Branch, Taichung Veterans General Hospital, Chiayi, Taiwan. The participants underwent screening that included their medical and psychiatric history, laboratory test results, illicit drug screening, and a physical examination. A psychiatric diagnosis of schizophrenia was established using the structured clinical interview from the DSM-IV and a semi-structured interview conducted by a research psychiatrist. After receiving a complete explanation of the study procedures, all participants provided written informed consent as approved by the institutional review board. This study was approved by the ethics committee of the Taichung Veterans General Hospital and was conducted in accordance with Good

Table 1 Comparison of demographic characteristics between normal, moderately, and markedly ill schizophrenic patients

Demographic variables	Group 1 Normal ($n = 10$)	Group 2 Moderately ill ($n = 17$)	Group 3 Markedly ill ($n = 17$)	Group 1 and 2 (p value)	Group 1 and 3 (p value)	Group 2 and 3 (p value)
Age (years)	41.7 ± 6.31	42.18 ± 7.07	42.47 ± 6.98	.862	.777	.904
Sex (male/female)	4/6	8/9	9/8	0.734	0.534	.741
Age of illness onset (y/o)	0	27 ± 8.75	23.82 ± 5.74	N/A	N/A	.220
Illness duration (years)	0	17.53 ± 6.86	19.65 ± 6.72	N/A	N/A	.370
Medication (e.g., chlorpromazine equivalent, mg)	0	190.59 ± 101.76	232.94 ± 91.09	N/A	N/A	.210
PANSS total	0	70.06 ± 4.25	95.88 ± 10.53	N/A	N/A	.000
PANSS positive	0	17.53 ± 3.28	24.24 ± 4.49	N/A	N/A	.000
PANSS negative	0	16.71 ± 2.57	23.82 ± 4.16	N/A	N/A	.000
PANSS global	0	35.82 ± 4.26	47.82 ± 5.23	N/A	N/A	.000

Clinical Practice procedures and the current revision of the Declaration of Helsinki [29].

Materials

In this study, we use three different types of pictures of IAPS as visual stimulations (45 pictures). The study participants [48 males (mean age 35.94 ± 12.38) and 52 females (mean age 37.45 ± 14.14), born and raised in Taiwan] filled out the questionnaires. These emotional pictures were divided into valence and arousal with two dimensions, and the nine-point Likert scale was used for the analysis. The resulting responses to those pictures were divided into three types. Specifically, there are HVLA (high valence low arousal; valence: 7.42 ± 0.51 arousal: 4.77 ± 0.37), LVLA (low valence low arousal; valence: 3.26 ± 0.53 arousal: 4.55 ± 0.86), and LVHA (low valence high arousal; valence: 1.21 ± 0.59 arousal: 6.45 ± 0.56). The relationship between the time and order of the images is shown in Fig. 1. We use three different types of emotional stimulations in this study. Among them, neutral control was not included because the subjects watched emotional pictures prior to the neutral pictures. The continuation time of human moods is different. Thus, we decided not to include the neutral control in this study.

Entropy calculation method

Entropy is a measure of unpredictability of information content. Therefore, it can display the characterization of the power spectrum. Entropy was first proposed by Shannon in 1940 to measure the unpredictability of information content, and this is now known as information entropy. Subsequently, many similar entropy calculation methods were proposed and applied in the analyses of EEG signals. In 1991, Pincus proposed the ApEn as a technique for measuring sequence complexity and statistical qualification [22]. Most importantly, it measures the probability of generating new models in the signal based on the aspect of measuring the complexity time series. The greater the probability, the more complex the sequence, and the greater the corresponding ApEn. If the EEG signals from a single location are represented as $x(i) = [u(i), u(i+1), \ldots, u(i+m-1)], i = 1, 2, \ldots, (N-m+1)$,

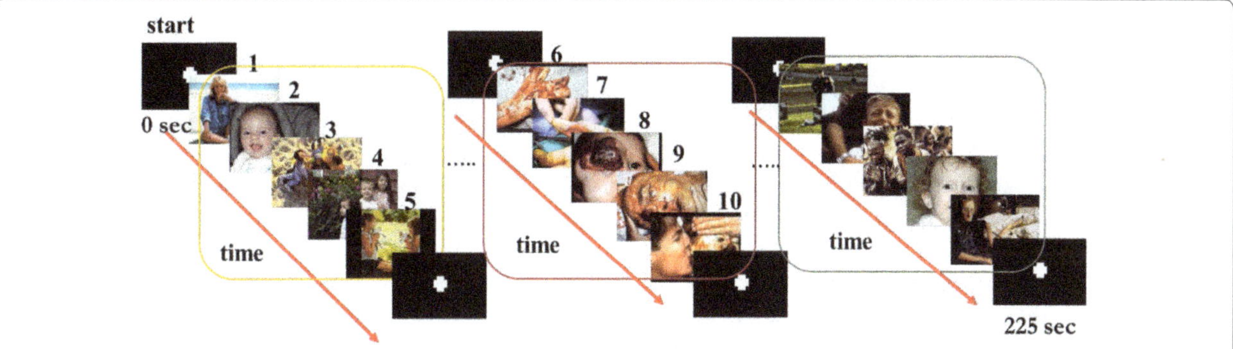

Fig. 1 Schematic diagram of the relationship between the time and the order of the images. During each test, each picture was displayed for 3 s, and the patients were allowed 10 s of rest after one stimulation unit that consisted of five pictures of the same emotion. The three types of emotion appeared three times over the course of the entire 225 s test time

where m specifies the pattern length and N represents the number of time points, then the ApEn definition can be rewritten as follows [22]:

$$\mathrm{ApEn}(m, r, N) = \Phi^{m}(r) - \Phi^{m+1}(r), \tag{1}$$

where

$$\Phi^{m}(r) = (N - m + 1)^{-1} \sum_{i=1}^{N-m+1} \log C_i^m(r),$$

r represents a predetermined tolerance value, (2)

$$C_i^m(r) = \frac{\left(\text{number of } j \text{ such that } \mathrm{d}\left[x(i), x(j)\right] \le r\right)}{(N - m + 1)}, \tag{3}$$

$$\mathrm{d}\left[x(i), x(j)\right] = \max_{k=1,2,\ldots,m} \left(\left|u(i + k - 1) - u(j + k - 1)\right|\right). \tag{4}$$

PE is a simple type of entropy calculation method that was proposed by Bandt in 2002, and it is able to amplify small detailed changes in the time series [30].

Because of the higher flexibility of the AAPE method compared with the classical PE method in the quantification of signal motifs, it is now straightforward to track changes in both the amplitude and frequency [26]. At the same time, it is important to take into consideration the mean value of amplitudes and the differences between the amplitude values in the AAPE algorithm. When the delay time is set to 1, the definition of PE may be rewritten as follows with m as the order of the patterns, x_t the time series, and N the time series of length [23]:

$$\mathrm{PE}(m) = -\sum_{\pi_i=1}^{m!} p(\pi_i) \log p(\pi_i). \tag{5}$$

$$p(\pi_i) = \frac{f(\pi_i)}{N - m + 1}, \tag{6}$$

$$f(\pi_i) = \left\{t \mid t \le N - m, (x_{t+1}, \ldots, x_{t+m}) \text{ has type } \pi_i\right\}, \tag{7}$$

where the relative frequency $p(\pi_i)$ is the probability of appearance of π_i in various arrangements in the signals. The AAPE method modifies the calculation method for the probability of $p(\pi_i)$ by taking the influence of amplitude into consideration to ensure that it is sensitive to the changes in amplitude. When A is set to 0.5, the definition of AAPE can be rewritten as follows [26]:

$$p_{\mathrm{AAPE}}(\pi_i) = \frac{-\sum_{t=1}^{N-m+1}\sum_{i=1}^{m!}\left(\frac{A}{m}\sum_{k=1}^{m}\left|x_{t+(k-1)}\right| + \frac{1-A}{m-1}\sum_{k=2}^{m}\left|x_{t+(k-1)} - x_{t+(k-2)}\right|\right)}{\sum_{t=1}^{N-m+1}\left(\frac{A}{m}\sum_{k=1}^{m}\left|x_{t+(k-1)}\right| + \frac{1-A}{m-1}\sum_{k=2}^{m}\left|x_{t+(k-1)} - x_{t+(k-2)}\right|\right)},$$
$$\text{if type } (X_t^m) = \pi_i. \tag{8}$$

$$\mathrm{AAPE}(m) = -\sum_{\pi_i=1}^{m!} p_{\mathrm{AAPE}}(\pi_i) \log p_{\mathrm{AAPE}}(\pi_i). \tag{9}$$

EEG signal processing

The brainwaves were captured using a Procomp Infiniti™ (Thought Technology Ltd, Montreal West, Quebec, Canada). The sampling rate was 256 Hz, the Fz, Cz, and Pz locations were used as electrode points. The power source has four 1.5 V AA batteries, thus the frequency noise of alternating current does not exist. Left ear (A1), right ear (A2), and (A1 + A2)/2 were used for the reference electrode. According to the studies of Huang et al. [31], the electrode sites were identified by Fp1, Fp2, AF3, AF4, F7, F3, Fz, F4, F8, FC5, FC1, FC2, FC6, T7, C3, Cz, C4, T8, CP5, CP1, CP2, CP6, P7, P3, Pz, P4, P8, PO3, PO4, O1, and O2. However, we found that the used statistical method with factor analysis supports electrode positions. Specifically, Fz, Cz, and Pz were indicators of schizophrenia. Therefore, Fz, Cz, and Pz electrode positions are used in this study. To avoid the sound and light interferences that happen during the experimental procedure, the room was surrounded by three layers of curtains. The subjects only needed to focus on the front visual-stimulation video during the test. They needed to prevent any unnecessary movements to avoid unnecessary noise. We stopped the test if the subjects felt uncomfortable. IAPS images in a specific time sequence were shown to the subjects while the EEG signals from Fz, Cz, and Pz points were recorded. To explore the reaction of brainwave, we proposed an EEG signal processing procedure, as shown in Fig. 2.

Results

Classification of different groups based on brainwaves

We used the ApEn method to calculate the preprocessing signals as features for the classification. For the normal and markedly ill groups, the identification rate was 81.5%. For the normal and moderately ill groups, the identification rate was 70.4%. For the markedly and moderately ill groups, the identification rate was 67%.

According to the abovementioned results, we observed the differences between the markedly and moderately ill groups. Table 2 shows the classification of moderately and markedly ill schizophrenic patients using the features

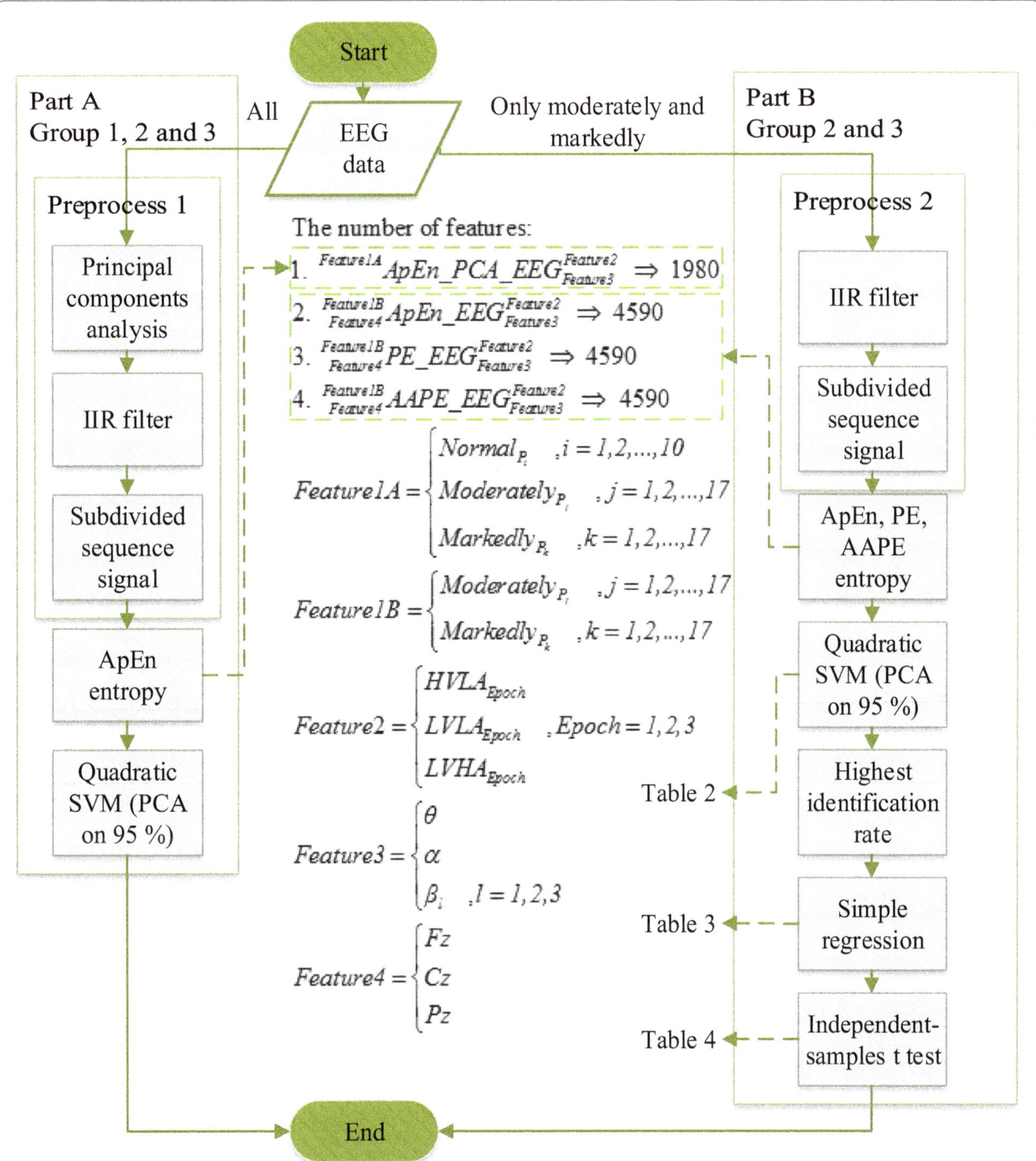

Fig. 2 Flowchart of EEG signal processing. First, we wanted to observe the differences between the brainwaves of normal, moderately, and markedly schizophrenic patients. Therefore, we put all signals into a matrix. The PCA method is used to decompose the matrix. Then, the signal is separated into five frequency bands using IIR filters (6-order Butterworth bandpass filters designed with the Matlab R2015b "Signal Processing Toolbox"): θ(4–8 Hz), α(8–12 Hz), β_1(12–15 Hz), β_2(15–18 Hz), and β_3(18–30 Hz). We separate all different frequency bands of the signals into nine signal fragments according to the timeline that evoked stimuli. Then, we calculate the signals using the ApEn entropy methods. Finally, the obtained features are placed into the SVM (PCA on 95%) for classification. The predictive accuracy was evaluated using the 27-fold cross validation method [32] with a quadratic kernel, in Part A. After that, we classify the features from three points of brainwaves, three types of visual stimuli (HVLA, LVLA, and LVHA), and three methods of entropy (ApEn, PE, and AAPE) in schizophrenic patients. Finally, using linear simple regression and independent-samples *t* test statistical analysis, we analyze the features of the highest identification degree in the classification results and the total scores of PANSS, in Part B

calculation methods at the Fz, Cz, and Pz points. The results indicate that the identification rate at the Fz point was the highest when using the ApEn method, and the identification rate was as high as 79.5% for the moderately and markedly ill schizophrenic patients under the HVLA stimulation.

Correlation analysis between the features of each frequency bands and the total scores of PANSS

The total scores in the PANSS test can specifically evaluate thoughts. As described above, for the signals recorded at the Fz point, the ApEn method is the best method to use to identify moderate and markedly ill schizophrenic patients. Therefore, the correlations test was performed based on the total scores of PANSS and the frequency bands that were calculated using the signals captured at the Fz point and processed using the ApEn method. The results are summarized in Table 3. The results show that the p value of the correlation analysis at β_1(12–15 Hz) and β_2(15–18 Hz) was less than .05, which indicates that the features of these frequencies significantly affect the identification.

Independent-samples *t* test between the features of beta frequency bands and the group 2 and 3

Based on the above results, there were significant differences in beta frequency bands. Therefore, using the features of beta frequency bands, the group 2 and 3 (moderately and markedly ill schizophrenic patients) were analyzed with independent-samples t test. The results are summarized in Table 4. The results show a significant difference between the group 2 and 3 at β_1(12–15 Hz) and β_2(15–18 Hz).

Discussion

EEG signals are complex nonlinear dynamic signals, and it is challenging to accurately extract the EEG signal characteristics. In this study, images from the IAPS were used to evoke emotional responses from subjects while

Table 2 Identification rates of entropy and emotion at different points (%)

Brainwave point	Entropy	Type			Avg. (%)
		HVLA (%)	LVLA (%)	LVHA (%)	
Fz	ApEn	79.5	73.5	73.5	75.5
	PE	52.9	73.5	58.8	61.7
	AAPE	64.7	64.7	70.6	66.7
Cz	ApEn	41.2	35.3	58.8	45.1
	PE	38.2	50	50	46.1
	AAPE	41.2	32.4	52.9	42.2
Pz	ApEn	38.2	50	58.8	49
	PE	67.6	55.9	73.5	65.7
	AAPE	52.9	67.6	61.8	60.8

Table 3 Correlation analysis between the total scores of PANSS and the frequency bands calculated using the ApEn method at the Fz point

	Type								
	HVLA			LVLA			LVHA		
Section:	1	2	3	1	2	3	1	2	3
Frequency									
θ(4–8 Hz)									
Pearson's r	.071	.153	.202	.023	.149	.43	−.070	.038	.088
p value	.692	.387	.252	.897	.401	.809	.696	.831	.620
α(8–12 Hz)									
Pearson's r	.224	.170	.188	.169	.182	.160	.130	.082	.094
p value	.202	.337	.288	.339	.304	.367	.464	.645	.595
β_1(12–15 Hz)									
Pearson's r	*.366*	*.472*	*.472*	*.366*	*.542*	*.505*	*.346*	*.454*	*.382*
p value	*.033**	*.005***	*.005***	*.033**	*.001***	*.002**	*.045**	*.007**	*.026***
β_2(15–18 Hz)									
Pearson's r	*.553*	*.548*	*.590*	*.582*	*.569*	*.555*	*.554*	*.561*	*.573*
p value	*.001****	*.001****	*.000*****	*.000*****	*.000*****	*.001****	*.001****	*.001****	*.000*****
β_3(18–30 Hz)									
Pearson's r	−.248	−.263	−.257	−.302	−.234	*−.342*	−2.37	−.339	−.230
p value	.157	.133	.142	0.83	.182	*.048**	.176	.050	.191

* $p < .05$, ** $p < .01$, *** $p < .001$

Table 4 Independent-samples *t* test between the group 2 and 3 and beta frequency bands calculated using the ApEn method at the Fz point

	Type								
	HVLA			LVLA			LVHA		
Section:	1	2	3	1	2	3	1	2	3
Frequency									
β_1(12–15 Hz)									
Moderately ill	.583	.597	.589	.587	.587	.590	.588	.587	.573
Mean (SD)	(.069)	(.040)	(.048)	(.055)	(.042)	(.043)	(.050)	(.046)	(.062)
Markedly ill	.625	.624	.627	.626	.627	.627	.621	.624	.622
Mean (SD)	(.009)	(.006)	(.005)	(.005)	(.004)	(.005)	(.025)	(.016)	(.018)
t value	−2.462	−2.801	−3.231	−2.860	−3.999	−3.616	−2.417	−3.126	−3.086
p value	*.025**	*.012**	*.005***	*.011**	*.001***	*.002***	*.024**	*.005***	*.006***
β_2(15–18 Hz)									
Moderately ill	.538	.543	.540	.538	.540	.540	.537	.536	.537
Mean (SD)	(.071)	(.067)	(.067)	(.064)	(.067)	(.065)	(.064)	(.067)	(.066)
Markedly ill	.608	.606	.609	.606	.606	.605	.602	.605	.607
Mean (SD)	(.013)	(.012)	(.008)	(.006)	(.013)	(.011)	(.016)	(.021)	(.014)
t value	−4.050	−3.812	−4.214	−4.325	−3.957	−4.014	−4.047	−4.052	−4.276
p value	*.001***	*.001***	*.001***	*.001***	*.001***	*.001***	*.001***	*.001***	*.000****
β_3(18–30 Hz)									
Moderately ill	.564	.575	.568	.569	.567	.570	.568	.573	.563
Mean (SD)	(.051)	(.044)	(.043)	(.047)	(.045)	(.045)	(.046)	(.045)	(.051)
Markedly ill	.554	.555	.557	.554	.558	.555	.556	.554	.552
Mean (SD)	(.015)	(.015)	(.015)	(.014)	(.012)	(.013)	(.019)	(.018)	(.014)
t value	.788	1.735	1.041	1.275	.821	1.381	.960	1.581	.897
p value	.441	.092	.310	.218	.422	.184	.344	.124	.381

* $p < .05$, ** $p < .01$ *** $p < .001$

the corresponding EEG signals were recorded. Then, the EEG signals at different frequency bands were analyzed, and different entropy calculation methods were used to explore the differences between normal, moderately, and markedly ill schizophrenic patients.

Based on the identification results, we can clearly determine that normal and schizophrenic patients have significant differences in the reaction of brainwaves. Therefore, further discussion about the schizophrenic patients in different situations is pending. PANSS is a medical scale for measuring symptom severity of schizophrenic patients. We separated schizophrenic patients into moderately and markedly ill based on the total scores of PANSS, and then calculated the features from the proposed preprocessing approach. The identification results are shown in Table 2. Firstly, we observed that the highest average identification rate was 75.5%, which was calculated using the ApEn method of the Fz point signal. Fz points belong to the frontal area. Therefore, this result corresponds with the research of fMRI [33, 34] and EEG [35, 36]. Then, for different types of emotion, the identification rate was 79.5% in HVLA, and 73.5% in LVHA and LVHA. The results showed that the calculated ApEn features at the Fz point when combined with the SVM identification can effectively classify moderately and markedly ill patients. This confirms that the differences in the EEG signal responses at the Fz point among the patients with different emotional stimulations were significant, and ApEn as features can be simplified for clear identification.

According to the abovementioned results, the ApEn features calculated from the Fz point is the best method for identifying moderately and markedly ill schizophrenic patients, and the total scores of the PANSS test can be specifically evaluated. Further, the correlation between the Fz point signal at five frequency bands and the total scores of PANSS was evaluated. The signals, which are separated into five frequency bands, are considered to be functionally significant by many researchers and correspond to general characteristics. Specifically, Theta is creativity, insight, deep states; Alpha is alertness, peacefulness, readiness; Beta is thinking, focusing, sustained attention [37]. In addition, some researchers divide Beta into three bands for observation and analysis [38]. It can be considered abnormal and leads to several neural diseases [39]. Table 3 shows that the p value for the features extracted from the β_1(12–15 Hz) and β_2(15–18 Hz) signals at the Fz point and the total scores of PANSS were less than .05 and .001, respectively, which indicates that there was some correlation between the features extracted from the signals at this frequency and the scale score. The result from Table 4 also showed that there were significant differences between the moderately and markedly ill schizophrenic patients at β_1(12–15 Hz) and β_2(15–18 Hz). The Beta wave tends to exhibit larger changes under external stimulation, and hence, with visual emotional stimulation, the features obtained from the Beta are able to better represent the differences between patients with different degrees of illness by applying visual emotional stimulation on schizophrenic patients.

Conclusions

The IAPS were used to evoke three different types of emotions in schizophrenic patients while the corresponding EEG signals were recorded. The SVM algorithm was used as the classifier for normal, moderately, and markedly ill schizophrenic patients. The identification result was as high as 81.5%. We further explore and classify moderately and markedly ill schizophrenic patients. The identification rate of the ApEn features calculated for the HVLA at the Fz point was as high as 79.5%. Thus, ApEn is better than PE and AAPE entropy calculation method. The correlation analysis between the ApEn features at the Fz point and the total scores of the PANSS test show that the p value was less than .001 at the beta band (15–18 Hz frequency range). The results indicate that the signal analysis method proposed in this study can provide reference information that can be used to determine the phases of schizophrenia symptoms in clinical applications.

Abbreviations

EEG: electroencephalography; IAPS: International Affective Picture System; IIR filter: infinite impulse response filter; PANSS: positive and negative syndrome scale; SVM: support vector machine; HVLA: high valence low arousal; LVLA: low valence low arousal; LVHA: low valence high arousal.

Authors' contributions

WLC conceived the study, designed the protocol, analyzed the data, and prepared the manuscript. KSC participated in the study design and made significant comments on the manuscript. MWH and BLJ participated in the study design and helped draft the manuscript. All authors contributed substantially to editing and refining the final draft of the manuscript. All authors read and approved the final manuscript.

Author details

[1] Department of Biomedical Engineering, National Cheng Kung University, Tainan 701, Taiwan. [2] Department of Psychiatry, Chiayi Branch, Taichung Veterans General Hospital, Chia-Yi 600, Taiwan. [3] Department of Aeronautics and Astronautics, National Cheng Kung University, Tainan 701, Taiwan.

Acknowledgements

We express our deep appreciation to Assistant Professor Chun-Ju Hou for her methodological support and instructions and Jia-Ying Zhou for her conscientious clinical work during the research phases of the project.

Competing interests

The authors declare that they have no competing interests.

Funding

Personal funds of the research.

References

1. McGlashan TH. Early detection and intervention of schizophrenia: rationale and research. Br J Psychiatry. 1998;172:3–6.
2. Whiteford HA, Degenhardt L, Rehm J, Baxter AJ, Ferrari AJ, Erskine HE, Charlson FJ, Norman RE, Flaxman AD, Johns N, et al. Global burden of disease attributable to mental and substance use disorders: findings from the Global Burden of Disease Study 2010. Lancet. 2013;382:1575–86.
3. Lett TA, Voineskos AN, Kennedy JL, Levine B, Daskalakis ZJ. Treating working memory deficits in schizophrenia: a review of the neurobiology. Biol Psychiatry. 2014;75:361–70.
4. Acharya UR, Sree SV, Swapna G, Martis RJ, Suri JS. Automated EEG analysis of epilepsy: a review. Knowl Based Syst. 2013;45:147–65.
5. Lin PF, Tsao JH, Lo MT, Lin C, Chang YC. Symbolic entropy of the amplitude rather than the instantaneous frequency of EEG varies in dementia. Entropy. 2015;17:560–79.
6. Linden M, Habib T, Radojevic V. A controlled study of the effects of EEG biofeedback on cognition and behavior of children with attention deficit disorder and learning disabilities. Biofeedback Self Regul. 1996;21:35–49.
7. Esposito M, Carotenuto M. Intellectual disabilities and power spectra analysis during sleep: a new perspective on borderline intellectual functioning. J Intellect Disabil Res. 2014;58:421–9.
8. Bachiller A, Romero S, Molina V, Alonso JF, Mananas MA, Poza J, Hornero R. Auditory P3a and P3b neural generators in schizophrenia: an adaptive sLORETA P300 localization approach. Schizophr Res. 2015;169:318–25.
9. Matsumoto A, Ichikawa Y, Kanayama N, Ohira H, Iidaka T. Gamma band activity and its synchronization reflect the dysfunctional emotional processing in alexithymic persons. Psychophysiology. 2006;43:533–40.
10. Jian BL, Chen CL, Chu WL, Huang MW. The facial expression of schizophrenic patients applied with infrared thermal facial image sequence. BMC Psychiatry. 2017;17(1):229.
11. Angelopoulos E, Koutsoukos E, Maillis A, Papadimitriou GN, Stefanis C. Brain functional connectivity during the experience of thought blocks in schizophrenic patients with persistent auditory verbal hallucinations: an EEG study. Schizophr Res. 2014;153:109–12.
12. Bachiller A, Lubeiro A, Diez A, Suazo V, Dominguez C, Blanco JA, Ayuso M, Hornero R, Poza J, Molina V. Decreased entropy modulation of EEG response to novelty and relevance in schizophrenia during a P300 task. Eur Arch Psychiatry Clin Neurosci. 2015;265:525–35.
13. Gregor S, Lin ACH, Gedeon T, Riaz A, Zhu DY. Neuroscience and a nomological network for the understanding and assessment of emotions in information systems research. J Manag Inf Syst. 2014;30:13–47.
14. Gross JJ, Levenson RW. Emotion elicitation using films. Cognit Emot. 1995;9:87–108.
15. Lang PJ, Bradley MM, Cuthbert BN. Motivated attention: affect, activation, and action. Atten Orienting Sens Motiv Process. 1997;97:135.
16. Palomba D, Sarlo M, Angrilli A, Mini A, Stegagno L. Cardiac responses associated with affective processing of unpleasant film stimuli. Int J Psychophysiol. 2000;36:45–57.
17. Kim KH, Bang SW, Kim SR. Emotion recognition system using short-term monitoring of physiological signals. Med Biol Eng Comput. 2004;42:419–27.
18. Mitchell JC, Ragsdale KA, Bedwell JS, Beidel DC, Cassisi JE. Sex differences in affective expression among individuals with psychometrically defined schizotypy: diagnostic implications. Appl Psychophysiol Biofeedback. 2015;40:173–81.

19. Pasparakis E, Koiliari E, Zouraraki C, Tsapakis EM, Roussos P, Giakoumaki SG, Bitsios P. The effects of the CACNA1C rs1006737 A/G on affective startle modulation in healthy males. Eur Psychiatry. 2015;30:492–8.
20. Azami H, Escudero J. Improved multiscale permutation entropy for biomedical signal analysis: interpretation and application to electroencephalogram recordings. Biomed Signal Process Control. 2016;23:28–41.
21. Li J, Yan JQ, Liu XZ, Ouyang GX. Using permutation entropy to measure the changes in EEG signals during absence seizures. Entropy. 2014;16:3049–61.
22. Pincus SM. Approximate entropy as a measure of system-complexity. Proc Natl Acad Sci USA. 1991;88(6):2297–301.
23. Wang X, Meng J, Tan G, Zou L. Research on the relation of EEG signal chaos characteristics with high-level intelligence activity of human brain. Nonlinear Biomed Phys. 2010;4(1):2.
24. Li X, Ouyang G, Richards DA. Predictability analysis of absence seizures with permutation entropy. Epilepsy Res. 2007;77:70–4.
25. Ouyang G, Li J, Liu X, Li X. Dynamic characteristics of absence EEG recordings with multiscale permutation entropy analysis. Epilepsy Res. 2013;104:246–52.
26. Azami H, Escudero J. Amplitude-aware permutation entropy: illustration in spike detection and signal segmentation. Comput Methods Programs Biomed. 2016;128:40–51.
27. Li X, Chen X, Yan Y, Wei W, Wang ZJ. Classification of EEG signals using a multiple kernel learning support vector machine. Sensors. 2014;14(7):12784–802.
28. Leucht S, Kane JM, Kissling W, Hamann J, Etschel E, Engel RR. What does the PANSS mean? Schizophr Res. 2005;79(2–3):231–8.
29. Association WM. World Medical Association Declaration of Helsinki: ethical principles for medical research involving human subjects. JAMA. 2013;310:2191.
30. Bandt C, Pompe B. Permutation entropy: a natural complexity measure for time series. Phys Rev Lett. 2002;88:174102.
31. Huang MW, Chou FHC, Lo PY, Cheng KS. A comparative study on long-term evoked auditory and visual potential responses between Schizophrenic patients and normal subjects. BMC Psychiatry. 2011;11:74.
32. Varma S, Simon R. Bias in error estimation when using cross-validation for model selection. BMC Bioinform. 2006;7:91.
33. Deserno L, Sterzer P, Wustenberg T, Heinz A, Schlagenhauf F. Reduced prefrontal-parietal effective connectivity and working memory deficits in schizophrenia. J Neurosci. 2012;32(1):12–20.
34. Dirnberger G, Fuller R, Frith C, Jahanshahi M. Neural correlates of executive dysfunction in schizophrenia: failure to modulate brain activity with task demands. Neuroreport. 2014;25(16):1308–15.
35. Yu Y, Zhao Y, Si Y, Ren Q, Ren W, Jing C, Zhang H. Estimation of the cool executive function using frontal electroencephalogram signals in first-episode schizophrenia patients. Biomed Eng Online. 2016;15(1):131.
36. Breakspear M. The nonlinear theory of schizophrenia. Aust N Z J Psychiatry. 2006;40(1):20–35.
37. Marzbani H, Marateb HR, Mansourian M. Methodological note: neurofeedback: a comprehensive review on system design, methodology and clinical applications. Basic Clin Neurosci. 2016;7(2):143–58.
38. Rangaswamy M, Porjesz B, Chorlian DB, Wang K, Jones KA, Bauer LO, Rohrbaugh J, O'Connor SJ, Kuperman S, Reich T, et al. Beta power in the EEG of alcoholics. Biol Psychiatry. 2002;52(8):831–42.
39. Schomer DL, Da Silva FL. Niedermeyer's electroencephalography: basic principles, clinical applications, and related fields. Philadelphia: Lippincott Williams & Wilkins; 2012.

3

Preventing involuntary admissions: special needs for distinct patient groups

Knut Hoffmann[1,2*], I. S. Haussleiter[1], F. Illes[1,2], J. Jendreyschak[1,2], A. Diehl[3], B. Emons[1], C. Armgart[1], A. Schramm[1] and G. Juckel[1,2]

Abstract

Background: Coercive measures in psychiatry are a controversial topic and raise ethical, legal and clinical issues. Involuntary admission of patients is a long-lasting problem and indicates a problematic pathway to care situations within the community, largely because personal freedom is fundamentally covered by the UN declaration of human rights and the German constitution.

Methods: In this study, a survey on a large and comprehensive population of psychiatric in-patients in the eastern part of North Rhine-Westphalia, Germany, was carried out for the years 2004–2009, including 230.678 treatment cases. The data were collected from the dataset transferred to health insurance automatically, which, since 2004 is available in an electronic form. In addition, a wide variety of information on treatment, sociodemographic and illness-related factors were collected and analysed. Data were collected retrospectively and analyses were calculated using statistical software (IBM SPSS Statistics 19.0®). Quantitative data are presented as mean and standard deviation. Due to the unequal group sizes, group differences were calculated by means of Chi-square tests or independent sample *t* tests. A Bonferroni correction was applied to control for multiple comparisons.

Results: We found an over-representation of involuntary admissions in young men (<21 years) suffering from schizophrenia and in female patients aged over 60 with a diagnosis of dementia. Most of our results are concordant with the previous literature. Also admission in hours out of regular out-patient services elevated the risk.

Conclusion: The main conclusion from these findings is a need for a fortification of ambulatory treatment offers, e.g. sociopsychiatric services or ward round at home for early diagnosis and intervention. Further prospective studyies are needed.

Keywords: Involuntary admission, Coercion, Legal basics

Background

Since Pinel, involuntary treatment is an important issue for discussion in psychiatry, and today, it is still widely accepted as a necessary part of psychiatric treatment. The highly sensitive and controversial nature of this issue meant that the legal regulations for involuntary treatment in most countries have become very strict. In Germany, there are two main acts that dictate the necessary criteria for involuntarily treatment: the first is the "Psychisch-KrankenGesetz" (PsychKG), and the second relates to guardianship, as defined by the civil law code. The PsychKG mental health act states that patients fulfilling the criteria for involuntary treatment must exhibit a highly acute symptomatology, which is expressed by a high risk of the patient being a danger to themselves or to their environment, including other people. The civil law code relating to guardianship also states that patients should exhibit highly acute symptomatology and thus be at a high risk of being a danger to themselves, but this does not apply to them being a danger to others. Both routes to involuntary admission to mental health services require a medical statement from a psychiatrist as well as an approval from a judge. In this study, we only refer to the PsychKG-based treatments.

*Correspondence: knut.hoffmann@lwl.org; knut.hoffmann@wkp-lwl.org
[2] Department of Psychiatry, LWL-University Hospital Bochum, Alexandrinenstr. 1, 44791 Bochum, Germany
Full list of author information is available at the end of the article

Unfortunately, there are appearing reports of increase in the number of involuntary admissions under PsychKG conditions in Germany; similarities are reported from other countries [1–3]. However, there are also reports from Germany which more recently found a large decline between 1988 and 2009 [4], and also [5] could demonstrate, that the overall percentage of involuntary admissions to inpatient wards across the country had stayed relatively stable between 1993 and 2003. Mostly, these findings were interpreted as a result of shortened treatment times and a higher frequency of admissions [6]. A European-wide comparison of compulsory admissions over a period of 8 years stated that Germany had the greatest overall percentage increase (75%), with the UK having the lowest (5%). Germany was also shown to have the second highest rate of involuntary admission per 100,000 inhabitants, with Portugal, France and Denmark having the lowest. According to this study, the most frequent diagnosis was schizophrenia (29.5–52.7%), followed by affective disorders (9.2–13.7%), then substance abuse (5.2–24.5%) and then dementia (2.2–12.6%) [7], which was similar for smaller regions [8–10]; sociodemographic risk factors were suggested to be a married status and living alone. Even in different German hospitals, there was a great variety of coercive measures (1.9–16.2%); also depending on the diagnosis [11], this could also been demonstrated for Switzerland [12]. The incidence of seclusion and restraint varied from 35.6% of all admissions in Austria, to 2.6% in Norway and around 0% in Iceland and the UK, though notably, coercion is legally prohibited in Norway and only 1:1 nursing is used instead [13]. Risk was also elevated on Fridays [14]. In terms of legal status, the change from primarily involuntary to voluntary treatment has been demonstrated to be dependent on a variety of certain sociodemographic factors, such as young age, higher education and being employed [15]. Also rehospitalisation has an effect on the rate of involuntary admission [16]. Severity of psychotic symptomatology, measured by PANSS-scale was a risk factor in two independent studies [17, 18]. In most studies, schizophrenia has the highest impact on involuntary admissions [19, 20], fortified by comorbid substance abuse [21]. Also organic psychosis, married status and young age showed an elevated rate of involuntary admission in New York [22]. Interestingly, in Greece, the F1 diagnosis group showed a reverse risk compared to the risk associated with immigration (53.2 vs. 14.5%), whereas all other diagnostic category groups demonstrated a greater risk [23]. A systematic literature review done in 2008 [24] compared 41 previous studies and concluded that involuntarily admitted patients had a higher suicide rate, but no increased mortality had equal levels of psychopathology and treatment compliance. The primary research goal of this study is to identify factors influencing the risk for involuntary psychiatric hospital admission. Due to the fact that reducing these rates is probably only possible on the background of certain knowledge of these risk factors and changing of supposed structural influence factors depends this knowledge.

Methods

Sample

A retrospective, large-scale multicentre comparative study of psychiatric admissions was carried out in the district of Westphalia-Lippe of the German federal state of North Rhine-Westphalia for the years 2004–2009. Data were collected from within the LWL Psychiatry Network that consists of 13 psychiatric hospitals for adults (3700 treatment places). The catchment area covers about 8.5 million inhabitants, thus covering nearly half of the inhabitants of North Rhine-Westphalia and about 10% of the whole German population.

The hospital registry data (§21, German hospital reimbursement law) are usually transferred to health insurance companies as part of the daily routine, thus leading to the accumulation of a reliable and comprehensive database of sociodemographic information on all patients treated in the district. The type of information that is recorded includes date of admission, time of admission, date of discharge, diagnosis, legal status, including changes of legal status during the treatment, all coercive measures used, number of treatments, name of the hospital, date of birth, gender, age, family status, postal code, nationality and religious denomination.

The whole sample ($n = 230.678$) was divided into two main subsamples: voluntary ($n = 196,389$, which was 85.14% of the whole sample) and involuntary ($n = 34.289$, 14.86% of the whole sample) admissions to hospital. The involuntary admissions were then further divided into the two subgroups: one that was admitted under the PsychKG act and the other that was admitted on the basis of the civil law code of "guardianship" (Fig. 1). Only the PsychKG cases (17.206 patients; 50.18% of the involuntary admissions, 8.05% of all admissions) were included in the analysis in which PsychKG involuntary admissions were compared to voluntary admissions. The separation of subgroups and the sample size of each subgroup are shown in Fig. 1.

Data analysis

Data were collected retrospectively and analyses were calculated using statistical software (IBM SPSS Statistics 19.0®). Quantitative data are presented as mean and standard deviation. Due to the unequal group sizes,

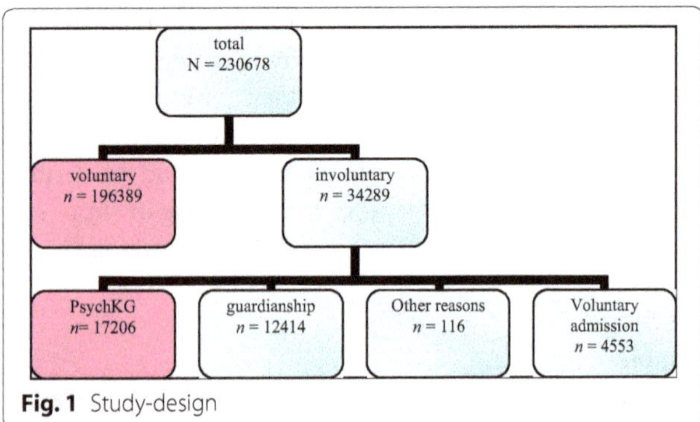

Fig. 1 Study-design

group differences were calculated by means of Chi-square tests or independent sample *t* tests. A Bonferroni correction was applied to control for multiple comparisons.

Results

Table 1 summarizes the full clinical and demographic data of the voluntary and involuntary subsamples, which are described in the following.

Demographic factors

Mean age was 4.12 years younger in the involuntary group ($p < .001$). Clustered age groups compared due to the legal implications showed a highly significant over-representation of the age groups 18–21, 61–70 and over 70 for involuntary admission. A comparison regarding the change of average age at time of both voluntary and involuntary admission over the time of study (Table 2) showed a steady rise from 43.73 years in 2004 (SD = 17.03) to 45.33 years (SD = 17.48) in 2009, demonstrating a 3.7% increase, but no significance ($p = .306$).

Married people appeared to display an increased risk for involuntary admission (married 28.4 vs. 30.7%, single 71.6 vs. 69.3%, $p < .001$).

Nationality showed no significant risk related to involuntary admissions. However, it is important to note that the data did not provide sufficient information to identify migration status, especially for those who were second or third generation migrants. Analysis of age-related subsamples showed that 38.5% of the patients with German origin were between 22 and 40 years old, and the fraction of patients from a non-German origin in this age group was higher than in other age groups (53.3% Italian, 54.3% Polish, 69.4% Turkish). From looking at the legal status of patients in the age group of 22–40, it appears that the portion of the voluntarily treated Germans and Italians was higher than those that were involuntarily treated (39.1 vs. 30.5% for the German population, 54.5 vs. 43.2% in the Italian group), 69.5% of the group with Turkish origin voluntarily treated were between 22 and 40 years old, whereas in the group of the involuntary treated patients, this amount was a little bit higher. A very clear difference between voluntary and involuntary admissions could be seen for the patients with Polish origin, whereby the proportion of those in this age group who were voluntarily treated was 53.3 and 69.6% in the involuntarily treated group.

Due to a large quantity of missing data, the influence of religious denomination is not interpretable.

Service-related factors

The total number of admissions for each month was calculated and a group comparison was made for the three months that had the highest number of admissions for each group. In the voluntary group, August (8.7%), July (8.6%) and March (8.6%) showed the highest number of admissions. The highest number of admissions in the involuntarily treated patients was in July (9.5%), followed by August (9.1%) and then June (9%). This difference showed high statistical significance ($p < .001$). One remarkable finding was that the most involuntary admissions happened during the summer months (24.7 vs. 27.6%, $p < .001$).

Further on, the day was divided into three parts: morning, afternoon and late afternoon and night. The greatest number of voluntary admissions (48%) occurred in the morning (8–12 a.m.), whereas only 16.2% of involuntary admissions occurred at this time of the day. The time of day in which the greatest number of involuntary admissions occurred was in the late afternoon and night, i.e. between 4 p.m. and 8 a.m. (57.5%), though only 24.8% of the voluntary admissions happened at this time ($p < .001$).

The groups differed also highly significant regarding the admitting profession: voluntary patients were primarily admitted by non-psychiatrists (54.5%, general practitioners: 46.1%, other specialities: 8.4%). In the involuntary group, general practitioners admitted 19.7% of the patients, other specialities for 14.7% (total 34.4%). Psychiatrists in practice have quite equal representation in both groups (31.5 vs. 31.8%). The involuntary group showed a higher amount of admissions initiated by hospital psychiatrist on call (33.5 vs. 13.7%, $p < .001$). Also the receiving department was of great importance for the investigated question. The largest proportion of the voluntarily treated patients was admitted to a department for addiction (41.3%), whereas most of the involuntary admissions were allocated to general psychiatry (48.2%). The voluntary admissions were allocated to gerontopsychiatry (11.8%) less than the involuntary admissions (20.9%, $p < .001$).

Table 1 Sociodemographic and illness-related data of voluntary and involuntary admissions, F0–G3: diagnostic groups according to ICD-10

	Variable	Voluntary ($N = 196{,}389$), data in %	Involuntary ($N = 17{,}206$), data in %	Group comparison	*p* value
Gender	Male	57.6	58.0	$\chi^2_{(1)} = 1.047$	$p = .306$
	Female	42.4	42.0		
Age	M (SD)	44.41 (17.04)	48.55 (19.52)	$t_{(19{,}561.444)} = -26.877$	$p < .001$
	<18	0.1	0.1	$\chi^2_{(7)} = 1263.41$	$p < .001$
	18–21	5.4	6.2		
	22–30	18.0	13.6		
	31–40	22.1	18.5		
	41–50	24.5	22.7		
	51–60	12.7	12.3		
	61–70	6.9	8.4		
	>70	10.2	18.1		
Marital status	Married	28.4	30.7	$\chi^2_{(2)} = 195.049$	$p < .001$
	Single	71.6	69.3		
Nationality	German	95.1	94.0	$\chi^2_{(4)} = 39.927$	$p < .001$
	Turkish	2.2	2.4		
	Polish	0.3	0.4		
	Italian	0.3	0.3		
	Other	2.1	2.8		
Religion	Roman-Catholic	49.6	54.2	Due to a high amount of missing data no statistics could be used	
	Protestant	34.4	32.7		
	Muslim	3.9	3.1		
	Other	12.1	10.0		
Month of admission (most frequent)	1	August: 8.7	July: 9.5	$\chi^2_{(11)} = 88.221$	$p < .001$
	2	July: 8.6	August: 9.1		
	3	March: 8.6	June: 9.0		
Time of day of admission	Morning (8–12 a.m.)	48.0	16.2	$\chi^2_{(2)} = 9704.74$	$p < .001$
	Afternoon (12 a.m.–4 p.m.)	27.2	26.3		
	Late afternoon and night (4 p.m.–8 a.m.)	24.8	57.5		
Admission type	Hospital doctor on call	13.7	33.5	$\chi^2_{(6)} = 3449.047$	$p < .001$
	(Psychiatrist)	31.5	31.8		
	General practitioner	46.1	19.7		
	Other specialist	8.4	14.7		
Service allocation	General psychiatry	40.4	48.2	$\chi^2_{(3)} = 2380.468$	$p < .001$
	Addiction psychiatry	41.3	28.0		
	Gerontopsychiatry	11.8	20.9		
	Other	6.5	3.0		
Main diagnosis (ICD-10)	F0	5.1	16.1	$\chi^2_{(10)} = 7709.130$	$p < .001$
	F1	36.7	22.8		
	F2	14.7	30.5		
	F3	28.2	14.9		
	F4	3.1	2.8		
	F5	0.2	0.1		
	F6	5.2	6.8		
	F7	1.7	1.8		
	F8	0.0	0.0		
	F9	0.2	0.5		
	G3	2.2	3.4		

Table 1 continued

	Variable	Voluntary ($N = 196{,}389$), data in %	Involuntary ($N = 17{,}206$), data in %	Group comparison	*p* value
Comorbidity	Psychiatric	47.4	43.6	$\chi^2_{(22)} = 1137.372$	$p < .001$
	Somatic	10.8	10.7	$\chi^2_{(40)} = 208.934$	$p < .001$
Duration of stay	M (SD)	22.60 (23.795)	24.84 (28.480)	$t_{(19{,}367.606)} = -10.005$	$p < .001$
	1 day	1.4	3.7	$\chi^2_{(8)} = 5922.69$	$p < .001$
	2 days	5.0	10.0		
	2 weeks	42.1	34.0		
	6 weeks	36.4	34.2		
	≥7 weeks	15.1	18.2		
Number of previous treatments	M (SD)	7.61 (12.79)	5.84 (10.12)	$t_{(22{,}316.321)} = 21.397$	$p < .001$
	1	24.5	33.5	$\chi^2_{(4)} = 786.410$	$p < .001$
	2	16.2	16.3		
	3	11.0	10.4		
	4–10	29.6	25.7		
	>10	18.8	14.1		

Table 2 The mean (M) age of admissions in the voluntary and involuntary group for each year over the study period of 2004–2009

Year of admittance	Age voluntary		Age involuntary	
	M	SD	M	SD
2004	46.66	18.569	43.73	17.025
2005	47.71	19.314	44.01	17.077
2006	48.06	19.571	44.22	16.936
2007	48.89	19.744	44.28	16.799
2008	50.16	19.805	44.65	16.862
2009	49.46	19.794	45.33	17.476

Illness-related factors

The most common diagnosis in the voluntary group was substances abuse (36.7%), while in the involuntary group, the most common diagnosis was in the schizophrenia (30.5%); schizophrenia was less than half as common in the voluntary group (14.7%). In the group of affective disorders (F3), there were quite reverse findings (28.2 vs. 14.9%), further differentiation (i.e. to F30, F31, F32, F33) showed an excess of bipolar affective disorder (18.9 vs. 7.2%) in the involuntary group.

In the ICD-10 F0/G3 diagnostic category (organic psychiatric disorders, in particular, dementia and other neurodegenerative diseases), a substantial difference was revealed between the groups. 19.5% of the involuntary group had a F0/G3 diagnosis, but only 7.3% of the voluntarily treated patients had this diagnosis.

For personality disorders (F6), a mild over-representation of involuntarily treated patients was found (6.8% involuntary vs. 5.2% voluntary). Group differences were highly significant for the main categories of diagnosis ($p < .001$).

Furthermore, the changes in percentages of diagnoses over the study period were different between the diagnostic categories (see Table 3). While most ICD-10 categories stayed quite stable (F0, F2, F5, F6, F7), a decline of ICD-10: F4-cluster could be demonstrated, whereas dementia (ICD-10: F0, G3) and affective disorder (ICD-10: F3) showed a clear increase (F0: 14.7% to 21.7%, F3 13.2% to 16.8%).

Psychiatric comorbidity was higher in the voluntarily treated group (47.4 vs. 43.6%, $p < .001$), whereas somatic comorbidity was quite equal (10.8 vs. 10.7%).

The duration of stay was compared in two different ways. First, a comparison of the median duration of stay was carried out, which revealed that the voluntarily treated patients had a generally shorter median duration of stay of 22.6 days (SD = 23.80) relative to the median duration of stay of the involuntary group (24.84 days, SD = 28.48, $p < .001$). In a second step, a comparison of both groups regarding different clusters of durations of stay was performed, looking at the proportion of patients that stayed for 1 day, 2 days, 2 weeks, 6 weeks and 7 or more weeks. The first notable result was that more than twice as many of the involuntarily admitted patients, as compared to the voluntary group, were discharged on the day of admission (3.7 vs. 1.4%). These findings were also very similar for duration of stay of 2 days (10 vs. 5%). However, medium-length stays were more common

Table 3 Percentage and number of admissions in each ICD-10 diagnostic category over study period, both groups

Main diagnosis	Year											
	2004		2005		2006		2007		2008		2009	
	N	%	*N*	%	*N*	%	*N*	%	*N*	%	*N*	%
F0	324	12.8	406	13.9	446	15.7	471	16.6	567	18.8	563	18.5
F1	683	26.9	693	23.7	646	22.7	604	21.3	630	20.9	659	21.6
F2	818	32.2	957	32.7	834	29.4	868	30.6	877	29.0	900	29.5
F3	336	13.2	408	13.9	453	16.0	426	15.0	436	14.4	512	16.8
F4	102	4.0	84	2.9	76	2.7	79	2.8	78	2.6	58	1.9
F5	1	0.0	3	0.1	4	0.1	1	0.0	3	0.1	2	0.1
F6	170	6.7	196	6.7	188	6.6	195	6.9	222	7.4	204	6.7
F7	34	1.3	52	1.8	53	1.9	49	1.7	59	2.0	56	1.8
F8	0	0.0	2	0.1	0	0.0	0	0.0	0	0.0	0	0.0
F9	13	0.5	10	0.3	23	0.8	21	0.7	17	0.6	9	0.3
G3	48	1.9	106	3.6	109	3.8	111	3.9	124	4.1	81	2.7
Not stated	9	0.4	10	0.3	8	0.3	7	0.2	7	0.2	5	0.2
Total	2538	100	2927	100	2840	100	2832	100	3020	100	3049	100

for the voluntary rather than involuntary admissions, as the proportion of the voluntary group that stayed for 2 and 6 weeks was 42.1 and 36.4%, respectively, whereas the proportion of stays for 2 and 6 weeks was 34.0 and 34.2% for involuntary admissions. For longer term stays (>7 weeks), the involuntary group was 18.2, 15.1% in the voluntary group. To sum up, it could be demonstrated that very short treatment times (1–2 days) were more common for involuntary admissions (6.4 vs. 13.7%, $p < .001$).

The mean number of previous treatments received by patients differed significantly in both groups [voluntary 7.61 (SD = 12.79), involuntary 5.84 (SD = 10.12), $p < .001$]. Looking at clustered numbers of pre-treatments, a further comparison of the groups was made. A substantially greater number of involuntary admissions were first hospitalized (24.5 vs. 33.5%), whereas the difference between the proportion of voluntary and involuntary groups for their second and third treatments was minimal (16.2 vs. 16.3% for 2nd treatment, and 11 vs. 10.4% for 3rd treatment). For the patients who had received 4–10 previous treatments, a greater proportion was represented by voluntary admissions (29.6 vs. 25.7%), which was also the case for those that had received more than ten previous treatments (18.8 vs. 14.1%).

Discussion

Analysis of the relationship between legal status, gender, age and diagnosis showed that the largest proportion of involuntary admissions was with men between 22 and 30 years old who suffered from an ICD-10: F2 diagnosis, which is concordant with the literature findings. It is likely that schizophrenia is a diagnosis that still has insufficient services for early recognition, and therefore schizophrenia appears in many cases with very impressive psychopathological features and thus may lead to a higher rate of emergency admittances. On the other hand, there is a large representation of women aged over 70 with an ICD-10: F0/G3 diagnosis. The predominance of females in this older group is likely to be an effect of the longer life expectancy of woman (actual data in Germany: woman: 82.73 years, man 77.72 years [25]. What also could be displayed was a clear decline in the ICD-10: F4-cluster which may be explained by an improvement of the out-patient service structure for people getting into acute psychiatric crisis situations.

The finding that being married is possibly associated with an increased risk for involuntary admission is also quite interesting and was not expected, particularly as stable social surroundings are generally thought to be protective. Possibly, additional problems that accompany being in a relationship (e.g. marital crisis, problems in education of children, deaths of close relatives) may act as stress factors which may worsen illness. Previous findings of the influence of being married on preventing involuntary admission are mixed in literature, and still not satisfactorily elucidated [22, 26, 27]. Further research on this topic is needed, especially as only a few studies on this topic exist until now [10, 20, 22]. Therefore, it is likely that the influence of family status has a multidimensional aspect and thus could only be clarified in a specific, prospective survey with a main focus on this topic.

Another quite interesting finding is that most of the voluntarily treated patients were admitted during regular hospital hours rather than on duty time. One explanation for this finding could be that the more severely ill patients are less able to admit themselves to hospital, and only the presentation of acute symptomatology like suicidal intent or aggressive behaviour would initiate an admission. This might indicate that the needs of severely affected psychiatric patients are not met by the current structures of psychiatric services. This was confirmed by other studies [28].

Regarding the migration background, the most interesting finding shows that the rate of patients with a non-German origin was higher in the involuntary than in the voluntary group, which is especially prominent for migrants coming from eastern European countries [9]. The high representation of young Polish people for involuntary admissions may be explained by the long history of immigration to this area for work in the coal mines over the past 100 or so years, which now has gone down. In general, the findings from our study show that young people who had immigrated to North Rhine-Westphalia seemed to be especially more often in psychiatric crisis. Problems of integration probably have an important influence on this effect, possibly also due to communication barriers [29, 30].

Due to the result that most of the involuntarily admitted patients were diagnosed with schizophrenia spectrum disorders (F2), and were also mostly admitted during the summer months, the question of whether there may be a relationship between environment, climate and psychosis should be raised again. Many authors have suggested that there is the potential for higher dopamine levels during the summer months due to higher environment temperatures [31–34]. Another possible explanation for this season-related finding could be that psychiatric services during summer months are not quite as well equipped as in other seasons, due to a higher number of staff taking holidays, and thus leading to a reduction in resources. It may be that access to the patients' support system, like guardianship, during the summer months may be reduced, as compared to the other seasons. However, this suggestion is highly speculative and would require confirmation from future studies looking more specifically into the effect of season on involuntary admissions.

Another main finding from this study was that a higher proportion of involuntary admissions fell under the category of short-term treatments, when compared to voluntary admissions. One possible explanation for the higher incidence of short-term treatments in the involuntary group may be due to the over-representation of the diagnosis of acute intoxication (ICD-10: F1X.0) in this group, which normally leads to only very short treatment times due to the short duration of the influence of intoxication on psychopathology.

Conclusion

Due to limitation of a retrospective study with a restricted and unswayable data pool, our findings have to be considered carefully. Our main findings, the risk for involuntary admissions for older women with dementia and younger man with schizophrenia lead to the necessity of special attention for these groups of people. Further on, a prospective study is needed to minimize the limitations reported below.

Limitations

To the best of the authors' knowledge, this study is the most extensive investigation on this topic related to a catchment area of this size, but was limited by the structure of the data, because the data structure had been already predefined for purposes other than research, and could not be adjusted for the use in such a study. This has to be taken into account when considering its results: the use of complete hospital admission and discharge registers enabled us to investigate the largest cohort of this kind in psychiatric hospitals so far published. However, at the same time, the retrospective nature of this study and the structure of the data only allowed for limited conclusions, partly as a result of the limited period in which the data covered, i.e. covering data on admissions between 2004 and 2009. This was due to the fact that these data had only been stored electronically since 2004. In addition to this, information on the potential risk of harm to self or others prior to the admission or the administration of medication throughout the hospital stay was not available, otherwise additional connections and conclusions could have been drawn out of such data. Other factors (e.g. family background, physical and cognitive development, suicidality, aggressiveness, treatment variables or past experiences regarding the health care system) that may have had an influence on the admission status were also not included. In order to draw a realistic picture of the current mental health care situation, and to consider the severity and course of certain diseases, all treatment data over the 6-year period were used, and as a result, it was not that data on single patients were included in the analysis, but rather treatment "cases". One patient might therefore have been included several times if they had been re-admitted during the study period. This might have thus caused a bias in the results on age, gender and diagnosis in the subgroups. The very important issue of patients' subjective perception towards coercion during admission could also not be assessed because of the retrospective nature of the data used and the large sample size. Further research on this topic is evidently needed, ideally in the form of a prospective study.

Despite the limitations, the following issues were identified as areas that could be addressed to reduce involuntary psychiatric treatments. The first issue highlighted by this study that could have an influence is the early recognition and prevention of psychotic disorders in young people, with a particular focus on improving these services for males. In addition, a greater involvement of government mental health services might be very useful in preventing acute psychiatric crises and thus also reducing consecutive involuntary admission. Secondly, this study highlights the importance of making service improvements for older people, especially females, suffering from delirium/dementia. Due to the overall increasing age of the population, it is inevitable that the number of older people with ICD-10 F0/G3 diagnosis will rise in both genders. Only an improvement of non-hospital psychiatric services in conjunction with early intervention services could help to prevent this group of patients from involuntary treatment. Thirdly, in terms of immigration, the data in this study particularly identify an over-representation of Polish people being involuntarily admitted. One step towards addressing this issue of immigration as being a possible risk factor for involuntary psychiatric treatment may be to have a closer look at improving the integration of immigrants, while also taking addiction and addiction prevention into special consideration.

Authors' contributions

GJ, KH, ISH, AD conceived of the study, and participated in its design and coordination. KH drafted the manuscript. FI, JJ, BE, CA and AS did the statistical analysis. All the authors helped in collecting the data and transferring them to SPSS. All authors read and approved the final manuscript.

Author details

[1] Dept. of Psychiatry, LWL Institute of Mental Health, LWL University Hospital, Ruhr-University Bochum, Alexandrinenstr.1, 44791 Bochum, Germany.
[2] Department of Psychiatry, LWL-University Hospital Bochum, Alexandrinenstr. 1, 44791 Bochum, Germany. [3] NRW Center for Health, Gesundheitscampus 9, 44801 Bochum, Germany.

Acknowledgements

The authors gratefully acknowledge the collaborative partners in the LWL-PsychiatryNetwork, especially: Leßmann J. (LWL-hospital Warstein and Lippstadt), Sprick U. (LWL-hospital Dortmund), Kronmüller KT (LWL-hospital Gütersloh), Holtmann M. (LWL-University hospital Hamm), Trenckmann U. (LWL-hospital Hemer), Turmes L. (LWL-hospital Herten), Chrysanthou C. (LWL-hospital Lengerich), Haas C. R. (LWL-hospital Marl-Sinsen), Bender S. (LWL-hospital Marsberg), Reker T (LWL-hospital Münster), Vieten B (LWL-hospital Paderborn), Bruchmann G. (LWL-Psychiatrieverbund), Schnieder H. (LWL-Psychiatrieverbund), Profazi T. (LWL-Psychiatrieverbund und LWL-IT), Schuhmann-Wessolek H. (LWL-Psychiatrieverbund), Höffler J. (Martin-Luther-hospital Bochum-Wattenscheid), Nyhuis P. W. (St. Marien-Hospital Herne-Eickel), Schulze-Mönking H. (Sankt-Rochus-Hospital Telgte), Massing P. (LVR-Dezernat Klinikverbund und Heilpädagogischen Hilfen), van Brederode M. (LVR-Dezernat Klinikverbund und Heilpädagogischen Hilfen), Gaebel W. (LVR-Klinikum Universität Düsseldorf) SpD Bochum (Kalthoff J), SpD Dortmund Mitte. SpD Dortmund Nord. SpD Kreis Gütersloh. SpD Hamm. SpD Hemer. SpD Herne. SpD Herten. SpD Lengerich. SpD Lippstadt. SpD Marl. SpD Marsberg. SpD Münster. SpD Paderborn. SpD Wanne-Eickel. SpD Kreis Warendorf. SpD Warstein.

Competing interests

G. J. received fees for consulting from AstraZeneca, Bristol-Myers-Squibb/Otsuka, Janssen, Lilly, Lundbeck, Pfizer. He was advisory board member of AstraZeneca, Bristol-Myers-Squibb/Otsuka, Janssen-Cilag. He received research funding from Jansen, AstraZeneca, Lundbek, BMS. All other authors declare that there are no competing interests.

Funding body agreements and policies

This study was supported by the NRW Center for Health LZG.NRW (SZ-01/2010).

References

1. Spengler A. Zwangseinweisungen in Deutschland—Basisdaten und Trends. Psychiatr Prax. 2005;34:191–5.
2. Spengler A, Dressing H, Koller M, Salize HJ. Zwangseinweisungen—bundesweite Basisdaten und Trends. Nervenarzt. 2005;76:363–70.
3. Darsow-Schütte KI, Müller P. Zahl der Einweisungen nach PsychKG in 10 Jahren verdoppelt. Psychiatr Prax. 2001;28:226–9.
4. Leßmann J. Zur Differenzierung von Zuweisungen und Unterbringungen nach PsychKG. Recht Psychiatr. 2010;8:132–6.
5. Salize HJ, Spengler A, Dressing H. Involuntary hospital admissions of mentally ill patients—how specific are differences among the German federal states? Psychiatr Prax. 2007;34((suppl 2)):196–202.
6. Haebler D, von Beuscher H, Fähndrich E, Kunz D, Priebe S, Heinz A. Wie offen kann die Psychiatrie sein? Zwangseinweisungen in zwei innerstädtischen Berliner Bezirken. Dtsch Arztebl t. 2007;104:A–1232/B–1096/C–1048.
7. Dressing H, Salize HJ. Compulsory admission of mentally ill patients in European Union Member States. Soc Psychiatry Psychiatr Epidemiol. 2004;39:797–803.
8. Oyffe I, Kurs R, Gelkopf M, Melamed Y, Bleich A. Revolving-door patients in a public psychiatric hospital in Israel: cross sectional study. Croat Med J. 2009;50:575–82.
9. Bruxner G, Burvill P, Fazio S, Febbo S. Aspects of psychiatric admission of migrants to hospitals in Perth, Western Australia. Aust N Z J Psychiatry. 1997;31:532–42.
10. Spengler A. Factors influencing assignment of patients to compulsory admission. Soc Psychiatry. 1986;21:113–22.
11. Steinert T, Martin V, Baur M, Bohnt U, Goebel R, Hermelink G, Kronstorfer R, Kuster W, Martinez-Funk B, Roser M, Schwink A, Voigtländer W. Diagnosis-related frequency of compulsory measures in 19 German psychiatric hospitals and correlates with hospital characteristics. Soc Psychiatry Psychiatr Epidemiol. 2007;42:140–5.
12. Lay B, Nordt C, Rössler W. Variation in use of coercive measures in psychiatric hospitals. Eur Psychiatry. 2011;26:244–51.
13. Steinert T, Lepping P, Bernhardsgrütter R, Conca A, Hatling T, Janssen W, Keski-Valkam A, Mayoral F, Whittington R. Incidence of seclusion and restraint in psychiatric hospitals: a literature review and survey of international trends. Soc Psychiatry Psychiatr Epidemiol. 2010;45:889–97.
14. Kropp S, Blanke U, Meiners-Emrich H. Involuntary hospitalisations in 2000 according to German PsychKG in the city of Hannover. Psychiatr Prax. 2005;32(1):18–22.
15. Nicholson RA. Characteristics associated with change in the legal status of involuntary psychiatric patients. Hosp Community Psychiatry. 1988;39:424–9.
16. Rosca P, Bauer A, Grinshpoon A, Khawaled R, Mester R, Ponizovsky AM. Rehospitalization among psychiatric patients whose first admission was involuntary; a 10-year follow-up. Isr Psychiatry Relat Sci. 2006;43:57–64.
17. Steinert T, Schmid P. Voluntariness and coercion in patients with schizophrenia. Psychiatr Prax. 2004;31:28–33.
18. Wheeler A, Robinson E, Robinson G. Admissions to acute psychiatric inpatient services in Auckland, New Zealand: a demographic and diagnostic review. N Z Med J. 2005;118:1752.

19. Opjordsmoen S, Friis S, Melle I, Haahr U, Johannessen JO, Larsen TK, Rossberg JI, Rund BR, Simonsen E, Vaglum P, McGlashan TH. A 2-year follow-up of involuntary admission's influence upon adherence and outcome in first-episode psychosis. Acta Psychiatr Scand. 2010;121:371–6.
20. Sanguinetti VR, Samuel SE, Schwartz SL, Robeson MR. Retrospective study of 2200 involuntary psychiatric admissions and readmissions. Am J Psychiatry. 1996;153:392–6.
21. Ng XT, Kelly BD. Voluntary and involuntary care: three-year study of demographic and diagnostic admission at an inner-city adult psychiatry unit. Int J Law Psychiatry. 2010;35:317–26.
22. Opsal A, Clausen T, Kristensen Ø, Elvik I, Joa I, Larsen TK. Involuntary hospitalization of first-episode psychosis with substance abuse during a 2-year follow-up. Acta Psychiatr Scand. 2011;124:198–204.
23. Rabinowitz J, Slyuzberg M, Salamon I, Dupler SE. Differential use of admission status in a psychiatric emergency room. Bull Am Acad Psychiatry Law. 1995;23:595–606.
24. Bilanakis N, Kalampokis G, Christou K, Peritogiannis V. Use of coercive physical measures in a psychiatric ward of a general hospital in Greece. Int J Soc Psychiatry. 2010;56:402–11.
25. Kallert TW, Glöckner M, Schützwohl M. Involuntary vs. voluntary hospital admission. A systematic literature review on outcome diversity. Eur Arch Psychiatry Clin Neurosci. 2008;258:195–209.
26. Statistisches Bundesamt. Lebenserwartung in Deutschland. 2013. www.destatis.de/De/ZahlenFakten/GesellschaftStaat/Bevoelkerung/Sterbefälle/Tabellen/Lebenserwartung/Deutschland.html. Accessed 07 Jan 2013.
27. Kelly BD, Clarke M, Brown S, Mc Tigue O, Gervin M, Kinsella A, Lane A, Larkin C, O'Callaghan E. Clinical predictors of admission status in first episode schizophrenia. Eur Psychiatry. 2004;19:67–71.
28. Feigon S, Hays JR. Prediction of readmission of psychiatric inpatients. Psychol Rep. 2003;93(3 Pt 1):816–8.
29. Hustoft K, Larsen TK, Auestad B, Johannessen JO, Ruud T. Predictors of involuntary hospitalizations to acute psychiatry. Int J Law Psychiatry. 2013;36:136–43.
30. Künzler N, Garcia-Brand E, Schmauss M, Messer T. German language skills among foreign psychiatric patients: influence of voluntariness and duration of hospital treatment. Psychiatr Prax. 2004;31(suppl 1):21–3.
31. Eisenberg DP, Kohn PD, Baller EB, Bronstein JA, Masdeu JC, Berman KF. Seasonal effects on human striatal presynaptic dopamine synthesis. J Neurosci. 2010;30:14691–4.
32. Chong TW, Castle DJ. Layer upon layer: thermoregulation in schizophrenia. Schizophr Res. 2004;69:149–57.
33. Amr M, Volpe FM. Seasonal influences on admission for mood disorders and schizophrenia in a teaching psychiatric hospital in Egypt. J Affect Disord. 2012;37:56–60.
34. Sung TI, Chen MJ, Lin CY, Lung SC, Su HJ. Relationship between mean daily ambient temperature range and hospital admissions for schizophrenia: results from a national cohort of psychiatric inpatients. Sci Total Environ. 2011;41:410–1.

4

Prevalence and effect of attention-deficit/hyperactivity disorder on school performance among primary school pupils in the Hohoe Municipality, Ghana

Kingsley Afeti and Samuel Harrenson Nyarko*

Abstract

Background: Attention-deficit/hyperactivity disorder (ADHD) is one of the most common disorders in early childhood. However, not many studies have been conducted on the prevalence and effect of ADHD on school performance in Ghana. This study sought to ascertain the prevalence of ADHD and its effect on school performance among primary school pupils in the Hohoe municipality of Ghana.

Methods: This is a cross-sectional descriptive study that included 400 primary school pupils in the Hohoe Municipality of Ghana. The study adopted the disruptive behaviour disorder rating scale which includes the three subtypes of ADHD among pupils in the form of a close-ended questionnaire for data collection.

Results: The results revealed the overall prevalence of ADHD to be 12.8%. The males had a higher prevalence (14.4%) compared to the females (10.5%). For the subtypes, the prevalence was 8.0% for attention-deficit disorder, 8.5% for hyperactivity disorder and 3.8% for the combined subtype. In terms of school performance, the results showed that there was a significant difference in the school performance between ADHD-positive pupils and the negative status pupils among the various core subjects.

Conclusions: Attention-deficit/hyperactivity disorder was quite prevalent among primary school pupils in the Hohoe Municipality, and has impacted negatively on their school performance. Screening of pupils for ADHD should be integrated into the school health services to enable early detection and management.

Keywords: Prevalence, Attention-deficit/hyperactivity disorder, Primary school pupils, Hohoe, Ghana

Background

Education is an important tool for national development. In the developing countries including Africa, where the literacy level is low, significant efforts are directed toward the need to increase the level of literacy through increasing priority for education [1]. In Ghana, there have been some initiatives to improve upon school work, including the introduction of the School Feeding Programme, provision of school uniforms and shoes to students and the awarding of scholarships to needy but brilliant children. In spite of these efforts, little is done to identify and eliminate the impediments to learning, especially among children. One of such impediments is attention-deficit/hyperactivity disorder (ADHD), which has been identified to affect 3–12% of primary school children [2].

Attention-deficit/hyperactivity disorder is one of the most common disorders in early childhood [3]. It is characterized by inattention, hyperactivity, and impulsivity, cognitive, behavioural, and emotional deficits. It is also closely related to learning disabilities, lack of self-control, and social skill deficits [4]. There are three subtypes of ADHD: predominantly inattentive type (attention-deficit disorder, ADD), predominantly hyperactive type (hyperactivity disorder) and the combined type [5]. It has been

*Correspondence: samharrenson@gmail.com
Department of Population and Behavioural Sciences, School of Public Health, University of Health and Allied Sciences, Hohoe, Ghana

estimated that more than 50% of children with ADHD are prone to experience other psychiatric disorders such as oppositional defiant disorder (ODD), depression and anxiety disorder [6]. The major etiological factor has been identified to be genetic [7].

While it was previously thought that children eventually outgrow ADHD, recent studies suggest that 30–60% of affected children continue to show significant symptoms of the disorder during adulthood [8]. ADHD can be counted as a major public health issue due to its prevalence and chronic nature, and its potential to interfere with different areas of developmental relevance [9]. Also, ADHD has effects on the school performance of children. Children with more symptoms of ADHD, including impulsiveness or restlessness, have significantly lower math and reading scores on standardized tests, increased probability of class repetition, enrollment in special education, and delinquency, which includes behaviours such as stealing, hitting people, or using drugs [10]. In adulthood, problems caused by ADHD may include lateness, absenteeism, excessive errors, and an inability to accomplish expected workloads. At home, relationship difficulties and breakups may be more common [11].

In spite of the fact that ADHD hinders school development in children and has adulthood negative effects, not much has been done on it. Little information also exists on the prevalence of ADHD and its effects on school children in Ghana. This study, therefore, sought to investigate the prevalence of ADHD and its effect on school performance by comparing the school performance of children diagnosed with ADHD and those without ADHD in the core subjects.

Methods

The study was conducted in the Hohoe Municipality of the Volta Region, Ghana. It was conducted among pupils in 10 public and private schools between the ages of 6 and 12 in the classes of primary 1 to 6. This target population had no pupils with intellectual disability and their culturally compatible IQ tests would place them in the normal range of intelligence. The study adopted a descriptive cross-sectional study design.

Simple random sampling (lottery method) was used to select ten schools for the study. The process was carried out by writing the names of all the primary schools in the municipality on sheets of paper that were folded and then randomly picking 10 out of them. Quota sampling technique was then used to select 400 respondents from all the classes in the schools selected.

This study used the parent/teacher disruptive behaviour disorder rating scale (DBDRS) in the form of a close-ended questionnaire for data collection. This explores the prevalence of all three subtypes of ADHD among the pupils. The parent/teacher DBDRS is a standard rating scale used to screen children for the presence of ADHD and other disruptive behaviours diagnosed in early childhood. This rating scale was completed by the class teacher because it was assumed that the teacher might have been with the child for more than 3 months and, therefore, knew the child well enough to complete the rating scale on his or her behalf. The school performance of each pupil in the core subjects such as Mathematics, Science and English was also obtained from the school registers. The performance was, therefore, classified based on a grading of 70–100% for good performance, 40–69 for average and 39 or below for poor performance.

The completed questionnaires were cleaned and checked for completeness. Stata version 12 was used to process the data. The results were presented in tables in the form of frequencies, percentages and proportions, while Chi square test was used to examine the effect of ADHD on school performance of the pupils. Pupils diagnosed with the disorder were labelled 'positive' while those without the disorder were labelled 'negative'.

Results

Background characteristics

A summary of the background characteristics of respondents has been presented in Table 1. The respondents were made up of 57.3% males and 42.7% females. The ages of the respondents ranged from 6 to 12 with an average age of 9.6. The highest representation of 40.5% was for respondents who were aged 11–12, while the least representation was for respondents aged 6–7 with 21.5%. The respondents were selected from classes 1–6 in primary schools. Class 1 was the most represented with 23.0%, followed by class 2 with 18.7%, while class 6 was the least represented with 11.5%.

Table 1 Background characteristics of respondents

Variables	Frequency	Percentages
Sex		
Male	229	57.3
Female	171	42.7
Age		
6–7	86	21.5
8–10	152	38.0
11–12	162	40.5
Classes		
1	92	23.0
2	75	18.7
3	64	16.0
4	61	15.3
5	62	15.5
6	46	11.5

Prevalence of ADHD

The total prevalence of ADHD has been presented in Table 2. Out of the 400 respondents who participated in the study, 51 met the criteria for the diagnosis of ADHD, which represents a total prevalence of 12.8%. The prevalence is presented as the prevalence for males (14.41%), the prevalence for females (10.53%) and the total prevalence (12.8%).

Results were also presented for the various subtypes of ADHD by the background characteristics of the respondents. The results for the first subtype, ADD, have been presented in Table 3. As indicated in the table, the total prevalence of the ADD subtype was 8.0%, the male and female prevalence were 9.6% and 5.9%, respectively. However, there was no significant association between sex of respondent and ADD. In terms of age, the prevalence for respondents aged 8–10 was 10.5% while that for respondents aged 6–7 was 4.7%, though there was no significant association between age of respondent and ADD. With regard to the classes, the highest prevalence was found in class four (14.7%), followed by class two (12.0%), and the least was class one (2.2%). In effect, there was a significant association between class of respondent and the ADD subtype (PV = 0.034).

A summary of the results for the second subtype, hyperactivity disorder (HD), is also presented in Table 4. The total prevalence of the HD subtype was 8.5%, the male and female HD prevalence were 9.6% and 7.0%, respectively, even though there was no significant association between sex of respondent and the HD subtype.

For age, the prevalence of the HD subtype was highest (11.7%) among respondents aged 11–12, but was lowest among respondents aged 8–10 (4.6%). However, there was no significant association between age of respondent and the HD subtype. With the classes, the highest (17.3%) prevalence was among class two pupils, followed by class six pupils (15.2%), while the least was observed among class one pupils (2.2%). As such, the results showed a significant association between class of respondent and the HD subtype (PV = 0.004).

Table 5 shows a summary of the results for the combined subtype. The total prevalence of the combined type observed was 3.8%, while prevalence for males was 4.8% and that for females was 2.3%. However, no significant association was observed between sex of respondent and the combined subtype. The highest prevalence of 4.0% was observed among pupils aged 8–10, while the lowest prevalence (3.5%) was observed among pupils aged 6–7, and there was no significant association between age of respondent and the combined subtype. Disparities were also observed among the different classes with the highest (6.7%) prevalence being among class two pupils and

Table 2 Total prevalence of attention-deficit/hyperactivity disorder

Variables	Negative	Positive	Total
Sex			
Male	196 (85.59%)	33 (14.41%)	229
Female	153 (89.47%)	18 (10.53%)	171
Total	349 (87.25%)	51 (12.75%)	400

Table 3 Prevalence of the attention-deficit disorder subtype

Prevalence of attention-deficit disorder (inattention symptoms)				Chi square (*P* value)
	Negative ADHD status *N* = 368 (%)	Positive ADHD Status *N* = 32 (%)	Total *N* = 400 (%)	
Sex				
Male	207 (90.4)	22 (9.6)	229 (57.3)	1.87 (0.170)
Female	161 (94.1)	10 (5.9)	171 (42.7)	
Age				
6–7	82 (95.3)	4 (4.7)	86 (21.5)	2.70 (0.258)
8–10	136 (89.5)	16 (10.5)	152 (38.0)	
11–12	150 (92.6)	12 (7.4)	162 (40.5)	
Class				
Class one	90 (97.8)	2 (2.2)	92 (23.0)	12.09 (0.034)
Class two	66 (88.0)	9 (12.0)	75 (18.8)	
Class three	59 (92.2)	5 (7.8)	64 (16.0)	
Class four	52 (85.3)	9 (14.7)	61 (15.2)	
Class five	60 (96.8)	2 (3.2)	62 (15.5)	
Class six	41 (89.1)	5 (10.9)	46 (11.5)	

Table 4 Prevalence of the hyperactivity disorder subtype

Prevalence of hyperactivity disorder (hyperactivity/impulsivity symptoms)				Chi square (*P* value)
	Negative ADHD status *N* = 366 (%)	Positive ADHD status *N* = 34 (%)	Total *N* = 400 (%)	
Sex				
Male	207 (90.4)	22 (9.6)	229 (57.3)	0.84 (0.358)
Female	159 (93.0)	12 (7.0)	171 (42.7)	
Age				
6–7	78 (90.7)	8 (9.3)	86 (21.5)	5.20 (0.074)
8–10	145 (95.4)	7 (4.6)	152 (38.0)	
11–12	143 (88.3)	19 (11.7)	162 (40.5)	
Class				
Class one	90 (97.8)	2 (2.2)	92 (23.0)	17.32 (0.004)
Class two	62 (82.7)	13 (17.3)	75 (18.8)	
Class three	62 (96.9)	2 (3.1)	64 (16.0)	
Class four	56 (91.8)	5 (8.2)	61 (15.2)	
Class five	57 (91.9)	5 (8.1)	62 (15.5)	
Class six	39 (84.8)	7 (15.2)	46 (11.5)	

Table 5 Prevalence of the combined subtype

Combined subtype				Chi square (*P* value)
	Negative ADHD status *N* = 385 (%)	Positive ADHD status *N* = 15 (%)	Total *N* = 400 (%)	
Sex				
Male	218 (95.2)	11 (4.8)	229 (57.3)	1.64 (0.199)
Female	167 (97.7)	4 (2.3)	171 (42.7)	
Age				
6–7	83 (96.5)	3 (3.5)	86 (21.5)	0.03 (0.983)
8–10	146 (96.0)	6 (4.0)	152 (38.0)	
11–12	156 (96.3)	6 (3.7)	162 (40.5)	
Class				
Class one	90 (97.8)	2 (2.2)	92 (23.0)	5.24 (0.387)
Class two	70 (93.3)	5 (6.7)	75 (18.8)	
Class three	63 (98.4)	1 (1.6)	64 (16.0)	
Class four	58 (95.1)	3 (4.9)	61 (15.2)	
Class five	61 (98.4)	1 (1.6)	62 (15.5)	
Class six	43 (93.5)	3 (6.5)	46 (11.5)	

the least being among classes two and five pupils (1.6%), though no significant association was observed between class of respondent and the combined subtype.

Effect of ADHD on school performance of pupils with ADHD

The study also sought to examine the possible effect of ADHD on the school performance of the respondents. Table 6, therefore, shows a summary of results on the performance of ADHD-positive respondents as compared to respondents who were ADHD negative. As indicated in the table, close to half (49.2%) of the respondents had an average performance in Mathematics and 42% had good performance while only 8.8% had poor performance. However, 26.7% of the ADHD positive pupils performed poorly compared to 8.1% of the ADHD-negative pupils. Also, 13.3% of the positive pupils had a good performance compared to 43.1% of the ADHD negative respondents. Consequently, the results showed a significant difference in performance in Mathematics between respondents

Table 6 School performance of pupils with the ADHD combined subtype

School performance of students with ADHD combined type				Chi square (*P* value)
	Negative ADHD status	Positive ADHD status	Total	
	N = 385 (%)	*N* = 15 (%)	*N* = 400 (%)	
Mathematics				
Poor performance	31 (8.1)	4 (26.7)	35 (8.8)	9.13 (0.010)
Average performance	188 (48.8)	9 (60.0)	197 (49.2)	
Good performance	166 (43.1)	2 (13.3)	168 (42.0)	
Science				
Poor performance	33 (8.6)	3 (20.0)	36 (9.0)	8.52 (0.014)
Average performance	186 (48.3)	11 (73.3)	197 (49.3)	
Good performance	166 (43.1)	1 (6.7)	167 (42.7)	
English				
Poor performance	33 (8.6)	2 (13.3)	35 (8.8)	12.22 (0.002)
Average performance	177 (46.0)	13 (86.7)	190 (47.5)	
Good performance	175 (45.4)	0 (0.0)	175 (43.7)	

diagnosed with ADHD and those without ADHD (PV = 0.010).

For science, 49.3% of the respondents performed averagely, 42% had good performance, and only 9.0% performed poorly. Twenty percent of the ADHD-positive respondents had poor performance compared to 8.6% of the ADHD-negative respondents. Likewise, 6.7% of the ADHD-positive respondents attained good performance compared to 43.1% of the ADHD-negative respondents. Therefore, the study found a significant difference in performance in the Science subject between ADHD-positive and the ADHD-negative respondents (PV = 0.014).

With regard to English language, 47.5% of the respondents were average performers while 43.7% were good performers with only 8.8% being poor performers. About 13% of the ADHD-positive respondents performed poorly compared to 8.6% for the ADHD-negative respondents who performed poorly. In the same way, none of the ADHD-positive respondents were good performers in English language compared to 45.4% of the ADHD-negative respondents who were good performers in the subject. The study, therefore, showed a significant difference in performance in the English language subject between the ADHD-positive and the negative respondents (PV = 0.002).

Discussion

This study found the total prevalence of ADHD among pupils in the Hohoe municipality to be 12.8%. In the context of the study area, this prevalence may be on the high side. On the other hand, a similar study also came out with a similar prevalence of 11.6% in Jeddah City, Saudi Arabia [12]. However, the prevalence of ADHD in this study is rather quite lower than the prevalence in other studies such as the 23.1% found in Benin Metropolis, Nigeria by Abikwi [13].

Furthermore, the findings of the study showed prevalence of the subtypes as ADD 8.0%, HD 8.5%, and the combined subtype of 3.8%. In a similar study conducted in Lebanon, Bathiche [14] found the prevalence of the subtypes of ADHD to be 11.4% for the ADD (inattentive), 8.7% for the HD (the hyperactive/impulsive), and 3.5% for the combined type. However, these results are quiet higher compared to findings from other studies such as Ofovwe et al. [15], where the prevalence of the various subtypes were 3.0% for ADD, 2.7% for HD, and 2.5% for the combined subtype. This implies that the prevalence of ADHD varies among studies due to a number of factors, some of which may be the study setting as well as the target population of the study.

The study showed a significantly higher prevalence among males compared to females in all the three subtypes of ADHD, making it a common disorder among the males than the females. Also, the results showed that sex and age of respondent had no association with all the three subtypes of the disorder. This could mean that the symptoms may not differ between the sexes and may not diminish as the child grows older. However, class of respondent had a significant association with two of the subtypes except the combined subtype. This may imply that regardless of the child's sex or age, there were some significant differences among the various classes in terms of the ADD and the HD. It may also mean that the prevalence or the symptoms of ADD and HD may persist with the increase in the class or age of the respondents.

The results further revealed that school performance in subjects such as Mathematics, Science and English was poorer among ADHD-positive respondents than the ADHD-negative respondents. Thus, not only was the school performance poor among the ADHD-positive respondents compared to the ADHD-negative respondents, but also, there were significant differences in the school performance of the two categories of respondents in all the three subjects. This means that ADHD has serious implications for the school performance of the respondents. A number of similar studies around the globe have, therefore, come out with similar findings. For instance, Daley and Birchwood [16] have come out that ADHD is associated with school underachievement across the developmental spectrum, from preschoolers to adults. In another study, Bolic et al. [17] indicate that students with ADHD had low satisfaction with computer use in school, which implied that pupils with ADHD are more likely to have poorer school performance in educational activities that require the use of computer than their counterparts. This may be explained as a result of lack of focus on school work due to the various obvious symptoms of the disorder among the respondents. However, a potential limitation of this study may be that since the class teacher is the only observer and respondent of the rating scale, it is possible for the teacher to be biased, which could influence the findings particularly at the lower classes. Nevertheless, this may not have any direct effect on the findings, since it has to do with school performance of pupils and not children in general.

Conclusions

The study showed that ADHD is quite a prevalent disorder among primary school pupils in the Hohoe Municipality, Ghana. The disorder has a dire implication for the school performance of the school pupils in the municipality. Hence, pupils with positive ADHD status are more likely to perform poorly in school compared to their counterparts with negative ADHD status. It is, therefore, imperative to integrate the screening of pupils for ADHD into the school health services in order to enable early detection and management of the disorder. Also, there is the need to intensively educate teachers on ADHD and how they can manage these pupils in order to help to improve their school performance. This can be done by the District Health Directorate through organizing workshops on ADHD for teachers.

Abbreviations

ADHD: attention-deficit/hyperactivity disorder; ADD: attention-deficit disorder; HD: hyperactivity disorder; DBDRS: disruptive behaviour disorder rating scale; IQ: intelligent quotient.

Authors' contributions

KA conceived, designed the study and performed the analysis. SHN drafted and edited the manuscript. Both authors read and approved the final manuscript.

Acknowledgements

The authors wish to show their sincerest appreciation to the teaching staff of the schools that participated in the study for their role in the data collection process.

Competing interests

The authors declare that they have no competing interests.

References

1. Meyer A, Eilertsen DE, Sundet JM, Tshifularo JG, Sagvolden T. Cross-cultural similarities in ADHD-like behaviour amongst South African primary school children. South Afri J Psych. 2004;34:123–39.
2. American Academy of Pediatrics. Clinical practice guideline: diagnosis and evaluation of the child with attention-deficit/hyperactivity disorder. Pediatrics. 2004;10:1158–70.
3. Breton JJ, Bergeron L, Valla JP, Berthiaume C, Gaudet N, Lambert J, St-Georges M, Houde L, Lépine S. Quebec child mental health survey: prevalence of DSM-III-R mental health disorders. J Child Psych Psychiat. 1999;40(3):375–84.
4. Khushabi K, Pour-Etemad H, Mohammadi M, Mohammad Khan P. The prevalence of ADHD in primary school students in Tehran. Med J Islamic Repub Iran. 2006;20(3):147–50.
5. American Psychiatric Association. Diagnostic and statistical manual of mental disorders: DSM-5. 5th ed. Washington, D.C: American Psychiatric Association; 2013.
6. Kaplan H, Sadock B. Synopsis of psychiatry. 3rd ed. Philadelphia: Williams & Wilkins; 2003.
7. Faraone SV, Perlis RH, Doyle AE, Smoller JW, Goralnick JJ, Holmgren MA, Sklar P. Molecular genetics of attention deficit/hyperactivity disorder. Bio Psychiat. 2005;57:1313–23.
8. Weiss G, Hechtman L. Hyperactive children grown up: ADHD in children, adolescents and adults. New York: Guildford; 1993.
9. Döpfner M, Breuer D, Wille N, Erhart M, Ravens-Sieberer U. How often do children meet ICD-10/DSM-IVcriteria of attention deficit-/hyperactivity disorder and hyperkinetic disorder? Parent-based prevalence rates in a national sample—results of the BELLA study. Euro Child Adol Psychiat. 2008;17(1):59–70.
10. Coile C. The effects of ADHD on educational outcomes. 2015. http://www.nber.org/bah/summer04/w10435.html. Accessed 5 Dec 2016.
11. Biederman J, Wilens TE, Mick E, Faraone SV, Spencer T. Does attention-deficit hyperactivity disorder impact the development course of drug and alcohol abuse and dependence? Bio Psychiat. 1998;44(4):269–73.
12. Homidi M, Obaidat Y, Hamaidi D. Prevalence of attention deficit and hyperactivity disorder among primary school students in Jeddah city, KSA. Life Sci J. 2013;3:10.
13. Abikwi EO. The prevalence of attention deficit/hyperactivity disorder (ADHD) among primary school pupils of Benin Metropolis, Nigeria. J Hum Ecol. 2007;22(2):317–22.
14. Bathiche M. The prevalence of ADHD symptoms in a culturally diverse and developing country: Lebanon. Montreal: McGill University; 2008.
15. Ofovwe CE, Ofovwe GE, Meyer A. The prevalence of attention-deficit/hyperactivity disorder among school-aged children in Benin City, Nigeria. J Child Adol Mental Health. 2006;18(1):1–5.
16. Daley D, Birchwood J. ADHD and academic performance: why does ADHD impact on academic performance and what can be done to support ADHD children in the classroom?: ADHD and academic performance. Child Care Health Dev. 2010;36(4):455–64.
17. Bolic V, Lidström H, Thelin N, Kjellberg A, Hemmingsson H. Computer use in educational activities by students with ADHD. Scand J Occup Ther. 2013;20(5):357–64.

5

A new technique to measure online bullying: online computerized adaptive testing

Shu-Ching Ma[1,2], Hsiu-Hung Wang[1] and Tsair-Wei Chien[3,4*]

Abstract

Background: Workplace bullying has been measured in many studies to investigate mental health issues. None uses online computerized adaptive testing (CAT) with cutting points to report bully prevalence at workplace.

Objective: To develop an online CAT to examine person being bullied and verify whether item response theory-based CAT can be applied online for nurses to measure exposure to workplace bullying.

Methods: A total of 963 nurses were recruited and responded to the 22-item Negative Acts Questionnaire-Revised (NAQ-R). All non-adaptive testing (NAT) items were calibrated with the Rasch rating scale model. Three scenarios (i.e., NAT, CAT, and the randomly selected method to NAT) were manipulated to compare their response efficiency and precision by comparing (i) item length for answering questions, person measure, (ii) correlation coefficients, (iii) paired *t* tests, and (iv) estimated standard errors (SE) between CAT and the random to its counterpart of NAT.

Results: The NAQ-R is a unidimensional construct that can be applied for nurses to measure exposure to workplace bullying on CAT. CAT required fewer items (=8.9) than NAT (=22, an efficient gain of 60% =1–8.9/22). Nursing measures derived from both tests (CAT and the random to NAT) were highly correlated ($r = 0.93$ and 0.96) and their measurement precisions were not statistically different (the percentage of significant count number less than 5%) as expected, but CAT earns smaller person measure SE than the random scenario. The prevalence rate for nurses was 1.5% (=15/963) when cutting points set at −0.7 and 0.7 logits.

Conclusion: The CAT-based NAQ-R reduces respondents' burden without compromising measurement precision and increases endorsement efficiency. The online CAT is recommended for assessing nurses using the criteria at −0.7 and 0.7 (or <30 and <60 in summed score) to identify bully grade as one of the three levels (high, moderate, and low). The bullied nurse can get help from a psychiatrist or a mental health expert at an earlier stage.

Keywords: Computerized adaptive testing, Non-adaptive testing, Item response theory, The Negative Acts Questionnaire-Revised, workplace bullying

Background

During the last 20 years, the prevalence rate of workplace bullying has been reported in a range of different studies to investigate mental health issues [1–3]. Despite all this attention on the bully phenomenon, the criteria of cutting points indeed influence the calculation of prevalence rate on workplace bullying.

The prevalence rate of bullying, using the same bully scale of the 22-item Negative Acts Questionnaire-Revised (NAQ-R) with examinee's self-labeling (i.e., with a single quest to answer whether she/he is a bullied victim [4, 5]), was, respectively, reported at 24% for hospital nurses [2], higher than seen in studies of Japanese nurses (19%) [3], and Italian employees (15.2%) [4], and workers in general services (2–17%) [1]. Nielsen et al. [6] addressed that self-labeling with definition studies yielded far lower estimates of bullying than self-labeling studies without definitions. The findings for the prevalence rate on workplace bullying would be thus biased and overestimated without definitions when self-labeling bullied perception.

*Correspondence: smile@mail.chimei.org.tw
[3] Research Department, Chi-Mei Medical Center, 901 Chung Hwa Road, Yung Kung Dist., Tainan 710, Taiwan
Full list of author information is available at the end of the article

Common cutting points are required

For studies using the behavioral method (i.e., with several items to respond with regard to encountered negative acts or behaviors in a workplace [1, 7], like the NAQ-R) with an operational criterion, prevalence rates seem to vary between 3 and 17%, depending on the cutoff criterion utilized [8]. Unfortunately, no such a common cutting point for calculating the bully prevalence rate was applied to the NAQ-R till now. A comparison between derived score levels and the suggested best cutoff points can help clinicians evaluate examinees at risk of an incidence [9, 10], and multiple cutoff points are usually more powerful and useful than one single cutoff point [11, 12]. How to determine appropriate cutting points for the NAQ-R is an issue of the current study.

Cutting points are required for computerized adaptive testing

The NAQ-R is evident of a unidimensional construct and can be applied to measure exposure to workplace bullying through the computerized adaptive testing (CAT) administration [2]. The CAT requires fewer items to answer than the traditional pen-and-paper approach (an efficiency gain of 32%), suggesting a reduced burden for respondents [2]. However, the CAT-based NAQ-R is just administered on a computerized nursing cart (i.e., not an online CAT version) and is not set with multiple cutting points to help clinicians evaluate examinees at risk of an incidence, especially because each person answers a different number of items on the CAT. Determining cutting points is thus a critical issue for the NAQ-R CAT.

Computerized adaptive testing

Computerized adaptive testing (CAT) is based on item response theory (IRT)_test that adapts to the examinee's ability level. The computer follows an IRT-based algorithm that offers the patient the next not-too-hard-and-not-too-easy item. So, only the fewest possible items are offered per patient, resulting in less respondent burden and even more accurate outcomes [2]. As with all forms of Web-based technology development, there is no *online* CAT assessment applied to the NAQ-R till now.

Objectives

First, we verify whether the NAQ-R is a unidimensional construct. Second, we determine a set of cutting points that can be used for computing a prevalence rate at workplace on CAT. Third, we compare CAT with non-adaptive testing (NAT) and the randomly selected method to NAT on efficiency and precision. Fourth, we developed an online CAT for nurses to measure exposure to workplace bullying.

Methods

Study participants

The study sample was recruited from three hospitals (Hospital A: 1236-bed medical center; B: 265-bed local hospital; C: 877-bed region hospital) in southern Taiwan in the summer of 2012. No incentive for participation was offered. A total of 970 copies of the bully questionnaire were validated with a return rate of 96.3%.

This study was approved and monitored by the Research Ethics Review Board of the Chi-Mei Medical Center. Demographic data were anonymously collected: gender, work tenure in hospitals of all types, age, marital status, and education level.

Scales used for reporting exposure to bullying

The 22-item NAQ-R with 5 response alternatives (1 = never, 2 = occasionally, 3 = monthly, 4 = weekly, 5 = daily) was used to measure exposure to workplace bullying within the past 6 months. With permission from the author [13], the NAQ-R was professionally translated into Chinese by authors in Taiwan using a back-translation technique (English–Chinese–English).

Dimensionality

Tennant and Pallant [14] suggested three steps that should be applied to assess scale unidimensionality: (1) conduct prior testing using Horn's parallel analysis [15] for ensuring that unidimensionality is retained, (2) use Rasch [16] fit statistics ranging from 0.5 to 1.5 [17, 18] to determine the usefulness of the one-dimensional scaling, and (3) run post hoc tests using Rasch standardized residual loading [19] (i.e., $|Z| < 2.0$) across items to inspect the convergent validity, and Smith [20] independent t tests to compare estimates of the percentages (<5%, within ±1.96) and verify invariance of Rasch model. A dimension coefficient (>0.67, DC) suggested by Chien [21] was used for identifying a single-dimensional scale. Point-biserial correlation coefficients on items (PTME, the Pearson correlation between the observations of an item and the item difficulties that is like factor loading in exploration factor analysis) >0.40 was reported to support scale dimensionality.

Cutting points used for the NAQ-R

According to the literature [22–24], as a scale's reliability (i.e., Cronbach's α) increases, so does the person-number of ranges that can be confidently distinguished. Measures with reliabilities of 0.67 will tend to vary within two groups that can be separated with 95% confidence; 0.80 will vary within three groups; 0.90, within four groups; 0.94, within five groups; 0.96, within six groups; 0.97, within seven groups; etc. [25].

More conservative to compute the number of the strata, the scale reliability was referred to the Rasch person separation reliability, and then referred to the Rasch threshold difficulty guideline [26] with an appropriate distance between two thresholds ranging from 1.4 to 5.0 logits.

An equal sample size in each stratum suggested by Maslach et al. [27] was applied to determine cutting points. Accordingly, a threshold at zero logits is suggested for two strata, -0.7 and 0.7 (=1.4 − logit difference with probabilities at 0.33 and $0.67 = 1 - \exp(-0.7)/[1 + \exp(-0.7)]$ for three strata, -1.1, 0.0, and 1.1 (=1.1 − logit difference with probabilities at 0.25, 0.50, and $0.75 = 1 - \exp(-1.1)/[1 + \exp(-1.1)]$ for four strata, and -1.4, -0.4, 0.4 and 1.4 (=1.0 − logit difference with probabilities at 0.20, 0.40, 0.60 and $0.80 = 1 - (-1.4)/[1 + \exp(-1.4)]$ for five strata.

Comparison of efficiency and precision using CAT algorithm

Three scenarios (i.e., NAT, CAT, and the randomly selected method to NAT) were manipulated to compare their response efficiency and precision by comparing (i) item length for answering questions, person measure, (ii) correlation coefficients and (iii) Smith's paired *t* tests [20], and (iv) estimated standard errors (SE) between CAT and the random to its counterpart of NAT (Fig. 1).

We ran an author-programed VBA (Visual Basic for Applications) module in Microsoft Excel. Rasch person separation reliability yielded from the NAQ-R of the study by Winsteps (i.e., excluding all extreme scores summed to zero) was used to determine the CAT termination criterion using the standard error of measurement ($SEM = SD * \sqrt{1 - reliability}$). Another termination criterion is the mean of the last five change differences between the pre- and post-estimated abilities on each CAT <0.05.

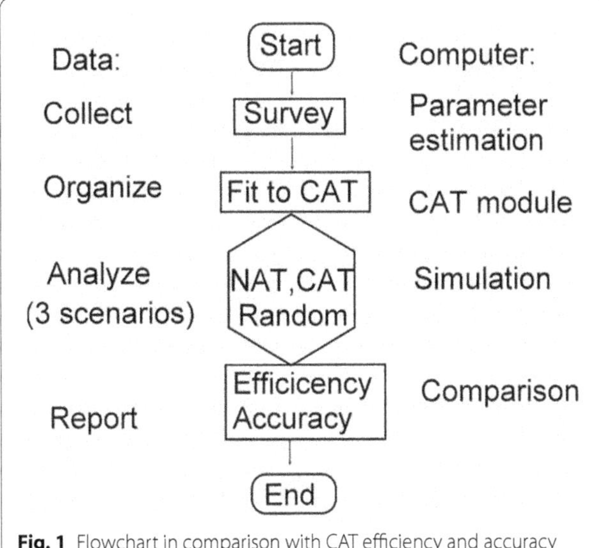

Fig. 1 Flowchart in comparison with CAT efficiency and accuracy

The minimum number of questions required for completion was set at 7 (7/22 items on NAQ-R item length = 30%). The first item was randomly selected from the 22 items when starting the CAT. The provisional measures were estimated by the maximum log-likelihood estimation (MLE). The next question selected was the one with the most information obtained from the remaining unanswered items, interacting with the previously provisional person measures.

An online CAT was designed for smart phones

An online CAT was designed for examinees to report their bully scores in a unit of logit (log odds). The 22 items with their threshold difficulties (calibrated by Rasch Winsteps) and their responsive audios and pictures were uploaded to the website. The rules of the first and the next selected CAT item and the termination criteria are like the aforementioned simulation method.

Statistical tools and data analyses

SPSS 15.0 for Windows (SPSS Inc., Chicago, IL) and MedCalc 9.5.0.0 for Windows (MedCalc Software, Mariakerke, Belgium) were used to calculate (1) Cronbach's α, (2) dimension coefficients, and (3) correlation coefficients between estimated person measures for CAT and the random to its counterpart of NAT. Independent *t* tests were used to compare (4) the ratios of the different paired person measures. Rasch Winsteps was used for producing (5) person separation reliability. The prevalence rate of workplace bully is calculated by the formula (=the number of bullied grade excluded from the low stratum divided by the sample).

Results

The sample of 963 nurses was obtained from the study. The mean age of the participants was 32.7 (±5.8) years, 96% ($n = 924$) were female, and >57.5% ($n = 554$) were unmarried (Table 1).

Dimensionality

The NAQ-R can be unidimensional because

(1) one factor was extracted using parallel analysis;
(2) all Infit and Outfit mean squares for the 22 items are in a range of 0.5–1.5 (in the Infit column in Table 2; Fig. 2);
(3) item loadings from the Rasch PCA of residuals on the first contrast are standardized (i.e., (loading − mean)/SD) within −1.24 and 1.57 (within ±2.0 in the Z column in Table 2); PTME are between 0.51 and 0.74 (in the PTME column in Table 2).

Table 1 Demographic characteristics of the participants ($n = 963$)

Variable	Category	Number	%
Hospital			
	Hospital A	543	56.4
	Hospital B	324	33.6
	Hospital C	96	10.0
Gender			
	Male	39	4.0
	Female	924	96.0
Education			
	High school	6	0.6
	College	465	48.3
	University	475	49.3
	Graduate school	17	1.8
Marriage			
	Unmarried	554	57.5
	Married	405	42.1
	Divorced	4	0.4
Nursing grade			
	N0	34	3.5
	N1	282	29.3
	N2	317	32.9
	N3	244	25.3
	N4	86	8.9
Title			
	Nurse	773	80.3
	Chief	170	17.7
	Leader	8	0.8
	Others	12	1.2
Age and tenure	**Mean**	**SD**	**Range**
Age (years)	32.7	5.8	23–55
Out of hospital (months)	21.9	34.7	0–240
Within hospital (months)	89.6	49.7	3–378

Rasch person separation reliability = 0.84, Cronbach $\alpha = 0.96$, DC = 0.88 (>0.67), and Smith's t test of proportions [20] is near to zero (=1.14% = 11/963) outside the range ±1.96. In addition, category structure for the NAQ-R displays the monotonically increasing threshold (−3.26, −0.71, 0.71, 3.25 logits) in compliance with Linacre's guidelines [26] at least distance ranging from 1.4 to 5.0 logits.

Cutting point determination

The person separation reliability for the NAQ-R is 0.84, indicating that three strata can be separated with thresholds at −0.7 and 0.7. Prevalence rate of workplace bully is 1.5% (=0.3% + 1.2%), see Fig. 2.

Comparison of efficiency and precision

The CAT required substantially fewer items (mean = 8.9; SD = 2.4; SE = 0.08; 95% CI 8.78–9.09) than did NAT (=22) and provided an efficient gain in test length of 0.60 (=1−8.9/22), see Fig. 3 in panel a. Person measures from CAT did not statistically differ from NAT because (1) Smith's t test of proportions [20] is 1.6% (=15/963 < 5%), see Fig. 3 in panel b, and (2) correlation coefficient = 0.93 ($=\sqrt{\hat{O}\text{R-square}} = \sqrt{0.87}$, see Fig. 3 in panel c). As compared to the random scenario, CAT earns a set of smaller SE, see Fig. 3 in panel d.

Online NAQ-R assessment

By scanning a QR-code (Fig. 4 at right bottom), the NAQ-R item appears on the smartphone. We developed an online CAT module to demonstrate the assessment in action. The CAT processed each nurse item-by-item with picture animations (Fig. 4 at top). Adaptive item selection is based on maximizing information across unanswered items. The measurement of standard error (MSE) for each subscale decreased when the number of the items increased (Fig. 4). The result with a person measure and the bully grade (i.e., low, moderate, or high) instantly shows on smartphone (Fig. 4).

Discussion

Key findings

The results from this study indicate that the 22-item NAQ-R is unidimensional. A set of cutting point at −0.7 and 0.7 logits were determined for future use in workplace bullying surveys. The prevalence of bullying for the study sample was 1.5%. The CAT is 60% more efficient for answering questions and achieved similar precision in measurements as did NAT. An available-for-download online CAT NAQ-R APP for nurses was suited for smartphones (Additional file 1).

What this adds to what was known

Consistent with the literature [2, 28–32], the 22-item NAQ-R can be unidimensional. The efficiency of CAT over NAT was supported. We confirm that CAT-based NAQ-R requires significantly fewer answered items to measure explosion of workplace bully than NAT without compromising its measurement precision.

What it implies and what should be changed?

Cutoff point recommended for calculating bully prevalence rate

According a study in Belgian employees [33], six different groups of respondents were identified based on their exposure to negative behaviors: (1) not bullied (35%), (2) limited work criticism (28%), (3) limited negative

Table 2 One factor extracted from the Negative Acts Questionnaire-Revised (NAQ-R) scale with mean square between 0.50 and 1.50

Item	Feature	Difficulty			MNSQ	loading
	Type[a]	Delta	SE	PTME	Infit	Z
During the last 6 months, how often have you been subjected to the following negative acts in the work place?						
21. Being exposed to an unmanageable workload	1	1.5	0.14	0.53	0.97	1.57
22. Threats of violence or physical abuse or actual abuse	3	1.5	0.14	0.51	0.95	0.26
9. Intimidating behaviors such as finger-pointing, invasion of personal space shoving, blocking your way	3	1.29	0.13	0.51	1.07	−0.41
8. Being shouted at or being the target of spontaneous anger	3	0.87	0.12	0.56	1	−0.26
19. Pressure not to claim something to which by right you are entitled	1	0.74	0.11	0.62	0.76	0.81
3. Being ordered to do work below your level of competence	1	0.5	0.11	0.59	1.04	−0.41
18. Excessive monitoring of your work	1	0.23	0.1	0.61	1.14	1.08
5. Spreading of gossip and rumors about you	2	0.16	0.1	0.61	1.09	−0.66
15. Practical jokes carried out by people you don't get along with	2	0.06	0.1	0.67	0.83	1.54
16. Being given tasks with unreasonable deadlines	1	−0.06	0.09	0.66	0.98	1.05
14. Having your opinions ignored	1	−0.08	0.09	0.68	0.87	0.78
20. Being the subject of excessive teasing and sarcasm	2	−0.11	0.09	0.67	0.93	1.17
2. Being humiliated or ridiculed in connection with your work	2	−0.17	0.09	0.62	1.21	−0.60
17. Having allegations made against you	2	−0.19	0.09	0.66	1.02	0.96
6. Being ignored or excluded	2	−0.24	0.09	0.68	0.92	−1.21
12. Being ignored or facing a hostile reaction when you approach	2	−0.39	0.09	0.7	0.94	−0.93
11. Repeated reminders of your errors or mistakes	2	−0.41	0.09	0.68	1.07	−1.24
10. Hints or signals from others that you should quit your job	2	−0.83	0.08	0.69	1.1	−0.84
1. Someone withholding information which affects your performance	1	−0.89	0.08	0.69	1.16	−1.08
13. Persistent criticism of your errors or mistakes	2	−0.9	0.08	0.74	0.83	0.75
4. Having key areas of responsibility removed or replaced with more trivial or unpleasant tasks	2	−1.29	0.08	0.71	1.11	−1.24
7. Having insulting or offensive remarks made about your person, attitudes, or your private life	2	−1.29	0.08	0.7	1.3	−1.11
Minimum		−1.29	0.08	0.51	0.76	−1.24
Maximum		1.50	0.14	0.74	1.30	1.57

Threshold difficulties are −3.26, −0.71, 0.71, 3.25

[a] Type: *1* work-related bullying; *2* Person-related bullying; *3* physically intimidating bullying

encounter (17%), (4) sometimes bullied (9%), (5) work-related bullying (8%), and (6) victims of bullying (3%). Too many grades is hard to help clinicians evaluate examinees at risk of an incidence [9, 10]. A single cut point of >−4.2 logits (or >30 in summation) for the NAQ-R was proposed [2]. However, multiple cutoff points are usually more powerful and useful than one single cutoff point [11, 12]. Maslach et al. [27] suggested setting an equal sample size in each stratum as a way to determine cutting points.

At the end of 2016, more than 10,977 papers were found in a search with keyword "cut point." None discussed the determination of cutting points used for CAT with different item lengths for a respondent. Frequently, we usually do not know the patient's true- and false-positive disease-specific status, like the NAQ-R. The issue we face in clinical settings is how to identify the degree of patient incident problems. Through this study, if cutting points at −0.7 and 0.7 logits are selected for the NAQ-R, the raw score in cutting points can be transformed by the formula (=total score × the probability at 0.33 and 0.67), whereas 0.33 comes from the equation exp (−0.7)/(1 + exp (−0.7)) and 0.67 is from the equation 1 − exp (−0.7)/(1 + exp (−0.7)), total score = 88 when 5-point (from 0 to 4) 22-item NAQ-R is defined beforehand. The cutting points in raw score can be set at <30 (=88 × 0.33), and ≥60 (=33 × 0.67) to separate three strata in bully degree. The prevalence rate is easy to calculated and compared either with paper-and-pen format or with CAT in future.

Online CAT assessment

At the end of 2016, 757 papers were collected in US National Library of Medicine National Institutes of Health (pubmed.org) when searching keywords: computer adaptive testing. None was applicable using an

Wright Map

<Person — Item>

Item Infit MNSO 0.5 — 1.0 — 1.5

Logit	Level	Items	Note	Person	item
2.6				0	0
2.4				0	0
2.2				0	0
2				0	0
1.8				0	0
1.6	Hight			1	0
1.4		21 22		1	2
1.2		9	0.3%	0	1
1				0	0
0.8		8	=3/963	1	1
0.6		19		1	1
0.4		3		2	1
0.2		18		2	1
0	Moderate	15 5		2	2
-0.2		14 20 16 17 2		4	5
-0.4		6 12	1.2%	0	2
-0.6		11	=12/963	1	1
-0.8				0	0
-1		13 10 1		0	3
-1.2				4	0
-1.4		4 7		5	2
-1.6				1	0
-1.8	Low			4	0
-2				6	0
-2.2				8	0
-2.4				24	0
-2.6				12	0
-2.8				2	0
-3				16	0
-3.2				6	0
-3.4				15	0
-3.6				23	0
-3.8				18	0
-4				22	0
-4.2				22	0
-4.4				27	0
-4.6				40	0
-4.8				39	0
-5				61	0
-5.2				0	0
-5.4				56	0
-5.6				0	0
-5.8				0	0
-6				67	0
-6.2				0	0
-6.4				0	0
-6.6				100	0
-6.8				0	0
-7				0	0
-7.2				0	0
-7.4				0	0
-7.6				0	0
-7.8				2	0
-8				368	0
				963	22

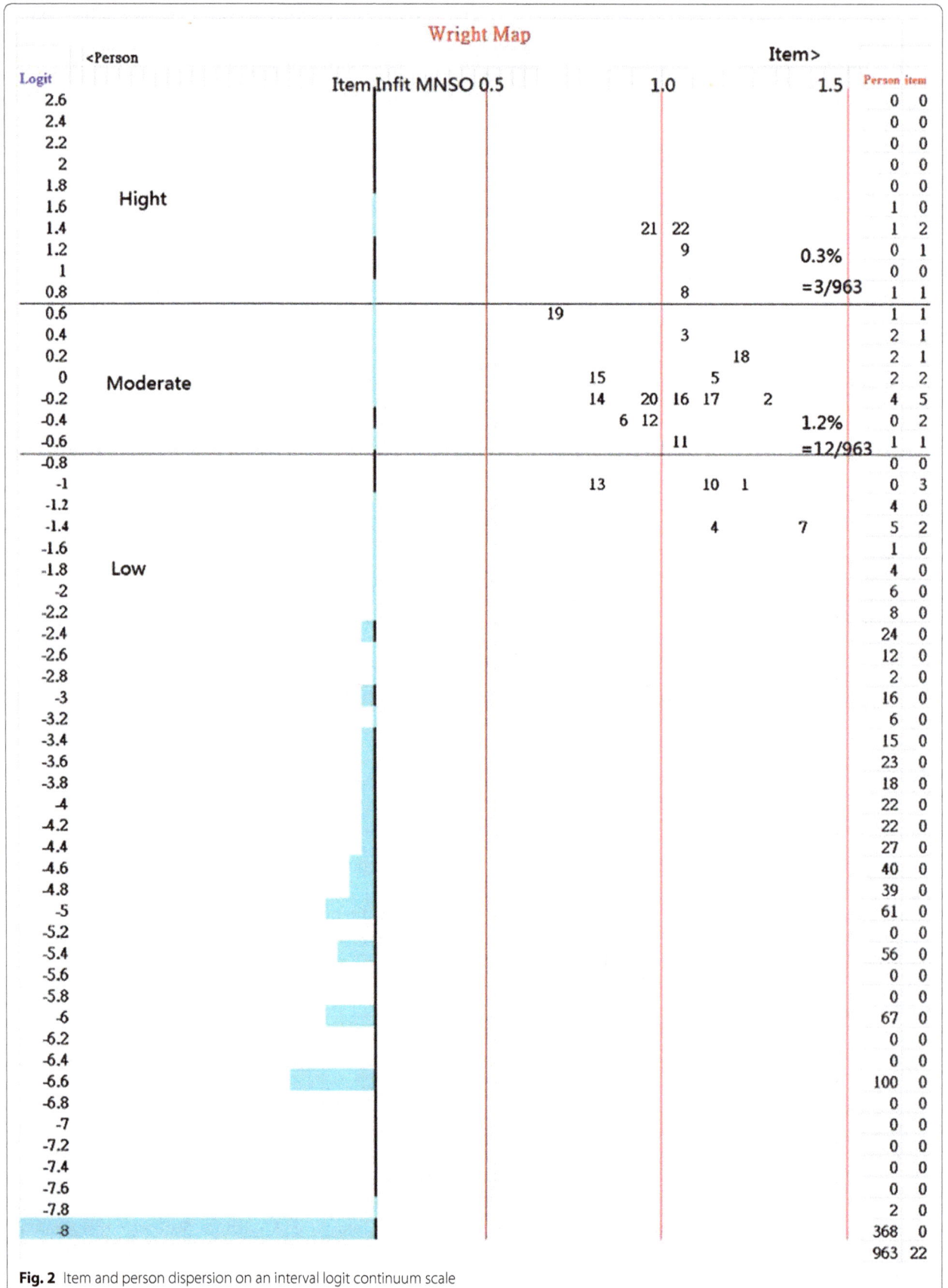

Fig. 2 Item and person dispersion on an interval logit continuum scale

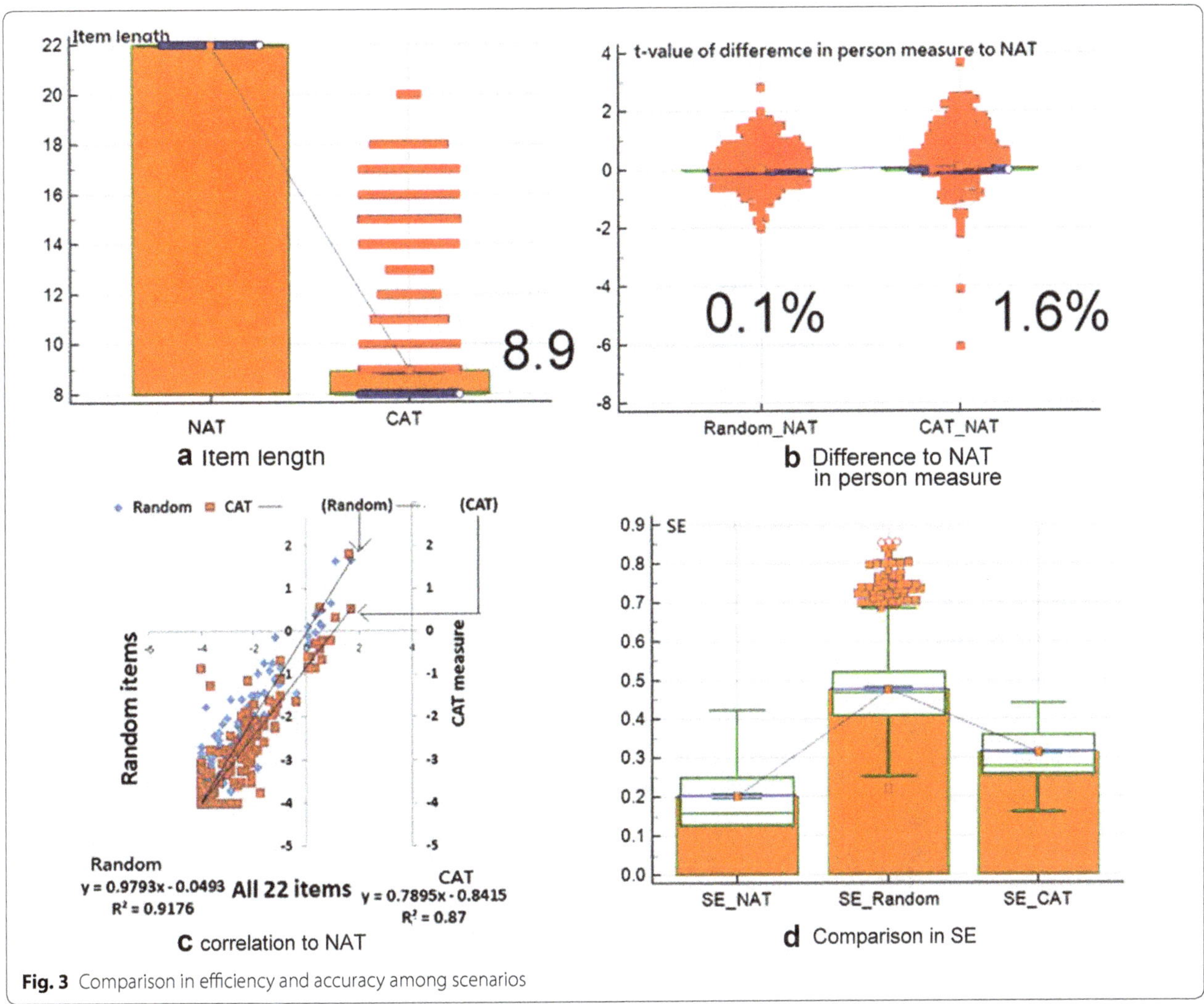

Fig. 3 Comparison in efficiency and accuracy among scenarios

online assessment suited for smartphones until the online skin cancer CAT was published [32]. We do ensure that more papers in future will be published on the usefulness of online CAT as with all forms of Web-based technology are rapidly increasing [34].

Unidimensional scale detection

Many studies [21, 35–38] reported the issue of scale unidimensionality detection. From the Library of PubMed and BioMed Central, we got 1005 and 333 papers with the keyword "unidimensionality," 4688 and 745 results for "bully." In the current study, we demonstrated the method Tennant and Pallant [14] suggested using three steps to assess scale unidimensionality: (1) conduct prior testing using Horn's parallel analysis, (2) use Rasch fit statistics, and (3) run post hoc tests using Rasch standardized residual loading, and Smith [20] independent t tests to compare estimates of the percentages (<5%, within ±1.96). In addition, the dimension coefficient (≥0.67, DC) and PTME (>0.40) included in detecting scale unidimensionality are recommended to readers.

Strengths of this study

Four goals have been reached in this study: (1) we verified the 22-item NAQ-R is unidimensional, (2) cutting points at −0.7 and 0.7 logits were recommended to future studies in computing bully prevalence rate at workplace, (3) CAT gains 60% efficient than did NAT, and (4) online CAT is applicable in practice. Among them, the reason for 60% efficient than did NAT is because we added another termination rule in CAT: the mean of the last five change differences between the pre- and post-estimated abilities on each CAT less than 0.05. The termination rule of detecting the last five change differences in estimated abilities less than 0.05 makes the item length less than that in other studies [2, 28–31]. It is because many low grade of workplace bully were found and led to short item length required to complete the CAT. Around 82.6%

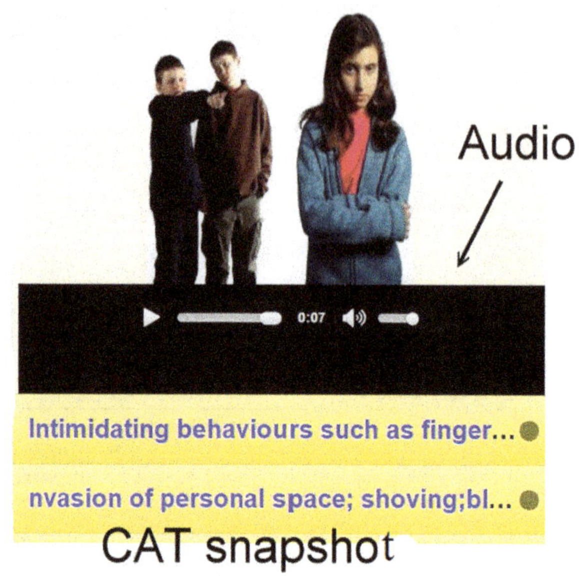

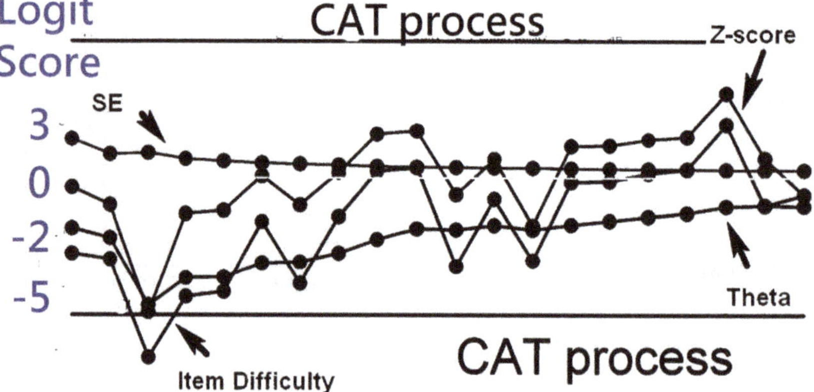

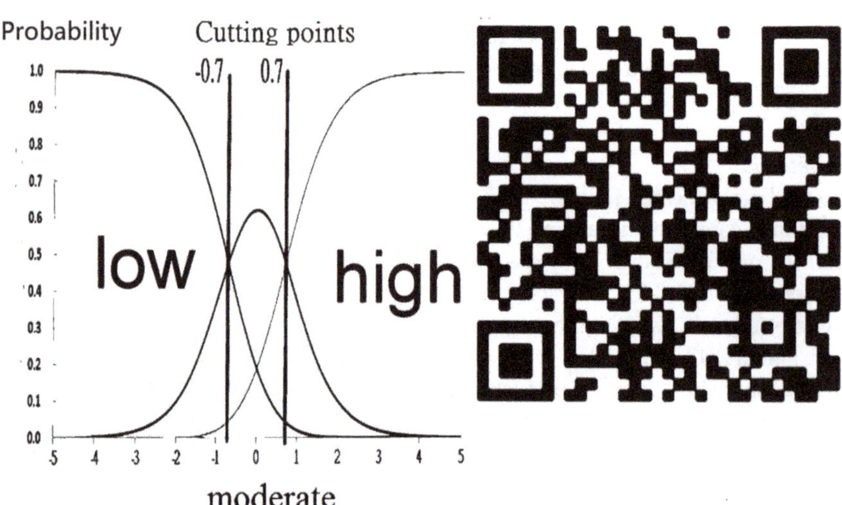

Fig. 4 A snapshot of online CAT-based NAQ-R assessment

(=795/964) terminated CAT at eight items. A total of 368 nurses responded to all items with zero (i.e., never). If all CAT cases are controlled by the only termination rule of SE less than 0.44 (=SQRT (1 − 0.8) = SQRT (1 − reliability)), the precision measured by SE on CAT (in panel D in Fig. 3) will be substantially higher than the dual stop conditions we did in this study.

In addition, the online CAT with audio and picture animations is available for interested readers to practice if scanned on the QR-code in Fig. 3, which is rare in any previously published articles.

Furthermore, cutting points set at −0.7 and 0.7 logits with an equal stratum member size might be generalized to other incidences or diseases when the patient's true- and false-positive disease-specific status is not known beforehand. Like the NAQ-R, we merely intend to identify the grade of the incidence and compare to the norm.

Limitations of the study

Several issues should be considered more thoroughly in further studies. First, many female nurses (96%) in sample let us not identify differential item functioning (DIF) on gender. Second, the low bully prevalence rate (1.5%) was reported here as compared to the previous papers at 24% for hospital nurses [2], higher than seen in studies of Greek nurses (30.2%) [39], Japanese nurses (19%) [3], Korean nurses (17.2%) [40], and Italian employees (15.2%) [4], and workers in general services (2–17%) [1]. One ensured reason is attributable to different cutting points and self-labeling definitions. For instance, one [40] defined a victim of workplace bullying if subjects had experienced at least 2 of the 22 negative acts from NAQ-R by a colleague every day or every week in the past 6 months. Another [39] used an additional question "Have you been bullied at work?". Valid criteria are thus urgently required to classify levels of incidence and to calculate the prevalence rate of workplace bully. Accordingly, the study cannot be generalized to others.

More studies are needed to assess the generalizability of the study with different samples using the same cutting points and the same version of NAQ-R. Third, the online CAT is not equipped with much functionality as we expected in practice, such as protecting cheating behaviors and detecting aberrant responses that are required to be in future advanced versions. Fourth, although the scale's Cronbach's α coefficients was 0.96, we conservatively determined that the scales' person strata were three according to Rasch separation reliability = 0.84 and the literature [22–25]. Multiple cutoff points are not limited to three strata if the separation index reaches an extremely higher level, which will affect the determination of appropriate cutting points for the NAQ-R.

Conclusions

The CAT-based NAQ-R forming a unidimensional construct reduces respondents' burden without compromising measurement precision and increases endorsement efficiency. The online NAQ-R module developed by the authors is recommended for assessing nurses or other workers using the criteria at −0.7 and 0.7 (or <30 and <60 in summed score) to identify bully grade as one of the three levels (high, moderate, and low). The bullied nurse can get help from a psychiatrist or a mental health expert at an earlier stage.

Abbreviations

APP: application; CAT: computer adaptive testing; CTT: classic test theory; DC: dimension coefficients; DIF: differential item functioning; IRT: item response theory; MLE: maximum likelihood estimation; MNSQ: mean square; MSE: mean-squared error; NAT: non-adaptive testing; NAQ-R: Negative Acts Questionnaire-Revised; PCA: principal component analysis; PTME: point-biserial correlation coefficients on measures; SD: standard deviation; SE: standard error; SEM: standard error measurement; VBA: visual basic for applications.

Authors' contributions

SCM developed the study concept and design. TWC and SCM analyzed and interpreted the data. HHW monitored the process of this study and help responded to the reviewers' advices and comments. TWC drafted the manuscript, and all authors provided critical revisions for important intellectual content. The study was supervised by TWC. All authors read and approved the final manuscript.

Authors' information

SCM is a nursing expert with Ph.D working at Chi-Mei Medical Center, Taiwan. HHW is a Professor teaching healthcare and nursing in College of Nursing, Kaohsiung Medical University, Kaohsiung, Taiwan. TWC is an assistant professor at Chi-Mei Medical Center, Taiwan. He is an expert in computer science and Rasch modeling, mainly in the field of data analysis using statistical technique.

Author details

[1] College of Nursing, Kaohsiung Medical University, Kaohsiung, Taiwan. [2] Nursing Department, Chi-Mei Medical Center, Tainan, Taiwan. [3] Research Department, Chi-Mei Medical Center, 901 Chung Hwa Road, Yung Kung Dist., Tainan 710, Taiwan. [4] Department of Hospital and Health Care Administration, Chia-Nan University of Pharmacy and Science, Tainan, Taiwan.

Competing interests

The authors declare that they have no competing interests.

Declarations

We thank Frank Bill who provided medical writing services to the manuscript.

References

1. Nielsen MB, Notelaers G, Einarsen S. Measuring exposure to workplace bullying. In: Einarsen S, Hoel H, Zapf D, Cooper CL, editors. Bullying and harassment in the workplace: developments in theory, research, and practice. Boca Raton: Boca Raton CRC Press; 2011. p. 149–76.
2. Ma SC, Chien TW, Wang HH, Li YC, Yui MS. Applying computerized adaptive testing to the negative acts questionnaire-revised: Rasch analysis of workplace bullying. J Med Internet Res. 2014;16(2):e50.
3. Abe K, Henly SJ. Bullying (ijime) among Japanese hospital nurses: modeling responses to the revised Negative Acts Questionnaire. Nurs Res. 2010;59(2):110–8.

4. Giorgi G, Arenas A, Leon-Perez JM. An operative measure of workplace bullying: the negative acts questionnaire across Italian companies. Ind Health. 2011;49(6):686–95.
5. Einarsen S. Bullying and harsassment at work: epidemiological and psychosocial aspects. Bergen: University of Bergen; 1996.
6. Nielsen MB, Mattjiesem SB, Einarsen S. The impact of methodological moderators on prevalence rates of workplace bullying: a meta-analysis. J Occup Org Psychol. 2010;83(4):955–79.
7. Einarsen S, Hoel H, Notelaers G. Measuring bullying and harassment at work: validity, factor structure, and psychometric properties of the Negative Acts Questionnaire-Revised. Work Stress. 2009;23(1):24–44.
8. Nielsen MB. Methodological issues in research on workplace bullying: operationalisations, measurements, and samples. Unpublished dictorial dissertation, University of Bergen, Norway, 2009.
9. Hwang AW, Chou YT, Hsieh CL, Hsieh WS, Liao HF, Wong AM. A developmental screening tool for toddlers with multiple domains based on Rasch analysis. J Formos Med Assoc. 2015;114:23–34.
10. Chien TW, Lin WS. Simulation study of activities of daily living functions using online computerized adaptive testing. BMC Med Inform Decis Mak. 2016;16(1):130.
11. Straus E, Richardson WS, Glaszion P, Haynes RB. Evidence-based medicine: how to practice and teach EBM. 3rd ed. London: Elsevier Churchill Livingstone; 2005.
12. Liao HF, Yao G, Chienc CC, Cheng LY, Hsiehe WS. Likelihood ratios of multiple cutoff points of the Taipei City Developmental Checklist for Preschoolers, 2nd version. Formosan J Med. 2014;113(3):179–86.
13. Einarsen S, Skogstad A. Bullying at work: epidemiological findings in public and private organizations. Eur J Work Org Psychol. 1996;5(2):185–201.
14. Tennant A, Pallant JF. Unidimensionality matters! (A tale of two Smiths?). Rasch Meas Trans. 2006;20(1):1048–51.
15. Horn JL. A rationale and test for the number of factors in factor analysis. Psychometrika. 1965;30(2):179–85.
16. Rasch G. Probabilistic models for some intelligence and achievement test. Copenhagen: Danish Institute for Educational Research, 1960. Expanded ed. Chicago: The University of Chicago Press; 1980.
17. Linacre JM. User's Guide to Winsteps. Chicago: Mesa Press; 2010.
18. Bond TG, Fox CM. Applying the Rasch model: fundamental measurement in human sciences. 2nd ed. Mahwah: Lawrence Erlbaum; 2007. p. 179.
19. Linacre JM. Structure in Rasch residuals: why principal components analysis (PCA). Rasch Meas Trans. 1998;12(2):636.
20. Smith EV. Detecting and evaluating the impact of multidimensionality using item fit statistics and principal component analysis of residuals. J Appl Meas. 2002;3(2):205–31.
21. Chien TW. Cronbach's alpha with the dimension coefficient to jointly assess a scale's quality. Rasch Meas Trans. 2012;26(3):1379.
22. Fisher W Jr. Reliability, separation, strata statistics. Rasch Meas Trans. 1994;6(3):238.
23. Wright BD, Masters GN. Number of person or item strata. Rasch Meas Trans. 2002;16(3):888.
24. Wright BD. Reliability and separation. Rasch Meas Trans. 1996;9(4):472.
25. Fisher WP Jr. The cash value of reliability. Rasch Meas Trans. 2008;22(1):1160–3.
26. Linacre JM. Optimizing rating scale category effectiveness. J Appl Meas. 2002;3(1):85–106.
27. Maslach C, Schaufeli WB, Leiter MP. Job burnout. Ann Rev Psychol. 2001;52:397–422.
28. Chien TW, Wang WC, Huang SY, Lai WP, Chow JC. A web-based computerized adaptive testing (CAT) to assess patient perception in hospitalization. J Med Internet Res. 2011;13(3):e61.
29. Chien TW, Wu HM, Wang WC, Castillo RV, Chou W. Reduction in patient burdens with graphical computerized adaptive testing on the ADL scale: tool development and simulation. Health Qual Life Outcomes. 2009;7:39.
30. Wainer HW, Dorans NJ. Computerized adaptive testing: a primer. Hillsdale: L Erlbaum Associates; 1990.
31. Embretson S, Reise S, Reise SP. Item response theory for psychologists. Mahwah: L Erlbaum Associates; 2000.
32. Djaja N, Janda M, Olsen CM, Whiteman DC, Chien TW. Estimating skin cancer risk: evaluating mobile computer-adaptive testing. J Med Internet Res. 2016;18(1):e22.
33. Notelaers G, Einarsen S, De Witte H, Vermunt J. Measuring exposure to bullying at work: the validity and advantages of the latent class cluster approach. Work Stress. 2006;20(4):288–301.
34. Mitchel SJ, Godoy L, Shabazz K, Horn IB. Internet and mobile technology use among urban African American parents: survey study of a clinical population. J Med Internet Res. 2014;16(1):e9.
35. Smith RM. A Comparison of methods for determining dimensionality in Rasch measurement. Struct Equ Model. 1996;3:25–40.
36. Zwick WR, Velicer WF. Comparison of the rules for determining the number of components to retain. Psychol Bull. 1986;99:432–42.
37. Wright BD. Unidimensionality coefficient. Rasch Meas Trans. 1994;8(3):385.
38. Linacre JM. Rasch measures and unidimensionality. Rasch Meas Trans. 2011;24(4):1310.
39. Karatza C, Zyga S, Tziaferi S, Prezerakos P. Workplace bullying and general health status among the nursing staff of Greek public hospitals. Ann Gen Psychiatry. 2016;15:7.
40. Yun S, Kang J, Lee YO, Yi Y. Work environment and workplace bullying among Korean intensive care unit nurses. Asian Nurs Res. 2014;8(3):219–25.

6

Resilience and burnout status among nurses working in oncology

Sevinc Kutluturkan[1*], Elif Sozeri[1], Nese Uysal[2] and Figen Bay[3]

Abstract

Background: This study aimed to identify the resilience and burnout status of nurses working in the field of oncology.

Methods: This descriptive study was conducted with 140 oncology nurses. The data were collected using a sociodemographic attributes form, Resilience Scale for Adults, and the Maslach's Burnout Inventory. Percentage ratios, mean and median values, Kruskal-Wallis test, Mann–Whitney *U* test, correlation analysis, and multiple stepwise linear regression analysis were used to evaluate the data.

Results: The Maslach's Burnout Inventory total median score was 49.00. The emotional exhaustion median score was 24.00, the depersonalization median score was 9.00, and the personal accomplishment median score was 16.00. The Resilience Scale for Adults total median score was 134.00. The median resilience subscale scores, such as structural style, perception of future, family cohesion, self-perception, social competence, and social resources, were 16.00, 16.00, 24.00, 25, 23, and 31, respectively. A relationship existed between emotional exhaustion and perception of future; depersonalization and structured style and self-perception; and personal accomplishment and structured style, perception of future, and self-perception. Multiple stepwise linear regression analysis revealed a significant relationship between the number of years in the field and emotional exhaustion and depersonalization scores. Moreover, a significant relationship between structured style variables and personal accomplishment scores was observed.

Conclusions: This study demonstrated the relationship between burnout and resilience situations among the oncology nurses. The results can be used to plan individual and organizational interventions to increase resilience and reduce the experience of burnout by developing measures such as improving communication skills, providing education on stress management and coping strategies, using social resources, and organizing programs that provide psychological support.

Keywords: Burnout, Oncology nursing, Resilience

Background

Burnout is an important problem frequently encountered in the scientific, social, and professional lives. One of the main factors that lead to burnout is exposure to stress for a long time. If the stress continues for a long time, the individual is negatively affected and experiences burnout. Some factors that lead to burnout in oncology include physical stressors (e.g., working under unsuitable conditions, long working hours, and insufficient tools and equipment as well as insufficient staff), psychological stressors (e.g., too many symptoms related to diseases and treatment, increased expectations of patients and families, and problems related to occupational safety), and administrational stressors (e.g., insufficient performance measures and unsatisfactory salaries) [1–3]. This burnout manifests in the form of emotional exhaustion, depersonalization, and a decrease in personal accomplishment. Emotional exhaustion represents the individual stress dimension of burnout. Depersonalization is the dimension where cold, uninterested, and strict and nonhuman attitudes develop toward the person's job or toward other people from work-related relations.

*Correspondence: skutlu1@yahoo.com
[1] Department of Nursing, Gazi University Faculty of Health Sciences, Besevler, 06500 Ankara, Turkey
Full list of author information is available at the end of the article

A diminished sense of personal accomplishment is the reduction in a person's sense of competence and feelings of success [4]. In the study conducted by Trufelliet et al. [5] emotional exhaustion was 36%, depersonalization was 34%, and low personal accomplishment was 25% in oncology professionals.

Burnout has negative effects on physical, emotional, and mental health. One of the most important factors to prevent burnout is the effective management of the sources of stress which lead to burnout. Individuals' personality traits and psychological functions are the most important factors in stress management and preventing burnout [6]. In recent years, the concept of psychological resilience has emerged as a personality trait that is protective against burnout [7–9]. Despite a number of descriptions focusing on different aspects of resilience, which has a multidimensional and learnable structure, resilience is defined as a person's adaptation to important stressful sources such as trauma, threat, tragedy, familial and relationship problems, and workplace and financial issues [8, 10]. Friborg et al. [10] emphasized six factors to explain the structure of resilience. These factors are self-perception, perception of future, structured style, social competence, family cohesion, and social resources. Self-perception is the state of a person being aware of himself or herself. Perception of future is the individual's perspective of the future. Structured style is the person's personal attributes such as self-confidence, strengths, and self-discipline. Social competence is where persons are supported socially. Family cohesion is the individual's harmony with those closest to them [10].

With the increase in resilience, the individual is able to cope with barriers, uncertainty, and many similar negative situations, and increase their ability to be successful. With the enhancement of resilience, the nurses are able to cope with the negative conditions better, their abilities of adaptation and achievement are increased, and they probably experience less burnout. The potential association between resilience and burnout in the oncology nurses is completely unexplored [9–11].

It is hypothesized that the presence of resilience in the oncology nurses might be associated with a lower prevalence of burnout. To test this hypothesis, a survey was conducted to determine (a) the burnout and resilience states, (b) the factors influencing burnout and resilience, and (c) the relationship between burnout and resilience in oncology nurses. Understanding the concept of resilience and burnout can assist in providing support and developing programs to help nurses become and stay resilient.

Methods

Study sample

This study was carried out with nurses actively working in the oncology–hematology clinic and the chemotherapy Administration Unit and Policlinic. The entire population was included in the study sample with no specific sample selection. Inclusion criteria for the study were experience in the oncology–hematology clinics and willingness to volunteer for the study. Exclusion criteria for the study were working in departments other than oncology–hematology clinic/polyclinic, not actively working as a nurse, and not accepting to participate in the study. Ten nurses who refused to participate and 20 nurses who did not complete the forms were not included in the study. The study was carried out with 140 oncology nurses.

Procedure and measures

The data for this study were collected using a socio-demographic attributes form, Resilience Scale for Adults, and Maslach's Burnout Inventory.

Socio-demographic attributes form

The socio-demographic attributes form contained two different sections. The first section contained socio-demographic features (age, sex, marital status, educational status, dependents they care for, family type, and the existence and the number of children), and the second section contained career attributes (years of professional experience, duty, and working hours).

Maslach's Burnout Inventory

The Maslach's Burnout Inventory was created by Maslach and Jackson in 1981. The inventory contained 22 items and 3 subscales of emotional exhaustion, depersonalization, and personal accomplishment. In the emotional exhaustion subscale, eight items were related to fatigue, being fed up, and the reduction of emotion energy. In the depersonalization subscale, six items were about the individual's behaviors that lacked emotion toward those who were cared for and were given service to. In the personal accomplishment dimension, eight items defined the situation where the person felt sufficient and successful [12].

The Maslach's Burnout Inventory was evaluated according to a 5-point Likert scale where 0 points denotes "never" and 4 points denotes "always." For this study, the minimum scores on the sub-dimensions were subtracted from the maximum scores, and then the scores were divided by three, which gave the cutoff points. It was expected that in individuals experiencing burnout, the emotional exhaustion (30 and above: high; 19–29: moderate; 8–18; low) and depersonalization scores (23 and above: high; 15–22: moderate; 6–14: low) would be high and the personal accomplishment scores (30 and above: high; 19–29: moderate; 8–18: low) would be lower.

The Inventory's Turkish reliability and validity study was conducted by Cam [13] and Ergin [14]. Cronbach's alpha coefficient was found to be 0.83 for emotional exhaustion, 0.71 for depersonalization, and 0.72 for personal accomplishment [13, 14]. In this study, Cronbach's alpha coefficient was 0.70 for emotional exhaustion, 0.78 for depersonalization, and 0.76 for personal accomplishment. The total score was 0.78.

Resilience Scale for Adults

The Resilience Scale for Adults was created by Friborg et al. [10]. The scale contained 33 items and 6 subscales measuring self-perception, perception of future, structured style, social competence, family cohesion, and social resources. In measuring resilience as high or low, scoring was left free. When scores on the scale increased and resilience was desired to increase, then from left to right, the answer boxes were evaluated as 1, 2, 3, 4, and 5. If the scores decreased and resilience was desired to increase, then the answer boxes were evaluated as 5, 4, 3, 2, and 1. The total score from the inventory was then divided into the number of items, and the median scores were evaluated. High scores obtained on the inventory indicate high resilience scores [10]. The reliability and validity study for the Turkish scale was conducted by Basım and Cetin [8]. Cronbach's alpha coefficients for the subscales were found to be between 0.66 and 0.81 [8]. In the present study, Cronbach's alpha coefficient was 0.71 for structural style, 0.71 for perception of future, 0.70 for self-perception, 0.64 for family cohesion, 0.70 for social competence, and 0.70 for social resources. The total score was 0.73.

Statistics

The data collected for this study were analyzed by the researchers using Statistical Package for Social Science (SPSS 21) for Windows package program. Demographic information for the nurses was reported as frequencies and percentages. Continuous variables were reported as mean ± standard deviation or median and interquartile range (IQR) as appropriate. Normality of the Maslach's Burnout Inventory and Resilience Scale for Adults scores were examined by the Shapiro–Wilk test. Scale scores were not normally distributed, and nonparametric tests were used. To examine the relationship between the Burnout Inventory subscales, the Resilience Scale for Adults subscales, and the socio-demographic attributes, the Mann–Whitney U (MU) test and the Kruskal–Wallis (KW) test were used. To examine whether a significant relationship existed between the Maslach's Burnout Inventory's subscales and the Resilience for Adults subscales, Spearman's correlation coefficient was evaluated. Central limit theorem was based on the regression analysis, although data source was not normally distributed. According to the law of large numbers, $n \to \infty$ the basis of knowledge of the distribution of the sample mean for normal distribution to approximate regression analysis was performed. Multiple stepwise linear regression analysis was conducted to explore the factors affecting the burnout. Cronbach's alpha was computed for the Maslach's Burnout Inventory and Resilience Scale for Adults instruments to assess the internal reliability of the questions. The level of significance was determined after the pairwise comparison Bonferroni correction.

Results

Nurses' socio-demographic and career attributes data are shown in Table 1.

Maslach's Burnout Inventory results

The total median score and interquartile range for Maslach's Burnout Inventory was 49.00: emotional exhaustion (EE), depersonalization (D), and personal accomplishment (PA) median scores of the oncology nurses were found to be 24.00, 9.00, and 16.00 respectively.

According to the nurses' demographic information, as per the median score distribution of the Maslach's Burnout Inventory, the nurses who did not have any dependents and worked in the field between 1 and 8 years had higher emotional exhaustion median scores and the difference between the median scores was found to be statistically significant ($p < 0.05$) (Table 2).

Resilience Scale for Adults results

The total median score and interquartile range for Resilience Scale for Adults was 134.00 (122.0; 146.0). The median scores of the nurses for structural style, perception of future, family cohesion, self-perception, social competence, and social resources were found to be 16.00, 16.00, 24.00, 25.00, 23.00, and 31.00 respectively.

The median score distribution for the Resilience Scale for Adults by nurses' demographic characteristics indicated that the nurses between the ages of 36 and 44 years had higher structured style and self-perception median scores compared with the other age groups, and the difference was statistically significant ($p < 0.05$).

The nurses who had children compared with the nurses who did not have children had higher self-perception median scores, and the difference between the median scores was statistically significant ($p < 0.05$) (Table 3).

The results of the analyses conducted with the other socio-demographic variables (gender, age, marital status, education level, family type, presence of any children, length of service in oncology, position and working hours) did not reveal any statistically significant differences ($p > 0.05$).

The median scores for the Resilience Scale for Adults and the nurses' education level suggested that the social

Table 1 Nurses' socio-demographic and career attributes

Socio-demographic characteristics	Number	%
Sex		
Female	126	90
Male	14	10
Age groups (years)		
19–27	23	16.2
28–35	55	39.4
36–44	49	35
45–53	13	9.4
Marital status		
Married	85	59.3
Single	55	40.7
Education status		
High school graduate	21	15
Associate's degree	27	19.3
Bachelor's degree	84	60
Higher education graduate	8	5.7
Family type		
Nuclear	126	90
Extended	11	7.9
Divorced	3	2.1
Any children		
Yes	78	56.1
No	62	43.9
Dependents		
Yes	73	52.5
No	67	47.5
People taken care of		
Child	45	61.6
Parents	21	28.8
Sibling	7	9.6
Number of children		
1	34	46.6
2	35	48
3 or more	4	5.4
Career attributes	Number	%
Number of years in the field (years)		
1–8	56	40
9–16	44	31.4
17–24	31	22.2
25–33	9	6.4
Number of years working in oncology	Mean ± SD 3.70 ± 3.69	
Clinic stationed at		
Oncology day treatment	68	48.6
Oncology/medical oncology clinic	48	34.3
Hematology clinic	12	8.6
Bone marrow transplantation clinic	6	4.3
Palliative care clinic	2	1.4
Internal medicine clinic	2	1.4
Hematology day treatment	2	1.4

Table 1 continued

Socio-demographic characteristics	Number	%
Duty at current clinic		
Clinical nurse	84	60
Chief nurse	40	28.5
Policlinic nurse	16	11.5
Working hours at the current clinic		
8–16	77	55
8–16 or 16–24	36	25.7
16–08 or 16–24	18	12.9
16–24 or 24–08	9	6.4
Previous clinics of practice		
Oncology/hematology clinics	91	34.9
Internal medicine clinics	68	26.1
Surgical clinics	47	18
Intensive care clinics	32	12.2
Pediatric clinics	16	6.1
Gynecology clinics	7	2.7

resources' median scores were significantly higher for the nurses who had an associate's degree (Table 3).

A statistically significant difference was reported between the median scores of structured style and self-perception based on the number of years the nurses had worked in the field. The significance tests conducted for multiple variables revealed a significant difference between the nurses working in the field for 17–24 years and the nurses working in the field for 1–8 years ($p < 0.05$) (Table 3). The results of the analyses conducted with the other socio-demographic variables (gender, marital status, family type, dependents they care for, length of service, position and working hours) did not reveal any statistically significant differences ($p > 0.05$).

Resilience Scale for Adults and Maslach's Burnout Inventory results

Spearman's correlation analysis of the median scores for the Resilience Scale for Adults and the Maslach's Burnout Inventory suggested a significantly negative correlation between emotional exhaustion and perception of future; depersonalization and structured style and self-perception; and personal accomplishment and structured style, perception of future, and self-perception (Table 4). The correlation analysis between the total scale scores showed that there was a negative and significant correlation.

Multiple regression analysis revealed a significant correlation between the number of years in the field, emotional exhaustion scores, and depersonalization ($p < 0.01$). This variable explained 4.97 and 3.49% of the total variance, respectively. A significant correlation was observed between structured style and personal

Table 2 Distribution of the Maslach's Burnout Inventory scores of oncology nurses according to their socio-demographic characteristics and career attributes

	Maslach's Burnout Inventory		
	Emotional exhaustion (median, IQR)	**Depersonalization (median, IQR)**	**Personal accomplishment (median, IQR)**
Dependents			
Yes	23.00 (20.0;28.0)	8.00 (5.0;10.0)	16.00 (12.2;19.0)
No	26.00 (21.0; 31.0)	10.00 (7.0;13.0)	16.00 (13.0;20.0)
	MU = 1951,000, $p = 0.039$*	MU = 1700,000, $p = 0.002$*	MU = 2366,500, $p = 0.857$
Years of professional experience (years)			
1–8	25.50 (22.0; 31.0)	9.50 (7.0; 13.0)	17.00 (13.0; 20.0)
9–16	24.00 (20.0; 29.7)	9.00 (6.0; 11.0)	16.00 (13.0; 18.0)
17–24	23.00 (19.0; 29.0)	8.00 (5.0; 11.0)	16.00 (12.0; 20.0)
25–33	20.00 (16.5; 22.5)	8.00 (5.5; 9.0)	14.00 (12.0; 17.0)
	KW = 9.841, $p = 0.020$*	KW = 5.294, $p = 0.151$	KW = 2.159, $p = 0.540$

* $p < 0.05$

Table 3 Distribution of the Resilience Scale for Adults scores of oncology nurses according to their socio-demographic characteristics and career attributes

	Resilience Scale for Adults					
	Structural style (median, IQR)	**Perception of future (median, IQR)**	**Family cohesion (median, IQR)**	**Perception of self (median, IQR)**	**Social competence (median, IQR)**	**Social resources (median, IQR)**
Age groups (years)						
19–27	17.00 (12.0;18.0)	17.00 (15.0; 20.0)	24.00 (20.0; 26.0)	24.00 (20.0; 26.0)	22.00 (19.0; 24.0)	29.00 (27.0; 32.0)
28–35	15.00 (13.0; 16.0)	15.00 (12.0; 19.0)	23.00 (20.0; 26.0)	24.00 (21.0; 27.0)	23.00 (20.0; 26.0)	31.00 (28.0; 34.0)
36–44	16.00 (15.0; 19.0)	16.00 (14.0; 19.0)	25.00 (21.0; 28.0)	26.00 (22.0; 28.0)	22.00 (20.0; 28.0)	31.00 (29.0; 33.0)
45–53	16.00 (14.0; 20.0)	17.00 (15.0; 19.5)	25.00 (21.0; 27.0)	26.00 (23.0; 29.5)	26.00 (23.0; 30.0)	32.00 (29.0; 35.0)
	KW = 12.268, $p = 0.007$*	KW = 3.854, $p = 0.278$	KW = 2.075, $p = 0.557$	KW = 8.008, $p = 0.046$*	KW = 4.938, $p = 0.176$	KW = 4.930, $p = 0.177$
Education status						
High school	16.00 (14.0; 18.5)	17.00 (14.5; 20.0)	25.00 (22.0; 28.0)	24.00 (22.0; 28.5)	22.00 (20.0; 27.0)	29.00 (27.0; 32.0)
Associate's degree	16.00 (15.0; 20.0)	16.00 (14.0; 20.0)	25.00 (22.0; 27.0)	26.00 (24.0; 29.0)	24.00 (20.0; 29.0)	32.00 (31.0; 35.0)
Bachelor's degree	16.00 (13.0; 18.0)	16.00 (13.2; 19.0)	23.00 (20.0; 26.7)	24.00 (21.0; 27.0)	23.00 (20.0; 26.7)	31.00 (28.0; 34.0)
Higher education	15.00 (12.0; 18.0)	15.00 (14.0; 17.0)	23.00 (20.0; 26.0)	21.00 (19.0; 26.2)	21.00 (19.0; 24.0)	30.00 (28.0; 33.0)
	KW = 2.733, $p = 0.435$	KW = 1.577, $p = 0.665$	KW = 3.632, $p = 0.304$	KW = 6.462, $p = 0.091$	KW = 2.726, $p = 0.436$	KW = 10.045, $p = 0.018$*
Have children						
Yes	16.00 (14.0; 18.5)	16.00 (14.0; 19.0)	25.00 (21.5.0; 27.0)	26.00 (22.0; 28.0)	23.00 (20.5; 27.5)	31.00 (29.0; 34.0)
No	15.50 (12.7; 17.7)	16.00 (13.0; 19.0)	23.00 (20.0; 26.0)	24.00 (21.0; 26.5)	22.00 (19.0; 26.0)	31.00 (28.0; 33.0)
	MU = 2054,000, $p = 0.155$	MU = 2321,50, $p = 0.780$	MU = 1980,50, $p = 0.084$	MU = 1880,00, $p = 0.044$*	MU = 2029,50, $p = 0.129$	MU = 2218,50, $p = 0.472$
Number of years in the field (years)						
1–8	16.00 (13.0; 17.0)	16.00 (13.0; 19.0)	24.00 (21.0; 26.0)	23.00 (20.2; 26.0)	22.00 (19.0; 25.7)	30.50 (22.2; 33.0)
9–16	15.00 (13.0; 17.0)	16.00 (13.0; 18.0)	23.50 (20.0; 27.0)	25.00 (21.0; 28.0)	22.00 (20.0; 26.0)	31.00 (28.0; 34.70)
17–24	18.00 (15.0; 20.0)	16.00 (14.0; 20.0)	24.00 (20.0; 27.0)	26.00 (24.0; 29.0)	25.00 (21.0; 28.0)	31.00 (30.0; 33.0)
25–33	18.00 (14.0; 20.0)	19.00 (15.5; 20.0)	25.00 (21.0; 28.5)	29.00 (24.5; 30.0)	26.00 (22.0; 30.0)	32.00 (28.0; 35.0)
	KW = 11.535, $p = 0.009$*	KW = 5.421, $p = 0.143$	KW = 0.773, $p = 0.856$	KW = 13.056, $p = 0.005$*	KW = 7.563, $p = 0.056$	KW = 2.936, $p = 0.402$

* $p < 0.05$

Table 4 Spearman's correlation between the Resilience Scale for adults and the Maslach's Burnout Inventory median scores

Resilience Scale for Adults subscales	Maslach's Burnout Inventory subscales			Total
	Emotional exhaustion	Depersonalization	Personal accomplishment	
Structural style	−.107	*−.195**	*−.300**	*−.258**
Perception of future	*−.222**	−.142	*−.272**	*−.287**
Family cohesion	0.029	−.049	−.095	−.045
Perception of self	*−.226*	*−.210**	*−.452**	*−.394**
Social competence	−.108	−.092	−.130	−.135
Social resources	−.013	−.072	−.155	−.107
Total	*−.191**	−.161	*−.350**	*−.320**

* $p < 0.01$

accomplishment scores. This variable explained approximately 6.12% of the total variance (Table 5).

Discussion

This section will be presented in three parts based on the findings of this study. The first part presents the status of having burnout and the variables that are influential on burnout. The second one is the state of resilience and the variables that are influential on resilience. The third one is the dimension of the correlation between burnout and resilience and the factors that are influential on this correlation.

Burnout

The total median score and interquartile range for Maslach's Burnout Inventory was 49.00 (43.0; 59.0). Many factors are effective in the manifestation of burnout. The literature reports a negative relationship between the level of burnout and the age, working time, and field experience [15–17]. While some factors have an effect on emotional exhaustion, other factors have an effect on depersonalization and personal accomplishment. An important fact related to emotional exhaustion is the time working in the field. Individuals with little field experience, wanting to be recognized in the field in a short period of time, believing that they will earn back all of their efforts very quickly, and experiencing disappointments when they do not reach their goals may emotionally burn out much faster [16–18]. In this study, emotional exhaustion was experienced much more, especially in nurses with less experience in the field. Similarly, the regression analysis revealed a negative correlation between the number of working years in the field and emotional exhaustion and depersonalization.

In this study, having dependents to care for as a socio-demographic variable was influential in oncology nurses experiencing emotional exhaustion. Akyüz [19] reported results similar to those observed in this study where individuals having dependents to care for had higher ratios of emotional exhaustion and depersonalization. The role of a caregiver leads to individuals experiencing emotional exhaustion more frequently and, as a result, increases the rate of developing burnout [20, 21]. Demir et al. [15] found that continuous day work reduced depersonalization, and the nurses in charge had high personal accomplishment levels. This study also found a negative correlation between working status and depersonalization.

Resilience

Resilience is the person's ability to successfully cope with barriers, uncertainty, and similar negative situations [22]. In this study, in terms of resilience, oncology nurses' scores on structured style, family cohesion and social competence, perception of future, self-perception, and social resource were close to the expected level. A person's resilience level is affected by individual, familial, and environmental factors. Individual factors such as

Table 5 Results of regression analysis of the effect of independent variables on burnout

Independent variables	Dependent variable	Beta	Standard error	R2	Standardize beta	*t*	*p*
Number of years in the field	EE	−1.792	0.0619	0.049	−.236	−2.846	*0.000*
Number of years in the field	D	−.748	0.308	0.034	−.203	−2.426	*0.017*
Structural style	PA	−.497	0.156	0.062	−.262	−3.179	*0.002*

Italic values indicate significance of *p* value ($p < 0.05$)

EE emotional exhaustion, *D* depersonalization, *PA* personal achievement

age either positively or negatively influence the individual's psychological development starting from childhood and continuing through adulthood [23]. In this study, the oncology nurses in the age group of 36–44 years had higher median scores for structured style and self-perception. Regarding the reasons for the relationship between age and structured style, which represents the person's strengths, it is thought that the adults in the age group of 36–44 years are in a period where they know themselves better and have more self-confidence. In this study, one factor affecting resilience in the oncology nurses was the number of working years. Demir et al. [15] found that the personal accomplishments increased with the number of working years. Finn [24] reported that as the nurses' field experience increased, they had stronger professional autonomy and higher job satisfaction.

Having children was another factor affecting resilience. In a study performed on radiation therapists and oncology nurses, 53.6% had children and their resilience levels were reported to be moderate [25]. In this study, nurses who had children had higher median scores for resilience indicator of self-perception.

Another factor affecting the oncology nurses' resilience was the level of education. In this study, compared with other nurses, nurses with an associate's degree had better levels of resilience, as they were thought to be using social resources in a much better way. The use of social resources is closely related to the education level. As the education level increases, the individuals realize the importance of social support resources, learn how to access resources, and increase their use [24]. One of the coping methods doctors and nurses, working with cancer patients, use to cope with work-related stresses is the use of social support [26]. Lim et al. [27] reported that nurses used spouse, friend, and family support as a coping strategy for stress. In a study conducted on pediatric oncology nurses aimed at determining their coping and resilience, it was found that to cope and increase their resilience, and the nurses needed to use their social support resources very well [28].

The number of working years in the field is another variable that influences resilience. As the number of working years increases, the oncology nurses' ability to cope with stress also increases and they become aware of themselves. A study conducted on health care professionals working with cancer patients reported that the nurses working between 1 and 10 years had higher stress scores compared with the nurses working for 11 years or more [26]. In this study, the nurses working in the field for 17–24 years had higher median scores for structured style and self-perception compared with the nurses working for 1–8 years. Another study reported that age, professional experience, education, and the number of working years had no effect on resilience [29]. It is estimated that as the nurses' professional experience increases, their self-confidence increases too, and they become more aware of their competence/lack of competence.

Burnout and resilience

Resilience, in general, refers to a success or adaptation period [8]. Burnout and resilience, which are influenced by personal and professional factors, are often seen when adaptation is not possible. Personal and professional factors can lead to the stress factors causing burnout. A person's self-perception is among the personal factors. If the person's self-awareness is low, their confidence that they will accomplish good things is also low. They exaggerate barriers and give up fighting with the barriers very quickly. The person focuses on their failures and not their successes, and their susceptibility to burnout increases [30, 31]. This study reported a negative correlation between the subscales of emotional exhaustion and self-perception. It has been noted that individuals with insufficient self-competence constitute high-risk groups in terms of burnout [32, 33]. Garrosa et al. [34] reported a negative relationship between the nurses' personal resources and control situations where they experience emotional exhaustion.

Having negative expections and perceptions about the future leads to burnout. Taorimo and Law [35] reported that burnout was significantly affected by perceptions of the future. Similarly, individuals experiencing burnout have not been very successful in the past and, with this perspective, assume that they will not be successful in the future either [36]. Coping with stress allows the person to know themselves better and, by establishing positive expectations regarding the future, their resilience increases and their burnout is better controlled. This study found a significant negative relationship between emotional exhaustion and perception of future.

In this study, personal accomplishments influenced structured style, perception of future, and self-perception. Moreover, the regression analysis indicated a relationship between the structured style, which represented the strong sides of a person, and personal accomplishment. While increasing resilience increases personal accomplishments, burnout reduces a person's personal accomplishments. A decrease in the feeling of personal success manifests when a person sees their job performance as weak and evaluates themselves negatively. When people feel insufficient and unsuccessful, it causes them to lose their self-respect. The person may think that their contributions to work and society are limited [17, 37]. A study conducted with health care personnel working in an oncology center reported that doctors had much higher levels of emotional exhaustion and depersonalization and nurses lacked much more in personal success [38].

Conclusions

This study demonstrated the relationship between burnout and resilience situations among the oncology nurses. It was found that to increase their resilience, the nurses should be supported in structured style, perception of future, and perception of self. For less experience of burnout, they should not experience emotional exhaustion and should increase their personal accomplishments. Hence, the results of this study can be used to plan individual and organizational interventions to increase resilience and reduce the experience of burnout by developing measures such as improving communication skills, providing education on stress management, organizing programs that provide psychological support, using psychodrama and relaxation techniques, establishing a positive work environment, and so forth.

This study had some limitations. The results of this study were limited by the small sample size. Also, the nurses were evaluated for burnout and resilience only once. However, the study reflected what nurses working in an oncology clinic actually experience. Another important limitation is that 20 nurses were excluded from the analysis part of the study since there was some missing information in their research forms. Statistical data analysis was performed on 140 nurses with no missing information.

Abbreviations

D: depersonalization; EE: emotional exhaustion; IQR: interquartile range; KW: Kruskal–Wallis; MU: Mann–Whitney *U*; PA: personal achievement.

Authors' contributions

SK is the first author of this manuscript. She owns the responsibility for study design, data acquisition, analysis, result interpretation, and drafting of the manuscript. ES first proposed the conception of this study and has substantial contribution in the design and implementation of the study, data collection, and statistical analysis, as well as drafting of the manuscript. NU has participated in data collection and statistical analysis, as well as drafting of the manuscript. FB has substantial contribution in the design and implementation of the study as well as data collection. All authors read and approved the final manuscript.

Author details

[1] Department of Nursing, Gazi University Faculty of Health Sciences, Besevler, 06500 Ankara, Turkey. [2] Yıldırım Beyazıt Üniversity Faculty of Health Science, Ankara, Turkey. [3] Gazi University Health Research and Application Center, Gazi Hospital, Ankara, Turkey.

Acknowledgements

We appreciate all the nurses who participated in this study.

Competing interests

The authors declare that they have no competing interests.

References

1. Onan N, Işıl Ö. Coping, stress, and burnout of nurses in the oncology department: literature review. Maltepe Univ J Nurs Sci Art. 2010;4:264–71.
2. Italia S, Favara-Scacco C, Di Cataldo A, Russo G. Evaluation and art therapy treatment of the burnout syndrome in oncology units. Psychooncology. 2008;17:676–80.
3. Pierce B, Dougherty E, Panzarella T, Le LW, Rodin G, Zimmermann C. Staffstress, work satisfaction, and death attitudes on an oncology palliative care unit, and on a medical and radiation oncology in patient unit. J Palliat Care. 2007;23:32–9.
4. Maslach C, Schaufeli WB, Leiter MP. Job burnout. Annu Rev Psychol. 2001;52:397–422.
5. Trufelli DC, Bensi CG, Garcia JB, Narahara JL, Abrão MN, Diniz RW, Miranda Vda C, Soares HP, Del Giglio A. Burnout in cancer professionals: a systematic review and meta-analysis. Eur J Cancer Care. 2008;17:524–31.
6. Antoniou AG, Davidson MJ, Cooper CL. Occupational stress, job satisfaction and health state in male and female junior hospital doctors in Greece. J Manag Psychol. 2003;18:592–621.
7. Curtis WJ, Cicchetti D. Moving research on resilience into the 21st century: theoretical and methodological considerations in examining the biological contributors to resilience. Dev Psychopathol. 2003;15:773–810.
8. Basım N, Cetin F. Reliability and validity studies of resilience scale for adults. Turk J Psychiatry. 2011;22:104–14.
9. Demirci S, Yildirim YK, Ozsaran Z, Uslu R, Yalman D, Aras AB. Evaluation of burnout syndrome in oncology employees. Med Oncol. 2010;27:968–74.
10. Friborg O, Barlaug D, Martinussen M, Rosenvinge JH, Hjemdal O. Resilience in relation to personality and intelligence. Int J Methods Psychiatr Res. 2005;14:29–42.
11. Ablett JR, Jones RSP. Resilience and well-being in palliative care staff: a qualitative study of hospice nurses' experience of work. Psycho-Oncol. 2007;16:733–40.
12. Maslach C, Jackson SE. Manuel Maslach Burnout Inventory. 2nd ed. California: Consulting Psychologists Press; 1986. p. 1–17.
13. Çam O. Examining the reliability and validity of the burnout inventory. VII National Psychological Congress (Congress Book). Ankara. 1992; 22-25:155–160.
14. Ergin C. The translation of the scale of burnout in physicians and nurses in addition to Maslach's Burnout Inventory. 1992 VII National Psychological Congress (Congress Book). Ankara. 1992; 22–25:143–54.
15. Demir A, Ulusoy M, Ulusoy MF. Investigation of factors influencing burnout levels in the Professional and private lives of nurses. Int J Nurs Stud. 2003;40:807–27.
16. Ersoy F, Yıldırım RC, Edirne T. Burnout syndrome. J Contin Med Educ. 2001;10:15–20.
17. Maslach C. Jackson SE The measurement of experienced burnout. J Occup Behav. 1981;2:99–113.
18. Brewer EW, Shapard L. Employee burnout: a meta-analysis of the relationship between age or years of experience. Hum Resour Dev Rev. 2004;3:102–23.
19. Akyüz İ. Investigation of level of nurses' burnout and depression in terms of working conditions and demographic characteristics. J Bus Econ Stud. 2015;3:21–34.
20. Özçakar N, Kartal M, Dirik G, Tekin N, Gülda D. Burnout and relevant factors in nursing staff: what affects the staff working in an elderly nursing home? Turk J Geriatr. 2012;15:266–72.
21. Götze H, Brähler E, Gansera L, Schnabel A, Köhler N. Exhaustion and overload of family caregivers of palliative cancer patients. Psychother Psychosom Med Psychol. 2015;65:66–72.
22. Youssef CM, Luthans F. Positive organizational behavior in the work place: the impact of hope, optimism, and resilience. J Manag. 2007;33:774–800.
23. Öz F, Yılmaz EB. A significant concept in protecting mental health: resilience. J Hacettepe Univ Fac Nurs. 2009;9:82–9.
24. Finn CP. Autonomy: an important component for nurses' job satisfaction. Int J Nurs Stud. 2001;38:349–57.
25. Poulsen MG, Poulsen AA, Baumann KC, McQuitty S, Sharpley CF. A cross-sectional study of stressors and coping mechanisms used by radiation therapists and oncology nurses: resilience in cancer care study. J Med Imaging Radiat Sci. 2014;61:225–32.

26. Isikhan V, Comez T, Danis MZ. Job stress and coping strategies in health care professionals working with cancer patients. Eur J Oncol Nurs. 2004;8:234–44.
27. Lim J, Hepworth J, Bogossian F. A qualitative analysis of stress, uplifts and coping in the personal and professional lives of Singaporean nurses. J Adv Nurs. 2011;67:1022–33.
28. Zander M, Hutton A, King L. Exploring resilience in paediatric oncology nursing staff. Collegian. 2013;20:17–25.
29. Gillespie BM, Chaboyer W, Wallis M, Grimbeek P. Resilience in the operating room: developing and testing of a resilience model. J Adv Nurs. 2007;59:427–38.
30. Aycock N, Boyle D. Interventions to manage compassion fatigue in oncology nursing. Clin J Oncol Nurs. 2009;13:183–91.
31. Kravits K, McAllister-Black R, Grant M, Kirk C. Self-care strategies for nurses : a psychoeducational intervention for stress reduction and the prevention of burnout. Appl Nurs Res. 2010;23:130–8.
32. Tuğrul B, Çelik E. Burnout in pre-school teachers working with normal children. Pamukkale Üniv J Educ. 2002;12:1–11.
33. Eren V, Durna U. Organizational burnout as a three dimensional approach. Selçuk Univ J EAS. 2006;10:40–51.
34. Garrosa E, Rainho C, Moreno-Jiménez B, Monteiro MJ. The relationship between job stressors, hardy personality, coping resources and burnout in a sample of nurses: a correlational study at two time points. Int J Nurs Stud. 2010;47:205–15.
35. Taormina RJ, Law CM. Approaches to preventing burnout: the effects of personal stress management and organizational socialization. J Nurs Manag. 2000;8:89–99.
36. Seta CE, Paulus PB, Baron RA. Effective human relations a guide to people at work. 4th ed. Alllynand Bacon; 2000.
37. Altay B, Gönener D, Demirkıran C. The level of burnout and influence of family support in nurses working in a university hospital. Fırat Med J. 2010;15:10–6.
38. Elit L, Trim K, Mand-Bains IH, Sussman J, Grunfeld E, Society of Gynecologic Oncology Canada. Job satisfaction, stress and burnout among Canadian gynecologic oncologists. Gynecol Oncol. 2004;94:134–9.

7

Serum prolactin levels and sexual dysfunction in patients with schizophrenia treated with antipsychotics: comparison between aripiprazole and other atypical antipsychotics

Eiji Kirino[1,2,3*]

Abstract

Objectives: Antipsychotics, even atypical ones, can induce hyperprolactinemia. Aripiprazole (APZ), a dopamine D2 partial agonist, has a unique pharmacological profile and few side effects. We investigated the incidence of hyperprolactinemia in patients with schizophrenia treated with APZ and other antipsychotics.

Methods: Serum prolactin levels were measured by ELISA (enzyme-linked immunosorbent assay). A questionnaire survey was used to evaluate subjective sexual dysfunction.

Results: Based on the results of the questionnaire, approximately half (48.1%) of the patients complained of sexual dysfunction. The serum prolactin levels were significantly higher in patients with sexual dysfunction than in those without. In patients treated with antipsychotic monotherapy, the serum prolactin levels were significantly lower in patients treated with APZ than with other antipsychotics. In patients receiving 2 or more antipsychotics, the serum prolactin levels were significantly lower in patients treated with APZ-containing regimens than in patients treated with APZ-free regimens.

Conclusions: Treatment with APZ did not influence the serum prolactin level, and adjunctive treatment with APZ may ameliorate the hyperprolactinemia that occurs during monotherapy with other antipsychotics.

Keywords: Schizophrenia, Hyperprolactinemia, Antipsychotics, Aripiprazole, Sexual dysfunction

Introduction

Antipsychotics are an effective pharmacological therapy for schizophrenia. Second-generation antipsychotics (SGAs) have been developed recently that have effects on positive symptoms that are similar to those of first-generation antipsychotics (FGAs) plus a lower incidence of adverse reactions, such as extrapyramidal symptoms (EPSs). Although SGAs are not a homogeneous group [1–4], some SGAs have more promising effects on negative symptoms than FGAs [5, 6]. However, even SGAs that have been demonstrated to be safe have been found to induce weight gain, disturb glucose/lipid metabolism, and cause hyperprolactinemia [7]. Hyperprolactinemia that is related to excessive blockage of funnel/pituitary gland system D2 receptors is closely associated with sexual dysfunction, including irregular menstruation and erectile insufficiency, decreases in bone density after long-term use, and the risk of breast cancer [8–10]. However, it can be difficult to detect side effects such as sexual dysfunction that may contribute to recurrent schizophrenia due to self-discontinuation of drug therapy. Although FGAs were initially thought to be

*Correspondence: ekirino@juntendo.ac.jp
[1] Department of Psychiatry, Juntendo University Shizuoka Hospital, 1129 Nagaoka, Izunokunishi, Shizuoka 4102211, Japan
Full list of author information is available at the end of the article

responsible for antipsychotic-induced hyperprolactinemia, SGAs have also been implicated. Leucht et al. [11] in a meta-analysis comparing the tolerability of 15 antipsychotics reported that most SGAs elevated serum prolactin levels significantly.

Aripiprazole (APZ) has a unique pharmacological profile and is a partial agonist of dopamine D2 and serotonin 5-HT1A receptors and an antagonist of the serotonin 5-HT2A receptor. This drug has few of the typical side effects of other antipsychotic drugs, such as EPSs, hyperprolactinemia, weight gain, metabolic disorders, and sedation [12]. APZ appropriates intrinsic activity at dopamine D2 receptors, thereby stabilizing dopamine D2 receptor-mediated neurotransmission without excessive blocking. Because of this, APZ is often called a dopamine system stabilizer [13].

Kapur et al. [14] proposed that antipsychotics with fast dissociation from the D2 receptor are more accommodating of physiological dopamine transmission, achieving an antipsychotic effect without motor side effects, prolactin elevation, or secondary negative symptoms. That group argued that the atypical antipsychotic effect, which they called "atypicality," can be produced by appropriate modulation of the D2 receptor alone and that the blockade of other receptors is neither necessary nor sufficient.

In line with these findings, Kane et al. [15] reported a multicenter, randomized, double-blind, placebo-controlled 16-week study of adjunctive APZ for patients with schizophrenia or schizoaffective disorder treated with quetiapine (QTP) or risperidone (RIS) monotherapy. Adjunctive APZ was associated with significantly greater decreases in mean serum prolactin levels compared to baseline versus the adjunctive placebo (− 12.6 ng/mL for APZ vs − 2.2 ng/mL for placebo; $P < 0.001$). This effect was seen in the RIS subgroup (− 18.7 ng/mL vs − 1.9 ng/mL; $P < 0.001$) but not in the QTP subgroup (− 3.01 ng/mL vs + 0.15 ng/mL; $P = 0.104$). Similar reductions in prolactin levels were seen following adjunctive use of APZ in haloperidol (HPD) treated patients with hyperprolactinemia [16].

The present study investigated the incidence of hyperprolactinemia in patients with schizophrenia treated with APZ and other antipsychotics. In addition, we conducted a survey about sexual dysfunction using an original questionnaire.

Subjects and methods

This non-blinded open study evaluated the serum prolactin level and subjective sexual dysfunction as well as the positive and negative syndrome scale (PANSS) score and the Clinical Global Impressions-Severity (CGI-S) score. The subjects were outpatients with schizophrenia (ICD-10, DSM-4-TR/DSM-5: schizophrenia, schizoaffective disorder, or schizotypal disorder, or schizoid personality) who were aged 17–60 years who were treated at the Department of Psychiatry at the Juntendo University Shizuoka Hospital between June 1, 2010 and May 31, 2017 and who received 1 or more antipsychotic medication. The subjects were serially registered during the entry period.

There were 87 subjects, including 36 males (41.4%) and 51 females (58.6%). The mean age was 39.16 ± 14.11 years (males: 38.81 ± 13.72; females: 39.41 ± 14.51). The patient age distribution was as follows: 10–19 years, 11 (12.6%); 20–29 years, 13 (14.9%); 30–39 years, 21 (24.1%); 40–49 years, 25 (28.7%); and others, 17 (19.5%). Of the 87 subjects, 67 (77.0%) were diagnosed with schizophrenia, 13 (14.9%) with schizoaffective disorder, and 7 (8.1%) with other disorders (schizotypal disorder, schizoid personality). A total of three patients (3.4%) had acute conditions, and 83 (95.4%) had chronic conditions. The mean duration of illness was 12.40 ± 10.58 years, and 19 patients (21.8%) had a history of hospital admission. Complications were noted in eight patients (Table 1). While 85 patients (97.7%) had received atypical agents, four had received (4.6%) typical agents (including combination therapy). The atypical agents included APZ in 60 patients (69.0%), QTP in 33 (37.3%), olanzapine (OLZ) in 19 (21.8%), and RIS in 12 (13.8%). Antipsychotic monotherapy had been prescribed to 53 patients (60.9%); of these, 32 (60.4%) had received APZ, the largest population for any agent (Fig. 1).

An ELISA kit (enzyme-linked immunosorbent assay) (Bioclone Australia Pty Limited, Marrickville NSW Australia) was used to measure serum prolactin levels. We prepared an original questionnaire survey about subjective sexual dysfunction to investigate whether each subject experienced erectile insufficiency, projectile ejaculation/semen, irregular menstruation, breast tension/phyma, breast milk production, or decreased sexual libido.

For statistical analysis, alpha values of 0.05 were considered significant in paired t tests and for Spearman's rank correlation coefficients.

Results

The mean serum prolactin level in females (18.57 ± 21.96 μg/mL) was significantly higher than in males (9.95 ± 14.08 μg/mL) ($P = 0.04508$). The normal range is 1.5–9.7 μg/mL in males and 1.4–14.6 μg/mL in females (Fig. 2). There were 10 males (27.8%) and 16 females (31.4%) with abnormal values, and some had a serum prolactin level > 100 μg/mL (1 female during OLZ 20 mg/day monotherapy and 1 female during RIS 3 mg/day monotherapy). The latter two patients reported irregular or no menstruation on the survey sheet. There were no significant correlations between serum prolactin level

Table 1 Demographic and clinical characteristics of the patient sample

Number of patients	87
Gender	Male: 36 (41.4%), Female: 51 (58.6%)
Age (mean ± SD)	39.16 ± 14.11 years Male: 38.81 ± 13.72 years, Female: 39.41 ± 14.51 years
Diagnosis	Schizophrenia: 67 (77.0%) Schizoaffective disorder: 13 (14.9%) Others: 7 (8.1%)
Acute/chronic phases	Acute phase: 3 (3.4%), chronic phase: 83 (95.4%), unclear: 1 (1.1%)
Duration of illness (mean ± SD)	12.40 ± 10.58 years
History of admission	Present: 19 (21.8%), absent: 67 (77.0%), unclear: 1 (1.1%) Previous admission, once: 11, twice: 5, 3 times: 2, 4 times: 1
Complication	Present: 8 patients (9.2%) Autoimmune hepatitis in 1 patient, lung cancer in 1, drug-induced hepatopathy in 1, breast cancer in 1, uterine cancer/A–V block in 1, sarcoidosis in 1, anomaly of the cerebral artery in 1, and congestive heart failure in 1

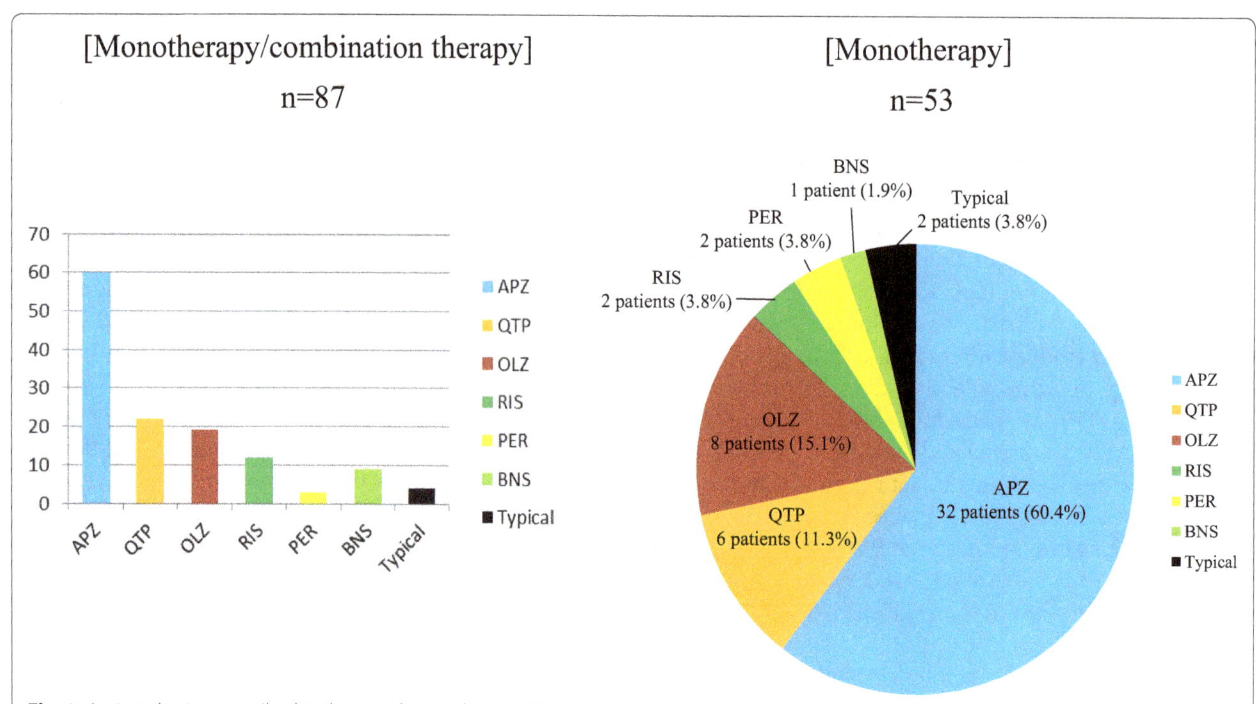

Fig. 1 Antipsychotics prescribed in the sample population. APZ was most frequently prescribed in patients treated with monotherapy or combination therapy. *APZ* aripiprazole, *BNS* blonanserin, *OLZ* olanzapine, *PER* perospirone, *RIS* risperidone, *QTP* quetiapine

and age, the number of antipsychotics, the dose of the antipsychotics (chlorpromazine equivalent), or the duration of illness when calculating Spearman's rank correlation coefficient.

Of the 81 patients (collection rate: 93.1%) from whom we collected survey sheets, 39 (48.1%) checked items indicating sexual dysfunction. In this sexual dysfunction group, the mean serum prolactin level (21.43 ± 31.57 μg/mL) was significantly higher than in subjects who did not check any items (non-sexual dysfunction group; 9.18 ± 9.66 μg/mL) ($P = 0.01647$) (Fig. 3). Although this was not statistically significant, the serum prolactin levels in females complaining of irregular menstruation tended to be higher than the levels in those without this problem (29.19 ± 43.7 vs 12.75 ± 10.34 μg/mL; $P = 0.05024$) (Fig. 4).

In patients receiving monotherapy, the mean serum prolactin level in patients treated with APZ was significantly lower than in those treated with other antipsychotics (9.60 ± 12.18 μg/mL vs 29.24 ± 41.89 μg/

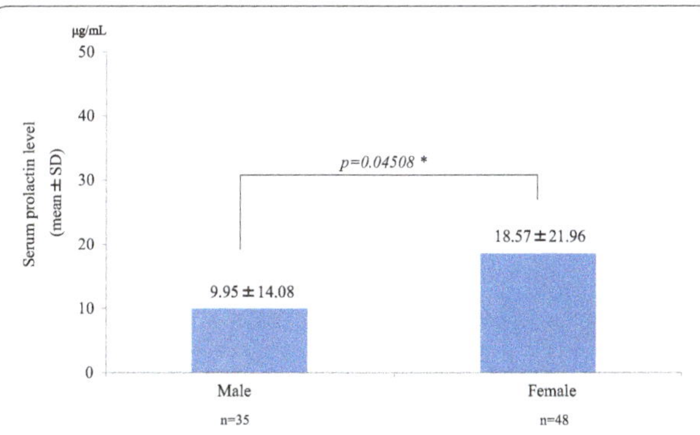

Fig. 2 Gender differences in serum prolactin levels. The mean serum prolactin level in females was significantly higher than the mean level in males

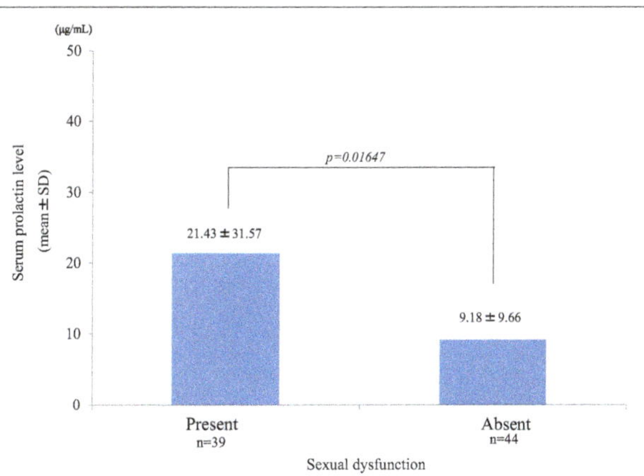

Fig. 3 The contribution of the presence of sexual dysfunction to serum prolactin levels. The serum prolactin levels were significantly higher in patients who checked at least 1 sexual dysfunction item on the questionnaire versus those who did not

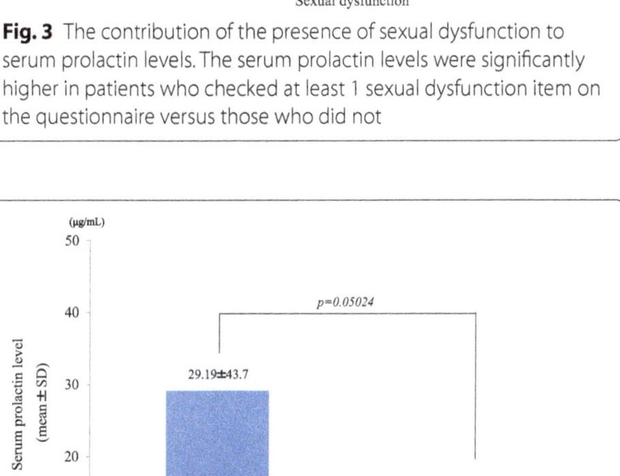

Fig. 4 The contribution of the presence of menstruation abnormalities to serum prolactin levels. Although not statistically significant, the serum prolactin levels in females who reported irregular menstruation tended to be higher than in those who did not

mL; $P = 0.01633$) (Fig. 5). There were no significant differences in the total mean PANSS scores in the APZ group vs the other antipsychotic group (65.61 ± 16.67 vs 70.76 ± 19.10; $P = 0.30772$). Similarly, there were no significant differences in the mean CGI-S score in the APZ group vs the other antipsychotic group (2.48 ± 0.85 vs 2.76 ± 0.70; $P = 0.21760$) (Fig. 6).

Regarding patients who were receiving 2 or more antipsychotics, the mean serum prolactin level in patients treated with APZ-containing regimens was significantly lower than in those treated with APZ-free regimens (8.10 ± 8.09 μg/mL vs 31.48 ± 18.60 μg/mL; $P = 0.00005$) (Fig. 7).

Discussion

This study found that the serum prolactin level increased in some patients with schizophrenia who were treated with antipsychotics. Approximately half of the patients who completed the study questionnaire reported sexual dysfunction. Antipsychotic-associated sexual dysfunction can reduce patient compliance; accordingly, it may be important to evaluate the presence of sexual dysfunction in the early phase of treatment by communicating with the patient. Notably, the serum prolactin level may have increased in patients complaining of sexual dysfunction.

Baggaley [17] reported that the incidence of sexual dysfunction ranged from 30 to 80% in patients with schizophrenia who were not treated or who were receiving treatment. The incidence was higher than in patients with other psychiatric disorders, suggesting that sexual dysfunction reduces the patient's quality of life. Fujii et al. [18] indicated that clinicians must consider the risk of sexual dysfunction because the incidence was

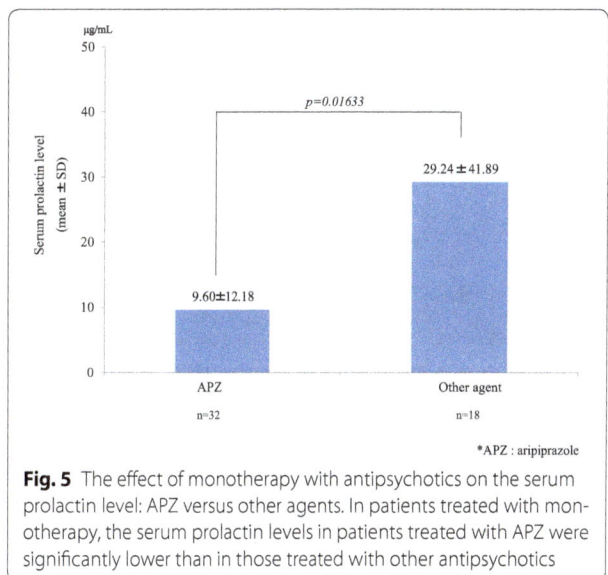

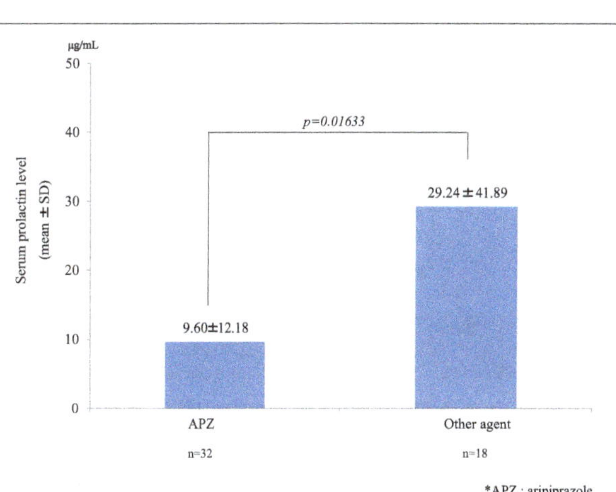

Fig. 5 The effect of monotherapy with antipsychotics on the serum prolactin level: APZ versus other agents. In patients treated with monotherapy, the serum prolactin levels in patients treated with APZ were significantly lower than in those treated with other antipsychotics

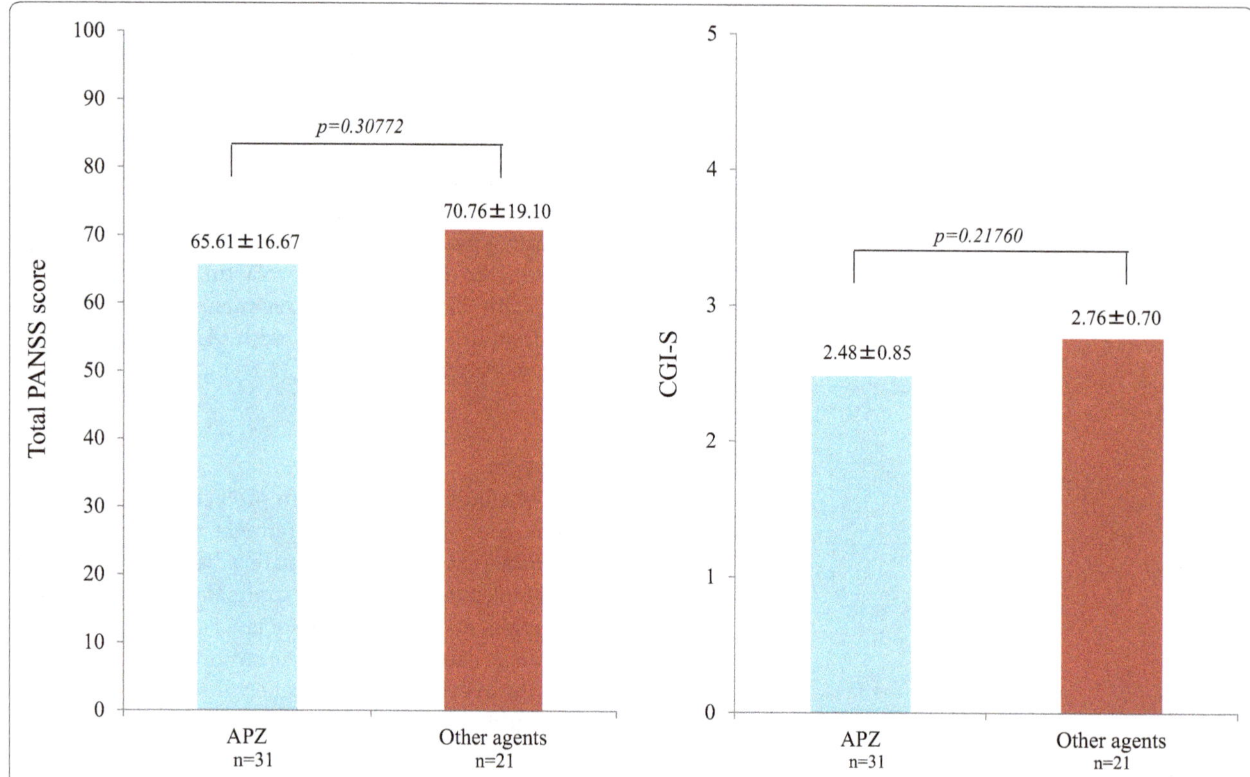

Fig. 6 The effect of monotherapy with antipsychotics on the total PANSS score and the CGI-S score: APZ versus other agents. There were no significant differences in the mean total PANSS score or CGI-S score between the APZ group versus other antipsychotic groups

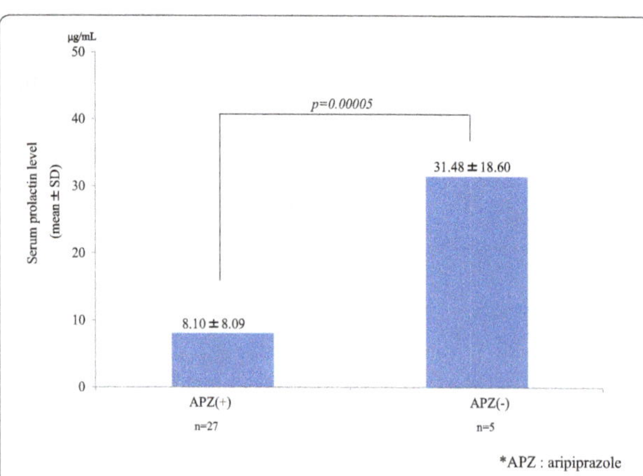

Fig. 7 The effect of APZ-containing regimens versus APZ-free regimens in combination therapies on the serum prolactin level. In patients receiving 2 or more antipsychotics, the serum prolactin levels in patients treated with APZ-containing regimens were significantly lower than the levels in those treated with APZ-free regimens

higher in patients with schizophrenia than in healthy adults in Asia. The Expert Consensus Guideline 2009 [19] emphasized that sexual dysfunction is an important side effect of antipsychotics that is associated with compliance.

In the present study, the serum prolactin level in females was significantly higher than in males. Kleinberg et al. [20] measured the serum prolactin level in patients with schizophrenia during RIS or HPD therapy and also found that the serum prolactin level was higher in females than in males, although the values for both sexes were higher than in the placebo group, regardless of dose. Jerrell et al. [21] reported that in patients receiving antipsychotics, the incidence of sexual dysfunction was higher in females, adolescent patients, patients receiving an SSRI or valproate, obese patients, and those with endocrine disturbances. Therefore, factors other than the type of antipsychotic, including gender, age, and concurrent agents, should be considered when treating schizophrenia as these factors may cause sexual dysfunction.

In this study, 48.1% of the patients indicated that at least 1 sexual dysfunction item was present during antipsychotic therapy. However, Cutler [22] reported that the incidence of sexual dysfunction that was predicted by the psychiatrists of patients with schizophrenia during antipsychotic therapy was 10–20% lower than the actual incidence of sexual dysfunction that patients subjectively experienced. In clinical practice, it may be necessary to investigate the presence of sexual dysfunction in patients treated with antipsychotics by asking them directly or by using a questionnaire. The serum prolactin level was significantly higher in patients who reported at least 1 sexual dysfunction item than in those who did not; therefore, the serum prolactin level should be measured in patients who complain of sexual dysfunction. Citrome [23] argued that there should be regular follow-up of the serum prolactin level after the start of antipsychotic therapy based on the patient's medical history and manifestation of symptoms. This is in accordance with at least 7 guidelines for the administration of any antipsychotic that may cause sexual dysfunction, i.e., the guidelines of the American Psychiatric Association; Mount Sinai Conference; Expert Consensus Survey; Canadian Psychiatric Association, Australia and New Zealand; UK National Institute for Health and Clinical Excellence 2006; and the Maudsley Prescribing Guidelines. Therefore, it is recommended that the baseline serum prolactin level should be measured initially and then monitored regularly [23].

The present study found that the serum prolactin level increased in the sexual dysfunction group. Furthermore, some of the patients in this study showed abnormally high prolactin levels that exceeded 100 μg/mL, and these patients reported irregular or no menstruation on the questionnaire. In the other patients, the serum prolactin levels in females who reported irregular menstruation tended to be higher than in those without this problem. However, there was no correlation between the number or dose of antipsychotics, duration of illness, or prolactin level, suggesting that follow-up of hyperprolactinemia or sexual dysfunction is necessary in both patients with long-term schizophrenia who receive massive doses of therapy with several antipsychotics and in patients with short-term schizophrenia who are receiving low-dose monotherapy.

Bostwick et al. [24] indicated that treatment should be switched to combination therapy with agents that do not influence the prolactin level, such as dopamine agonists, when there is an antipsychotic-related increase in the prolactin level, although this may compromise antipsychotic efficacy. In addition, the doses of agents that cause an elevation in prolactin should be decreased in patients that show a high serum prolactin level. Otherwise, agents that decrease the prolactin level, such as cabergoline and bromocriptine, should be added, or the patient should be treated with an agent such as APZ that does not influence the serum prolactin level, as reported by this study as well as others [15, 16, 25, 26]. Both strategies of switching to APZ [27–29] and addition of APZ [15, 30–32] to previous antipsychotics have been reported to be effective in resolving antipsychotic-induced hyperprolactinemia and hyperprolactinemia-related adverse events [33]. However, APZ being a partial agonist has a lower intrinsic activity at the D2 receptor than dopamine, allowing it to act as both, a functional agonist and antagonist, depending on the surrounding levels of dopamine [34]. Hence, it should be reminded in clinical scenes that APZ could act as a functional antagonist and thus elevate prolactin levels in the absence of a competing D2 antagonist and the presence of dopamine (the natural agonist) in some cases [34, 35].

We found a significant difference in the prolactin levels in patient groups treated with APZ-containing regimens vs APZ-free regimens, which is in line with previous findings [15, 16]. Adjunctive APZ with RIS may optimize D2 receptor activity and, hence, diminish the risk for EPS associated with RIS [36] as well as decrease prolactin elevation resulting from high D2 receptor occupancy by a full antagonist [16]. Thus, adjunctive APZ may potentially ameliorate the side effects that occur during monotherapy with other antipsychotics [15].

This study had some limitations. Our present findings are underpowered due to our relatively small sample. Furthermore, the sampling was biased in that the number of patients treated with APZ was much higher than the number of those treated with other antipsychotics. We should be prudent in interpreting our results although some of the analyses were statistically significant. Elucidating the clinical implications of our present findings will require further randomized or blinded studies in a larger sample.

Conclusions

Treatment with APZ did not influence the serum prolactin level, and adjunctive treatment with APZ may ameliorate the hyperprolactinemia that occurs during monotherapy with other antipsychotics.

Competing interests
The author declares that he has no competing interests.

Author details
[1] Department of Psychiatry, Juntendo University Shizuoka Hospital, 1129 Nagaoka, Izunokunishi, Shizuoka 4102211, Japan. [2] Department of Psychiatry, Juntendo University School of Medicine, 2-1-1 Hongo, Bunkyoku, Tokyo 1138421, Japan. [3] Juntendo Institute of Mental Health, 700-1 Fukuroyama, Koshigayashi, Saitama 3430032, Japan.

Consent for publication
Consent for publication was obtained from all subjects.

Funding
The author received an honorarium and research funding from Otsuka Pharmaceutical Co. The sponsor had no control over the interpretation, writing, or publication of this work.

References

1. Leucht S, Kissling W, Davis JM. Second-generation antipsychotics for schizophrenia: can we resolve the conflict? Psychol Med. 2009;39:1591–602.
2. Leucht S, Corves C, Arbter D, Engel RR, Li C, Davis JM. Second-generation versus first-generation antipsychotic drugs for schizophrenia: a meta-analysis. Lancet. 2009;373:31–41.
3. Leucht S, Komossa K, Rummel-Kluge C, Corves C, Hunger H, Schmid F, Asenjo Lobos C, Schwarz S, Davis JM. A meta-analysis of head-to-head comparisons of second-generation antipsychotics in the treatment of schizophrenia. Am J Psychiatry. 2009;166:152–63.
4. Leucht S, Arbter D, Engel RR, Kissling W, Davis JM. How effective are second-generation antipsychotic drugs? A meta-analysis of placebo-controlled trials. Mol Psychiatry. 2009;14:429–47.
5. Tandon R, Marcus RN, Stock EG, Riera LC, Kostic D, Pans M, McQuade RD, Nyilas M, Iwamoto T, Crandall DT. A prospective, multicenter, randomized, parallel-group, open-label study of aripiprazole in the management of patients with schizophrenia or schizoaffective disorder in general psychiatric practice: Broad Effectiveness Trial With Aripiprazole (BETA). Schizophr Res. 2006;84:77–89.
6. Wolf J, Janssen F, Lublin H, Salokangas RK, Allain H, Smeraldi E, Bernardo M, Millar H, Pans M, Adelbrecht C, et al. A prospective, multicentre, open-label study of aripiprazole in the management of patients with schizophrenia in psychiatric practice in Europe: Broad Effectiveness Trial with Aripiprazole in Europe (EU-BETA). Curr Med Res Opin. 2007;23:2313–23.
7. Weiden PJ, Miller AL. Which side effects really matter? Screening for common and distressing side effects of antipsychotic medications. J Psychiatr Pract. 2001;7:41–7.
8. Abraham G, Paing WW, Kaminski J, Joseph A, Kohegyi E, Josiassen RC. Effects of elevated serum prolactin on bone mineral density and bone metabolism in female patients with schizophrenia: a prospective study. Am J Psychiatry. 2003;160:1618–20.
9. Halbreich U, Kinon BJ, Gilmore JA, Kahn LS. Elevated prolactin levels in patients with schizophrenia: mechanisms and related adverse effects. Psychoneuroendocrinology. 2003;28(Suppl 1):53–67.
10. Kishimoto T, Watanabe K, Shimada N, Makita K, Yagi G, Kashima H. Antipsychotic-induced hyperprolactinemia inhibits the hypothalamo-pituitary-gonadal axis and reduces bone mineral density in male patients with schizophrenia. J Clin Psychiatry. 2008;69:385–91.
11. Leucht S, Cipriani A, Spineli L, Mavridis D, Orey D, Richter F, Samara M, Barbui C, Engel RR, Geddes JR, et al. Comparative efficacy and tolerability of 15 antipsychotic drugs in schizophrenia: a multiple-treatments meta-analysis. Lancet. 2013;382:951–62.
12. Stahl SM. Dopamine system stabilizers, aripiprazole, and the next generation of antipsychotics, part 2: illustrating their mechanism of action. J Clin Psychiatry. 2001;62:923–4.
13. Tadori Y, Miwa T, Tottori K, Burris KD, Stark A, Mori T, Kikuchi T. Aripiprazole's low intrinsic activities at human dopamine D2L and D2S receptors render it a unique antipsychotic. Eur J Pharmacol. 2005;515:10–9.
14. Kapur S, Seeman P. Does fast dissociation from the dopamine d(2) receptor explain the action of atypical antipsychotics?: a new hypothesis. Am J Psychiatry. 2001;158:360–9.
15. Kane JM, Correll CU, Goff DC, Kirkpatrick B, Marder SR, Vester-Blokland E, Sun W, Carson WH, Pikalov A, Assuncao-Talbott S. A multicenter, randomized, double-blind, placebo-controlled, 16-week study of adjunctive aripiprazole for schizophrenia or schizoaffective disorder inadequately treated with quetiapine or risperidone monotherapy. J Clin Psychiatry. 2009;70:1348–57.
16. Shim JC, Shin JG, Kelly DL, Jung DU, Seo YS, Liu KH, Shon JH, Conley RR. Adjunctive treatment with a dopamine partial agonist, aripiprazole, for antipsychotic-induced hyperprolactinemia: a placebo-controlled trial. Am J Psychiatry. 2007;164:1404–10.
17. Baggaley M. Sexual dysfunction in schizophrenia: focus on recent evidence. Hum Psychopharmacol. 2008;23:201–9.
18. Fujii A, Yasui-Furukori N, Sugawara N, Sato Y, Nakagami T, Saito M, Kaneko S. Sexual dysfunction in Japanese patients with schizophrenia treated with antipsychotics. Prog Neuropsychopharmacol Biol Psychiatry. 2010;34:288–93.
19. Velligan DI, Weiden PJ, Sajatovic M, Scott J, Carpenter D, Ross R, Docherty JP, Expert Consensus Panel on Adherence Problems in S, Persistent Mental I. The expert consensus guideline series: adherence problems in patients with serious and persistent mental illness. J Clin Psychiatry. 2009;70(Suppl 4):1–46 **(quiz 7–8)**.
20. Kleinberg DL, Davis JM, de Coster R, Van Baelen B, Brecher M. Prolactin levels and adverse events in patients treated with risperidone. J Clin Psychopharmacol. 1999;19:57–61.
21. Jerrell JM, Bacon J, Burgis JT, Menon S. Hyperprolactinemia-related adverse events associated with antipsychotic treatment in children and adolescents. J Adolesc Health. 2009;45:70–6.
22. Cutler AJ. Sexual dysfunction and antipsychotic treatment. Psychoneuroendocrinology. 2003;28(Suppl 1):69–82.
23. Citrome L. Current guidelines and their recommendations for prolactin monitoring in psychosis. J Psychopharmacol. 2008;22:90–7.
24. Bostwick JR, Guthrie SK, Ellingrod VL. Antipsychotic-induced hyperprolactinemia. Pharmacotherapy. 2009;29:64–73.
25. Byerly MJ, Marcus RN, Tran QV, Eudicone JM, Whitehead R, Baker RA. Effects of aripiprazole on prolactin levels in subjects with schizophrenia during cross-titration with risperidone or olanzapine: analysis of a randomized, open-label study. Schizophr Res. 2009;107:218–22.
26. Hanssens L, L'Italien G, Loze JY, Marcus RN, Pans M, Kerselaers W. The effect of antipsychotic medication on sexual function and serum prolactin levels in community-treated schizophrenic patients: results from the Schizophrenia Trial of Aripiprazole (STAR) study (NCT00237913). BMC Psychiatry. 2008;8:95.
27. Bakker IC, Schubart CD, Zelissen PM. Successful treatment of a prolactinoma with the antipsychotic drug aripiprazole. Endocrinol Diabetes Metab Case Rep. 2016;2016:160028.
28. Curran RL, Badran IA, Peppers V, Pedapati EV, Correll CU, DelBello MP. Aripiprazole for the treatment of antipsychotic-induced hyperprolactinemia in an adolescent boy. J Child Adolesc Psychopharmacol. 2016;26:490–1.
29. Naono-Nagatomo K, Naono H, Abe H, Takeda R, Funahashi H, Uchimura D, Ishida Y. Partial regimen replacement with aripiprazole reduces serum prolactin in patients with a long history of schizophrenia: a case series. Asian J Psychiatry. 2017;25:36–41.
30. Fujioi J, Iwamoto K, Banno M, Kikuchi T, Aleksic B, Ozaki N. Effect of adjunctive aripiprazole on sexual dysfunction in schizophrenia: a preliminary open-label study. Pharmacopsychiatry. 2017;50:74–8.
31. Qiao Y, Yang F, Li C, Guo Q, Wen H, Zhu S, Ouyang Q, Shen W, Sheng J. Add-on effects of a low-dose aripiprazole in resolving hyperprolactinemia induced by risperidone or paliperidone. Psychiatry Res. 2016;237:83–9.
32. Raghuthaman G, Venkateswaran R, Krishnadas R. Adjunctive aripiprazole in risperidone-induced hyperprolactinaemia: double-blind, randomised, placebo-controlled trial. Br J Psychiatry Open. 2015;1:172–7.
33. Yoon HW, Lee JS, Park SJ, Lee SK, Choi WJ, Kim TY, Hong CH, Seok JH, Park IH, Son SJ, et al. Comparing the effectiveness and safety of the addition of and switching to aripiprazole for resolving antipsychotic-induced hyperprolactinemia: a multicenter, open-label, prospective study. Clin Neuropharmacol. 2016;39:288–94.
34. Joseph SP. Aripiprazole-induced hyperprolactinemia in a young female with delusional disorder. Indian J Psychol Med. 2016;38:260–2.
35. Sogawa R, Shimomura Y, Minami C, Maruo J, Kunitake Y, Mizoguchi Y, Kawashima T, Monji A, Hara H. Aripiprazole-associated hypoprolactinemia in the clinical setting. J Clin Psychopharmacol. 2016;36:385–7.
36. Marder SR, Meibach RC. Risperidone in the treatment of schizophrenia. Am J Psychiatry. 1994;151:825–35.

8

Insomnia severity and its relationship with demographics, pain features, anxiety, and depression in older adults with and without pain: cross-sectional population-based results from the PainS65+ cohort

Elena Dragioti[1*], Lars-Åke Levin[2], Lars Bernfort[2], Britt Larsson[1] and Björn Gerdle[1]

Abstract

Background: Insomnia is a major cause of concern in the elderly with and without pain. This study set out to examine the insomnia and its correlates in a large sample of community adults aged ≥65 years.

Methods: A cross-sectional postal survey was completed by 6205 older individuals (53.8% women; mean age = 76.2 years; SD = 7.5). The participants also completed the Insomnia Severity Index (ISI) and questionnaires assessing pain intensity, pain spreading, anxiety, depression, and basic demographic information. The sample was divided into three groups based on the presence and duration of pain: chronic pain (CP; $n = 2790$), subacute pain (SP; $n = 510$), and no pain (NP; $n = 2905$).

Results: A proportion of each of the groups had an ISI score of 15 or greater (i.e., clinical insomnia): CP = 24.6%; SP = 21.3%; and NP = 13.0%. The average scores of ISI differed significantly among CP, SP, and NP groups ($p < 0.001$). Stratified regression analyses showed that pain intensity, pain spreading, anxiety, and depression were independently related to insomnia in the CP group. Anxiety and depression were independently related to insomnia in the SP group, but only anxiety was significantly associated with insomnia in the NP group. Age and sex were not associated with insomnia.

Conclusions: This study confirms that insomnia is not associated with chronological aging per se within the elderly population. Although the possible associations of insomnia with pain are complex, ensuing from pain intensity, pain spreading, anxiety, and depression, our results highlighted that anxiety was more strongly associated with insomnia in all groups than the depression and pain characteristics. Therapeutic plans should consider these relations during the course of pain, and a comprehensive assessment including both pain and psychological features is essential when older people are seeking primary health care for insomnia complaints.

Keywords: Pain, Chronic, Anxiety, Depression, Elderly, Insomnia, Insomnia Severity Index

Background

One of the most common sleep disturbances among older adults is insomnia [1–5]. Insomnia is defined as a "complaint of insufficient and non-restorative sleep described by the inability to initiate and/or maintain sleep" [6]. In older adults, the overall prevalence of insomnia ranges from 30 to 48% [7, 8] with an annual incidence of near 5% [9]. Furthermore, the prevalence of clinical insomnia in this population is estimated to be over 20% [10], and the incidence of insomnia symptoms

*Correspondence: elena.dragioti@liu.se
[1] Pain and Rehabilitation Centre, Department of Medical and Health Sciences (IMH), Linköping University, 581 85 Linköping, Sweden
Full list of author information is available at the end of the article

is expected to be even higher among men 85 years and older [9].

The impact of insomnia is particularly high in the elderly [2, 11, 14–26]. Insomnia incurs substantial adverse consequences for the individual and for society [8]. Hence, insomnia in older adults is associated with decreased quality of life [11, 12], impaired concentration and memory [13], cognitive decline [14–16], increased incidence of medical and psychiatric disorders [8, 17–19], and increased risk of falls, fractures, and mortality [20–22]. Moreover, large societal costs and increased health care resource use have been noted [8, 23]. For example, an overview study reported that the total direct, indirect, and related annual costs of insomnia in United States were estimated to be between 30 and 35 billion US dollars [23].

Traditionally, it has been argued that certain alterations in the circadian rhythm are connected to insomnia as people age [19]. The most significant demographic predictors of insomnia are older age and female sex [7, 9, 17, 24, 25]. However, insomnia in older adults is probably the result of morbidity rather than aging per se [26–28]. Thus, in the majority of older adults, insomnia is believed to be due to medical disorders (especially chronic pain and respiratory and neurological disorders), psychiatric disorders (especially depression and/or anxiety), and medications (especially anticholinergics and antidepressants) [8, 17, 19, 26, 27, 29, 30]. Older adults with chronic pain seem to be a group with a high risk of being afflicted by insomnia [27, 31, 32] with a prevalence of various sleep problems including insomnia ranging from 13 to 62% [32]. In addition, impaired sleep quality is associated with higher pain intensity [33, 34]. In this vein, a recent article has suggested that insomnia in older adults should be considered a "multifactorial geriatric syndrome" [35]. Because sleep complaints are influenced by a combination of medical, physical, cognitive, psychological, and social issues, diagnostic assessments and treatment plans should take into account all these issues rather than considering insomnia as an inevitable consequence of aging [35].

Considering all of this evidence, it is imperative that investigations of insomnia in older adults should account for level of pain. Although extensive research has been conducted on the relationship between insomnia and pain in older adults, to the best of our knowledge, no study has examined insomnia severity with respect to different pain groups or duration and course of pain. In addition, these studies have produced contradicting results as the definition of insomnia varies between studies [7, 36, 37]. Some studies have also emphasized that emotional symptoms like depression and anxiety have a stronger association with insomnia in pain populations than the psychical symptoms like the pain itself [34, 38–40]. However, little is known about the relationship between depression, anxiety, and pain symptoms that contribute to insomnia in the elderly people. Hence, this study evaluates the severity of insomnia and its relationship with, age, sex, pain intensity, pain spreading, anxiety, and depression in a large-scale population-based study in older adults with pain (i.e., chronic and subacute pain) and without pain.

Methods

This cross-sectional study used data from the PainS65+ cohort [41] and based on a sampling frame from the Swedish Total Population Register (TPR). From this registry, 10,000 subjects aged 65 years and older, were randomly selected for the following age strata: 65–69; 70–74; 75–79; 80–84; and 85 years and older. The data were collected during 1 year period (from October 2012 to January 2013) using a postal survey, as a part of a larger project in which the health status of the elderly individuals in the general population was investigated in various domains [41, 42]. The parts of the instrument used in this study are described below. An overview of all parts of the survey and the details of the subsequent procedure are described elsewhere [41, 42]. The study was approved by the Regional Ethics Research Committee in Linköping, Sweden (Dnr: 2012/154-31).

Measurements

Insomnia

Insomnia was assessed using the Insomnia Severity Index (ISI), a reliable and valid instrument with excellent internal consistency [43]. The ISI is a seven-item self-report instrument that assesses the nature, severity, and impact of insomnia [43, 44] using a five-point Likert scale (0 = no problem and 4 = very severe problem), yielding a total score ranging between 0 and 28. A higher score indicates greater insomnia severity. The total score is further divided into four categories: no clinically significant insomnia (ISI = 0–7); sub-threshold insomnia (ISI = 8–14); moderate clinical insomnia (ISI = 15–21); and severe clinical insomnia (ISI = 22–28). Clinical insomnia was defined as the sum of moderate clinical insomnia and severe clinical insomnia [39, 40]. This study presents the ISI total score as well as the subcategory scores.

Definition of pain categories

The pain was defined by a single question and one follow-up question with respect to the presence and time course of pain: "Do you usually have pain?" (yes/no) and "If yes, has your pain lasted fewer than 3 months or more than 3 months?" The subjects who responded "no" were assigned to the no pain (NP) group. Subjects who responded "yes, with more than 3 months" were assigned to the chronic pain (CP) group. Accordingly, the subjects who responded "yes, with fewer than 3 months" were assigned to the subacute pain (SP) group.

Pain intensity

The average pain intensity for the previous 7 days was registered using an 11-point numeric rating scale (NRS7d) with the anchors 0 (no pain) and 10 (worst imaginable pain) [45]. The subjects in the NP group marked 0 in this scale.

Pain spreading

Pain spreading (i.e., spatial extent) was assessed by having the respondents' mark where they experience pain on a body manikin with 45 predefined anatomical areas. The subjects marked the anatomical areas where they experienced either subacute or chronic pain during the previous 7 days [46]. The subjects in the NP group did not mark any anatomical areas. Thus, the number of sites associated with pain ranged between 0 and 45; higher values indicated higher pain spreading.

Anxiety and depression

Two subscales of the General Well-Being Schedule (GWBS) were used to assess anxiety (items 2, 5, 8, 16) and depression (items 4, 12, 18): GWBS-anxiety (range 0–25) and GWBS-depression (range 0–20). The GWBS is a common instrument for assessing life satisfaction and level of psychological distress [47]. It consists of 18 items yielding a total score ranging from 0 to 110 (high score indicating positive well-being and low distress). The first 14 questions use a six-point rating scale (anchors 0 and 5) that represents either intensity or frequency, and the remaining four items use an 11-point rating scale with the anchors 0 (very concerned) and 10 (not concerned). The GWBS has good internal consistency, test–retest reliability, and validity [47]. Four subscales of the instrument are not used in this study: GWBS-positive well-being: items 1, 6, 11; range 0–15; GWBS-self-control: items 3, 7, 13; range 0–15; GWBS-vitality: items 9, 14, 17; range 0–20; and GWBS-general health: items 10, 15; range 0–15 [48].

Data analysis

The statistics were performed using the statistical package IBM SPSS Statistics (version 23.0; IBM Inc., New York, USA). In all tests, a p value of ≤ 0.05 (two-tailed) was considered significant. Continuous data are reported as the mean and standard deviation (SD), and the categorical data are represented as n (%). Both analysis of variance (ANOVA) and Student's independent t test were used for the continuous variables and Chi-square t tests were used for the categorical variables. Post hoc comparisons (Bonferroni criterion used for the total score of ISI and Dennett's test used for the subcategories of ISI) were also performed when significant differences ($p < 0.05$) in ANOVA tests were identified. Pearson correlation analysis was used for bivariate correlations (i.e., investigating the correlations between total score of ISI and the other examined variables). Multiple linear regression (MLR) analyses were performed to regress insomnia (a dependent variable treated as a continuous variable) using age, female sex, pain intensity, pain spreading, and anxiety and depression (exploratory variables) with each pain group. Multicollinearity was assessed by examining tolerance and the variance inflation factor (VIF). A tolerance of less than 0.20 or 0.10 and/or a VIF of 5 or 10 and above indicate multicollinearity [49].

In addition, ordinal logistic regression (OLR) models were used with the ISI categories and these categories were treated as ordinal outcome variables. Odds ratios (OR) and 95% confidence intervals (CI) are reported. All analyses were stratified by the three pain groups.

Results

Sample characteristics

The CP group included 2790 individuals (61.1% women; average age 76.2 years [SD 7.5]), the SP group included 510 individuals (54.1% women; average age 75.6 years [SD 6.9]), and the NP group included 2905 individuals (46.1% women; average age 75.9 years [SD 7.6]). Age distribution did not differ among the three pain groups ($p = 0.47$), but there was a significant difference in gender distribution ($p < 0.001$). There were more women than men in the two pain groups (CP group: 61.1 vs 38.9% and SP group: 54.1 vs 45.9%) and more men than women in the NP group (53.9 vs 46.1%). Details of the socio-demographic characteristics and response rates of the total sample are described elsewhere [42].

Insomnia severity and its relationship with other variables in the total sample

The average ISI total score was 9.8 ± 5.5. The distribution in the different categories of ISI showed that 35.7% had no clinically significant insomnia, 44.3% had subthreshold insomnia, 17.8% had moderate clinical insomnia, and 2.2% had severe clinical insomnia (Fig. 1). That is, 20% of the total sample had clinical insomnia (ISI $\geq$ 15). A significant difference in the total score of ISI existed between the two sexes (men 9.4 ± 5.5; women 10.1 ± 5.5; $p = 0.003$), but this difference was not confirmed when we compared the distribution of the four categories of ISI between the two sexes (Fig. 2).

The four categories of ISI with respect to the other investigated variables are presented in Table 1, part a.

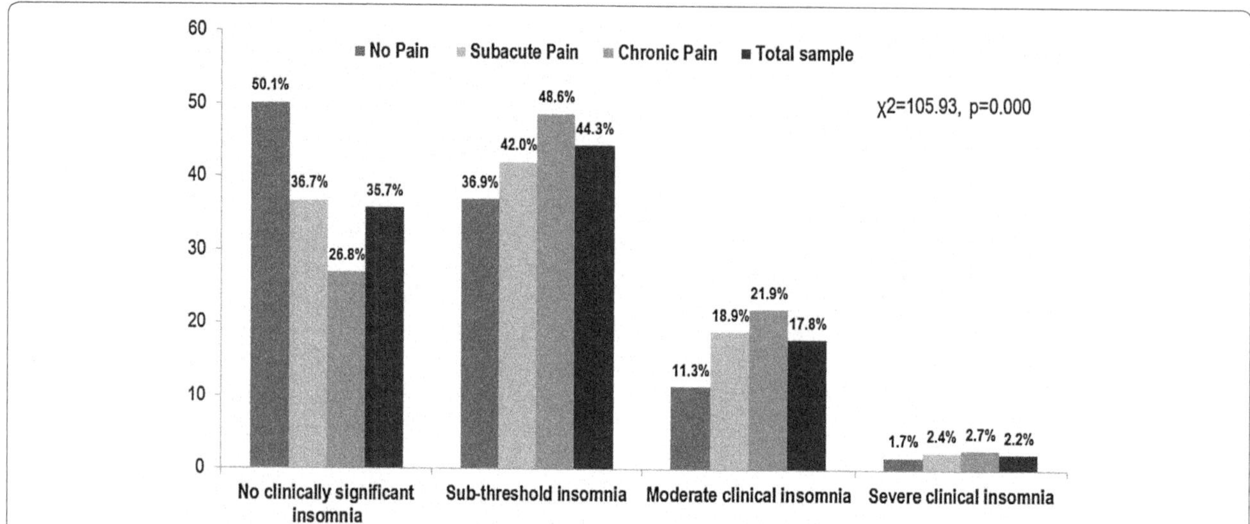

Fig. 1 Prevalence of insomnia severity in older adults with and without pain. The *x axis* represents the proportions of the study sample %; the *y axis* represents the categories of insomnia by the three pain groups and the total sample

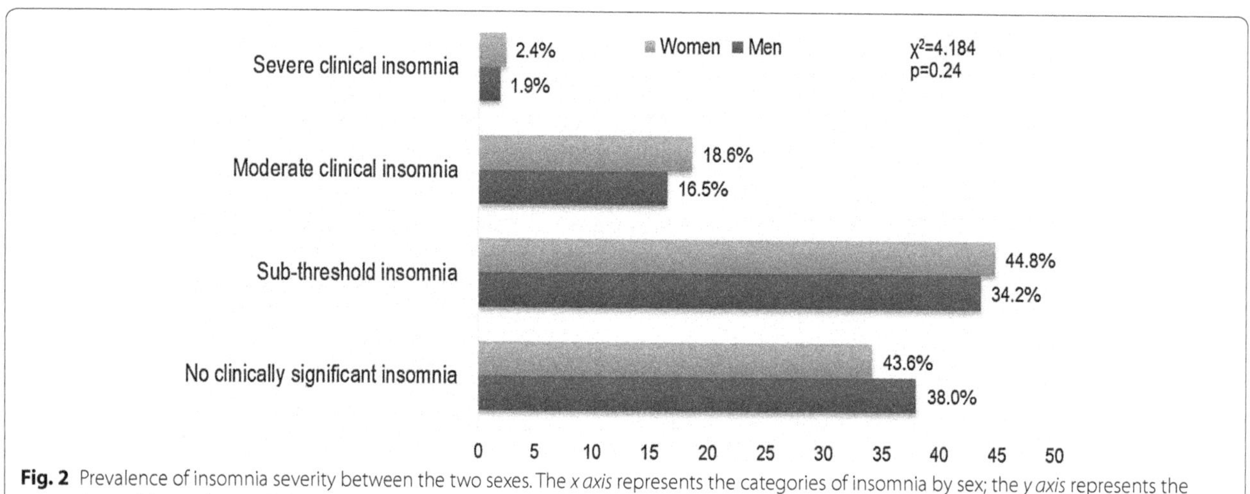

Fig. 2 Prevalence of insomnia severity between the two sexes. The *x axis* represents the categories of insomnia by sex; the *y axis* represents the proportions of the study sample %

Prominent and significant differences were found for all investigated variables except for age. More specifically, higher pain intensity, pain spreading, anxiety, and depression were more common in severe clinical insomnia (ISI $\geq$ 22) compared to no clinically significant insomnia.

Insomnia severity in the chronic pain group and comparisons with subacute pain and no pain group

The average score of ISI in individuals with CP was 10.9 $\pm$ 5.4. The average scores of ISI differed very clearly between CP, SP, and NP groups ($p < 0.001$) (Fig. 3). Post hoc comparisons found that the average ISI in the NP group was significantly lower compared to the SP and CP groups ($p < 0.001$). No significant differences between CP and SP groups were found ($p = 0.12$).

The distribution in the different ISI categories showed that in the CP group 26.8% had no clinically significant insomnia, 48.6% had sub-threshold insomnia, 21.9% had moderate clinical insomnia, and 2.7% had severe clinical insomnia. That is, about 25.0% of older individuals with chronic pain had clinical insomnia (ISI $\geq$ 15). The overall fraction of clinical insomnia was 21.3% in SP group and 13.0% in NP group (Fig. 1). Within the CP group, a significant difference in the total score of ISI between the two sexes was found (men 10.4 $\pm$ 5.3; women 11.1 $\pm$ 5.4; $p = 0.03$), but this was not the case for SP ($p = 0.86$) and NP groups ($p = 0.56$).

Table 1 Insomnia severity in individuals with and without pain and the categories of insomnia related to age, pain intensity, pain spreading, anxiety, and depression

Subgroup of ISI	All	No clinically significant insomnia (NCSI)	Sub-threshold insomnia (S-TI)	Moderate clinical insomnia (MCI)	Severe clinical insomnia (SCI)	Statistics (ANOVA)	Post hoc comparisons (Dunnett t)[a]		
Variables	Mean ± SD	Mean ± SD	Mean ± SD	Mean ± SD	Mean ± SD	*p* value	S-TI vs NCSI	MCI vs NCSI	SCI vs NCSI
a. Total sample ($n = 6205$)									
Age (years)	76.3 ± 7.4	76.5 ± 7.2	76.0 ± 7.4	76.5 ± 7.6	78.1 ± 8.3	0.175	NA	NA	NA
Pain intensity	4.2 ± 2.6	3.2 ± 2.6	4.5 ± 2.4	5.3 ± 2.5	6.0 ± 2.7	<0.001	***	***	***
Pain spreading	5.6 ± 5.4	4.4 ± 4.6	5.3 ± 4.7	7.7 ± 7.1	7.4 ± 7.1	<0.001	*	***	***
GWBS-anxiety	6.4 ± 4.5	4.1 ± 3.7	6.6 ± 4.3	9.7 ± 5.2	12.8 ± 5.9	<0.001	***	***	***
GWBS-depression	5.8 ± 3.8	4.1 ± 3.2	5.9 ± 3.3	8.2 ± 3.9	10.5 ± 4.8	<0.001	***	***	***
b. Chronic pain ($n = 2790$)									
Age (years)	76.2 ± 7.5	76.6 ± 7.6	75.6 ± 7.2	76.9 ± 7.8	78.7 ± 7.6	0.015	ns	ns	**
Pain intensity	5.1 ± 2.1	4.4 ± 2.1	5.1 ± 1.9	5.7 ± 2.2	6.5 ± 2.48	<0.001	***	***	***
Pain spreading	6.2 ± 5.6	5.1 ± 4.9	5.8 ± 4.8	8.3 ± 7.2	8.0 ± 7.2	<0.001	ns	***	***
GWBS-anxiety	7.4 ± 4.9	5.0 ± 4.1	7.2 ± 4.3	10.0 ± 5.1	13.5 ± 6.7	<0.001	***	***	***
GWBS-depression	6.3 ± 3.8	4.8 ± 3.4	6.1 ± 3.3	8.2 ± 3.8	10.7 ± 5.1	<0.001	***	***	***
c. Subacute pain ($n = 510$)									
Age (years)	75.6 ± 6.9	75.2 ± 6.9	75.4 ± 6.8	76.3 ± 7.3	76.0 ± 6.9	0.890	NA	NA	NA
Pain intensity	4.4 ± 1.8	4.1 ± 1.6	4.4 ± 1.9	4.8 ± 1.8	5.5 ± 0.7	0.304	NA	NA	NA
Pain spreading	3.1 ± 2.1	2.9 ± 2.1	3.1 ± 2.2	3.4 ± 2.2	2.0 ± 0.0	0.683	NA	NA	NA
GWBS-anxiety	6.5 ± 4.8	4.4 ± 3.5	6.6 ± 4.4	10.0 ± 5.3	13.7 ± 2.5	<0.001	**	***	***
GWBS-depression	5.8 ± 3.7	4.3 ± 3.1	5.7 ± 3.4	8.5 ± 3.7	10.0 ± 3.6	<0.001	*	***	***
d. No pain ($n = 2905$)									
Age (years)	75.9 ± 7.6	76.5 ± 6.9	76.4 ± 7.8	75.6 ± 7.4	77.1 ± 10.7	0.911	NA	NA	NA
Pain intensity	0.0 ± 0.0	0.0 ± 0.0	0.0 ± 0.0	0.0 ± 0.0	0.0 ± 0.0	NA	NA	NA	NA
Pain spreading	0.0 ± 0.0	0.0 ± 0.0	0.0 ± 0.0	0.0 ± 0.0	0.0 ± 0.0	NA	NA	NA	NA
GWBS-anxiety	4.8 ± 4.2	3.3 ± 3.3	5.3 ± 4.1	8.6 ± 4.8	10.9 ± 4.3	<0.001	***	***	***
GWBS-depression	4.7 ± 3.6	3.4 ± 2.9	5.2 ± 3.3	7.7 ± 4.2	9.9 ± 4.2	<0.001	***	***	***

NCSI no clinically significant insomnia, *S-TI* sub-threshold insomnia, *MCI* moderate clinical insomnia, *SCI* severe clinical insomnia, *ISI* Insomnia Severity Index, *GWBS* general well-being schedule, *NA* not applicable

[a] Dunnett *t* tests treat one group as a control (No clinically significant insomnia as control group), and compare all other groups against it; *ns* non-significant at $p < 0.05$; *NA* not applicable

* $p < 0.05$, ** $p < 0.01$, *** $p < 0.001$

Comparisons of ISI categories with the examined variables stratified by the three pain groups

The four ISI categories with respect to the other investigated variables and the three pain groups are presented in Table 1, parts b–d. In the CP group, prominent and significant differences emerged for all investigated variables. In the SP group and NP group, significant differences were found between ISI subgroups and anxiety and depression. In general, severe clinical insomnia (ISI ≥ 22) was associated with the worst situation with respect to the examined variables compared to no clinically significant insomnia.

Associations of ISI total scores and ISI categories with the examined variables stratified by the three pain groups

Correlation and multiple linear regression (MLR) analyses were conducted to examine the relationship between ISI total score and the other possible regressor variables; Table 2 summarizes the stratified correlations and the MLR analysis results by each pain group. Multicollinearity was rejected: the average tolerance was 0.70 and the average VIF was 1.42 for all independent variables.

In the CP group, both correlation and MLR analyses showed that pain intensity, pain spreading, anxiety, and depression were positively and significantly correlated with the ISI scores (Table 2; Model 1). Hence, older individuals with CP and higher scores on these variables were expected to have higher ISI scores. Anxiety was more important as a regressor than pain intensity, pain spreading, and depression. The MLR model with all six regressors explained 24% of the total variance [$R^2 = 0.24$, $F(6337.8) = 57.81, p < 0.001$]. Age and female sex did not contribute significantly to the model. In the SP group,

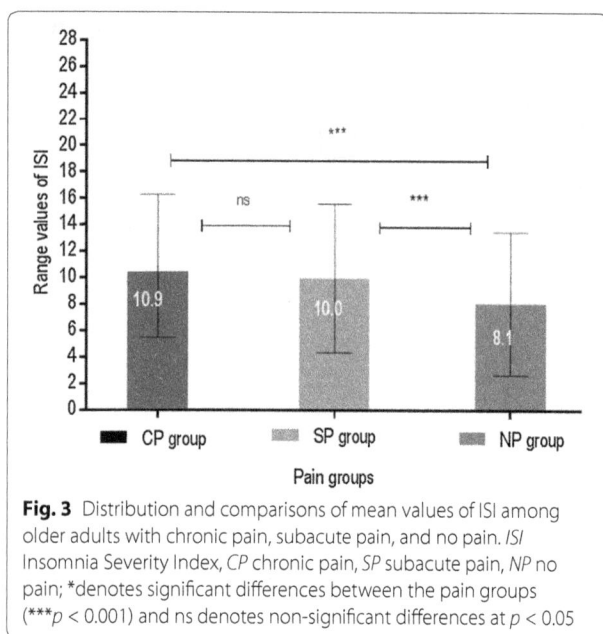

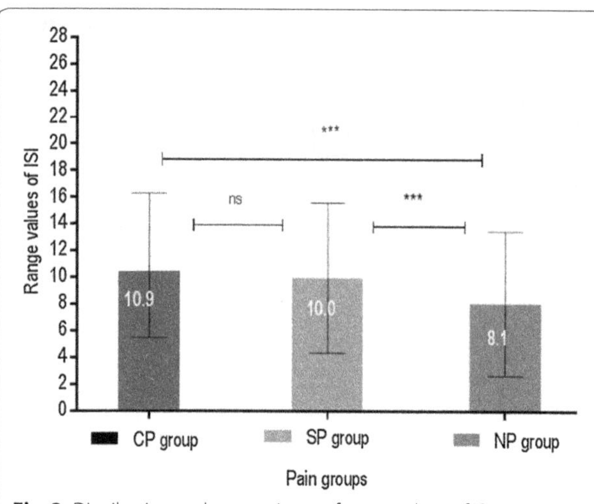

Fig. 3 Distribution and comparisons of mean values of ISI among older adults with chronic pain, subacute pain, and no pain. *ISI* Insomnia Severity Index, *CP* chronic pain, *SP* subacute pain, *NP* no pain; *denotes significant differences between the pain groups (***$p < 0.001$) and ns denotes non-significant differences at $p < 0.05$

Table 2 Correlations among variables and results from the linear regression models of ISI total score (continue variable) stratified by the three pain groups

Variable	Correlations with ISI (*r*)	Multiple regression weights		R^2
		B	*β*	
a. Model 1 Chronic pain ($n = 2790$)				0.24
Age (years)	0.43	−0.017	−0.023	
Female sex	0.19	0.235	0. 021	
Pain intensity	0.27***	0.356***	0.138***	
Pain spreading	0.20***	0.069*	0.075*	
GWBS-anxiety	0.43***	0.259***	0.237***	
GWBS-depression	0.40***	0.261***	0.132***	
b. Model 2 Subacute pain ($n = 510$)				0.26
Age (years)	0.01	−0.039	−0.053	
Female sex	0.07	0.188	0.018	
Pain intensity	0.16*	0.246	0.086	
Pain spreading	0.06	0.010	0.004	
GWBS-anxiety	0.48***	0.294*	0.274*	
GWBS-depression	0.46***	0.344*	0.246*	
c. Model 3 No pain ($n = 2905$)				0.44
Age (years)	0.21	0.045	0.056	
Female sex	−0.05	−0.061	−0.057	
Pain intensity	NA	NA	NA	
Pain spreading	NA	NA	NA	
GWBS-anxiety	0.66***	0.747***	0.581***	
GWBS-depression	0.53***	0.136	0.099	

ISI Insomnia Severity Index, *GWBS* general well-being schedule, *r* correlation coefficient, *B* unstandardized regression coefficients, *β* standardized regression coefficients, R^2 multiple correlation coefficient squared, *NA* not applicable

* $p < 0.05$, ** $p < 0.01$, *** $p < 0.001$

anxiety and depression had a clear association with ISI scores, but age, female sex, pain intensity, and pain spreading did not significantly contribute to the model. The MLR model with all six regressors explained 26% of the total variance [$R^2 = 0.26$, $F\,(923.1) = 9.21$, $p < 0.001$] (Table 2; Model 2). In the NP group, only anxiety was significantly associated with the ISI scores. In this model, both pain variables (i.e., pain intensity and spreading) were not entered in the model because the mean score on those variables was zero. The MLR model with the four relevant regressors explained 44% of the total variance [$R^2 = 0.44$, $F\,(601.6) = 11.61$, $p < 0.001$] (Table 2; Model 3). After we regressed the ISI categories (no clinically significant insomnia vs. sub-threshold insomnia, moderate insomnia, and severe clinical insomnia) as ordinal outcomes, we found identical results with respect to the most important variables (Table 3; Models 1–3).

Discussion

The main findings of this study were as follows:

- The overall prevalence of clinical insomnia in the total sample was 20.0%. Older adults with CP had the highest prevalence of clinical insomnia (24.6%).
- Age and sex were not associated with either total ISI score or ISI categories, regardless of pain group.
- Higher pain intensity, pain spreading, anxiety, and depression were more common in severe insomnia, moderate clinical insomnia, and sub-threshold insomnia compared to no clinically significant insomnia.
- The multivariate stratified analyses revealed the following associations: pain intensity, pain spreading, anxiety, and depression were independently related to insomnia in the CP group. Anxiety and depression were independently related to insomnia in the SP group, but only anxiety was significantly associated with insomnia in the NP group.

Overall, 20% of the participants reported clinical insomnia (ISI $\geq$ 15) [44], a rate lower compared to that reported in most other studies of elderly populations [1, 4, 11, 50]. Foley et al., for example, in a large sample of 9000 participants aged 65 years and older found that the estimated insomnia symptoms ranged between 23 and 34% [4]. Our study found a higher prevalence of insomnia than the findings of an investigation of 47,700 individuals in Norway (i.e., a similar geo-cultural environment to Sweden) where the prevalence rate of insomnia

Table 3 Results of ordinal logistic regression models of categories of ISI treated as an ordinal outcome stratified by the three pain groups

Variable	Multiple regression weights		
	Wald	OR (95% CI)	Nagelkerke R^2
a. Model 1			0.22
Chronic pain ($n = 2790$)			
Age (years)	1.013	0.99 (0.97–1.01)	
Female sex	1.116	1.03 (0.80–1.33)	
Pain intensity	15.501	1.13 (1.06–1.20)***	
Pain spreading	8.930	1.04 (1.01–1.06)**	
GWBS-anxiety	29.452	1.11 (1.06–1.15)***	
GWBS-depression	11.475	1.09 (1.03–1.14)***	
b. Model 2			0.23
Subacute pain ($n = 510$)			
Age (years)	1.189	0.98 (0.93–1.02)	
Female sex	0.398	0.99 (0.51–1.57)	
Pain intensity	0.979	1.10 (0.91–1.34)	
Pain spreading	0.052	1.01 (0.97–1.15)	
GWBS-anxiety	6.547	1.15 (1.03–1.28)*	
GWBS-depression	3.398	1.08 (1.01-1.25)*	
c. Model 3			0.41
No pain (n = 2905)			
Age (years)	0.057	0.99 (0.96–1.01)	
Female sex	0.187	0.99 (0.76–1.43)	
Pain intensity	NA	NA	
Pain spreading	NA	NA	
GWBS-anxiety	6.059	1.13 (1.06–1.18)*	
GWBS-depression	0.594	1.10 (0.99–1.24)	

ISI Insomnia Severity Index, *GWBS* general well-being schedule, *OR* odds ratio, R^2 multiple correlation coefficient squared, *NA* not applicable

* $p < 0.05$, ** $p < 0.01$, *** $p < 0.001$

symptoms was 13.5% [17]. That study, however, did not report results specifically for the elderly. Consistent with previous reports [24–27, 29, 30], we also found that the respondents in CP reported higher prevalence (24.6%) of clinical insomnia than respondents in the SP and NP groups. Indeed, there is evidence that patients with CP tended to demonstrate more sleep fragmentation, longer sleep latency, lower sleep quality, and shorter sleep duration [54]. Explanations for the observed differences of prevalence estimates may include the great variability of measurements and definitions of insomnia [7, 36, 51]. Studies using DSM-5 [52] criteria for insomnia reveal lower prevalence of insomnia in the elderly (4–12%). This discrepancy may also be the result of the age range of the studied population, pain definitions, and socioeconomic and cultural differences of the participants [7, 17, 24, 35].

In contradiction to some previous research findings [4, 9, 17, 24, 25], age and sex were not associated with insomnia symptoms or clinical insomnia. Although we found that in the CP group severe clinical insomnia compared to no clinically significant insomnia was more common in the older ages (Table 1, part b), this difference was not confirmed in the regression analysis. Nevertheless, our results are similar to some prospective studies that found no age effect related to insomnia [53, 54]. Moreover, our results (Tables 2, 3) suggest that insomnia cannot be explained by the chronologically age-related changes in the elderly population, but rather is explained by aging-related changes due to various mental and physical morbidities including pain [10, 11, 21, 27, 28, 30, 31, 48]. Therefore, as recently suggested, insomnia should be considered a "multifactorial geriatric syndrome" [32]. Similarly, we found that the total scores of insomnia were higher in women compared to men in the whole sample and in the CP group, but these sex differences were not confirmed in the regression analyses (Tables 2, 3). This finding is consistent with the suggestion that the relationship between female sex and insomnia (especially in the elderly) may be explained by an array of other factors such as depression, chronic diseases, living alone, marital status, occupational status, and social support deficits [35, 55].

The stratified multivariate analysis of the three pain groups revealed that in the CP group higher levels of pain intensity, pain spreading, anxiety, and depression had direct links to higher severity of insomnia. The most important regressors for both total ISI score and clinical insomnia were pain intensity and anxiety. This result is somewhat consistent with previous reports [24, 33, 34, 38, 56]. Our results, however, are not in line with some studies that report that insomnia in CP is more strongly related to depression and low mood than to pain intensity [38, 39], but in line with studies reporting that anxiety is more strongly related to insomnia than to pain intensity [34, 40]. Generally, the results of the regressions are consistent with previous reports that found strong relationships between both pain and psychological strain and the variability of sleep duration and fragmentation in various populations, including older adults [17, 24, 29, 34, 57].

In the SP group, both anxiety and depression had clear positive associations with total ISI score and clinically significant insomnia, whereas in the NP group only anxiety was significantly associated with insomnia. Hence, in these two groups, anxiety also had a stronger relationship with insomnia than depression, a finding that is not substantiated in previous studies [4, 26, 38, 39, 58]. One possible explanation for the stronger impact of anxiety in the present population could be the fact that in elderly depression symptoms are conflated with somatic complaints, and probably those symptoms are being underestimated and unreported by the respondents [59]. On the other hand, anxiety may more likely be the result of stressful events associated with aging, and perhaps this anxiety increases the likelihood of insomnia via increased levels of arousal [60]. It is also possible that anxiety and depression are interrelated with insomnia through different paths. According to previous prospective research, anxiety may more likely act as a pathway to insomnia while depression may more likely act as a consequence of insomnia [61, 62]. In any case, the relationship between insomnia and pain as well as other morbidities is difficult to interpret [27, 31, 32] and more studies, especially longitudinal studies, concerning the nature and the direction of these associations are needed.

To our best knowledge, this is the first study to evaluate insomnia severity in a large random sample of older adults with and without pain. This study's limitations include the issues associated with collecting data via a self-reported instrument and the inherent limitations of a cross-sectional study design. In addition, this study evaluated a limited set of variables. We did not examine the role of other factors such as medications, especially hypnotics or other physical comorbidities; life-style factors such as nicotine, caffeine, and alcohol use; or stressful life traumatic events that might be independently related to insomnia [25].

Conclusions

In conclusion, this study suggests that the relationship between insomnia severity and chronic pain in older adults is very complex, ensuing from pain intensity, pain spreading, anxiety, and depression. In subacute pain, pain symptoms seem to have no effect while a predominance of a psychological strain may account for higher levels of insomnia and clinical insomnia. Conversely, in older individuals without pain, anxiety had a clear positive relationship to both insomnia and clinical insomnia. Taken together, these results indicate that ongoing specific attention from health care providers on this topic is required to ensure that the best possible insomnia treatment modalities are made available to the elderly. For example, approaches including both psychological and pain management components would be beneficial for individuals with CP, whereas psychological approaches targeting depression and/or anxiety might be suitable for individuals who experience short durations of pain or no pain. This study also suggests that a comprehensive assessment including both pain and psychological aspects are essential when older people are seeking primary health care for insomnia complaints. Further research is also needed that defines these multifactorial relations so that elderly patients suffering from insomnia receive the most effective insomnia treatments regardless of their pain level.

Abbreviations

ANOVA: one way analysis of variance; CP: chronic pain; GWBS: the general well-being schedule; ISI: Insomnia Severity Index; MLR: multiple linear regression; NP: no pain; NRS7d: numeric rating scale for the previous 7 days; OLR: ordinal logistic regression; SD: standard deviation; SP: subacute pain; TPR: total population register.

Authors' contributions

L-ÅL, LB, BL, and BG were involved in study conception and study design. ED and BG performed the data analyses and drafted the manuscript. All authors discussed the results and commented on the manuscript. All authors read and approved the final manuscript.

Author details

[1] Pain and Rehabilitation Centre, Department of Medical and Health Sciences (IMH), Linköping University, 581 85 Linköping, Sweden. [2] Division of Health Care Analysis, Department of Medical and Health Sciences, Linköping University, 581 85 Linköping, Sweden.

Acknowledgements

Not applicable.

Competing interests

The authors declare that they have no competing interests.

Ethical approval

This study has been approved by the Regional Ethics Research Committee in Linköping, Sweden (Dnr: 2012/154-31).

Funding

The present study was sponsored by a grant from Grünenthal Sweden AB. The sponsor of the study had no role in study design, data collection, data analysis, data interpretation, writing of the report, or the decision to submit for publication. The authors had full access to all the data in the study and had final responsibility for the decision to submit for publication.

References

1. Morin CM, Benca R. Chronic insomnia. Lancet. 2012;379(9821):1129–41.
2. Sukying C, Bhokakul V, Udomsubpayakul U. An epidemiological study on insomnia in an elderly Thai population. J Med Assoc Thai. 2003;86(4):316–24.
3. Shochat T, Loredo J, Ancoli-Israel S. Sleep disorders in the elderly. Curr Treat Options Neurol. 2001;3(1):19–36.
4. Foley DJ, Monjan AA, Brown SL, Simonsick EM, Wallace RB, Blazer DG. Sleep complaints among elderly persons: an epidemiologic study of three communities. Sleep. 1995;18(6):425–32.
5. Monane M. Insomnia in the elderly. J Clin Psychiatry. 1992;53(Suppl):23–8.
6. Roth T. Insomnia: definition, prevalence, etiology, and consequences. J Clin Sleep Med. 2007;3(5 Suppl):S7–10.
7. Ohayon MM. Epidemiology of insomnia: what we know and what we still need to learn. Sleep Med Rev. 2002;6(2):97–111.
8. Hillman DR, Murphy AS, Pezzullo L. The economic cost of sleep disorders. Sleep. 2006;29(3):299–305.
9. Foley DJ, Monjan A, Simonsick EM, Wallace RB, Blazer DG. Incidence and remission of insomnia among elderly adults: an epidemiologic study of 6800 persons over three years. Sleep. 1999;22(Suppl 2):S366–72.
10. Mellinger GD, Balter MB, Uhlenhuth EH. Insomnia and its treatment. Prevalence and correlates. Arch Gen Psychiatry. 1985;42(3):225–32.
11. Barbar SI, Enright PL, Boyle P, Foley D, Sharp DS, Petrovitch H, Quan SF. Sleep disturbances and their correlates in elderly Japanese

American men residing in Hawaii. J Gerontol A Biol Sci Med Sci. 2000;55(7):M406–11.
12. Schubert CR, Cruickshanks KJ, Dalton DS, Klein BE, Klein R, Nondahl DM. Prevalence of sleep problems and quality of life in an older population. Sleep. 2002;25(8):889–93.
13. Weinger MB, Ancoli-Israel S. Sleep deprivation and clinical performance. JAMA. 2002;287(8):955–7.
14. Yaffe K, Falvey CM, Hoang T. Connections between sleep and cognition in older adults. Lancet Neurol. 2014;13(10):1017–28.
15. Pistacchi M, Gioulis M, Contin F, Sanson F, Marsala SZ. Sleep disturbance and cognitive disorder: epidemiological analysis in a cohort of 263 patients. Neurol Sci. 2014;35(12):1955–62.
16. Hauri PJ. Cognitive deficits in insomnia patients. Acta Neurol Belg. 1997;97(2):113–7.
17. Sivertsen B, Krokstad S, Overland S, Mykletun A. The epidemiology of insomnia: associations with physical and mental health. The HUNT-2 study. J Psychosom Res. 2009;67(2):109–16.
18. Neckelmann D, Mykletun A, Dahl AA. Chronic insomnia as a risk factor for developing anxiety and depression. Sleep. 2007;30(7):873–80.
19. Kamel NS, Gammack JK. Insomnia in the elderly: cause, approach, and treatment. Am J Med. 2006;119(6):463–9.
20. Helbig AK, Doring A, Heier M, Emeny RT, Zimmermann AK, Autenrieth CS, Ladwig KH, Grill E, Meisinger C. Association between sleep disturbances and falls among the elderly: results from the German Cooperative Health Research in the Region of Augsburg-Age study. Sleep Med. 2013;14(12):1356–63.
21. Mahgoub N, Majdak P, Friedman DB, Klimstra S. Insomnia and risk of falling in older adults. J Neuropsychiatry Clin Neurosci. 2012;24(3):E5–6.
22. Manabe K, Matsui T, Yamaya M, Sato-Nakagawa T, Okamura N, Arai H, Sasaki H. Sleep patterns and mortality among elderly patients in a geriatric hospital. Gerontology. 2000;46(6):318–22.
23. Chilcott LA, Shapiro CM. The socioeconomic impact of insomnia. An overview. Pharmacoeconomics. 1996;10(Suppl 1):1–14.
24. Taylor DJ, Lichstein KL, Durrence HH, Reidel BW, Bush AJ. Epidemiology of insomnia, depression, and anxiety. Sleep. 2005;28(11):1457–64.
25. Gu D, Sautter J, Pipkin R, Zeng Y. Sociodemographic and health correlates of sleep quality and duration among very old Chinese. Sleep. 2010;33(5):601–10.
26. Smagula SF, Stone KL, Fabio A, Cauley JA. Risk factors for sleep disturbances in older adults: evidence from prospective studies. Sleep Med Rev. 2016;25:21–30.
27. Vitiello MV, McCurry SM, Shortreed SM, Baker LD, Rybarczyk BD, Keefe FJ, Von Korff M. Short-term improvement in insomnia symptoms predicts long-term improvements in sleep, pain, and fatigue in older adults with comorbid osteoarthritis and insomnia. Pain. 2014;155(8):1547–54.
28. Foley D, Ancoli-Israel S, Britz P, Walsh J. Sleep disturbances and chronic disease in older adults: results of the 2003 National Sleep Foundation Sleep in America Survey. J Psychosom Res. 2004;56(5):497–502.
29. Taylor DJ, Mallory LJ, Lichstein KL, Durrence HH, Riedel BW, Bush AJ. Comorbidity of chronic insomnia with medical problems. Sleep. 2007;30(2):213–8.
30. Ancoli-Israel S. Insomnia in the elderly: a review for the primary care practitioner. Sleep. 2000;23(Suppl 1):S23–30.
31. Tang NK, McBeth J, Jordan KP, Blagojevic-Bucknall M, Croft P, Wilkie R. Impact of musculoskeletal pain on insomnia onset: a prospective cohort study. Rheumatology. 2015;54(2):248–56.
32. Lindstrom V, Andersson K, Lintrup M, Holst G, Berglund J. Prevalence of sleep problems and pain among the elderly in Sweden. J Nutr Health Aging. 2012;16(2):180–3.
33. Raymond I, Nielsen TA, Lavigne G, Manzini C, Choiniere M. Quality of sleep and its daily relationship to pain intensity in hospitalized adult burn patients. Pain. 2001;92(3):381–8.
34. Alfoldi P, Wiklund T, Gerdle B. Comorbid insomnia in patients with chronic pain: a study based on the Swedish quality registry for pain rehabilitation (SQRP). Disabil Rehabil. 2014;36(20):1661–9.
35. Vaz Fragoso CA, Gill TM. Sleep complaints in community-living older persons: a multifactorial geriatric syndrome. J Am Geriatr Soc. 2007;55(11):1853–66.
36. Buysse DJ, Ancoli-Israel S, Edinger JD, Lichstein KL, Morin CM. Recommendations for a standard research assessment of insomnia. Sleep. 2006;29(9):1155–73.
37. Lichstein KL, Durrence HH, Taylor DJ, Bush AJ, Riedel BW. Quantitative criteria for insomnia. Behav Res Ther. 2003;41(4):427–45.
38. O'Donoghue GM, Fox N, Heneghan C, Hurley DA. Objective and subjective assessment of sleep in chronic low back pain patients compared with healthy age and gender matched controls: a pilot study. BMC Musculoskelet Disord. 2009;10:122.
39. Smith MT, Perlis ML, Carmody TP, Smith MS, Giles DE. Presleep cognitions in patients with insomnia secondary to chronic pain. J Behav Med. 2001;24(1):93–114.
40. Schuh-Hofer S, Wodarski R, Pfau DB, Caspani O, Magerl W, Kennedy JD, Treede RD. One night of total sleep deprivation promotes a state of generalized hyperalgesia: a surrogate pain model to study the relationship of insomnia and pain. Pain. 2013;154(9):1613–21.
41. Dragioti E, Larsson B, Bernfort L, Levin LÅ, Gerdle B. Prevalence of different pain categories based on pain spreading on the bodies of older adults in Sweden: a descriptive level and multilevel association with demographics, comorbidities, medications and certain life style factors (PainS65+). J Pain Res. 2016;9:1131–41.
42. Bernfort L, Gerdle B, Rahmqvist M, Husberg M, Levin LA. Severity of chronic pain in an elderly population in Sweden—impact on costs and quality of life. Pain. 2015;156(3):521–7.
43. Morin CM, Belleville G, Belanger L, Ivers H. The Insomnia Severity Index: psychometric indicators to detect insomnia cases and evaluate treatment response. Sleep. 2011;34(5):601–8.
44. Bastien CH, Vallieres A, Morin CM. Validation of the Insomnia Severity Index as an outcome measure for insomnia research. Sleep Med. 2001;2(4):297–307.
45. Ferreira-Valente MA, Pais-Ribeiro JL, Jensen MP. Validity of four pain intensity rating scales. Pain. 2011;152(10):2399–404.
46. Grimby-Ekman A, Gerdle B, Bjork J, Larsson B. Comorbidities, intensity, frequency and duration of pain, daily functioning and health care seeking in local, regional, and widespread pain—a descriptive population-based survey (SwePain). BMC Musculoskelet Disord. 2015;16:165.
47. Fazio AF. A concurrent validational study of the NCHS general well-being schedule. Vital Health Stat. 1977;2(73):1–53.
48. McDowell I. Measuring health: a guide to rating scales and questionnaires. 3rd ed. In: McDowell I, editor. Oxford: Oxford University Press; 2006.
49. O'brien RM. A caution regarding rules of thumb of variance inflation factors. Qual Quant. 2007;41:673–90.
50. Ford DE, Kamerow DB. Epidemiologic study of sleep disturbances and psychiatric disorders. An opportunity for prevention? JAMA. 1989;262(11):1479–84.
51. Ohayon MM, Reynolds CF 3rd. Epidemiological and clinical relevance of insomnia diagnosis algorithms according to the DSM-IV and the International Classification of Sleep Disorders (ICSD). Sleep Med. 2009;10(9):952–60.
52. American Psychiatric Association (APA). Diagnostic and statistical manual of mental disorders: DSM-5. 5th ed. Washington, DC: American Psychiatric Association; 2013.
53. Morgan K, Clarke D. Risk factors for late-life insomnia in a representative general practice sample. Br J Gen Pract. 1997;47(416):166–9.
54. Roberts RE, Shema SJ, Kaplan GA. Prospective data on sleep complaints and associated risk factors in an older cohort. Psychosom Med. 1999;61(2):188–96.
55. Kim JM, Stewart R, Kim SW, Yang SJ, Shin IS, Yoon JS. Insomnia, depression, and physical disorders in late life: a 2-year longitudinal community study in Koreans. Sleep. 2009;32(9):1221–8.
56. Call-Schmidt TA, Richardson SJ. Prevalence of sleep disturbance and its relationship to pain in adults with chronic pain. Pain Manag Nurs. 2003;4(3):124–33.
57. Mezick EJ, Matthews KA, Hall M, Kamarck TW, Buysse DJ, Owens JF, Reis SE. Intra-individual variability in sleep duration and fragmentation: associations with stress. Psychoneuroendocrinology. 2009;34(9):1346–54.
58. Roth T, Jaeger S, Jin R, Kalsekar A, Stang PE, Kessler RC. Sleep problems, comorbid mental disorders, and role functioning in the national comorbidity survey replication. Biol Psychiatry. 2006;60(12):1364–71.

59. Allan CE, Valkanova V, Ebmeier KP. Depression in older people is underdiagnosed. Practitioner. 2014;258(1771):19–22.
60. Morin CM, Rodrigue S, Ivers H. Role of stress, arousal, and coping skills in primary insomnia. Psychosom Med. 2003;65(2):259–67.
61. Breslau N, Roth T, Rosenthal L, Andreski P. Sleep disturbance and psychiatric disorders: a longitudinal epidemiological study of young adults. Biol Psychiatry. 1996;39(6):411–8.
62. Jansson M, Linton SJ. The role of anxiety and depression in the development of insomnia: cross-sectional and prospective analyses. Psychol Health. 2006;21(3):383–97.

Suicidal thoughts among university students in Ethiopia

Berihun Assefa Dachew[1*], Berhanu Boru Bifftu[2], Bewket Tadesse Tiruneh[2], Degefaye Zelalem Anlay[2] and Meseret Adugna Wassie[3]

Abstract

Background: Suicide is a serious public health problem, responsible for 1.48% of all deaths worldwide, with suicidal ideation an important precursor. University and college students are among highly affected groups. This study aimed to determine the prevalence of suicidal ideation and to identify factors associated with suicidal ideation among university students in Ethiopia.

Methods: A random selection of 836 students was surveyed. Binary and multivariable logistic regression models were fitted, adjusting for potential confounders. Associations were measured using odds ratios (OR) and 95% confidence intervals (95% CI). Analyses were carried out using the SPSS version 20 software.

Results: The prevalence of suicidal ideation was 19.9% (95% CI 17.1–22.4%). The odds of suicidal ideation was higher among students who had mental distress (adjusted odds ratio (AOR) = 2.0, 95% CI 1.38–2.91), a family history of mental illness (AOR = 3.05, 95%, 1.89–4.92) and for those who had low social support (AOR = 2.0, 95% CI 1.35–2.82). Financial distress (AOR = 1.59, 95% CI 1.09–2.33), Khat chewing (AOR = 1.78, 95% CI 1.05–3), and alcohol use (AOR = 1.6, 95% CI 1.05–2.42) were also significantly associated with suicidal ideation. We found no evidence of associations between suicidal ideation and gender, age, relationship status, or year of study.

Conclusions: One in five students reported suicidal ideation. There was strong evidence of associations between suicidal ideation and mental distress, family history of mental illness, low social support, financial distress, and substance use. It is, therefore, important to develop suicide prevention strategies targeting these risk factors for university students in Ethiopia.

Keywords: University students, Suicidal ideation, Risk factors

Background

Suicide is a serious public health problem, responsible for 1.48% of deaths worldwide [1]. The burden is much higher in adolescents and young adults, accounting for 8.64% of deaths among 20–24 years [1] and is the third leading cause of death among 15–24 years [2].

University and college students are among groups affected more than the general population. Suicide is the second leading cause of death among college students [3]. This may be due to the broad range of challenges faced by university students, such as academic and social pressures [4] adaptation to a new social environment [5], and financial burdens [6, 7]. Moreover, common risk factors for suicide such as mental and substance use disorders are very common among university students [6, 8–12].

Suicidal thoughts, also known as suicidal ideation, are considered to be an important precursor to suicide [2]. At one American university, 12% of students had experienced suicidal thoughts during their studies, with 2.6% reporting persistent suicidal ideation [13]. Another study among medical students in Austria and Turkey revealed that 11% of Austrian students and 12% of Turkish students reported suicidal ideation during the 12 months prior to the survey [14]. Furthermore, a meta-analysis of studies conducted among college students in China

*Correspondence: berihunassefa21@gmail.com
[1] Department of Epidemiology and Biostatistics, Institute of Public Health, College of Medicine and Health Sciences, University of Gondar, Gondar, Ethiopia
Full list of author information is available at the end of the article

reported an overall pooled prevalence of suicidal ideation of 10.72% (95%CI 8.41–13.28%) [15].

Higher prevalence of suicide ideation has been reported among university students in Africa, reaching 47.5% among Botswana students [16] and 32.3% among South African medical students [17]. However, there have been no reports of the prevalence of suicidal ideation among university students in Ethiopia.

Suicide prevention efforts depend largely on early identification and adequate treatment of high-risk populations. Although studies report depression as a significant risk factor for suicidal ideation among university students [18], other mental disorders (such as anxiety, adjustment disorder, schizophrenia, and affective dysregulation), substance use or dependence, family history of suicide or psychiatric illness, low social support, sexual violence, loss of close friends or family, and conflict have also been linked [2, 13, 18–22].

Although there are some studies among university students in other African countries, the results are limited by study design issues such as small sample size and the use of convenience samples. In addition, risk factors may vary between countries. Therefore, this study aimed to determine the prevalence of suicidal ideation and to identify factors associated with suicidal ideation among university students in Ethiopia. Results from this study will help in developing evidence based mental health promotion and suicide prevention programs.

Methods

Study design: Institution-based cross-sectional study.

Study setting: The study was conducted at University of Gondar, in Northwest Ethiopia.

Sampling size and sampling technique: Systematic random sampling was used to select study participants Eight hundred and thirty-six undergraduate students were included in the study.

Data collection tools and procedures

A self-administered questionnaire was used to collect data from participants. Suicidal thought was recoded into a binary variable to denote the presence or absence of suicide ideation in the 12 months prior to the survey. The self-reporting questionnaire (SRQ-20) was used to determine the magnitude of mental distress over the previous month; this was dichotomised using a cut-off score of 8 or more to indicate mental distress. The tool is validated in Ethiopia [23]. The 12-item Multidimensional Scale of Perceived Social Support tool (MSPSS) was used to assess level of social support (none/low or medium/high) in students [24].

Current use (at least once in the month preceding the study) of alcohol, cigarettes, and khat was self-reported by participants.

Data analyses

Descriptive statistics (frequencies, percentages, means, and standard deviations) were used to present socio-demographic data and the prevalence of suicidal ideation. Binary logistic regression was used to identify factors associated suicidal thought. Multivariable logistic regression models were then fitted to control for the possible contribution of confounders. A significance level of $p < 0.05$ was used as the cut-off value for all statistical significance tests. The associations were measured using Odds Ratios (OR) and 95% confidence intervals (95% CI). All the analyses were carried out using the SPSS version 20 software.

Results

Socio-demographic characteristics of the respondents

A total of 836 students participated in the study, of whom 538 (64.4%) were male. The mean (± SD) age of respondents was 20 (± 1.54) years. Nearly, 65% of the respondents were from urban backgrounds (Table 1).

Prevalence of suicidal ideation

The prevalence of suicidal ideation in the total sample was 19.9% (95% CI 17.1–22.4%). The prevalence for

Table 1 Sociodemographic characteristics of the respondents

Socio-demographic characteristics	n	%
Sex		
Male	538	64.4
Female	298	35.6
Age (in years)		
≤19	160	19.1
20–24	658	78.7
25 and above	18	2.2
Residence		
Urban	544	65.1
Rural	292	34.9
Year of study		
1st	286	34.2
2nd	250	29.9
3rd and above	300	35.9
Relation ship		
Single	339	40.6
In relation	497	59.4

females (21.5%) was not significantly different to that for males (19%; $p = 0.72$).

Suicidal ideation among students with mental and substance use disorders

Of the total sample, 342 (41%) received SRQ-20 scores indicative of mental distress and 97 (11.6%) reported a family history of mental illness. Among individuals with suicidal ideation, 57.8% reported mental distress in the previous month. The prevalence of suicidal ideation was higher among those with a family history of mental illness (24.7%, $p < 0.0001$).

Among the respondents, 272 (32.5%) used alcohol, 114 (13.6%) chewed khat and 55 (6.6%) smoked cigarette in the month preceding the study. The prevalence of suicidal ideation was higher for those who chewed khat (29.8%; $p = 0.03$) and drink alcohol (27.7%; $p = 0.05$) (Table 2).

Factors associated with suicidal ideation among university students

The multivariate logistic regression analysis revealed that the odds of suicidal ideation was higher among students who had mental distress (adjusted odds ratio (AOR) = 2.0, 95% CI 1.38–2.91), family history of mental illness (AOR = 3.05, 95% 1.89–4.92), and for those who had low social support (AOR = 2.0, 95% CI 1.35–2.82). Financial distress (AOR = 1.59, 95% CI 1.09–2.33), Khat chewing (AOR = 1.78, 95% CI 1.05–3), and alcohol use (AOR = 1.6, 95% CI 1.05–2.42) were also significantly associated with suicidal ideation. We found no evidence of associations between suicidal ideation and gender, age, relationship status, or years of study (Table 3).

Table 2 Prevalence of suicidal ideation among Ethiopian university students, by mental distress, family history of mental illness, and current substance use

Variables	Suicidal ideation		*p* value
	Yes, number (%)	No, number (%)	
Mental distress			
Yes	96 (28.1)	246 (71.9)	< 0.0001
No	70 (14.2)	424 (85.8)	
Family history of mental illness			
Yes	41 (42.3)	56 (57.7)	< 0.0001
No	125 (16.9)	614 (83.1)	
Current alcohol user			
Yes	64 (23.5)	208 (76.5)	0.05
No	102 (18.1)	462 (81.9)	
Current cigarette smoker			
Yes	15 (27.3)	40 (72.7)	
No	151 (19.3)	630 (80.7)	0.16
Current khat chewer			
Yes	34 (29.8)	80 (70.2)	0.005
No	132 (18.3)	590 (81.7)	

Discussion

This is the first study assessing suicidal ideation and suicidal risk among University students in Ethiopia. One in five students reported suicidal ideation in the 12 months preceding the study, which is almost two times higher than the existing literature analysing suicidal ideation during the same period of time in other non African student populations. For example, a study among medical students in Austria and Turkey reported prevalence of 11.3 and 12%, respectively [14]. Furthermore, the prevalence of 10.7% was reported for university students in China [15] and Portugal [25]. However, this finding was low compared with results of similar studies in Africa. For example, it was much lower than the prevalence of suicidal ideation reported among Botswana students (47.5%) [16]. Similarly, higher prevalence suicidal ideation has been reported among South African medical students (32.3%) [17]. These variations may be attributed to the difference on factors influencing suicide such as socioeconomic, culture, and lifestyle factors [26].

In this study, mental distress was strongly associated with suicidal ideation. The odd of suicidal ideation was two times higher among students who had mental distress than those without. This aligns with numerous research findings, where mental health problems significantly correlated with suicidal thought [10, 18, 19, 27]. This may be due to the impact of mental disorders on the individual's daily performance and social relationships, which may in turn lead to suicidal ideation [27]. Moreover, the odds of suicidal ideation were three times higher for respondents with a family history of mental illness. This finding is in line with another study in which family history of psychiatric illness increased the risk of suicidal ideation [22]. However, it is important to note that the family history of mental illness is reported using a single question, rather than using formal diagnostic instruments.

The study also found that suicidal ideation was significantly associated with current substance use. Those students who chewed khat or use alcohol were 1.8 and 1.6 times, respectively, more likely to have had suicidal thought than to those who did not. This may be that students who drink alcohol or chew khat have characteristics that also dispose them towards suicidal ideation or that the use of alcohol and khat may contribute to depression and/or suicidal ideation. Associations between substance use and suicidal behaviour have been well documented [2, 10, 13, 28].

In agreement with the previous findings [2, 20, 29–31], the current study also found that lack of social support

Table 3 Bivariate and multivariate logistic regression models of suicidal ideation in Ethiopian university students

Variables	COR, 95% CI	AOR, 95% CI	*p* value
Gender			
Male	Ref		
Female	1.17 (0.82–1.66)	1.07 (0.73–1.58)	0.72
Age (years)			
17–19	Ref		
20–24	2.46 (0.85–7.14)	2.62 (0.83–8.22)	0.11
≥25	1.97 (0.73–5.36)	2.41 (0.84–6.91)	0.10
Residence			
Rural	Ref		
Urban	1.22 (0.85–1.76)	1.49 (0.99–2.21)	0.52
Year of study			
1st year	Ref		
2nd year	1.18 (0.78–1.79)	1.09 (0.69–1.73)	0.71
3rd year	0.87 (0.58–1.31)	0.87 (0.56–1.34)	0.52
Relationship status			
Single	0.7 (0.5–0.98)	0.71 (0.49–1.02)	0.06
In relationship	Ref		
Religious practice			
Yes	Ref		
No	1.23 (0.74–2.03)	1.54 (0.89–2.67)	0.13
Mental distress			
Yes	2.36 (1.67–3.34)	2.0 (1.38–2.91)	< 0.0001***
No	Ref		
Family history of mental illness			
Yes	3.60 (2.30–5.62)	3.05 (1.89–4.92)	< 0.0001***
No	Ref		
Social support			
Non or low	2.21 (1.56–3.1)	2.0 (1.35–2.82)	< 0.001**
Moderate or high	Ref		
Current cigarette smoker			
Yes	1.56 (0.84–2.91)	1.09 (0.52–2.31)	0.82
No	Ref		
Current kaht chewer			
Yes	1.9 (1.22–2.90)	1.78 (1.05–3.0)	0.03*
No	Ref		
Current alcohol user			
Yes	1.39 (0.91–1.93)	1.60 ((1.05–2.42)	0.03*
No	Ref		

Ref reference category, *COR* crude odds ratio, *AOR* adjusted odds ratio

* $p < 0.05$, **$p < 0.001$, ***$p < 0.0001$

was an important risk factor for suicidal ideation. Those students with no or low social support were two times at high risk of suicidal thought than those with high social support. This may be through social support increasing a feeling of belonging and thus reducing the risk of suicidal thought [31]. Conversely, students who feel loneliness may have thoughts of suicide.

Finally, this study showed that suicidal ideation was associated with financial distress. Similar studies conducted among university students in the United States and Poland found that financial burden was significantly related to suicidal thoughts [32, 33].

To our knowledge, this is the first study to assess suicidal ideation among university students in Ethiopia. Importantly, the study also measures important risk factors for suicidal ideation, such as mental distress, poor social support, substance use, and family history of mental disorders. Furthermore, it addresses some of the limitations of previous research (i.e., the use of convenience sampling and small sample sizes). Despite these strengths, the study has some limitations. As the study was cross section, causal relationships could not be determined. Furthermore, this study was based on self-reported data, which may reduce objectivity and introduce the possibility of reporting bias. Finally, the use of retrospective items in the questionnaire may have incurred recall bias

Conclusions

Suicidal ideation was found to be high. Future research efforts could be directed towards replicating these results. There was strong evidence of associations between suicidal ideation and mental distress, family history of mental illness, low social support, financial distress, and substance use. It is, therefore, important to develop suicide prevention programs and strategies for university students in Ethiopia. Programs aimed at preventing suicide should address these significant risk factors.

Abbreviations

AOR: adjusted odds ratio; COR: crude odds ratio; OR: odds ratio; SRQ-20: self-reporting questionnaire; SPSS: statistical package for the social sciences; MSPSS: multidimensional scale of perceived social support; 95% CI: 95% confidence interval.

Authors' contributions

BAD conceived and designed the study. DZA collected the data as a member of the research project. BAD and MAW performed the statistical analysis and drafted the original paper. BBB, BTT, and DZA critically reviewed the manuscript. All authors read and approved the final manuscript.

Author details

[1] Department of Epidemiology and Biostatistics, Institute of Public Health, College of Medicine and Health Sciences, University of Gondar, Gondar, Ethiopia. [2] School of Nursing, College of Medicine and Health Sciences, University of Gondar, Gondar, Ethiopia. [3] Department of Health Informatics, Teda Health Science College, Gondar, Ethiopia.

Acknowledgements

The authors would like to acknowledge the study participants for their dedicated cooperation. We would like to thank the University of Gondar for providing ethical clearance. We would like to extend our heartfelt gratitude to Dr. Caroline Salom for editing the manuscript.

Competing interests
The authors declare that they have no competing interests.

Consent for publication
Not applicable.

Funding
The authors received no specific funding for this work.

References

1. Institute for Health Metrics and Evaluation (IHME). GBD compare data visualization. Seattle: IHME, University of Washington; 2016. (http://vizhub.healthdata.org/gbd-compare). Accessed 27 Feb 2017.
2. Arria AM, O'Grady KE, Caldeira KM, Vincent KB, Wilcox HC, Wish ED. Suicide ideation among college students: a multivariate analysis. Arch Suicide Res. 2009;13(3):230–46.
3. Schwartz AJ. College student suicide in the United States: 1990–1991 through 2003–2004. J Am Coll Health. 2006;54(6):341–52.
4. Sreeramareddy CT, Shankar PR, Binu VS, Mukhopadhyay C, Ray B, Menezes RG. Psychological morbidity, sources of stress and coping strategies among undergraduate medical students of Nepal. BMC Med Educ. 2007;7:26.
5. Clinciu AI. Adaptation and stress for the first year university students. Proced Soc Behav Sci. 2013;78:718–22.
6. Dachew BA, Azale Bisetegn T, Berhe Gebremariam R. Prevalence of mental distress and associated factors among undergraduate students of University of Gondar, northwest Ethiopia: a cross-sectional institutional based study. PLoS ONE. 2015;10(3):e0119464.
7. Goodman E, Huang B, Wade TJ, Kahn RS. A multilevel analysis of the relation of socioeconomic status to adolescent depressive symptoms: does school context matter? J Pediatr. 2003;143(4):451–6.
8. Atwoli L, Mungla PA, Ndung'u MN, Kinoti KC, Ogot EM. Prevalence of substance use among college students in Eldoret, western Kenya. BMC Psychiatry. 2011;11:34.
9. Dachew BA, Bifftu BB, Tiruneh BT. Khat use and its determinants among university students in northwest Ethiopia: a multivariable analysis. Int J Med Sci Public Health. 2015;4(3):319–23.
10. Dvorak RD, Lamis DA, Malone PS. Alcohol use, depressive symptoms, and impulsivity as risk factors for suicide proneness among college students. J Affect Disord. 2013;149(1–3):326–34.
11. Stallman HM. Prevalence of psychological distress in university students–implications for service delivery. Aust Fam Physician. 2008;37(8):673–7.
12. Tavolacci MP, Ladner J, Grigioni S, Richard L, Villet H, Dechelotte P. Prevalence and association of perceived stress, substance use and behavioral addictions: a cross-sectional study among university students in France, 2009–2011. BMC Public Health. 2013;13:724.
13. Wilcox HC, Arria AM, Caldeira KM, Vincent KB, Pinchevsky GM, O'Grady KE. Prevalence and predictors of persistent suicide ideation, plans, and attempts during college. J Affect Disord. 2010;127(1–3):287–94.
14. Eskin M, Voracek M, Stieger S, Altinyazar V. A cross-cultural investigation of suicidal behavior and attitudes in Austrian and Turkish medical students. Soc Psychiatry Psychiatr Epidemiol. 2011;46(9):813–23.
15. Li ZZ, Li YM, Lei XY, Zhang D, Liu L, Tang SY, Chen L. Prevalence of suicidal ideation in Chinese college students: a meta-analysis. PLoS ONE. 2014;9(10):e104368.
16. Korb I, Plattner IE. Suicide ideation and depression in university students in Botswana. J Psychol Afr. 2014;24(5):420–6.
17. Van Niekerk L, Scribante L, Raubenheimer PJ. Suicidal ideation and attempt among South African medical students. S Afr Med J. 2012;102(6 Pt 2):372–3.
18. Cash SJ, Bridge JA. Epidemiology of youth suicide and suicidal behavior. Curr Opin Pediatr. 2009;21(5):613–9.
19. Garlow SJ, Rosenberg J, Moore JD, Haas AP, Koestner B, Hendin H, Nemeroff CB. Depression, desperation, and suicidal ideation in college students: results from the American Foundation for Suicide Prevention College Screening Project at Emory University. Depress Anxiety. 2008;25(6):482–8.
20. Peltzer K. Social support and suicide risk among secondary school students in Cape Town, South Africa. Psychol Rep. 2008;103(3):653–60.
21. Osama M, Islam MY, Hussain SA, Masroor SM, Burney MU, Masood MA, Menezes RG, Rehman R. Suicidal ideation among medical students of Pakistan: a cross-sectional study. J Forensic Leg Med. 2014;27:65–8.
22. Qin P, Agerbo E, Mortensen PB. Suicide risk in relation to family history of completed suicide and psychiatric disorders: a nested case-control study based on longitudinal registers. Lancet. 2002;360(9340):1126–30.
23. Youngmann R, Zilber N, Workneh F, Giel R. Adapting the SRQ for Ethiopian populations: a culturally-sensitive psychiatric screening instrument. Transcultural Psychiatry. 2008;45(4):566–89.
24. Zimet GD, Powell SS, Farley GK, Werkman S, Berkoff KA. Psychometric characteristics of the multidimensional scale of perceived social support. J Pers Assess. 1990;55(3–4):610–7.
25. Pereira A, Cardoso F. Suicidal ideation in university students: prevalence and association with school and gender. Paidéia. 2015;25(62):299–306.
26. Eshun S. Sociocultural determinants of suicide ideation: a comparison between American and Ghanaian college samples. Suicide Life Threat Behav. 2003;33(2):165–71.
27. Izadiniaa N, Amiria M, Jahromia R, Hamidia S. A study of relationship between suicidal ideas, depression, anxiety, resiliency, daily stresses and mental health among Tehran university students. Proced Soc Behav Sci. 2010;5:1515–9.
28. Zhang X, Wu LT. Suicidal ideation and substance use among adolescents and young adults: a bidirectional relation? Drug Alcohol Depend. 2014;142:63–73.
29. Whatley SL, Clopton JR. Social support and suicidal ideation in college students. Psychol Rep. 1992;71(3 Pt 2):1123–8.
30. Endo G, Tachikawa H, Fukuoka Y, Aiba M, Nemoto K, Shiratori Y, Matsui Y, Doi N, Asada T. How perceived social support relates to suicidal ideation: a Japanese social resident survey. Int J Soc Psychiatry. 2014;60(3):290–8.
31. Kleiman EM, Liu RT. Social support as a protective factor in suicide: findings from two nationally representative samples. J Affect Disord. 2013;150(2):540–5.
32. Eisenberg D, Gollust SE, Golberstein E, Hefner JL. Prevalence and correlates of depression, anxiety, and suicidality among university students. Am J Orthopsychiatry. 2007;77(4):534–42.
33. Mojs E, Warchol-Biederman K, Samborski W. Prevalence of depression and suicidal thoughts amongst university students in Poznan, Poland, preliminary report. Psychology. 2012;3(2):132–5.

10

A pilot study exploring the association of morphological changes with 5-HTTLPR polymorphism in OCD patients

Shinichi Honda[1*], Tomohiro Nakao[1*], Hiroshi Mitsuyasu[1], Kayo Okada[1], Leo Gotoh[2], Mayumi Tomita[3], Hirokuni Sanematsu[1], Keitaro Murayama[1], Keisuke Ikari[1], Masumi Kuwano[1], Takashi Yoshiura[4], Hiroaki Kawasaki[1,5] and Shigenobu Kanba[1]

Abstract

Background: Clinical and pharmacological studies of obsessive-compulsive disorder (OCD) have suggested that the serotonergic systems are involved in the pathogenesis, while structural imaging studies have found some neuroanatomical abnormalities in OCD patients. In the etiopathogenesis of OCD, few studies have performed concurrent assessment of genetic and neuroanatomical variables.

Methods: We carried out a two-way ANOVA between a variable number of tandem repeat polymorphisms (5-HTTLPR) in the serotonin transporter gene and gray matter (GM) volumes in 40 OCD patients and 40 healthy controls (HCs).

Results: We found that relative to the HCs, the OCD patients showed significant decreased GM volume in the right hippocampus, and increased GM volume in the left precentral gyrus. 5-HTTLPR polymorphism in OCD patients had a statistical tendency of stronger effects on the right frontal pole than those in HCs.

Conclusions: Our results showed that the neuroanatomical changes of specific GM regions could be endophenotypes of 5-HTTLPR polymorphism in OCD.

Keywords: Hippocampus, Precentral gyrus, Frontal pole, Imaging genetics, Obsessive-compulsive disorder (OCD), Serotonin transporter gene, 5-HTTLPR, Voxel-based morphometry (VBM)

Background

Obsessive-compulsive disorder (OCD) was made a disease independent of anxiety disorder in DSM-5. One of the reasons for this separation is that the biological bases of OCD and anxiety disorder are different [1].

Structural imaging studies have found neuroanatomical abnormalities in the cortico–striatal–thalamo–cortical (CSTC) circuits in OCD patients [2]. A recent voxel-based morphometry (VBM) systematic review suggested that widespread structural abnormalities may contribute to neurobiological vulnerability to OCD [3]. We previously found the presence of regional gray matter (GM) and white matter (WM) volume abnormalities in OCD patients [4].

Furthermore, positron emission tomography (PET) and functional magnetic resonance imaging (fMRI) have revealed abnormal activities in different nodes of the CSTC circuits in OCD patients compared with healthy controls (HCs) [2, 5]. In our previous fMRI study, we found decreased activations in several brain regions including the orbitofrontal cortex (OFC) [6] and a specific relationship between fMRI activation and symptom subtypes [7].

Meanwhile, family and twin studies have provided evidence for the involvement of a genetic factor in OCD. However, many linkage, association, and genome-wide

*Correspondence: shinhonn@npsych.med.kyushu-u.ac.jp; tomona@npsych.med.kyushu-u.ac.jp
[1] Department of Neuropsychiatry, Graduate School of Medical Sciences, Kyushu University, 3-1-1 Maidashi Higashi-ku, Fukuoka, Japan
Full list of author information is available at the end of the article

association studies have failed to identify responsible genes [8, 9].

Molecular genetic studies have focused on some structures, including receptor and transporter proteins, in the serotonergic and dopaminergic system.

Based on transporter imaging findings, a PET study [10] found a decrease of serotonin transporter binding in the insular cortex in OCD patients. They suggested that dysfunction of the serotonergic system in the limbic area might be involved in the pathophysiology of OCD.

It is possible to hypothesize that a polymorphism in the transcriptional control region upstream of the 5-hydroxytryptamine (serotonin) transporter (5-HTT) coding sequence could be an important factor in conferring susceptibility to OCD [8, 11, 12]. The 5-HTTLPR consists of a 44-bp deletion/insertion yielding a 14-repeat allele (short; S) and a 16-repeat allele (long; L). The S allele reduces the transcriptional efficiency of the 5-HTT gene promotor, resulting in decreased 5-HTT expression and availability. Bloch et al. [11]. suggested the possibility that the L allele is associated with specific OCD subgroups such as childhood-onset OCD. In contrast, Lin et al. [12] found that OCD was associated with the SS homozygous genotype. Some researchers suggested that this L allele could be subdivided further to L_A and L_G alleles [13]. The L_G allele, which is the L allele with an $A \rightarrow G$ substitution (rs25531), is thought to be similar to the S allele in terms of reuptake efficiency [14]. Rocha et al. [15] found that the L_A allele was associated to OCD. Hu et al. [14] found that the L_AL_A genotype was approximately twice as common in 169 whites with OCD than in 253 ethnically matched controls, and the L_A allele was twofold overtransmitted to the patients with OCD.

Despite the genetic and neuroanatomical importance, few studies of the etiopathogenesis of OCD have concurrently assessed genetic and neuroanatomical variables. We hypothesized that the widespread structural brain changes in OCD indicate the endophenotype of the 5-HTTLPR polymorphism. Therefore, the aim of this study was to investigate the association of genetic variations of the 5-HTTLPR with neuroanatomical changes in OCD.

Methods

Subjects

We studied 40 OCD patients (20 females and 20 males) who met DSM-IV [16] criteria for OCD and had no DSM-IV Axis I disorders except OCD and major depressive disorder as screened by the Structured Clinical Interview for DSM-IV (SCID). Patients who displayed a comorbid axis I diagnosis, neurological disorder, head injury, serious medical condition, or history of drug/alcohol addiction were excluded. We determined psychiatric diagnoses by a consensus of at least two psychiatrists after screening by SCID. Patients were recruited from among outpatients and inpatients of the Department of Neuropsychiatry, Kyushu University Hospital, Japan. Severity of OCD symptoms was assessed with the Yale-Brown Obsessive Compulsive Scale (Y-BOCS) [17]. Patients were also screened for the presence of depressive symptoms through the administration of the 17-item Hamilton Depression Rating Scale (HDRS) [18]. Forty HCs (26 females and 14 males) who were matched to the patients in age and sex were recruited from the staff of Kyushu University Hospital and related agencies. They had no DSM-IV Axis I disorders as determined by the SCID. They also had no current medical problems, psychiatric histories, neurological disorders, or mental retardation. Handedness was determined according to the Edinburgh Handedness Inventory for both OCD patients and HCs [19].

The study was approved by the local ethics committee <22-111, 491-01>, and each participating patient provided written informed consent after receiving a complete description of the study, which was approved by the institutional review board.

MRI procedures

All imaging examinations were performed on a 3.0-T MRI scanner (Achieva TX, Philips Healthcare, Best, The Netherlands) with a standard head coil at the Department of Radiology, Kyushu University. T1-weighted images were acquired with a 3D T1-weighted turbo field echo sequence with the following parameters: repetition time (TR) = 8.2 ms, echo time (TE) = 3.8 ms, flip angle = 8°, matrix = 240 × 240, T1 inversion time = 1026 ms, field of view (FOV) = 240 × 240 mm, NSA = 1, slice thickness = 1 mm, number of slices = 190, and scan time = 320 s.

VBM data processing

Acquired images were first converted from DICOM to NifTI-1 format using dcm2nii software (http://www.mccauslandcenter.sc.edu/mricro/mricron/dcm2nii.html). Data processing and examinations were performed with SPM8 software (developed under the auspices of the Functional Imaging Laboratory, The Wellcome Trust Centre for Neuroimaging at the Institute of Neurology at University College London, UK, http://www.fil.ion.ucl.ac.uk/spm/) in the environment of MATLAB (2011b ver., http://www.mathworks.co.jp/products/matlab/). AC–PC orientation was conducted on all T1-weighted data by an automatic process. Then, we applied the VBM8 toolbox (http://dbm.neuro.uni-jena.de/467/) for preprocessing the structural images by the VBM procedure. This VBM8 algorithm involves image bias correction, tissue classification, and normalization to the standard Montreal Neurological Institute (MNI) space using linear (12-parameter affine) and non-linear transformations. High-dimension DARTEL normalization, which is rather unbiased in its segmentation process, was used as anatomical registration with the default template provided in the VBM8 toolbox. Gray matter (GM) and white matter (WM) segments were modulated only by non-linear components, which allowed comparing the absolute amount of tissue corrected for individual brain volume, that is, correction for total brain volume.

Finally, modulated images were smoothed with a Gaussian kernel of 8 mm full width at half maximum. Although we used the East Asian Brains template in the process of affine regularization instead of European Brains, the default parameters were used in all other steps. Finally, 40 OCD patients and 40 HCs were assessed by structural MRI examinations with a 3.0-T MRI scanner.

Genotyping

A 10-ml venous blood sample was collected in EDTA vacuum tubes. Samples were immediately frozen at −80 °C until extraction of genomic DNA from nucleated white blood cells. Genomic DNA was extracted from peripheral blood leukocytes using a Promega DNA Purification Kit (Promega, Madison, WI, USA).

The polymerase chain reaction (PCR) was used to amplify 5-HTTLPR polymorphism. Forward (5′-GGCGTTGCCGCTCTGAATGC-3′) and reverse (5′-GAGGGACTGAGCTGGACAACCAC-3′) primers were used to amplify a fragment including 5-HTTLPR [20]. These primers amplify a 529-bp fragment for the S allele and a 575-bp fragment for the L allele.

PCR amplification was carried out in a final volume of 15 μl consisting of 50–100 ng genomic DNA, 2.5 mM deoxyribonucleotides, 0.2 μM of forward and reverse primers, PCR buffer (2× GC Buffer I, Takara Bio Inc., Shiga, Japan), and 1.25 U of DNA polymerase (TaKaRa LA Taq, Takara Bio Inc.). Denaturation was carried out at 94 °C for 30 s, annealing at 64 °C for 30 s, and extension at 72 °C for 3 min for 40 cycles.

To identify L_A and L_G alleles, a two-step protocol was performed. Step I: determination of the L or S allele, as described above; and step II: digestion of this amplicon with *Hap*II (Takara Bio Inc.) restriction endonuclease. The assay was designed to include an invariant *Hap*II digest site located 94 bp from the end of the amplicon to provide an internal control for digestion/partial digestion. Products were separated on a 4.0% agarose gel (Agarose-LE, Classic Type, Nacalai Tesque, Inc., Kyoto, Japan) supplemented with ethidium bromide (0.01%, Nacalai Tesque) and visualized under ultraviolet light. After separation of the digestion products by electrophoresis, the following restriction fragment allele sizes were obtained: L_A (341, 126, 62 bp) and L_G (174, 167, 126, 62 bp).

Statistical analysis

We conducted a two-sample *t* test, Chi square test, and Fisher's exact test to test for differences in demographic variables between OCD patients and HCs as well as between different variants of the alleles of 5-HTTLPR in OCD patients.

The genotype frequencies of OCD patients and HCs were compared using Chi square test after checking the Hardy–Weinberg equilibrium.

We divided the patients into L_A allele carriers (SL_A, L_AL_G, and L_AL_A) and non-L_A allele carriers (SS, SL_G, and L_GL_G). Hu et al. [14] noted that the normalized (to SS genotype) expression value of the L_A allele was approximately double the values of the S and L_G alleles. Thus, we thought that expressions of genotypes including the L_A allele were higher than those of other genotypes.

Statistical analysis was performed with SPM8, which implemented a general linear model. First, we performed a two-sample *t* test to detect the difference in GM volume between patients with OCD and HCs. The initial voxel threshold was set to $P < 0.001$ uncorrected. Clusters were considered significant that fell below a cluster-corrected family-wise error (FWE), $P = 0.05$. Next, we performed a two-way factorial analysis of variance between the 5-HTTLPR polymorphism and GM volumes in the OCD patients and HCs. A two-way ANOVA test was applied to assess the relationship between 5-HTTLPR polymorphism (L_A or non-L_A allele carriers) and GM brain volume changes in the OCD patients and HCs. If a statistical difference was present, a post hoc *t* test was performed to detect the inter-group difference of brain regions. Age and sex were set as covariates in the statistical analysis. We used a threshold of $P < 0.05$ cluster-corrected family-wise error (FWE) and $P < 0.001$ uncorrected with expected voxels per clusters. The $P < 0.001$ value is commonly used in VBM-based OCD studies [21–23].

Results

In demographic variables of age, gender, and handedness, OCD patients and HCs did not show any significant differences (Table 1). These variables also showed no significant difference between the genotypes of L_A allele carriers or non-L_A allele carriers in OCD patients (Table 2). OCD patients had significantly fewer years of education than HCs (Table 1). Non-L_A allele carriers, furthermore, had significantly fewer years of education than those of L_A allele carriers (Table 2). No significant differences were shown between the two genotypes in OCD

Table 1 Clinical and demographic characteristics of OCD patients and HCs

	OCD patients ($n = 40$)	HCs ($n = 40$)	P value
Age (years, mean ± SD)[a]	35.40 ± 12.07	39.70 ± 12.97	0.129
Gender (female/male)[b]	20/20	26/14	0.175
Handedness (right/left)[b]	37/3	39/1	0.305
Education (years, mean ± SD)[a]	13.69 ± 2.43	15.15 ± 1.35	0.001
Illness duration (years, mean ± SD)	11.33 ± 10.10		
Age of onset (years, mean ± SD)	23.98 ± 11.24		
Total Y-BOCS (total score, mean ± SD)	21.95 ± 6.32		
HDRS (17 items)[a]	6.08 ± 6.87	0.55 ± 0.88	0.000
5-HTTLPR[a]			
14/14	26	17	0.040
14/16	13	22	
16/16	1	1	
L_A allele carriers (SL_A, L_AL_G, L_AL_A)[b]	10	20	0.021
Non-L_A allele carriers (SS, SL_G, L_GL_G)[b]	30	20	

We found a significant difference between the OCD patients and HCs in the distribution of L_A allele carriers or non-L_A allele carriers of 5-HTTLPR polymorphism

[a] *T* test

[b] Chi square test

regarding illness duration, age of onset, total Y-BOCS, or the 17-item HDRS (Table 2).

The genotype frequencies of our samples did not deviate significantly from the values predicted by the Hardy–Weinberg equation.

As for the genotypic distribution, 1/40 OCD patients (2.5%) and 1/40 HCs (2.5%) were LL homozygotes, 13/40 OCD patients (32.5%) and 22/40 HCs (55.0%) were LS heterozygotes, 26/40 OCD patients (65%) and 17/40 HCs (42.5%) were SS homozygotes, and 10/40 OCD patients (25.0%) and 20/40 HCs (50.0%) were L_A allele carriers. We found a significant difference between the OCD patients and HCs in the distribution of L_A allele carriers or non-L_A allele carriers of 5-HTTLPR polymorphism (χ^2=5.333, 1 *df*, $P = 0.021$; Table 1).

In morphological changes in OCD, compared to the HCs, the OCD patients showed significant decreased GM volumes in the right hippocampus (extent threshold; $k = 763$ voxels, $P < 0.05$, FWE; Table 3; Fig. 1a) and increased GM volume in the left precentral gyrus (extent threshold; $k = 797$ voxels, $P < 0.05$, FWE; Table 3; Fig. 1b). In morphological changes associated with the 5-HTTLPR polymorphism, compared to L_A allele carriers, non-L_A allele carriers showed no significant GM volume difference.

As of genotype–diagnosis interaction, although no voxels survived multiple comparison, we observed a tendency that 5-HTTLPR polymorphism in OCD patients had stronger effects on the right frontal pole than those in HCs ($P < 0.001$, uncorrected; Table 3; Fig. 2). The OCD patients with the L_A allele carriers of 5-HTTLPR polymorphism exhibited a statistical tendency of reduction of GM volumes in the right frontal pole compared to the HCs with the L_A allele carriers.

Discussion

In the present study, we found that the OCD patients showed significant decreased GM volume in the right hippocampus and increased GM volume in the left precentral gyrus. Moreover, our study suggested that L_A allele carriers of the 5-HTTLPR polymorphism in OCD patients are associated with decreased GM volume in the right frontal pole.

Functional neuroimaging studies have been suggested that hippocampus might have an important role in the

Table 2 Clinical and demographic characteristics of non-L_A allele carriers and L_A allele carriers in OCD patients

	Non-L_A allele carriers ($n = 30$) (SS, SL_G, L_GL_G)	L_A allele carriers ($n = 10$) (SL_A, L_AL_G, L_AL_A)	P value
Age (years, mean ± SD)[a]	36.77 ± 12.50	31.30 ± 10.15	0.219
Gender (female/male)[b]	15/15	5/5	1.000
Handedness (right/left)[b]	27/3	10/0	0.411
Education (years, mean ± SD)[a]	13.23 ± 2.46	15.00 ± 1.70	0.042
Illness duration (years, mean ± SD)[a]	12.27 ± 10.75	8.50 ± 7.61	0.313
Age of onset (years, mean ± SD)[a]	24.53 ± 11.90	22.30 ± 9.30	0.593
Total Y-BOCS (total score, mean ± SD)[a]	22.75 ± 6.53	19.44 ± 5.15	0.176
HDRS (17 items)[a]	6.76 ± 7.61	4.10 ± 3.70	0.157

[a] *T* test

[b] Chi square test

Table 3 VBM analysis including association of variance between 5-HTTLPR polymorphisms and GM volumes in OCD patients and HCs

Regions	Brodmann area	Cluster size	*Z*	Talairach coordinates *x*, *y*, *z* (mm²)
Main effects				
Diagnosis effects ($P < 0.05$, FWE, $\langle k \rangle = 77.666$)				
R hippocampus (OCD patients < HCs)		763	5.08	33, −16, −18
L precentral gyrus (OCD patients > HCs)	4	797	4.88	−28, −27, 64
Genotype effects				
No suprathreshold clusters				
Genotype-diagnosis interaction effects ($P < 0.001$, uncorrected, $\langle k \rangle = 63.146$)				
R frontal pole	10	112	4.35	26, 50, −6

R right, *L* left, *FWE* family-wise error, $\langle k \rangle$ expected voxels per clusters

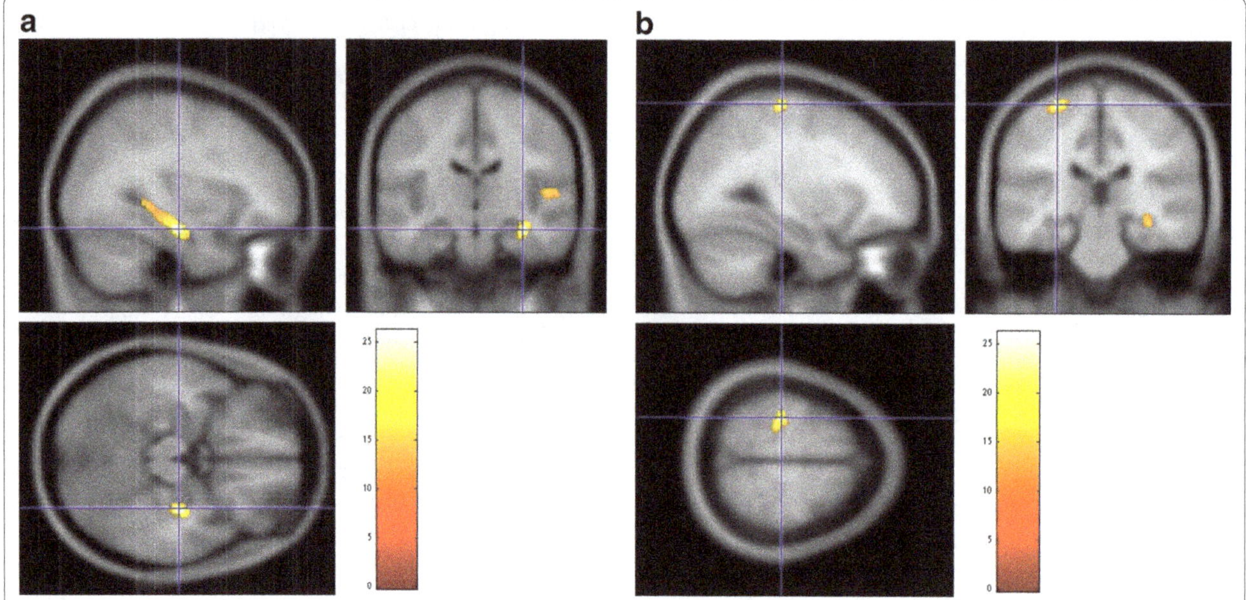

Fig. 1 **a** OCD patients showed decreased GM volume in the right hippocampus compared to HCs. **b** OCD patients showed increased GM volume in the left precentral gyrus compared to HCs [$P < 0.005$, cluster-corrected family-wise error (FWE), $\langle k \rangle = 77.666$]

pathophysiology of OCD [24, 25]. On the other hand, structural imaging studies have been suggested that hippocampal alteration may play an important role in the pathophysiology of OCD [26, 27].

The precentral gyrus is a prominent structure on the surface of the posterior frontal lobe. It is the site of the primary motor cortex (Brodmann area 4). Several researchers have suggested that the precentral gyrus may be involved in the pathophysiology of OCD [28, 29]. Russo et al. [30] suggested that OCD might be considered as a sensory motor disorder where a dysfunction of sensory–motor integration might play an important role in the release of motor compulsions. Our results also showed that the precentral gyrus might be involved in the pathophysiology of OCD.

The frontal pole comprises the most anterior part of the frontal lobe that approximately covers BA10. During human evolution, the functions in this area resulted in its expansion relative to the rest of the brain [31]. Specifically, the functions include multi-tasking [32], cognitive branching [33], prospective memory [34], conflict resolution [35], and selection of sub-goals [36]. It is suggested that such a highly advanced cognitive function is affected in OCD [37, 38].

In the field of imaging genetics, many researchers reported [39–42] an association between the serotonin transporter gene and brain structure. Regarding OCD, Atmaca et al. [43] found a significant genotype-by-side interaction for the OFC.

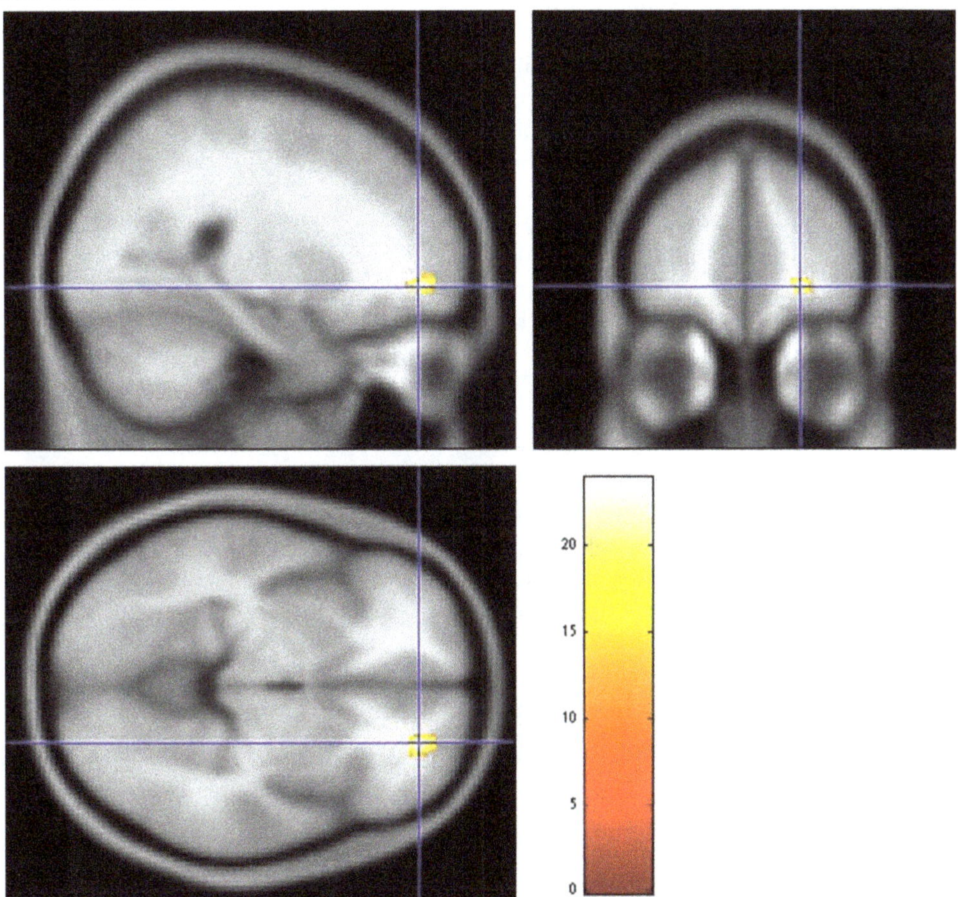

Fig. 2 Results of genotype–diagnosis interaction effects on brain morphology. The stronger effects of 5-HTTLPR polymorphism on brain morphology in OCD patients than those in HCs were noted in the right frontal pole ($P < 0.001$, uncorrected, $\langle k \rangle = 63.146$)

In contrast to the previous result reported by Atmaca et al. [43], our result suggested that a liability in development of the central nervous system might have occurred in OCD patients who are L_A allele carriers. Frodl et al. [44] suggested that the high-activity L_A allele with its increased number of 5-HTT transporter proteins, concomitant decrease in serotonin levels, and reduced effects on neuroplastic processes might cause structural changes during major depression. With similar mechanism, the volume decrease in the right frontal pole might have occurred in OCD patients who are L_A allele carriers.

There are some limitations to this study. First, we divided the patients into L_A allele carriers (SL_A, L_AL_G, and L_AL_A) and non-L_A allele carriers (SS, SL_G, and L_GL_G). In the view of expression activity, it might be better to divide samples into L_AL_A and others. Although we could not employ this division because our study included few L_AL_A genotypes, the difference between L_AL_A and other genotypes should be explored with larger samples in the future. In addition, our sample size was too small to identify the difference between the effects of L_A and non-L_A alleles on the brains of OCD patients and HCs. Thus, these findings should be considered preliminary until replicated in a larger sample.

The OCD patients had significantly fewer years of education than HCs, and non-L_A allele carriers had significantly fewer than L_A allele carriers. Education years might affect the difference in GM volumes if education years were proportional to high intelligence. In this study, we did not measure the intelligence quotient (IQ). Larger gray matter volumes are associated with higher IQ [45]. Ideally, the IQ should be measured and set as a covariate in the statistical analysis.

Although we examined 5-HTTLPR polymorphism as the sole candidate gene in this study, many other polymorphisms such as glutamate system genes and dopamine system genes [46, 47] may affect the brain morphology of OCD patients. We hope to explore an association between more candidate genetic polymorphisms and brain morphology in the future.

Moreover, the OCD patients were concurrently on medication. Our study was not designed to investigate medication effects. Thus, analyses of the effects of different medication types on the hippocampus, precentral gyrus, and frontal pole volumes did not reveal a significant difference. Further studies are necessary to explore possible effects of medication.

Finally, the uncorrected threshold used in the present study may not fully protect against results due to chance and the results may include false positives. Therefore, the significant clusters found in the present study need to be validated further.

Conclusions

We found that relative to the HCs, the OCD patients showed significant decreased GM volume in the right hippocampus, and increased GM volume in the left precentral gyrus. The OCD patients with the L_A allele carriers of 5-HTTLPR polymorphism exhibited a statistical tendency of reduction of GM volumes in the right frontal pole compared to the HCs with the L_A allele carriers. Our preliminary findings suggest that a variation of the 5-HTTLPR polymorphism might affect brain morphology differently in OCD patients and HCs in the right frontal pole volumes.

Abbreviations

OCD: obsessive-compulsive disorder; CSTC: cortico–striatal–thalamo–cortical; VNTR: a variable number of tandem repeat; 5-HTTLPR: serotonin transporter polymorphism; GM: gray matter; HCs: healthy controls; VBM: voxel-based morphometry; OFC: orbitofrontal cortex; DLPFC: dorsolateral prefrontal cortex; FEF: frontal eye fields; ACC: anterior cingulate cortex; PET: positron emission tomography; fMRI: functional magnetic resonance imaging; SCID: structured clinical interview for DSM-IV; Y-BOCS: Yale-Brown Obsessive Compulsive Scale; HDRS: Hamilton Depression Rating Scale; MNI: Montreal Neurological Institute; WM: white matter; PCR: polymerase chain reaction; FWE: family-wise error; IQ: intelligence quotient.

Authors' contributions

Study conception and design: TN, HS. Acquisition of data and clinical assessments: KM, SH, KO, KI, MK, TY, OT. Analysis and interpretation of data: LG, HM, MT. Drafting of manuscript: SH. Supervisors of this study: TN, HM, HK, SK. Critical revision: TN. All authors read and approved the final manuscript.

Author details

[1] Department of Neuropsychiatry, Graduate School of Medical Sciences, Kyushu University, 3-1-1 Maidashi Higashi-ku, Fukuoka, Japan. [2] Department of Mental Retardation and Birth Defect Research, National Institute of Neuroscience, National Center of Neurology and Psychiatry, Tokyo, Japan. [3] Kurume University Graduate School of Psychology, Fukuoka, Japan. [4] Department of Radiology, Graduate School of Medical and Dental Sciences, Kagoshima University, Kagoshima, Japan. [5] Department of Psychiatry, Faculty of Medicine, Fukuoka University, Fukuoka, Japan.

Acknowledgements

We would like to thank OCD patients and HCs who agreed to participate in this study. This study was supported by a Grant-in-Aid for Scientific Research (C) (22591262) (25461732) (16K10253) from the Japanese Ministry of Education, Culture, Sports, Science and Technology, and by the SENSHIN Medical Research Foundation. We were supported by a Grant-in-Aid for Scientific Research on Innovative Areas (Comprehensive Brain Science Network) from the Ministry of Education, Science, Sports and Culture of Japan in terms of the analysis technique, especially Dr. Kiyotaka Nemoto, who assisted in the VBM analysis technique. Katherine Ono provided assistance with language.

Competing interests

The authors declare that they have no competing interests.

Consent for publication

All the authors have read the manuscript and have approved this submission.

Funding

This study was supported by a Grant-in-Aid for Scientific Research (C) (22591262) (25461732) from the Japanese Ministry of Education, Culture, Sports, Science and Technology, and by the SENSHIN Medical Research Foundation.

References

1. American Psychiatric Association. American Psychiatric Association: DSM-5 Task Force: Diagnostic and statistical manual of mental disorders: DSM-5. 5th ed. Washington: American Psychiatric Association; 2013.
2. Milad MR, Rauch SL. Obsessive-compulsive disorder: beyond segregated cortico–striatal pathways. Trends Cogn Sci. 2012;16(1):43–51.
3. Piras F, Piras F, Chiapponi C, Girardi P, Caltagirone C, Spalletta G. Widespread structural brain changes in OCD: a systematic review of voxel-based morphometry studies. Cortex. 2015;62:89–108.
4. Togao O, Yoshiura T, Nakao T, Nabeyama M, Sanematsu H, Nakagawa A, Noguchi T, Hiwatashi A, Yamashita K, Nagao E, et al. Regional gray and white matter volume abnormalities in obsessive-compulsive disorder: a voxel-based morphometry study. Psychiatry Res. 2010;184(1):29–37.
5. Maia TV, Cooney RE, Peterson BS. The neural bases of obsessive-compulsive disorder in children and adults. Dev Psychopathol. 2008;20(4):1251–83.
6. Nakao T, Nakagawa A, Yoshiura T, Nakatani E, Nabeyama M, Yoshizato C, Kudoh A, Tada K, Yoshioka K, Kawamoto M, et al. Brain activation of patients with obsessive-compulsive disorder during neuropsychological and symptom provocation tasks before and after symptom improvement: a functional magnetic resonance imaging study. Biol Psychiatry. 2005;57(8):901–10.
7. Murayama K, Nakao T, Sanematsu H, Okada K, Yoshiura T, Tomita M, Masuda Y, Isomura K, Nakagawa A, Kanba S. Differential neural network of checking versus washing symptoms in obsessive-compulsive disorder. Prog Neuropsychopharmacol Biol Psychiatry. 2013;40:160–6.
8. Taylor S. Molecular genetics of obsessive-compulsive disorder: a comprehensive meta-analysis of genetic association studies. Mol Psychiatry. 2013;18(7):799–805.
9. Mattheisen M, Samuels JF, Wang Y, Greenberg BD, Fyer AJ, McCracken JT, Geller DA, Murphy DL, Knowles JA, Grados MA et al. Genome-wide association study in obsessive-compulsive disorder: results from the OCGAS. Mol Psychiatry. 2014;20(3):337–44
10. Matsumoto R, Ichise M, Ito H, Ando T, Takahashi H, Ikoma Y, Kosaka J, Arakawa R, Fujimura Y, Ota M, et al. Reduced serotonin transporter binding in the insular cortex in patients with obsessive-compulsive disorder: a [11C]DASB PET study. NeuroImage. 2010;49(1):121–6.
11. Bloch MH, Landeros-Weisenberger A, Sen S, Dombrowski P, Kelmendi B, Coric V, Pittenger C, Leckman JF. Association of the serotonin transporter polymorphism and obsessive-compulsive disorder: systematic review. Am J Med Genet B Neuropsychiatr Genet. 2008;147B(6):850–8.
12. Lin PY. Meta-analysis of the association of serotonin transporter gene polymorphism with obsessive-compulsive disorder. Prog Neuropsychopharmacol Biol Psychiatry. 2007;31(3):683–9.
13. Nakamura M, Ueno S, Sano A, Tanabe H. The human serotonin transporter gene linked polymorphism (5-HTTLPR) shows ten novel allelic variants. Mol Psychiatry. 2000;5(1):32–8.

14. Hu XZ, Lipsky RH, Zhu G, Akhtar LA, Taubman J, Greenberg BD, Xu K, Arnold PD, Richter MA, Kennedy JL, et al. Serotonin transporter promoter gain-of-function genotypes are linked to obsessive-compulsive disorder. Am J Hum Genet. 2006;78(5):815–26.
15. Rocha FF, Marco LA, Romano-Silva MA, Correa H. Obsessive-compulsive disorder and 5-HTTLPR. Revista brasileira de psiquiatria. 2009;31(3):287–8.
16. American Psychiatric Association. Diagnostic and statistical manual of mental disorders: DSM-IV. 4th ed. Washington: American Psychiatric Association; 1995.
17. Goodman WK, Price LH, Rasmussen SA, Mazure C, Delgado P, Heninger GR, Charney DS. The Yale-Brown Obsessive Compulsive Scale. II. Validity. Arch General Psychiatry. 1989;46(11):1012–6.
18. Hamilton M. A rating scale for depression. J Neurol Neurosurg Psychiatry. 1960;23:56–62.
19. Oldfield RC. The assessment and analysis of handedness: the Edinburgh inventory. Neuropsychologia. 1971;9(1):97–113.
20. Kaiser R, Muller-Oerlinghausen B, Filler D, Tremblay PB, Berghofer A, Roots I, Brockmoller J. Correlation between serotonin uptake in human blood platelets with the 44-bp polymorphism and the 17-bp variable number of tandem repeat of the serotonin transporter. Am J Med Genet. 2002;114(3):323–8.
21. Valente AA Jr, Miguel EC, Castro CC, Amaro E Jr, Duran FL, Buchpiguel CA, Chitnis X, McGuire PK, Busatto GF. Regional gray matter abnormalities in obsessive-compulsive disorder: a voxel-based morphometry study. Biol Psychiatry. 2005;58(6):479–87.
22. Yoo SY, Roh MS, Choi JS, Kang DH, Ha TH, Lee JM, Kim IY, Kim SI, Kwon JS. Voxel-based morphometry study of gray matter abnormalities in obsessive-compulsive disorder. J Korean Med Sci. 2008;23(1):24–30.
23. Kim JJ, Lee MC, Kim J, Kim IY, Kim SI, Han MH, Chang KH, Kwon JS. Grey matter abnormalities in obsessive-compulsive disorder: statistical parametric mapping of segmented magnetic resonance images. Br J Psychiatry. 2001;179:330–4.
24. McGuire PK, Bench CJ, Frith CD, Marks IM, Frackowiak RS, Dolan RJ. Functional anatomy of obsessive-compulsive phenomena. Br J Psychiatry. 1994;164(4):459–68.
25. Adler CM, McDonough-Ryan P, Sax KW, Holland SK, Arndt S, Strakowski SM. fMRI of neuronal activation with symptom provocation in unmedicated patients with obsessive compulsive disorder. J Psychiatr Res. 2000;34(4–5):317–24.
26. Atmaca M, Yildirim H, Ozdemir H, Ozler S, Kara B, Ozler Z, Kanmaz E, Mermi O, Tezcan E. Hippocampus and amygdalar volumes in patients with refractory obsessive-compulsive disorder. Prog Neuropsychopharmacol Biol Psychiatry. 2008;32(5):1283–6.
27. Hong SB, Shin YW, Kim SH, Yoo SY, Lee JM, Kim IY, Kim SI, Kwon JS. Hippocampal shape deformity analysis in obsessive-compulsive disorder. Eur Arch Psychiatry Clin Neurosci. 2007;257(4):185–90.
28. Hashimoto N, Nakaaki S, Kawaguchi A, Sato J, Kasai H, Nakamae T, Narumoto J, Miyata J, Furukawa TA, Mimura M. Brain structural abnormalities in behavior therapy-resistant obsessive-compulsive disorder revealed by voxel-based morphometry. Neuropsychiatr Disease Treat. 2014;10:1987–96.
29. Chen J, Silk T, Seal M, Dally K, Vance A. Widespread decreased grey and white matter in paediatric obsessive-compulsive disorder (OCD): a voxel-based morphometric MRI study. Psychiatry Res. 2013;213(1):11–7.
30. Russo M, Naro A, Mastroeni C, Morgante F, Terranova C, Muscatello MR, Zoccali R, Calabro RS, Quartarone A. Obsessive-compulsive disorder: a "sensory-motor" problem? Int J Psychophysiol. 2014;92(2):74–8.
31. Semendeferi K, Armstrong E, Schleicher A, Zilles K, Van Hoesen GW. Prefrontal cortex in humans and apes: a comparative study of area 10. Am J Phys Anthropol. 2001;114(3):224–41.
32. Burgess PW, Veitch E, de Lacy Costello A, Shallice T. The cognitive and neuroanatomical correlates of multitasking. Neuropsychologia. 2000;38(6):848–63.
33. Koechlin E, Hyafil A. Anterior prefrontal function and the limits of human decision-making. Science. 2007;318(5850):594–8.
34. Okuda J, Fujii T, Ohtake H, Tsukiura T, Yamadori A, Frith CD, Burgess PW. Differential involvement of regions of rostral prefrontal cortex (Brodmann area 10) in time- and event-based prospective memory. Int J Psychophysiol. 2007;64(3):233–46.
35. Posner MI, Sheese BE, Odludas Y, Tang Y. Analyzing and shaping human attentional networks. Neural Netw. 2006;19(9):1422–9.
36. Fletcher PC, Henson RN. Frontal lobes and human memory: insights from functional neuroimaging. Brain. 2001;124(Pt 5):849–81.
37. Cavedini P, Zorzi C, Piccinni M, Cavallini MC, Bellodi L. Executive dysfunctions in obsessive-compulsive patients and unaffected relatives: searching for a new intermediate phenotype. Biol Psychiatry. 2010;67(12):1178–84.
38. Olley A, Malhi G, Sachdev P. Memory and executive functioning in obsessive-compulsive disorder: a selective review. J Affect Disord. 2007;104(1–3):15–23.
39. Selvaraj S, Godlewska BR, Norbury R, Bose S, Turkheimer F, Stokes P, Rhodes R, Howes O, Cowen PJ. Decreased regional gray matter volume in S' allele carriers of the 5-HTTLPR triallelic polymorphism. Mol Psychiatry. 2011;16(5):472–3.
40. Eker MC, Kitis O, Okur H, Eker OD, Ozan E, Isikli S, Akarsu N, Gonul AS. Smaller hippocampus volume is associated with short variant of 5-HTTLPR polymorphism in medication-free major depressive disorder patients. Neuropsychobiology. 2011;63(1):22–8.
41. Frodl T, Zill P, Baghai T, Schule C, Rupprecht R, Zetzsche T, Bondy B, Reiser M, Moller HJ, Meisenzahl EM. Reduced hippocampal volumes associated with the long variant of the tri- and diallelic serotonin transporter polymorphism in major depression. Am J Med Genet B Neuropsychiatr Genet. 2008;147B(7):1003–7.
42. Frodl T, Meisenzahl EM, Zill P, Baghai T, Rujescu D, Leinsinger G, Bottlender R, Schule C, Zwanzger P, Engel RR, et al. Reduced hippocampal volumes associated with the long variant of the serotonin transporter polymorphism in major depression. Arch Gen Psychiatry. 2004;61(2):177–83.
43. Atmaca M, Onalan E, Yildirim H, Yuce H, Koc M, Korkmaz S, Mermi O. Serotonin transporter gene polymorphism implicates reduced orbitofrontal cortex in obsessive-compulsive disorder. J Anxiety Disord. 2011;25(5):680–5.
44. Frodl T, Koutsouleris N, Bottlender R, Born C, Jager M, Morgenthaler M, Scheuerecker J, Zill P, Baghai T, Schule C, et al. Reduced gray matter brain volumes are associated with variants of the serotonin transporter gene in major depression. Mol Psychiatry. 2008;13(12):1093–101.
45. Haier RJ, Jung RE, Yeo RA, Head K, Alkire MT. Structural brain variation and general intelligence. NeuroImage. 2004;23(1):425–33.
46. Wu K, Hanna GL, Easter P, Kennedy JL, Rosenberg DR, Arnold PD. Glutamate system genes and brain volume alterations in pediatric obsessive-compulsive disorder: a preliminary study. Psychiatry Res. 2013;211(3):214–20.
47. Olver JS, O'Keefe G, Jones GR, Burrows GD, Tochon-Danguy HJ, Ackermann U, Scott A, Norman TR. Dopamine D1 receptor binding in the striatum of patients with obsessive-compulsive disorder. J Affect Disord. 2009;114(1–3):321–6.

11

Effect of mirtazapine versus selective serotonin reuptake inhibitors on benzodiazepine use in patients with major depressive disorder: a pragmatic, multicenter, open-label, randomized, active-controlled, 24-week trial

Tasuku Hashimoto[1,9*], Akihiro Shiina[2,8], Tadashi Hasegawa[2,8], Hiroshi Kimura[1,7], Yasunori Oda[1], Tomihisa Niitsu[1,4], Masatomo Ishikawa[1], Masumi Tachibana[4], Katsumasa Muneoka[5], Satoshi Matsuki[3,6], Michiko Nakazato[3,7] and Masaomi Iyo[1]

Abstract

Background: This study aimed to evaluate whether selecting mirtazapine as the first choice for current depressive episode instead of selective serotonin reuptake inhibitors (SSRIs) reduces benzodiazepine use in patients with major depressive disorder (MDD). We concurrently examined the relationship between clinical responses and serum mature brain-derived neurotrophic factor (BDNF) and its precursor, proBDNF.

Methods: We conducted an open-label randomized trial in routine psychiatric practice settings. Seventy-seven MDD outpatients were randomly assigned to the mirtazapine or predetermined SSRIs groups, and investigators arbitrarily selected sertraline or paroxetine. The primary outcome was the proportion of benzodiazepine users at weeks 6, 12, and 24 between the groups. We defined patients showing a $\geq$50 % reduction in Hamilton depression rating scale (HDRS) scores from baseline as responders. Blood samples were collected at baseline, weeks 6, 12, and 24.

Results: Sixty-five patients prescribed benzodiazepines from prescription day 1 were analyzed for the primary outcome. The percentage of benzodiazepine users was significantly lower in the mirtazapine than in the SSRIs group at weeks 6, 12, and 24 (21.4 vs. 81.8 %; 11.1 vs. 85.7 %, both $P < 0.001$; and 12.5 vs. 81.8 %, $P = 0.0011$, respectively). No between-group difference was observed in HDRS score changes. Serum proBDNF levels were significantly decreased ($\chi^2 = 8.5$, $df = 3$, $P = 0.036$) and serum mature BDNF levels were temporarily significantly decreased ($F = 3.5$, $df = 2.4$, $P = 0.027$) in the responders of both groups at week 24.

Conclusion: This study demonstrated mirtazapine as the first-choice antidepressant for current depressive episodes may reduce benzodiazepine use in patients with MDD.

Trial registration UMIN000004144. Registered 2nd September 2010. The date of enrolment of the first participant to the trial was 24th August 2010. This study was retrospectively registered 9 days after the first participant was enrolled

Keywords: Depression, Mirtazapine, Benzodiazepines, Brain-derived neurotrophic factor, Serum

*Correspondence: t-hashimoto@faculty.chiba-u.jp
[1] Present Address: Department of Psychiatry, Graduate School of Medicine, Chiba University, 1-8-1 Inohana, Chuo-ku, Chiba 260-8670, Japan
Full list of author information is available at the end of the article

Background

Benzodiazepines and benzodiazepine-like drugs such as zolpidem and zopiclone are widely prescribed to improve insomnia and anxiety symptoms in combination with antidepressants for the pharmacological treatment of major depressive disorder (MDD) [1–3]. Evidence indicates that using benzodiazepines in conjunction with antidepressants in the first short-term treatment of MDD is effective [4, 5] and useful in preventing patients from dropout [4]. However, long-term use of benzodiazepines should be avoided because they elicit cognitive dysfunction, tolerance, dependence, and increase the risk of dementia in patients with MDD [5, 6], although a recent study has reported negative findings for the relationship between benzodiazepine use and the risk of dementia [7]. Therefore, it is important to establish a strategy for improving depression without using benzodiazepines from an early stage.

Mirtazapine is recognized as one of the first-line antidepressants for the treatment of MDD in addition to other antidepressants including selective serotonin reuptake inhibitors (SSRIs) [8, 9]. Mirtazapine has a unique pharmacological profile with not only α_2-adrenaline receptor antagonist activity but also histamine H_1 and serotonin $(5\text{-HT})_{2A}$ receptor antagonism, and it has hypnotic-like effects compared to the SSRIs and other first-line antidepressants [10]. In addition, mirtazapine has 5-HT_{2c} receptor antagonist activity, which is thought to be effective in the treatment of anxiety [11]. Moreover, it has been reported that the onset of clinical antidepressant responses to mirtazapine is faster than the onset with SSRIs [12, 13]. Considering that the actions of mirtazapine include hypnotic-like and fast-acting antidepressant effects, we hypothesized that selecting mirtazapine over other antidepressants including SSRIs as the first choice for a current depressive episode could reduce benzodiazepine use in patients with MDD.

Therefore, the primary purpose of this study was to determine whether treatment of current depressive episodes with mirtazapine could reduce the use of benzodiazepine in patients with MDD more than the representative SSRIs, sertraline and paroxetine could. Furthermore, the secondary purpose of this study was to compare the efficacy and safety of these three antidepressants in patients with MDD.

Accumulating preclinical and clinical studies have suggested that the brain-derived neurotrophic factor (BDNF) plays an important role in the pathophysiology of MDD and serum levels of BDNF may have the relationship with clinical responses to treatments for depression [14]. Moreover, recent studies have shown that serum levels of mature BDNF and proBDNF, which is a precursor form of mature BDNF, are successfully measured separately [15–17]. Furthermore, mature BDNF and proBDNF are reported to play different roles in neurophysiological functions via the tropomyosin receptor kinase B (TrkB) and p75 neurotrophin receptors, respectively [14, 18, 19]. Meta-analysis studies have shown that antidepressant treatments influence serum levels of BDNF in patients with MDD [20, 21]. However, the effects of antidepressant treatments on serum levels of mature BDNF and proBDNF in patients who are depressed are not well known. Therefore, we also determined whether serum levels of mature BDNF and proBDNF could be potential biomarkers of clinical responses to antidepressant treatments in patients with MDD.

Methods

Study design and participants

We conducted an open-label, randomized, and active-controlled 24-week trial in outpatients with current depressive episodes in routine psychiatric practice settings. The study participants were recruited from 13 sites in Japan, and the study was conducted from September 2010 to March 2014. This study was approved by the Institutional Review Boards and Ethics Committees of all the participating institutes and was performed in accordance with the ethical standards of the Helsinki Declaration of 1975, as revised in 2013. The trial was registered with the Clinical Trials Registry of the University Hospital Medical Information Network (UMIN, Tokyo, Japan, registration number UMIN000004144). All subjects provided written informed consent for their participation in the study after the procedure had been fully explained to them.

The inclusion criteria for prospective participants were: (1) age 20–75 years; (2) diagnosed according to the *Diagnostic and Statistical Manual of Mental Disorders, 4th Edition, Text Revision* criteria for MDD; (3) a $\geq$12 total score on the 17-item Hamilton depression rating scale (HDRS) [22]; (4) considered to require antidepressant treatment based on the judgment of the consulting psychiatrist. The exclusion criteria for participants were the following: (1) previous history of the use of mirtazapine or both sertraline and paroxetine; (2) pregnant or breast-feeding; (3) at significant risk for suicide; (4) diagnosed with a primary condition including dementia as well as bipolar, obsessive–compulsive, or eating disorders, schizophrenia, or alcohol or substance dependence except for tobacco dependence; (5) experiencing any medical conditions judged to render the patient ineligible to participate in the study.

Procedures

The participants in this study were treatment-seeking outpatients who personally visited each investigating hospital or clinic to consult about their current depressive symptoms. The participants were provided with the full details of the study modality and were informed that they were responsible for the usual consultation and medicine fees because the study was conducted in the routine psychiatric practice setting. The participants were randomly assigned to the mirtazapine or SSRIs groups in a 1:2 ratio. The computerized randomization program provided by EPS Associates Co., Ltd. (Tokyo, Japan) had a minimization algorithm with two prognostic factors, sex and sleep-related scores of the HDRS (i.e., low 0–3 or high 4–6). The investigators overseeing the SSRIs groups were free to choose either sertraline or paroxetine. If the participant had been taking other antidepressants before participating in this study, the drugs were tapered off during the first 4 weeks. The titration and tapering of the dosage of the investigational antidepressants were flexible and based on the clinical judgment of each investigator throughout the study.

Furthermore, each investigator prescribed benzodiazepines or benzodiazepine-like drugs such as zolpidem and zopiclone for insomnia or anxiety symptoms from the first day of the study after providing a sufficient explanation of the risks involved including dependence and sedation. In principle, the investigators were to prescribe the designated drugs of benzodiazepines for insomnia and anxiety symptoms of the participants. At the same time, they were also free to prescribe other benzodiazepines, zolpidem or zopiclone other than the designated benzodiazepines on the basis of the clinical judgement of each investigator-in-charge. In addition, the participants were provided with directions on how to administer the benzodiazepines according to the drug prescribing information and the original study instructions. Alternatively, the investigators were also allowed to avoid prescribing benzodiazepines when the patients did not wish to take them. The patients were directed to take the benzodiazepines when needed, similar to the pill-in-the-pocket approach according to each patient's judgment and not on a fixed schedule. The participants were required to maintain a daily record of taking the medication using specific notebooks, which were copied at every visit to check their compliance with the medication use and the use of the benzodiazepines. The patients were not informed that taking the benzodiazepines was one of the clinical outcomes of the study. Furthermore, they were provided with the usual medical consultation but were not treated with the specific psychotherapy for the purpose of reducing benzodiazepine use.

Blood samples were collected between 10:00 a.m. and 4:00 p.m. at baseline and weeks 6, 12, and 24 to measure the serum mature BDNF and proBDNF levels. The serum samples were rapidly delivered to the Department of Psychiatry, Chiba University Graduate School of Medicine in anticoagulant tubes at 4 °C and stored at −80 °C until analyzed.

Measurements of serum mature and precursor proBDNF levels

The mature BDNF and precursor proBDNF levels were measured using a human proBDNF enzyme-linked immunosorbent assay (ELISA) kit (Biosensis, Thebarton, SA, Australia) and the human mature BDNF ELISA Kit (Aviscera Bioscience, Santa Clara, CA, USA). All experiments were performed in duplicate according to the manufacturer's instructions. The optical density of the resulting reaction solutions in each well was measured using an automated microplate reader (Emax, Molecular Devices, Sunnyvale, CA, USA).

Assessments of clinical outcomes

The primary outcome of this study was the proportion of patients using benzodiazepines, denoted as "benzodiazepine users", at weeks 6, 12, and 24, which was compared for the two (mirtazapine and SSRIs) or three (mirtazapine, sertraline, and paroxetine) investigational groups. The benzodiazepine users and non-users were defined as patients who took benzodiazepine drugs once or more during the 1-week period prior to each assessment points (6, 12 and 24 weeks) or did not, respectively. Based on the frequencies of benzodiazepine use, the participants were distinguished into non-use, 1–6 days per week usage, and everyday usage and benzodiazepine users were defined as those in the 1–6 days per week usage or daily usage categories. To clarify the effect of each antidepressant on the use of benzodiazepines, we determined the number of patients in each group who were prescribed benzodiazepines from the first prescription day of the study and compared the proportion of benzodiazepine users between the groups. Therefore, the patients who did not want benzodiazepine prescriptions on the first day of the study were excluded from the primary outcome assessment.

The secondary outcomes were the efficacy and safety assessments of each antidepressant treatment, which were compared between the groups of patients prescribed benzodiazepines on the first day, and between the groups regardless of benzodiazepine prescription using an intent-to-treat analysis. To assess the severity of depressive symptoms, we used the HDRS and defined patients showing a ≥50 % reduction in HDRS scores from baseline to assessment day as responders, and those who did not as non-responders. We also assessed the self-reported inventory of depression using the Zung self-rating depression scale (SDS) questionnaire [23]. To assess the severity of sleep disturbances, we used the Athens insomnia scale (AIS) [24] and also administered the clinical global impressions-severity (CGI-S) scale [25]. The HDRS, SDS, AIS, and CGI-S scores were measured at baseline and weeks 1, 2, 6, 12, and 24. For the safety assessments, we collected information on all the adverse events (AEs) observed during this study, which were defined as serious AEs such as those leading to death, life-threatening conditions, hospitalizations, or persistent disability.

Assessments of relationship between clinical responses and serum BDNF levels

To explore the clinical applicability of serum mature BDNF and proBDNF measurements as biomarkers in depression treatment, we specifically examined the relationship between the clinical responses to antidepressant treatments and serum BDNF levels in both antidepressant groups using the following two approaches. One approach involved examining whether the measured baseline serum levels of mature BDNF and proBDNF would be adequate predictors of clinical responses to antidepressant treatments during the acute phase (e.g., 6–8 weeks) of depression treatment. Specifically, we examined the baseline levels of serum mature BDNF and proBDNF between responders and non-responders who were assessed at week 6. The other strategy was to evaluate the long-term effectiveness of antidepressant treatments by examining the associated changes in serum levels of mature BDNF and proBDNF in responders who achieved clinical responses by the final assessment day, week 24. Moreover, we also examined the ratio of the levels of mature BDNF and proBDNF according to a previous study [17].

Statistical analyses

The analyses of the primary outcome were performed in proportions of the benzodiazepine users at weeks 6, 12, and 24, between the groups of patients who were prescribed benzodiazepines from the first study day using a two-tailed Chi-square test or the Fisher's exact test.

The analyses of the efficacy outcomes were conducted on an intent-to-treat basis, and using a linear mixed-effects model for repeated measures (MMRM) with treatment group, week, and treatment group-by-week interaction as fixed effects and subject as a random effect. The Bonferroni adjustment was used for the multiple comparisons. The safety analyses were performed for the three groups of patients who took at least one dose of the prescribed antidepressant.

We used parametric tests to analyze the data of the serum mature BDNF levels while non-parametric tests were used for the serum proBDNF levels and the ratio of serum mature BDNF and proBDNF levels because these data did not follow a normal distribution although that of the mature BDNF did. We conducted an independent t test or the Mann–Whitney U test to compare the baseline levels of BDNF between the responders and non-responders. We used a repeated analysis of variance (ANOVA) for the serum mature BDNF levels while the Friedman's test was used for the proBDNF levels and the ratio of both proteins to examine the long-term effects of antidepressant treatments on continuous changes in serum BDNF levels.

A $P < 0.05$ was considered statistically significant in all analyses, which were conducted using the statistical package for the social sciences (SPSS) version 23.0 (IBM, NY, US).

We expected the proportions of benzodiazepine users to be 30.0 and 60.0 % in mirtazapine and SSRIs groups, respectively, according to a previous study [1] with an alpha error and power of 5.0 and 80.0 %, respectively. The total sample size of 120 participants was estimated with a consideration of a 20.0 % withdrawal. We allowed this study to be completed ahead of schedule when the result of the primary outcome was obviously confirmed by an interim analysis that was used to detect the difference in the proportions of benzodiazepine users at week 6 between the groups, which showed that the analysis achieved a $P < 0.001$ in the Chi-square test.

Results

Participants and clinical course outline

Of the 368 patients screened, 81 were enrolled in this study (Fig. 1). We perform an interim analysis of the data of 77 participants (Table 1) who were ready to be assessed by week 6 and subsequently terminated participant recruitment. The termination was instituted because we confirmed that the primary outcome results of the analysis had achieved a $P < 0.001$, and the proportions of benzodiazepine users in the mirtazapine and SSRIs groups were clearly distinct from each other. This indicated that we required a lower sample size than we originally expected.

Of the 18 patients assigned to receive paroxetine, ten and eight were prescribed the standard and controlled-release (CR) tablets, respectively. The daily mean peak doses of the antidepressants in this study were 27.2 ± 11.8, 73.4 ± 28.4, 24.0 ± 8.0, and 37.5 ± 10.8 mg in the mirtazapine and sertraline groups as well as paroxetine standard and paroxetine CR subgroups, respectively. The dose ranges of the mirtazapine, sertraline, paroxetine standard, and paroxetine CR antidepressants were as follows: 15.0–45.0, 25–100, 10–40, and 25–50 mg, respectively. Table 2 shows the breakdown of benzodiazepines prescribed to the 65 patients who were prescribed them from prescription day 1.

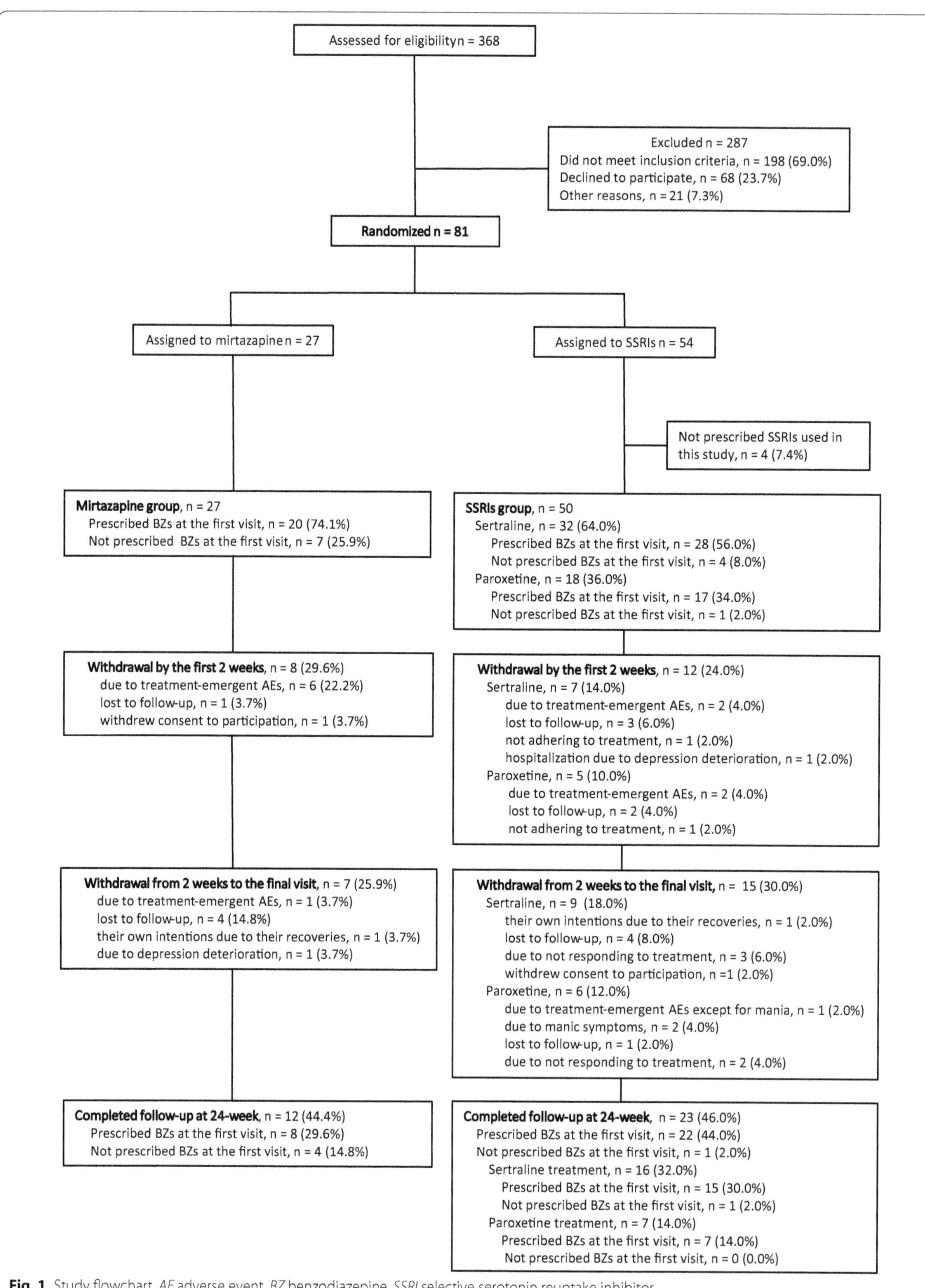

Fig. 1 Study flowchart. *AE* adverse event, *BZ* benzodiazepine, *SSRI* selective serotonin reuptake inhibitor

Table 1 Patient characteristics at baseline

Variable	Mirtazapine (*n* = 27)	SSRIs (*n* = 50)	*P*	Sertraline (*n* = 32)	Paroxetine (*n* = 18)	*P*
Male patients, *n* (%)	18 (66.7)	32 (64.0)	ns[c]	20 (62.5)	12 (66.7)	ns[c]
Age, mean (SD), years	38.9 (10.5)	40.4 (13.8)	ns[a]	39.7 (13.3)	41.7 (14.9)	ns[b]
Age at onset, mean (SD), years	38.1 (10.5)	39.3 (13.1)	ns[a]	39.0 (12.5)	39.8 (14.5)	ns[b]
Duration of illness, median [quartiles], week	30.0 [8.0–104.0]	20.0 [12.0–71.0]	ns[a]	20.0 [8.0–58.5]	19.0 [12.0–117.0]	ns[b]
Duration of current episode, median [quartiles], week	12.0 [7.0–40.0]	12.0 [8.0–34.0]	ns[a]	14.0 [7.3–44.0]	12.0 [12.0–21.0]	ns[b]
Depressive episodes			ns[c]			ns[c]
Single, *n* (%)	22 (81.5)	42 (84.0)		28 (87.5)	14 (77.8)	
Recurrent, *n* (%)[d]	5 (18.5)	8 (16.0)		4 (12.5)	4 (22.2)	
Past history of using any psychiatric services, *n* (%)	4 (14.8)	15 (30.0)	ns[c]	11 (34.4)	4 (22.2)	ns[c]
Past history of any psychotropic medication, *n* (%)	11 (40.7)	18 (36.0)	ns[c]	14 (43.8)	4 (22.2)	ns[c]
Treatments of the current episode, *n* (%)	4 (14.8)	5 (10.0)	ns[c]	5 (15.6)	0 (0.0)	ns[c]
Antidepressant treatment of the current episode, *n* (%)	3 (11.1)	3 (6.0)	ns[c]	3 (9.4)	0 (0.0)	ns[c]
Benzodiazepine treatment of the current episode, *n* (%)	1 (3.7)	1 (2.0)	ns[c]	1 (3.1)	0 (0.0)	ns[c]
HDRS, mean (SD)	23.0 (5.2)	23.1 (6.1)	ns[a]	23.2 (6.2)	22.9 (6.0)	ns[b]
SDS, mean (SD)	55.9 (5.4)	57.9 (7.8)	ns[a]	57.9 (7.4)	57.9 (7.1)	ns[b]
AIS, mean (SD)	11.2 (3.7)	12.9 (4.4)	ns[a]	12.8 (4.3)	13.1 (4.7)	ns[b]
CGI-S, median [quartiles]	4.0 [4.0–5.0]	4.0 [4.0–5.0]	ns[a]	4.5 [4.0–5.0]	4.0 [4.0–5.0]	ns[b]

SSRI selective serotonin reuptake inhibitor, *SD* standard variation, *HDRS* 17-item Hamilton depression rating scale, *SDS* Zung self-rating depression scale, *AIS* Athens insomnia scale, *CGI-S* clinical global impressions-severity

[a] Unpaired *t* test or Mann–Whitney *U* test

[b] One-way analysis of variance (ANOVA) or Kruskal–Wallis test

[c] Chi-square test or Fisher exact test

[d] Maximum number of recurrent episodes is two

Table 2 Breakdown of prescribed benzodiazepines

Benzodiazepines	Mirtazapine (*n* = 20)[a]	SSRIs (*n* = 45)[a]	Sertraline (*n* = 28)[a]	Paroxetine (*n* = 17)[a]
As hypnotics				
Brotizolam	12	22	9	13
Estazolam	1	0	0	0
Flunitrazepam	0	5	4	1
Nitrazepam	1	1	1	0
Rilmazafone	0	1	1	0
Triazolam	0	4	3	1
Zopiclone	0	1	1	0
Zolpidem	1	0	0	0
As anxiolytics				
Alprazolam	2	7	1	6
Bromazepam	0	5	5	0
Etizolam	2	5	5	0
Clotiazepam	0	2	2	0
Lorazepam	7	16	9	7

[a] Patients prescribed benzodiazepines at baseline (day 1) were only counted in numbers in this table

Primary outcome: group proportions of benzodiazepine users

Table 3 shows the frequencies of the benzodiazepine users for the groups at each assessment point. As shown in Fig. 2, the percentage of benzodiazepine users at week 6 in the mirtazapine group (21.4 %) was significantly lower than that in the SSRIs group (81.8 %, Fig. 2a). Similarly, the percentage of benzodiazepine users at weeks 12 and 24 was significantly lower in the mirtazapine group (11.1 and 12.5 %) than it was in the SSRIs group (85.7 and 81.8 %, Fig. 2b, c), respectively. Comparing the three antidepressant groups, the percentage of benzodiazepine users in the mirtazapine group was significantly lower than that sertraline and paroxetine groups were at weeks 6, 12, and 24 (Fig. 3a–c). Conversely, there were no significant differences in the percentages of benzodiazepine users between the mirtazapine and SSRIs groups at weeks 1 and 2 (52.9 vs. 72.1 and 53.3 vs. 66.7 %, respectively).

Table 3 Frequencies of benzodiazepine use in participants

	Baseline[a]	Week 1	Week 2	Week 6	Week 12	Week 24
Mirtazapine	*n* = 20	***n* = 17**	***n* = 15**	***n* = 14**	***n* = 9**	***n* = 8**
Non-use, *n* (%)		8 (47.1)	7 (46.7)	11 (78.6)	8 (88.9)	7 (87.5)
1–6 days per week, *n* (%)		5 (29.4)	4 (26.7)	1 (7.1)	0 (0.0)	0 (0.0)
Every day, *n* (%)		4 (23.5)	4 (26.7)	2 (14.3)	1 (11.1)	1 (12.5)
SSRIs	*n* = 45	***n* = 43**	***n* = 42**	***n* = 33**	***n* = 28**	***n* = 22**
Non-use, *n* (%)		12 (27.9)	14 (33.3)	6 (18.2)	4 (14.3)	4 (18.2)
1–6 days per week, *n* (%)		15 (34.9)	8 (19.0)	12 (36.4)	9 (32.1)	4 (18.2)
Every day, *n* (%)		16 (37.2)	20 (47.6)	15 (45.5)	15 (53.6)	14 (63.6)
Sertraline	*n* = 28	***n* = 26**	***n* = 26**	***n* = 22**	***n* = 19**	***n* = 15**
Non-use, *n* (%)		7 (26.9)	9 (34.6)	5 (22.7)	3 (15.8)	3 (20.0)
1–6 days per week, *n* (%)		8 (30.8)	4 (15.4)	7 (31.8)	5 (26.3)	2 (13.3)
Every day, *n* (%)		11 (42.3)	13 (50.0)	10 (45.5)	11 (57.9)	10 (66.7)
Paroxetine	*n* = 17	***n* = 17**	***n* = 16**	***n* = 11**	***n* = 9**	***n* = 7**
Non-use, *n* (%)		5 (29.4)	5 (31.3)	1 (9.1)	1 (11.1)	1 (14.3)
1–6 day per week, n (%)		7 (41.2)	4 (25.0)	5 (45.5)	4 (44.4)	2 (28.6)
Every day, *n* (%)		5 (29.4)	7 (43.8)	5 (45.5)	4 (44.4)	4 (57.1)

SSRI selective serotonin reuptake inhibitor

[a] Patients prescribed benzodiazepines at baseline (day 1) were only counted in numbers in this table

Efficacy

Regardless of whether the participants received benzodiazepine prescriptions from day 1, the average HDRS, SDS, AIS, and CGI-S total scores for each group were significantly decreased compared with those at the baseline, as determined using the MMRM ($P < 0.05$). Table 4 shows the sequential measurements of the efficacy outcomes for all participants. The difference in the changes in the HDRS scores were not statistically significant between the mirtazapine and SSRIs groups ($F = 0.37$, $df = 1, 78$; mean difference, 95 % confidence interval [CI] −0.78 [−3.31 to 1.76], $P = 0.54$) or among the three groups ($F = 0.49$, $df = 2, 76$, $P = 0.62$). In addition, there was no statistical difference in the changes in the AIS and CGI-S scores between the mirtazapine and SSRIs groups (AIS: $F = 2.23$, $df = 1, 73$; mean difference, 95 % CI −1.32 [−3.07 to 0.44], $P = 0.14$; CGI-S: $F = 1.11$, $df = 1, 78$; mean difference, 95 % CI −0.19 [−0.56 to 0.17], $P = 0.30$), and among the three groups (AIS: $F = 3.10$, $df = 2, 70$, $P = 0.051$; CGI-S: $F = 0.80$, $df = 2, 76$, $P = 0.45$). Regarding the SDS, the difference in the changes in SDS scores was not statistically significant between the mirtazapine and SSRIs groups ($F = 3.40$, $df = 1, 79$; mean difference, 95 % CI −3.30 [−6.86 to 0.26], $P = 0.069$); however, there was a significant difference among the three groups ($F = 3.29$, $df = 2, 76$, $P = 0.043$). Specifically, there were significantly different changes in the SDS scores between the mirtazapine and paroxetine groups (mean difference 95 % CI −5.74 [−11.22 to −0.25], $P = 0.038$), indicating that the SDS scores of the mirtazapine group had improved more significantly than those of the paroxetine group. Similarly, the analyses of the data of patients who were prescribed benzodiazepines from day 1 revealed that the differences in the changes from the baseline HDRS, AIS, and CGI-S scores were not statistically significant between the mirtazapine and SSRIs groups as well as among the three groups (data not shown). In contrast to the analysis of the data of all the participants, there were no significant differences in the HDRS, AIS, and CGI-S (data not shown) as well as the SDS between the mirtazapine and SSRIs groups (SDS: $F = 3.05$, $df = 1, 67$, $P = 0.085$) and among the three groups (SDS: $F = 2.45$, $df = 2, 64$, $P = 0.095$) in the patients who were prescribed benzodiazepines from day 1.

Safety analysis

Table 5 shows the details of all treatment-emergent AEs observed in this study. The AEs that led to the discontinuation of study participation appeared within the first 2 weeks except for the case of abnormal liver function tests, which was observed at week 6. However, the affected patients recovered after withdrawing from the study except for the patients with the SAEs. The analysis of the incidence rate of AEs revealed that the proportions of the patients with any AEs differed among the three antidepressant groups ($\chi^2 = 12.5$, $df = 2$, $P = 0.0019$). Specifically, the percentage of patients with any AEs was significantly lower in the sertraline (7/32, 21.9 %) group

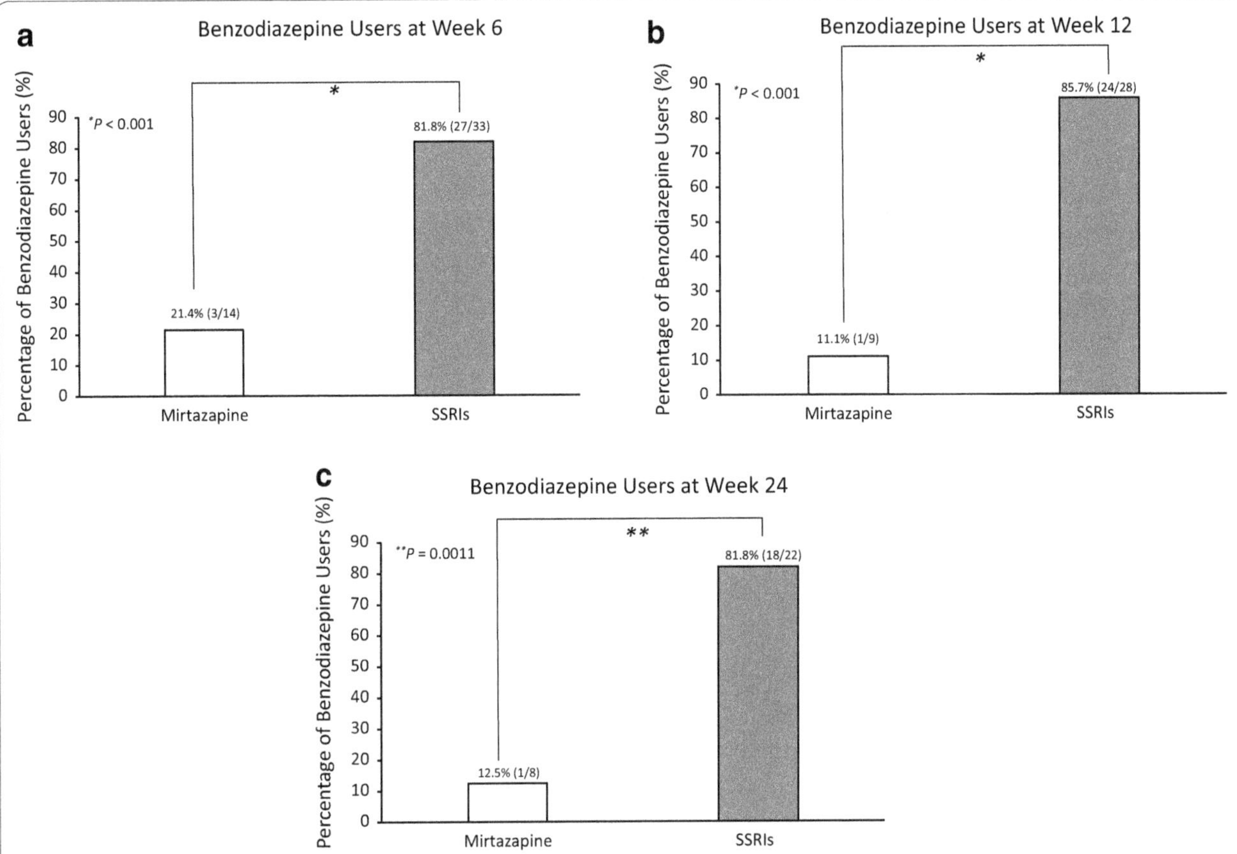

Fig. 2 Proportions of benzodiazepine users in mirtazapine and selective serotonin reuptake inhibitors (SSRIs) groups. *Numbers in parentheses* above *bars* are actual numbers of benzodiazepine users and group participants assessed each week. Benzodiazepine users are defined as patients who took benzodiazepine drugs once or more during the 1-week period prior to each assessment point (weeks 6, 12, and 24). Patients were prescribed benzodiazepines from study day 1. *P* values are based on analyses of Chi-square (**a**) and Fisher's exact test (**b**, **c**). *SSRI* selective serotonin reuptake inhibitor

than in the mirtazapine (16/27, 59.3 %, $\chi^2 = 8.6$, $df = 1$, $P = 0.034$) and paroxetine (12/18, 66.7 %, $\chi^2 = 9.8$, $df = 1$, $P = 0.0017$) groups.

Relationship between clinical responses and serum BDNF levels

Table 6 shows the comparisons of the baseline levels of mature BDNF, proBDNF, and their ratios between the responders and non-responders in both groups at week 6. There were no significant differences in the baseline levels of each BDNF protein between the two groups (Table 6).

Table 7 shows the long-term effectiveness of the antidepressant treatments on serum BDNF levels in 27 responders of both groups on the final assessment day at week 24. Of the 35 patients who completed the study, there were technical failures in the samples of five while three did not achieve a clinical response by week 24. The serum levels of the mature BDNF decreased significantly between weeks 6 and 12 from the baseline levels but the change did not persist (Table 7). Furthermore, the serum proBDNF levels of the responders who achieved clinical responses by week 24 were statistically significantly decreased when compared to the baseline levels (Table 7).

Discussion

Three interesting results in this study are of particular significance and worth expounding. First, among the patients with depression who were prescribed both an antidepressant and benzodiazepines from the beginning of the treatment, our results showed that there was a significantly smaller proportion of benzodiazepine users in the mirtazapine treatment group than there was in the SSRIs treatment group. However, the efficacy of mirtazapine in treating depression was not different from that of the SSRIs. Second, the safety assessment revealed that the proportion of patients who experienced treatment-emergent AEs was significantly lower in the sertraline group than it was in the mirtazapine and paroxetine

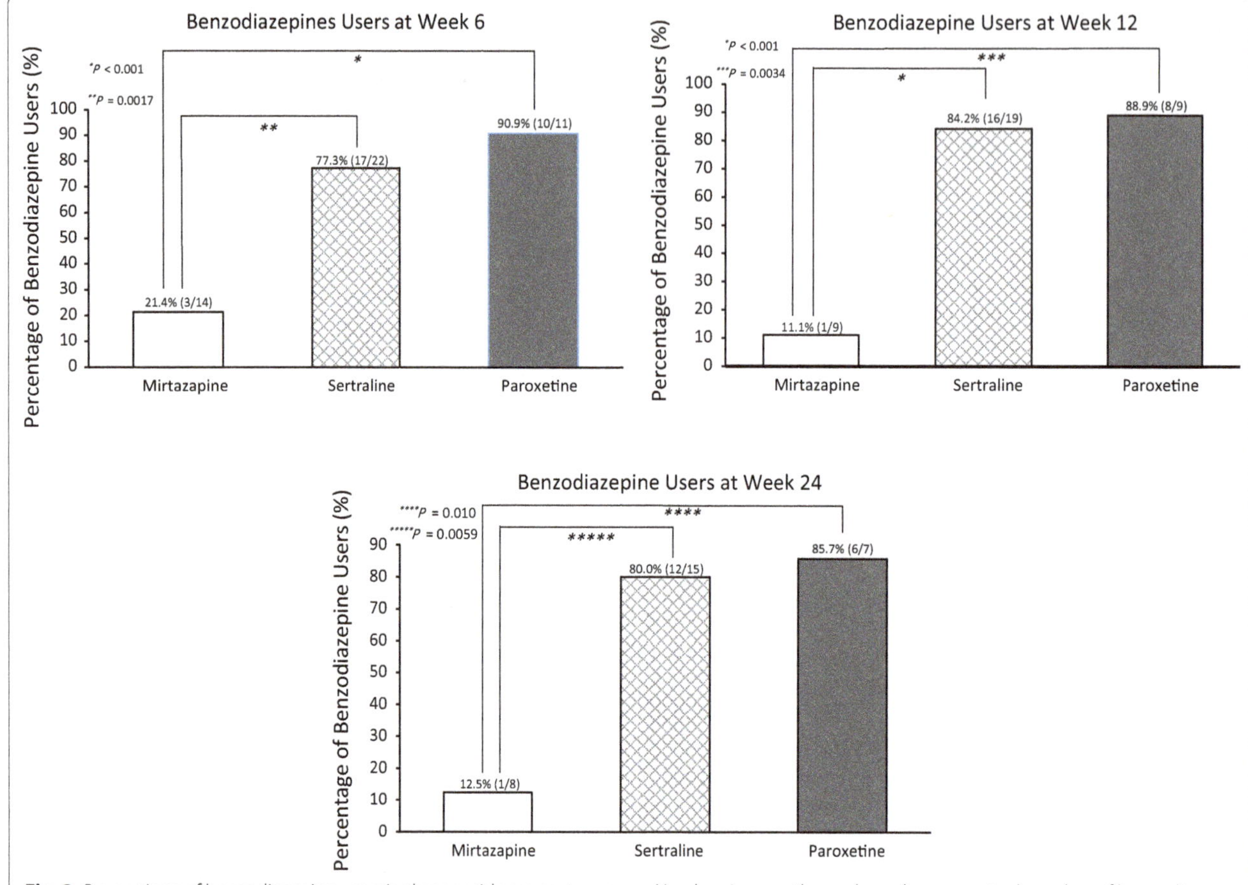

Fig. 3 Proportions of benzodiazepine users in three antidepressants groups. *Numbers in parentheses* above *bars* are actual number of benzodiazepine users and group participants assessed each week. Benzodiazepine users are defined as patients who took benzodiazepine drugs once or more during the 1-week period prior to each assessment point (weeks 6, 12, and 24). Patients were prescribed benzodiazepines from study day 1. We analyzed differences in the proportions in two groups using Chi-square test at week 6 (**a**) and Fisher's exact test at week 12 and 24 (**b**, **c**), after the analyses were conducted among the three groups using Chi-square test at week 6 and the Fisher's exact test at week 12 and 24. *P* values are based on analyses of Chi-square (**a**) and the Fisher exact test (**b**, **c**)

groups. Third, the present study showed that the serum proBDNF levels of the responders who achieved clinical responses in both antidepressant groups at the final assessment day, at week 24, were significantly decreased compared to the baseline levels, while the serum mature BDNF levels significantly decreased from week 6 to 12, but only temporarily, and this effect did not persist till week 24.

The results of our analysis revealed that among the depressed patients prescribed both an antidepressant and benzodiazepines at the beginning of treatment, there was a significantly smaller proportion of benzodiazepine users that were treated with mirtazapine than were treated with SSRIs. However, the efficacy of mirtazapine in depression treatment was not different from that of the SSRIs. These results are compatible with our hypothesis. A previous meta-analysis of the discontinuation of benzodiazepine use demonstrated that the effective strategies are mainly psychological interventions combined with regimens such as a gradual reduction in the dose of prescribed benzodiazepines [26–28]. Although numerous studies have indicated the benefits of discontinuing benzodiazepine use in pharmacotherapy, effective pharmacological interventions have not yet been established to replace them [26–29]. Although restricting or discontinuing the use of benzodiazepines is strongly recommended in the treatment of depression, this has been challenging to achieve in routine clinical practice [26]. Therefore, antidepressant treatments without benzodiazepines from the acute phase or the first stage of treatment of major depression are considered useful for reducing the number of benzodiazepine users. Furthermore, the findings of the present study have identified the antidepressant from the first-line recommended agents that

Table 4 Sequential measurements of clinical efficacy outcomes

Variables	Baseline	Week 1	Week 2	Week 6	Week 12	Week 24
	Estimated marginal means (SE)					
HDRS						
Mirtazapine	23.0 (1.2)	19.0 (1.3)	15.5 (1.3)	9.6 (1.4)	9.3 (1.5)	5.9 (1.6)
SSRIs	23.1 (0.9)	19.2 (0.9)	16.9 (0.9)	12.9 (1.0)	9.5 (1.0)	5.4 (1.1)
Sertraline	23.2 (1.1)	19.1 (1.2)	16.3 (1.1)	12.1 (1.2)	8.7 (1.3)	5.3 (1.4)
Paroxetine	22.9 (1.5)	19.4 (1.5)	17.8 (1.5)	14.6 (1.7)	11.2 (1.8)	5.8 (2.0)
SDS						
Mirtazapine	56.0 (1.7)	52.4 (1.8)	46.6 (1.8)	44.0 (1.9)	43.7 (2.1)	38.0 (2.2)
SSRIs	57.6 (1.3)	54.8 (1.3)	52.8 (1.3)	48.7 (1.4)	44.9 (1.5)	41.8 (1.6)
Sertraline	57.4 (1.6)	54.1 (1.7)	51.2 (1.6)	47.2 (1.7)	42.4 (1.8)	40.3 (1.9)
Paroxetine	57.9 (2.1)	56.1 (2.1)	55.0 (2.1)	51.4 (2.3)	49.8 (2.5)	44.5 (2.8)
AIS						
Mirtazapine	11.5 (0.9)	8.4 (0.9)	6.6 (0.9)	5.8 (1.0)	6.8 (1.1)	5.0 (1.1)
SSRIs	12.9 (0.6)	10.2 (0.6)	9.3 (0.6)	7.5 (0.7)	6.6 (0.7)	5.5 (0.8)
Sertraline	12.8 (0.8)	10.0 (0.8)	8.1 (0.8)	6.9 (0.8)	5.3 (0.9)	4.6 (1.0)
Paroxetine	13.1 (1.0)	10.5 (1.0)	11.3 (1.0)	8.8 (1.2)	9.2 (1.2)	7.2 (1.4)
CGI-S						
Mirtazapine	4.4 (0.2)	3.8 (0.2)	3.2 (0.2)	2.8 (0.2)	2.6 (0.2)	1.8 (0.2)
SSRIs	4.3 (0.1)	4.0 (0.1)	3.6 (0.1)	3.1 (0.1)	2.7 (0.1)	2.1 (0.2)
Sertraline	4.4 (0.2)	4.0 (0.2)	3.6 (0.2)	3.0 (0.2)	2.6 (0.2)	2.1 (0.2)
Paroxetine	4.2 (0.2)	4.1 (0.2)	3.6 (0.2)	3.5 (0.2)	3.0 (0.3)	2.0 (0.3)

All values are based on estimated marginal means using a linear mixed effects model for repeated measures data

SSRI selective serotonin reuptake inhibitor, *HDRS* 17-item Hamilton depression rating scale, *SDS* Zung self-rating depression scale, *AIS* Athens insomnia scale, *SE* standard error

influence the persistent use of benzodiazepines in the treatment of patients with MDD. Specifically, our results suggest that prescribing mirtazapine as the first antidepressant to be administered could potentially prevent patients who are depressed from having to continuously take benzodiazepines. Further comprehensive, double-blind studies would be required to confirm this finding.

The efficacy analysis of this study revealed there were no statistically significant differences in the changes in the HDRS scores between the mirtazapine and the SSRIs groups as well as between the three groups. These results are consistent with the findings of a meta-analysis study of mirtazapine versus other antidepressants including SSRIs [13]. Additionally, the mirtazapine group improved more than the paroxetine group did in the change in SDS scores. It is difficult to explain the discrepancy between the HDRS and SDS scores of the mirtazapine and paroxetine groups in this study because two meta-analysis studies previously demonstrated a lack of difference in the efficacy of mirtazapine and paroxetine [13, 30]. A plausible explanation is that the paroxetine group had a smaller size than the mirtazapine group did, which might have influenced the results. The efficacy of ameliorating sleep disturbances, as determined by the AIS assessment, showed no statistically significant differences between the groups. Considering that the efficacy of mirtazapine in treating depressive symptoms and sleep disturbances is not different from that of the SSRIs, the present findings could support mirtazapine as the first choice for the treatment of major depression because of its advantage of decreasing the benzodiazepine requirement compared to the SSRIs.

The safety analysis demonstrated that the proportion of patients who experienced treatment-emergent AEs was significantly lower in the sertraline group than it was in the mirtazapine and paroxetine groups. These results are consistent with the findings of a previous meta-analysis study [31] that demonstrated the high tolerability of sertraline and relatively low tolerability of mirtazapine and paroxetine in patients with MDD.

Focusing on the AEs of mirtazapine, our results showed that sedation, including somnolence, very likely caused the discontinuation of the drug in the early stage of the treatment of major depression. Although it has been reported that the effectiveness of mirtazapine on sleep disturbance appears very quickly [32], sedation caused by mirtazapine occurs with high frequency (50 % or more) [9]. The improvement of sleep disturbance and sedation

Table 5 Summary of treatment-emergent adverse events (AEs)

	Mirtazapine, $n = 27$ *n* (%)	Sertraline, $n = 32$ *n* (%)	Paroxetine, $n = 18$ *n* (%)
Total number of patients with AEs	16 (59.3)	7 (21.9)	12 (66.7)
Serious AEs (SAEs)	0 (0.0)	2 (6.3)	0 (0.0)
Brain hemorrhage[a]	0 (0.0)	1 (3.1)	0 (0.0)
Hospitalization due to depression deterioration	0 (0.0)	1 (3.1)	0 (0.0)
AEs leading to discontinuation except for SAEs	7 (25.9)	1 (3.1)	5 (27.8)
Sedation including somnolence	3 (11.1)	0 (0.0)	0 (0.0)
Insomnia	1 (3.7)	0 (0.0)	0 (0.0)
Abnormal liver function test	1 (3.7)	0 (0.0)	0 (0.0)
Eruption	1 (3.7)	0 (0.0)	0 (0.0)
Dysgeusia	1 (3.7)	0 (0.0)	0 (0.0)
Nausea	0 (0.0)	1 (3.1)	1 (5.6)
Sexual dysfunction (erection failure)	0 (0.0)	0 (0.0)	1 (5.6)
Mania	0 (0.0)	0 (0.0)	2 (11.1)
Panic attack	0 (0.0)	0 (0.0)	1 (5.6)
Specific symptoms of AEs except for SAEs			
Sedation including somnolence	9 (33.3)	0 (0.0)	3 (16.7)
Insomnia	2 (3.7)	1 (3.1)	0 (0.0)
Akathisia	1 (3.7)	0 (0.0)	2 (11.1)
Irritability	1 (3.7)	1 (3.1)	1 (5.6)
Mania	0 (0.0)	0 (0.0)	2 (11.1)
Weight increased	3 (11.1)	0 (0.0)	0 (0.0)
Increased appetite	1 (3.7)	0 (0.0)	0 (0.0)
Headache	0 (0.0)	0 (0.0)	2 (11.1)
Dizziness	0 (0.0)	0 (0.0)	1 (5.6)
Nausea	1 (3.7)	5 (15.6)	4 (22.2)
Fatigue	3 (11.1)	0 (0.0)	2 (11.1)
Eruption	1 (3.7)	0 (0.0)	0 (0.0)
Abnormal liver function test	1 (3.7)	0 (0.0)	0 (0.0)
Dysgeusia	1 (3.7)	0 (0.0)	0 (0.0)
Sexual dysfunction (erection failure)	0 (0.0)	0 (0.0)	1 (5.6)
Hyperhidrosis	0 (0.0)	0 (0.0)	2 (11.1)
Constipation	0 (0.0)	0 (0.0)	1 (5.6)

AE adverse event, *SAE* serious adverse event

[a] Brain hemorrhage was unrelated to sertraline administration according to the diagnosis by the neurosurgeon. All AEs were treatment emergent

Table 6 Baseline serum brain-derived neurotrophic factor (BDNF) levels of responders and non-responders at week 6

	Responders, $n = 24$	Non-responders, $n = 29$	Statistics	*P*
Levels at baseline				
Mature BDNF (ng/mL), mean (SD)	12.8 (3.8)	13.4 (3.4)	$t = -0.67, df = 51$	0.51
ProBDNF (pg/mL), median [quartiles]	607.5 [84.4, 5158.3]	135.0 [45.6, 2803.5]	$Z = -1.3$	0.18
Ratio of mature BDNF/proBDNF[a]	25.7 [2.3, 146.8]	105.7 [4.7, 309.2]	$Z = -1.3$	0.21

Responders and non-responders were assessed at week 6

BDNF brain-derived neurotrophic factor, *SD* standard deviation

[a] Ratio is serum level of mature BDNF (pg/mL) divided by that of proBDNF (pg/mL) in each individual. Serum mature BDNF levels were analyzed using Student *t* test. Serum proBDNF and ratio of mature BDNF/proBDNF were analyzed using Mann–Whitney *U* test

Table 7 Long-term changes in serum levels of brain-derived neurotrophic factor (BDNF) in responders at week 24

	Baseline	Week 6	Week 12	Week 24	Statistics	P
Mature BDNF (ng/mL), EMS (SE)	12.7 (0.7)	11.2 (0.7)[a]	11.8 (0.7)[a]	12.1 (0.7)	$F = 3.5, df = 2.4$	0.027*
ProBDNF (pg/mL), median [quartiles]	634.7 [92.4, 5381.8]	507.9 [95.6, 4975.8]	484.5 [82.5, 4471.0]	463.5 [109.5, 4018.4][b]	$\chi^2 = 8.5, df = 3$	0.036*
Ratio of mature BDNF/proBDNF, median [quartiles]	22.7 [2.1, 135.6]	27.0 [2.3, 115.5]	29.3 [2.7, 127.8]	30.4 [3.1, 153.6]	$\chi^2 = 1.6, df = 3$	0.67

Serum mature BDNF levels were analyzed using repeated measure analysis of variance (ANOVA). Adjustment for multiple comparisons was Bonferroni. Serum proBDNF levels and ratio of mature BDNF/proBDNF levels were analyzed using Friedman's test followed by Wilcoxon signed rank test

BDNF brain-derived neurotrophic factor, *EMS* estimated marginal means, *SE* standard error, *CI* confidence interval

[a] Mean differences in serum mature BDNF levels at week 6 (−1.4 ng/mL, SE = 0.5, 95 % CI −2.7 to −0.07, $P = 0.035$) and at week 12 (−0.8 ng/mL, SE = 0.3, 95 % CI −1.7 to −0.01, $P = 0.045$) were significantly decreased compared to the baseline levels

[b] Serum proBDNF levels at week 24 were significantly decreased compared to the baseline levels ($Z = -2.4, P = 0.019$). *$P < 0.05$, $n = 27$

with mirtazapine treatment is thought to be inextricably linked. Therefore, mirtazapine as the first-choice agent in depression treatment could be expected to effectively treat depression without the use of benzodiazepines by its rapid onset of clinical action and improvement of sleep disturbance [12, 13, 32, 33]. However, it would be necessary to implement considerations and strategies to reduce the risk of early dropout due to sedation.

The present study showed that serum proBDNF levels of the responders who achieved clinical responses in both antidepressant groups at the final assessment day were significantly decreased at week 24 compared to the baseline levels. Furthermore, the serum mature BDNF levels significantly decreased from week 6 to 12, but the change did not persist up to week 24. To the best of our knowledge, this is the first report to show the changes in serum levels of mature BDNF and proBDNF following antidepressant treatment in patients who are depressed and achieved clinical responses. A previous study by Yoshimura et al. [16] reported there were no changes in the serum levels of mature BDNF and proBDNF in patients with MDD, who were administrated fluvoxamine for 4 weeks. Our findings are inconsistent with their results, and a plausible reason is that the experimental conditions of these two studies differed. Specifically, our present study focused on clinical responders, and the duration was 24 weeks, which differed from that of Yoshimura et al. [16] that had a 4-week duration. The present results may not have provided practical biomarkers as predictors of clinical responses because the serum levels of mature BDNF changed erratically and the decrease in serum proBDNF levels was too slow. However, our present findings may contribute to the understanding of the physiological roles of mature BDNF and proBDNF in the timing of the clinical responses and effectiveness of antidepressant treatments in patients with MDD. The physiological mechanisms and dynamics of serum mature BDNF and proBDNF levels in mood disorders such as major depression and bipolar disorder are still unclear and remain to be elucidated. Furthermore, a recent meta-analysis reports that the peripheral blood levels of BDNF in patients with bipolar disorder with manic and depressive episodes are decreased, but those with euthymia are not altered compared to healthy controls [34]. In contrast, Södersten et al. [17] reported that the serum levels of mature BDNF are higher in patients with bipolar disorder than they are in the controls. Further studies are needed to identify the effects of antidepressants on blood levels of mature BDNF and proBDNF using larger sample sizes, to clarify their physiological mechanisms in mood disorders such as major depression and bipolar disorder.

In addition, there were no differences in the level of mature BDNF, proBDNF, and the ratio of mature BDNF/proBDNF at the baseline between the responders and non-responders assessed at week 6. Previous studies, which did not distinguish between mature BDNF and proBDNF, showed incongruous findings that serum BDNF levels would be useful as a predictor of responses to antidepressant treatments in patients who are depressed [35–37]. Our results do not support measuring mature BDNF and proBDNF at pre-treatment as a useful predictor of responses to antidepressant treatment in patients with MDD.

There are four main limitations to this study, which are worth mentioning. First, as a prospective, randomized, open-label, blinded endpoint (PROBE) procedure, the investigators were aware of the primary endpoint in this study. Therefore, there was a possibility that the investigators emphasized to the patients the effect of mirtazapine on sleep disturbance. This could have led to a potential placebo effect on those who took mirtazapine. Furthermore, this issue is a technical inevitability in an open study. Therefore, a double-blind, randomized clinical trial (RCT) would be needed to confirm our results. Second, the numbers of dropouts were too numerous to accurately assess the effects of antidepressant treatments in this study. Regarding the pragmatic aspects of conducting clinical trials, Rutherford et al. [38] reported that the frequency of patient visits influences the dropout rate in antidepressant treatment [38]. The assessment intervals in this study were 1 week or more even in the first 4 weeks because the priority was to ensure a routine psychiatric practice setting was maintained above the experimental considerations. Previous survey studies of antidepressant prescriptions for treating depression in general clinical practice demonstrated that patients discontinue an initial antidepressant in the first 4 weeks at a rate of 26.2–42.4 % [39–42]. The present results of the dropout rate evaluation were similar to the previously reported rates in general clinical practice [39–42]. To elucidate the effectiveness of antidepressants on the continuous use of benzodiazepines further, the rate of visit frequencies of future studies should be higher than they were in this study. Third, sertraline and paroxetine were not randomized in this study. The patients randomly assigned to the SSRIs group were prescribed sertraline or paroxetine according to each investigator's assessment and judgment. We incorporated a pragmatic trial design into real-life practice settings rather than an exploratory study design [43]. To clarify the findings of the present study, further studies that are strictly designed, such as a double-blind RCT, are necessary. Fourth, the sample size of this study was small and, therefore, we were unable to examine the potential applicability of the serum BDNF level as a biomarker of clinical antidepressant drug responses. Further studies with a larger sample size would be required to verify this.

Conclusions

This study showed the possibility of mirtazapine as the first-choice antidepressant for current depressive episodes by revealing its potential as an effective strategy to reduce the use of benzodiazepines in patients with major depression.

Abbreviations

SSRI: selective serotonin reuptake inhibitor; MDD: major depressive disorder; BDNF: brain-derived neurotrophic factor; HDRS: Hamilton depression rating scale; TrkB: tropomyosin receptor kinase B; UMIN: University Hospital Medical Information Network; ELISA: enzyme-linked immunosorbent assay; SDS: Zung self-rating depression scale; AIS: Athens insomnia scale; CGI-S: global impressions-severity; AE: adverse event; MMRM: mixed effects model for repeated measures; ANOVA: repeated analysis of variance; SPSS: statistical package for the social sciences; CR: controlled release; SAE: serious adverse event; PROBE: prospective, randomized, open-label, blinded endpoint; RCT: randomized clinical trial.

Authors' contributions

THash, MIshi and MIyo contributed to the design of this study. THash, AS, THase, HK, TN, MT, KM, SM, and MN recruited and assessed the patients enrolled in this study. YO contributed to measurement of serum levels of BDNF. THash, TN, and MIyo conducted the statistical analysis. THash was the principal investigator of this study. All authors read and approved the final manuscript.

Author details

[1] Present Address: Department of Psychiatry, Graduate School of Medicine, Chiba University, 1-8-1 Inohana, Chuo-ku, Chiba 260-8670, Japan. [2] Department of Psychiatry, Chiba University Hospital, 1-8-1 Inohana, Chuo-ku, Chiba 260-0856, Japan. [3] Research Center for Child Mental Development, Graduate School of Medicine, Chiba University, 1-8-1 Inohana, Chuo-ku, Chiba 260-8670, Japan. [4] Fujita Hospital, 3292-Ho Yokaichiba, Sosa-shi, Chiba 289-2146, Japan. [5] Kimura Hospital, 6-19 Higashihoncho, Chuo-ku, Chiba 260-0004, Japan. [6] Kisarazu Hospital, 2-3-1 Iwane, Kisarazu-shi, Chiba 292-0061, Japan. [7] Kokoronokaze Funabashi Clinic, 1-26-2 Motomachi, Funabashi-shi, Chiba 273-0005, Japan. [8] Kokoronokenko Tsudanuma Clinic, 2-13-13 Maebaranishi, Funabashi-shi, Chiba 274-0825, Japan. [9] Sodegaura Satsukidai Hospital, 5-21 Nagauraekimae, Sodegaura-shi 299-0246, Japan.

Acknowledgements

We would like to thank Editage (http://www.editage.jp) for the English language editing of our manuscript. We would like to thank all the patients and doctors who participated in this study. In particular, we are grateful to the doctors and medical staff at the Asahi General Hospital, Kohei Yoshino, Tsutomu Aoki; Chiba Medical Center, Daiji Sakurai, Miwako Kaiho; Choshi Kokoro Clinic, Tsuneo Senba, Rumiko Ishigami; Fujita Hospital, Atsushi Kimura, Motoki Watanabe; Kameda Medical Center, Toshihiko Okami, Hiraki Koishikawa; Kimura Hospital, Sho Kimura; Kisarazu Mental Clinic, Hiroyuki Endo; Kisarazu Hospital, Tatsuki Hata, Masaru Kuno, Aiko Sato, Hidetoshi Ino, Keijiro Koseki; Kokoronokaze Funabashi Clinic, Yutaka Hosoda, Hajime Sasaki; Kokoronokenko Tsudanuma Clinic, Taisuke Yoshida, Naoya Komatsu; Sodegaura Satsukidai Hospital, Hitoshi Suzuki, Shuichi Kikuchi; Soga Nishiguchi Clinic, Tamami Furuta for cooperating in this study. We also thank the researchers at the Division of Clinical Neuroscience Chiba University Centre for Forensic Mental Health, Tamaki Ishima, Yuko Fujita, Kenji Hashimoto and the Department of Psychiatry, Chiba University Graduate School of Medicine, Miwako Nakamura for assisting in this work. We further thank the clinical research nurses for supporting this work at Chiba University Hospital, Junko Goto, Kaoru Ikeda, Komako Ito, Chisako Fujishiro.

Competing interests

Dr. Tasuku Hashimoto has received honoraria as a speaker/consultant from Astellas, GlaxoSmithKline, Meiji Seika Pharma, Mochida, Otsuka, Tanabe Mitsubishi, Yoshitomiyakuhin, and received grants/research supports from Astellas, Chugai, Otsuka, and Shionogi. Dr. Akihiro Shiina has received research supports from Ministry of Health, Labour and Welfare, Non-Profit Organization of dependence research, General Association for Justice, and the Japan Science Society, lecture fees from Dainippon-Sumitomo and Chiba-ken Bengoshi-kai (Chiba Lawyers Association). Dr. Tadashi Hasegawa has received honoraria as a speaker/consultant from Meiji Seika Pharma, Mochida, Otsuka, Yoshitomiyakuhin, Shionogi, Eli Lilly, Dainippon-Sumitomo, and received a grant/research support from Novartis. Dr. Hiroshi Kimura has received honoraria as a speaker/consultant from Janssen, Meiji Seika Pharma, and Otsuka. Dr. Tomihisa Niitsu has received speakers' honoraria from Eli Lilly and Dainippon-Sumitomo. Dr. Masumi Tachibana has received honoraria as a speaker from Mochida, Eli Lily, and Dainippon-Sumitomo. Dr. Katsumasa Muneoka has received honoraria as a speaker/consultant from Meiji Seika Pharma, Mochida, Otsuka, Janssen, and Eli Lilly. Prof. Masaomi Iyo has received consultant fees from Eli Lilly, Dainippon-Sumitomo, Pfizer and Abbott and honoraria from Janssen, Eli Lilly, Otsuka, Meiji Seika Pharma, Astellas, Dainippon-Sumitomo, Ono, GlaxoSmithKline, Takeda, Mochida, Kyowa Hakko, MSD, Eisai, Daiichi-Sankyo, Novartis, Teijin, Shionogi, Hisamitsu and Asahi Kasei. Dr. Yasunori Oda, Dr. Masatomo Ishikawa, Dr. Satoshi Matsuki and Prof. Michiko Nakazato have no potential competing interests to report.

Funding

We declare that this work was financially supported by The Chiba University Psychiatry Doumonkai (Chiba, Japan) and Management Expenses Grants from Chiba University Graduate School of Medicine (Chiba, Japan). There was no financial support from any other companies. This study was materially supported by medical information, printing services, and the provision of meeting venues by Meiji Seika Pharma (Tokyo, Japan). Meiji Seika Pharma had no role in the study design, patient recruitment, analysis, data interpretation, and writing of the manuscript.

References

1. Uchida H, Suzuki T, Mamo DC, Mulsant BH, Tsunoda K, Takeuchi H, et al. Survey of benzodiazepine and antidepressant use in outpatients with mood disorders in Japan. Psychiatry Clin Neurosci. 2009;63:244–6.
2. van Dijk KN, de Vries CS, ter Huurne K, van den Berg PB, Brouwers JR, de Jong-van den Berg LT. Concomitant prescribing of benzodiazepines during antidepressant therapy in the elderly. J Clin Epidemiol. 2002;55:1049–53.
3. Valenstein M, Taylor KK, Austin K, Kales HC, McCarthy JF, Blow FC. Benzodiazepine use among depressed patients treated in mental health settings. Am J Psychiatry. 2004;161:654–61.
4. Furukawa TA, Streiner D, Young LT, Kinoshita Y. Antidepressants plus benzodiazepines for major depression. Cochrane Database Syst Rev. 2001;(3):CD001026. doi:10.1002/14651858.CD001026.
5. Baldwin DS, Aitchison K, Bateson A, Curran HV, Davies S, Leonard B, et al. Benzodiazepines: risks and benefits. A reconsideration. J Psychopharmacol. 2013;27:967–71.
6. Billioti de Gage S, Begaud B, Bazin F, Verdoux H, Dartigues JF, Peres K, et al. Benzodiazepine use and risk of dementia: prospective population based study. BMJ. 2012;345:e6231.
7. Gray SL, Dublin S, Yu O, Walker R, Anderson M, Hubbard RA, et al. Benzodiazepine use and risk of incident dementia or cognitive decline: prospective population based study. BMJ. 2016;352:i90.
8. Bauer M, Pfennig A, Severus E, Whybrow PC, Angst J, Moller HJ, et al. World Federation of Societies of Biological Psychiatry (WFSBP) guidelines for biological treatment of unipolar depressive disorders, part 1: update 2013 on the acute and continuation treatment of unipolar depressive disorders. World J Biol Psychiatry. 2013;14:334–85.
9. Lam RW, Kennedy SH, Grigoriadis S, McIntyre RS, Milev R, Ramasubbu R, et al. Canadian Network for Mood and Anxiety Treatments (CANMAT) clinical guidelines for the management of major depressive disorder in adults. III. Pharmacotherapy. J Affect Disord. 2009;117(Suppl 1):S26–43.
10. de Boer T. The pharmacologic profile of mirtazapine. J Clin Psychiatry. 1996;57(Suppl 4):19–25.
11. Berg KA, Harvey JA, Spampinato U, Clarke WP. Physiological and therapeutic relevance of constitutive activity of 5-HT 2A and 5-HT 2C receptors for the treatment of depression. Prog Brain Res. 2008;172:287–305.
12. Thompson C. Onset of action of antidepressants: results of different analyses. Hum Psychopharmacol. 2002;17(Suppl 1):S27–32.
13. Watanabe N, Omori IM, Nakagawa A, Cipriani A, Barbui C, McGuire H, et al. Mirtazapine versus other antidepressants in the acute-phase treatment of adults with major depression: systematic review and meta-analysis. J Clin Psychiatry. 2008;69:1404–15.
14. Hashimoto K. Brain-derived neurotrophic factor as a biomarker for mood disorders: an historical overview and future directions. Psychiatry Clin Neurosci. 2010;64:341–57.
15. Yoshida T, Ishikawa M, Niitsu T, Nakazato M, Watanabe H, Shiraishi T, et al. Decreased serum levels of mature brain-derived neurotrophic factor (BDNF), but not its precursor proBDNF, in patients with major depressive disorder. PLoS One. 2012;7:e42676.
16. Yoshimura R, Kishi T, Hori H, Atake K, Katsuki A, Nakano-Umene W, et al. Serum proBDNF/BDNF and response to fluvoxamine in drug-naive first-episode major depressive disorder patients. Ann Gen Psychiatry. 2014;13:19.
17. Sodersten K, Palsson E, Ishima T, Funa K, Landen M, Hashimoto K, et al. Abnormality in serum levels of mature brain-derived neurotrophic factor (BDNF) and its precursor proBDNF in mood-stabilized patients with bipolar disorder: a study of two independent cohorts. J Affect Disord. 2014;160:1–9.
18. Lu B, Pang PT, Woo NH. The Yin and Yang of neurotrophin action. Nat Rev Neurosci. 2005;6:603–14.
19. Teng HK, Teng KK, Lee R, Wright S, Tevar S, Almeida RD, et al. ProBDNF induces neuronal apoptosis via activation of a receptor complex of p75NTR and sortilin. J Neurosci. 2005;25:5455–63.
20. Sen S, Duman R, Sanacora G. Serum brain-derived neurotrophic factor, depression, and antidepressant medications: meta-analyses and implications. Biol Psychiatry. 2008;64:527–32.
21. Brunoni AR, Lopes M, Fregni F. A systematic review and meta-analysis of clinical studies on major depression and BDNF levels: implications for the role of neuroplasticity in depression. Int J Neuropsychopharmacol. 2008;11:1169–80.
22. Hamilton M. A rating scale for depression. J Neurol Neurosurg Psychiatry. 1960;23:56–62.
23. Zung WW. Depression in the normal aged. Psychosomatics. 1967;8:287–92.
24. Soldatos CR, Dikeos DG, Paparrigopoulos TJ. Athens insomnia scale: validation of an instrument based on ICD-10 criteria. J Psychosom Res. 2000;48:555–60.
25. Guy W. The clinician global severity and impression scales. In: ECDEU assessment manual for psychopharmacology. Rockville: National Institute of Mental Health; 1976. p. 218–222. DHEW Publication No. 76–338.
26. Parr JM, Kavanagh DJ, Cahill L, Mitchell G, Mc D, Young R. Effectiveness of current treatment approaches for benzodiazepine discontinuation: a meta-analysis. Addiction. 2009;104:13–24.
27. Gould RL, Coulson MC, Patel N, Highton-Williamson E, Howard RJ. Interventions for reducing benzodiazepine use in older people: meta-analysis of randomised controlled trials. Br J Psychiatry. 2014;204:98–107.
28. Oude Voshaar RC, Couvee JE, van Balkom AJ, Mulder PG, Zitman FG. Strategies for discontinuing long-term benzodiazepine use: meta-analysis. Br J Psychiatry. 2006;189:213–20.
29. Baandrup L, Lindschou J, Winkel P, Gluud C, Glenthoj BY. Prolonged-release melatonin versus placebo for benzodiazepine discontinuation in patients with schizophrenia or bipolar disorder: a randomised, placebo-controlled, blinded trial. World J Biol Psychiatry. 2016;17(7):514–24. doi:10.3109/15622975.2015.1048725.
30. Purgato M, Papola D, Gastaldon C, Trespidi C, Magni LR, Rizzo C, et al. Paroxetine versus other anti-depressive agents for depression. Cochrane Database Syst Rev. 2014;4:CD006531.
31. Cipriani A, Furukawa TA, Salanti G, Geddes JR, Higgins JP, Churchill R, et al. Comparative efficacy and acceptability of 12 new-generation antidepressants: a multiple-treatments meta-analysis. Lancet. 2009;373(9665):746–58.
32. Nutt DJ. Efficacy of mirtazapine in clinically relevant subgroups of depressed patients. Depress Anxiety. 1998;7(Suppl 1):7–10.
33. Behnke K, Sogaard J, Martin S, Bauml J, Ravindran AV, Agren H, et al. Mirtazapine orally disintegrating tablet versus sertraline: a prospective onset of action study. J Clin Psychopharmacol. 2003;23:358–64.
34. Fernandes BS, Molendijk ML, Kohler CA, Soares JC, Leite CM, Machado-Vieira R, et al. Peripheral brain-derived neurotrophic factor (BDNF) as a biomarker in bipolar disorder: a meta-analysis of 52 studies. BMC Med. 2015;13:289.
35. Umene-Nakano W, Yoshimura R, Ueda N, Suzuki A, Ikenouchi-Sugita A, Hori H, et al. Predictive factors for responding to sertraline treatment: views from plasma catecholamine metabolites and serotonin transporter polymorphism. J Psychopharmacol. 2010;24:1764–71.
36. Yoshimura R, Mitoma M, Sugita A, Hori H, Okamoto T, Umene W, et al. Effects of paroxetine or milnacipran on serum brain-derived neurotrophic factor in depressed patients. Prog Neuropsychopharmacol Biol Psychiatry. 2007;31:1034–7.
37. Wolkowitz OM, Wolf J, Shelly W, Rosser R, Burke HM, Lerner GK, et al. Serum BDNF levels before treatment predict SSRI response in depression. Prog Neuropsychopharmacol Biol Psychiatry. 2011;35:1623–30.
38. Rutherford BR, Cooper TM, Persaud A, Brown PJ, Sneed JR, Roose SP. Less is more in antidepressant clinical trials: a meta-analysis of the effect of visit frequency on treatment response and dropout. J Clin Psychiatry. 2013;74:703–15.
39. Furukawa TA, Onishi Y, Hinotsu S, Tajika A, Takeshima N, Shinohara K, et al. Prescription patterns following first-line new generation antidepressants for depression in Japan: a naturalistic cohort study based on a large claims database. J Affect Disord. 2013;150:916–22.
40. Milea D, Guelfucci F, Bent-Ennakhil N, Toumi M, Auray JP. Antidepressant monotherapy: a claims database analysis of treatment changes and treatment duration. Clin Ther. 2010;32:2057–72.
41. Olfson M, Marcus SC, Tedeschi M, Wan GJ. Continuity of antidepressant treatment for adults with depression in the United States. Am J Psychiatry. 2006;163:101–8.
42. Sawada N, Uchida H, Suzuki T, Watanabe K, Kikuchi T, Handa T, et al. Persistence and compliance to antidepressant treatment in patients with depression: a chart review. BMC Psychiatry. 2009;9:38.
43. Patsopoulos NA. A pragmatic view on pragmatic trials. Dialogues Clin Neurosci. 2011;13:217–24.

12

Suicide ideation and attempts among people with epilepsy in Addis Ababa, Ethiopia

Kelelemua Haile[1], Tadesse Awoke[2], Getinet Ayano[1], Minale Tareke[3*], Andargie Abate[3] and Mulugeta Nega[4]

Abstract

Background: Suicidal ideation and attempts are more frequent in people with epilepsy than in general population and suicide attempt increases the chance of later completed suicide. The aim of this study was to assess the prevalence and associated factors of suicidal ideation and attempt among people with epilepsy in Amanuel Mental Specialized Hospital, Addis Ababa, Ethiopia.

Methods: Institution-based cross-sectional study was conducted from May to June 2014 at Amanuel Mental Specialized Hospital among people with epilepsy. The pre-tested semi-structured questionnaire was used for interviewing the study participants. Logistic regression analysis was used to assess predictors of suicidal ideation and attempt.

Results: The study indicated that the prevalence of suicidal ideation and attempt among people with epilepsy were 29.8 and 14.1%, respectively. Poor social support, drug treatment for mental illness, had co-morbid depression, no seizure free within 1 year and family history committed suicide were significantly associated with suicidal ideation and attempt.

Conclusion: The prevalence of suicidal ideation and attempt in people with epilepsy found to be higher when compared to general population. Therefore, screening all epilepsy patients should be done for early diagnosis and treatment.

Keywords: Epilepsy, Suicidal ideation, Suicidal attempt

Introduction

Diagnostic and statistical manual of mental disorders, fifth edition (DSM-5) defines suicidal ideation as thoughts about self-harm with deliberate consideration or planning of possible techniques of causing one's own death, while suicide is the act of intentionally causing one's own death and suicide attempt is an attempt to end one's own life, which may lead to one's death [1]. There is a big difference between thinking about suicide and acting it out. Some persons may have ideas of suicide, but they will never act on. Some plan for days, weeks, or even years before acting, whereas others take their lives seemingly on impulse without advance planning [2].

*Correspondence: minale23@gmail.com
[3] College of Medicine and Health Science, Bahir Dar University, Bahir Dar, Ethiopia
Full list of author information is available at the end of the article

Fifty percent of all violent deaths in men and 71% of women were accounted for suicides globally. Suicide rates are highest in persons aged 70 and older years for both men and women in almost all regions of the world [3]. Every year, more than 800,000 people die due to suicide (one person every 40 s) ranking as the second leading cause of death next to traffic accidents among 15–29 years of age [3].

The burden of suicide constitutes a serious public health issue worldwide that needs mental health professionals increase their awareness towards suicide warning signs. Suicide warning signs are associated with acute factors that inform clinicians about observable signs, expressed emotions, and important for saving lives by early detection and intervention for those at risk [4].

Epilepsy is a chronic neurological disorder affecting people of all ages, race and social class with more than 50 million global distribution [5]. It is commonly associated with brain dysfunction, social isolation and vocational difficulty making it a complex disorder [6]. Living with epilepsy affects relationships with family and friends, school, employment and leisure activities. Each of these effects may contribute to the high magnitude of psychiatric illness among people with epilepsy [7]. Patients with epilepsy have a higher risk of suicide compared to the general population giving that suicide is highly common co-morbid psychiatric illness [8].

Different studies indicated that people with epilepsy are at higher risk for suicidal thoughts and attempts [9, 10] with an estimated lifetime prevalence rate ranged from 3.3 to 14.3% [11] or even up to 35% [12]. This rate has been reported to be 6–25 times higher with temporal lobe epilepsy (TLE) compared to 1.4–6.9% in general population [13, 14].

Around 11% deaths in epilepsy are due to suicide, and a suicide attempt increased the chance of later completed suicide by 38% [15]. According to Centers for Disease Control and Prevention report, the suicide rate among people with epilepsy is 22% higher than the general population [16].

Despite this burden and consequences, there is a limited study on suicidal ideation and attempt in people with epilepsy in Ethiopia. Therefore, this study was intended to assess the magnitude and associated factors of suicidal ideation and attempt among people with epilepsy at Amanuel Mental Specialized Hospital.

Methods

Study settings and population

The institution-based cross-sectional study design was done from May to June 2014 at Amanuel Mental Specialized Hospital in Addis Ababa, Ethiopia. It is one of the oldest hospitals established in 1930E.C and the only mental Hospital in Ethiopia which is located in western part of Addis Ababa. The hospital has 255 beds and 18 outpatient departments that give serve for all types of mental disorder cases. Of which, two outpatient departments provide services for an average 2200 people with epilepsy monthly. People living with epilepsy ($\geq$ 18 year) who have been clinically diagnosed with epilepsy and had follow-up treatment in outpatient epilepsy clinic in the Amanuel Mental Specialized Hospital were included in the study. However, patients unable to communicate and seriously ill were excluded from the study.

Sample size and sampling procedures

Sample size was calculated using single population proportion formula [$n = ((z\alpha/2)2p(1-p))/d2$]. By considering an assumption of 50% (0.5) proportion of suicidal ideation and attempt among people with epilepsy since it is unknown in our country, $Z_{\alpha/2}$ at 95% CI (1.96), and tolerable margin of error (0.05), the minimum sample size was 384. After adjusting for 10% contingency for non-response rate, a total of 423 study populations were involved in the study.

Sampling interval was determined by dividing total study population who had follow up during 1-month data collection period (2200) by total sample size (423). The sampling fraction is: 2200/423 $\approx$ 5. Hence, the sample interval is 5. The first study participant was selected by lottery method and the next study participants were chosen at regular intervals (every 5th) and interviewed by data collectors.

Data collection and quality assurance

Data were collected by interviewing patients and reviewing charts using semi-structured questionnaire. World health organization composite international diagnostic interview (CIDI) was used to assess suicidal ideation and attempt among people with epilepsy [17]. Depression and social support were assessed using patient health questionnaire (PHQ-9) [18] and Oslo-3-item, respectively. Probable depression symptoms (PHQ-9 score $\geq$ 5) [19] and the individual who scored greater than or equal to 9 on Oslo 3 item consider as good social support [20]. Data were collected by four psychiatric nurses for 1-month period.

Semi-structured questionnaire for socio-demographic data and clinical related variables were developed in English and translated to local language (Amharic) to be understandable by all participants and translated back to English again to ensure its consistency. Training was given for four data collectors and one supervisor for 2 days. Pre-test was done at black lion hospital 2 weeks before the beginning of actual data collection. The data collectors were supervised daily and the filled questionnaires were checked properly by the supervisor and principal investigator to ensure its completeness.

Data management and processing

The coded data were checked, cleaned and entered into epi.info version 3.5 and then exported into Statistical Package for the Social Sciences (SPSS) window version 20 for analysis. Descriptive statistic was used to explain the study participants in relation to study variable. Bivariate and multivariate logistic regression analyses were conducted to identify associated factors of suicidal ideation and attempt. The strength of the association was interpreted using odds ratio and 95% CI, and p value less than 0.05 was considered as statistically significant.

Ethical consideration

Ethical clearance was obtained from the Institutional Review Board (IRB) of the College of Medicine and Health Sciences, University of Gondar, and from Amanuel Mental Specialized Hospital. The data collectors had clearly explained the aims of the study for study participants. We obtained written consent from each participant. The right was given to the study participants to refuse or discontinue participation at any time. Confidentiality was maintained throughout the study. Those study participants suffering from recurrent severe suicidal thought were treated by communicating with case team.

Results

Descriptions of socio-demographic characteristics of the respondents

A total of 410 respondents were enrolled and participated in the study which yields the response rate of 97%. The mean (± SD) age of respondents was 32.95 (± 11.87) year. There were more males 245 (59.8%) than females 165 (40.2%) (Table 1).

Table 1 Distribution of people with epilepsy disorder by their socio-demographic characteristics

Variables	Frequency ($n = 410$)	Percent (%)
Sex		
Male	245	59.8
Female	165	40.2
Age group		
18–24	110	26.8
25–31	113	27.6
32–38	68	16.6
39–45	59	14.4
> 45	60	14.6
Occupation		
Government employee	80	19
Merchant	73	17.8
Farmer	77	18.8
Student	52	12.9
Daily laborer	72	17.8
House wife	56	13.7
Educational level		
No education	61	14.9
Primary	178	43.4
Secondary	130	31.7
Diploma and above	41	10.0
Income (ETB*)		
< 750	254	62
750–1199	81	19.7
≥ 1200	75	18.3
Marital status		
Single	206	50.2
Married	141	34.4
Divorce/widowed	63	15.4
Living arrangement		
With family	351	85.6
Alone	59	14.4
Social support		
Poor	166	40.5
Good	244	59.5

ETB*, Ethiopian Birr

Clinical characteristics and substance use

Regarding the onset of illness, 218 (53.2%) of the respondents were 18 years and above. Out of the total study participants, 18 (4.4%) and 19 (4.6%) had a family history of suicidal attempt and committed suicide, respectively (Table 2).

Table 2 Frequency distribution of clinical factors

Variables	Frequency ($n = 410$)	Percentage (%)
Age on set of epilepsy		
Under 18	192	46.8
18 and above	218	53.2
Duration of treatment (years)		
Up to 1	45	11.0
1–6	152	37.1
7–12	107	26.0
More than 12	106	25.9
Duration of illness (years)		
Up to 5	167	40.8
6–10	116	28.5
11–15	53	12.9
16–20	43	10.5
More than 20	30	7.3
Drug control on AED		
Seizure free/year	272	66.3
No seizure free/year	138	33.7
Co-morbid medical illness		
Yes	12	2.9
No	398	97.1
Drug taking for mental illness		
Yes	28	6.8
No	382	93.2
Co-morbid depression status		
Yes	116	28.3
No	294	71.7
Family history of epilepsy		
Yes	55	13.4
No	355	86.6
Family history of attempted suicide		
Yes	18	4.4
No	392	95.6
Family history of committed suicide		
Yes	19	4.6
No	391	95.4
Ever use substance		
Yes	129	31.4
No	281	68.6
Current substance use		
Yes	83	20.2
No	327	79.8

Prevalence of suicidal ideation and suicidal attempt

The lifetime prevalence of suicidal ideation among respondents was 122 (29.8%); of whom, 80 (65.6%) reported suicidal ideation in less than 12 months and 73 (17.8%) had planned to commit suicide. Regarding suicidal attempt, the lifetime prevalence of suicidal attempt in this study was 58 (14.1%). Out of those who attempt suicide, 50 (86.2%) report to have suicidal attempt within the last 12 months and 36 (63.2%) of them attempt suicide once in their life (Table 3).

Different methods were used to attempt suicide (Fig. 1)

Table 3 Frequency distribution of life time prevalence suicide ideation and attempt

Variable	Frequency ($n = 410$)	Percentage (%)
Ever suicidal ideation		
Yes	122	29.8
No	288	70.2
Duration of ever seriously thought suicide		
≤ 12	80	65.6
> 12	42	34.4
Suicidal thought in 1 month		
Yes	30	7.3
No	380	92.7
Ever plan of suicide		
Yes	73	17.8
No	337	82.2
Duration of suicidal plan		
≤ 12	58	79.4
> 12	15	20.6
Suicidal attempt		
Yes	58	14.1
No	352	85.9
Duration ever suicidal attempt		
≤ 12	50	86.2
> 12	8	13.7
Number of suicide attempt		
One	36	62.1
Two	16	27.6
More than two	6	10.3
Reason for suicide Attempt		
Family conflict	33	31.3
Economic problem	18	16.5
Related to current illness	33	31.3
Death of family	11	10.1
Physical illness	2	1.8
Relate to hopelessness	12	11

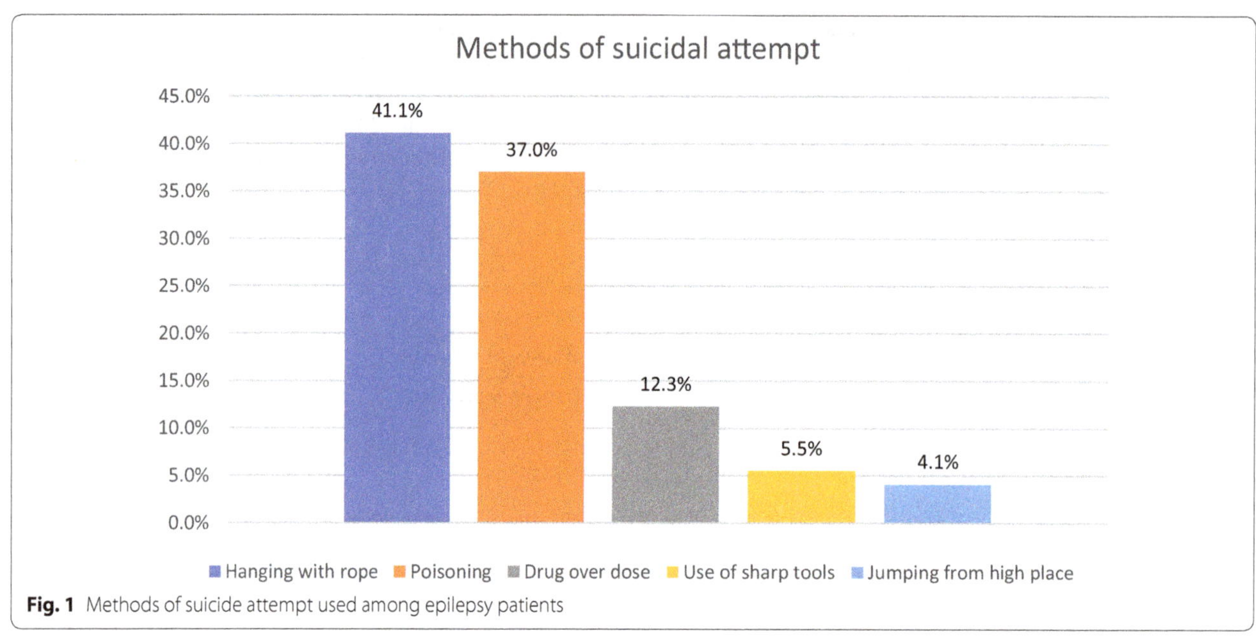

Fig. 1 Methods of suicide attempt used among epilepsy patients

Factors associated with suicidal ideation among people with epilepsy

The result of multivariate logistic regression revealed that those who live alone were 3.2 times more likely to have suicidal ideation than those who live with family (AOR 3.16, 95% CI 1.54, 6.46).

Respondents who had poor social support were 3.3 times more likely to have suicidal ideation as compared to those who had good social support (AOR 3.28, 95% CI 190, 5.68). In addition, those who had co-morbid depressive symptoms were 5.5 times more likely to have suicidal ideation compared to those who had no co-morbid depressive symptoms [AOR 5.47, 95% CI (3.12, 9.62)]. Taking drug treatment for mental illness also had a significant effect on suicidal ideation, indicating that those who were taking treatment were 4.2 times more likely to have suicidal ideation than those who had no history of mental illness and drug treatment for mental illness (AOR 4.16, 95% CI 1.42, 12.24). On the other hand, participants with no seizure free within 1 year were 2.6 times more likely to have suicidal ideation as compared to those with seizure free within 1 year (AOR 2.62. 95% CI 1.51, 4.56).

Concurrently, respondents who report family history of suicidal attempt were 4.4 times more likely to have suicidal ideation when compared to those who did not report a family history (AOR 4.36 95% CI 1.07, 17.80) (Table 4).

Factor associated with suicidal attempt among people with epilepsy

The result of multivariate logistic regression model revealed that clients who had poor social support, those on drug treatment for mental illness, had co-morbid depressive symptoms, no seizure free within 1 year and family history committed suicide were significantly associated with suicidal attempt (Table 5).

Discussion

In this study, the prevalence of lifetime suicidal ideation and attempt among people living with epilepsy and their possible associations with different variables were assessed. The prevalence of suicidal ideation was 29.8% which is higher than the result reported in Egypt (23.5%) [12], in Washington tertiary epilepsy clinics (11.9%) [21]. These might be due to the difference in sample size, study design, study participants, culture, time variation, and settings. In addition, in Washington, it was current suicide ideation but this study was lifetime prevalence.

However, the current finding is lower than from Bosnia and Herzegovina reported (38%) [22], Brazil (36.7%) [23], Cuba Havana (45.2%) [24]. The discrepancy might be due to the difference in settings, sample size, and study participants. The other possible reason might be the difference in study design since we used institution-based cross-sectional study design, but Brazilian study was community-based case–control study. Furthermore, in Cuba Havana, study subjects were patients with temporal lobe epilepsy, but our study included all people living with epilepsy.

Regarding suicidal attempt, the current study found that the prevalence of lifetime suicidal attempt among people with epilepsy was 14.1% which is closely consistent with many other reports in Egypt (11.5%) [12], Croatia (14.6%) [25], and Brazil (12.1%) [26]. However, this result was higher than the study done in Bosnia and

Table 4 Bivariate and multivariate analysis between some of selected factors and suicidal ideation

Explanatory variables	Suicide ideation Yes	Suicide ideation No	Crude OR (95% CI)	Adjusted OR (95% CI)
Sex				
Male	62	183	1.00	1.00
Female	60	105	1.69 (1.12, 2.59)	1.46 (0.78, 2.12)
Living arrangement				
Family	91	260	1.00	1.00
Alone	31	28	3.20 (1.585, 7.56)	3.16 (1.54, 6.46)*
Marital status				
Married	35	125	1.00	1.00
Single	66	140	1.684 (1.046, 2.709)	0.64 (0.28, 1.46)
Separate/divorced/widowed	21	23	3.261 (1.619, 6.569)	1.33 (0.59, 3.02)
Social support				
Good	41	203	1.00	1.00
Poor	81	85	4.72 (2.99, 7.42)	3.28 (1.90, 5.68)*
Co-morbid depressive symptoms				
Yes	75	41	9.61 (5.877, 15.73)	5.47 (3.12, 9.62)*
No	47	247	1.00	1.00
Family history of attempted suicide				
Yes	14	4	9.20 (2.96, 28.57)	4.36 (1.07, 17.80)*
No	108	284	1.00	1.00
Drug control on AED				
Seizure free/year	55	217	1.00	1.00
No seizure free/year	67	71	3.72 (2.38, 5.82)	2.62 (1.51, 4.56)*
Drug taking for mental illness				
Yes	19	9	5.72 (2.51, 13.04)	4.16 (1.42, 12.24)*
No	103	279	1.00	1.00

* *p* value < 0.05

Table 5 Bivariate and multivariate logistic regression analysis between some of selected factors and suicidal attempt

Explanatory variables	Suicide attempt Yes	Suicide attempt No	COR	AOR
Sex				
Male	27	218	1.00	
Female	31	134	1.87 (1.07, 3.27)	1.63 (0.76, 3.51)
Living arrangement				
Family	44	307	1.00	
Alone	14	45	2.17 (1.10, 4.28)	1.02 (0.38, 2.76)
Social support				
Yes	16	228	1.00	1.00
No	42	124	4.83 (2.61, 8.94)	3.48 (1.96.6.16)*
Co-morbid depressive symptoms				
Yes	45	71	13.70 (7.01, 26.77)	7.84 (3.58, 15.21)*
No	13	281	1.00	1.00
Family history committed suicide				
Yes	10	9	7.94 (3.07, 20.53)	5.32 (1.55, 18.20)*
No	48	343	1.00	1.00
Drug taking for mental illness				
Yes	16	12	10.79 (4.78, 24.37)	6.81 (3.00, 22.45)*
No	42	340	1.00	1.00
Drug control on AED				
Seizure free/year	22	250	1.00	1.00
No seizure free/year	36	102	4.01 (2.25, 7.15)	3.19 (1.48, 6.86)*

* *p* value < 0.05

Herzegovina (18%) [22], Cuba Havana (28.6%) [24]. The difference might be due to sample size, study participants, and study design described above.

The most commonly used method for suicidal attempt in people with epilepsy in this study was hanging (41%) which is inconsistent with the study findings from different countries. For instance, 34.9% of Korean [27] and 87.5% of Japanese [28] study participants used drug overdose especially Phenobarbital. This discrepancy might be due to cultural difference, availabilities of methods and knowledge of participants. Poisoning by pesticide is common in many Asian countries and in Latin America while poisoning by drugs is common in northern Europe countries and the United Kingdom. Hanging is the preferred method of suicide in Eastern Europe and using gun shooting is common in the United States and jumping from a high place in cities and urban societies such as Hong Kong Special Administrative Region, China [29].

In this study, those participants living alone were more likely to have suicidal ideation. The possible reason could be those who live alone could not share the problem nearby family on time; this increases hopelessness and may lead to suicidal ideation which is supported by study done in Washington [21].

Those respondents who had poor social support, no seizure free within 1 year were predictors for suicidal ideation in this study. The previous study done in Ethiopia revealed that frequent seizure attacks were associated with depression and increased perceived stigma [30, 31]. This may, in turn, increase suicidal ideation and attempt in people with epilepsy. WHO report in 2004 showed that weak social ties and low support from friends or relatives have been significantly associated with suicidal ideation [32]. The reason may be repeated seizure attack, increased lesion in the brain with neuron-chemical involvement, and the increased frequency could be again low coping mechanism contributing to suicidal ideation [12].

Those study participants who were taking drug for mental illness in addition to epilepsy drug and having co-morbid depressive symptoms were highly exposed for suicidal ideation. This was in line with study done in Denmark, Sweden, Croatia and Washington [25, 33, 34]. The possible reason could be presence of mental illness by itself and drug treatment for longer time may make negative view of life.

Respondents who had family history of suicidal attempt were found to have suicidal ideation. This was in line with the study in Chicago and Denmark [15, 35]. The possible reason might be from biological perspective; environmental and non-genetic such as shared exposure to the family stress and common life style could contribute to the suicidal ideation.

Furthermore, social support and co-morbid depressive symptoms among people with epilepsy were significantly associated with suicidal attempt which is consistent with study done in Finland, Japan and Cuba [28, 36]. These factors might be due to misunderstanding of the disorders, avoidance from family and workplace lead to unemployment, poor social ties and low support increases patients' suicidal attempt. Depression increase suicidality due to the effect in neuron-transmitter alteration in people with epilepsy [37]. On another hand, those depressed patients have hopelessness and suicidal ideation making them attempt suicide [38].

Participants having drug treatment for mental illness and no seizure free within 1 year were associated with suicidal attempt which is in line with study done in Sweden and Egypt [12, 34]. Since the presence of mental illness like mood disorder, schizophrenia and anxiety can increase suicidality. Some psychotropic drugs may lower seizure threshold which makes it easier for patient to experience seizure [39]. The co-existing of two chronic illnesses and drug treatment for longer time may make negative attitude for life leading to suicidal attempt. Fear of having seizure attack in public place can affect their performance and contribute to poor self-esteem, social isolation, negatively influence on their ability to work and finally may result in suicidal attempt [40].

It is the first study in Ethiopia that determined the prevalence and associated factors for both suicidal ideation and attempt. However, the discussion was done by considering the limitations of not addressing types of medication and types of epilepsy because it was difficult to get specific diagnosis in the patient's chart.

Conclusion

The prevalence of suicidal ideation and attempt among people living with epilepsy were found to be high. Social support, living alone, co-morbid depression, partially controlled seizure, drug taking for mental illness, family history of suicidal attempt and committed suicide were significantly associated with suicidal ideation and attempt independently. Screening of suicidal ideation and attempt for all epilepsy patients should be done for early diagnosis and treatment. It is better to conduct a further longitudinal study among epilepsy and co-morbid mental illness with their specific drug treatment for suicidal ideation and attempt.

Authors' contributions

KH conceived the study and was involved in the study design, reviewed the article, analysis, report writing, and drafted the manuscript, TA, GA, MT, AA, and MN were involved in the study design and analysis and drafted the manuscript. All authors read and approved the final manuscript.

Author details

[1] Department of Psychiatry, Amanuel Mental Specialized Hospital, Addis Ababa, Ethiopia. [2] Department of Epidemiology and Biostatistics, University of Gondar, Gondar, Ethiopia. [3] College of Medicine and Health Science, Bahir Dar University, Bahir Dar, Ethiopia. [4] College of Medicine and Health Science, Haramaya University, Harer, Ethiopia.

Acknowledgements

The authors acknowledge University of Gondar and AMSH for funding the study. We are grateful to all data collectors, supervisors and study participants for their important contribution in this study.

Competing interests

The authors declare that they have no competing interests.

Consent for publication

Not applicable.

Funding

This research work is funded by University of Gondar and Amanuel Mental Specialized Hospital.

References

1. American Psychiatric Association. Diagnostic and statistical manual of mental disorders. 5th ed. Washington, DC: American Psychiatric Association; 2013.
2. Sadock BJ, Sadock VA. Kaplan & Sadock's synopsis of psychiatry: behavioral sciences/clinical psychiatry. 11th ed. Alphen aan den Rijn: Wolters Kluwer; 2015.
3. World Health Organization. Preventing suicide. A global imperative. Geneva: World Health Organization; 2014. p. 7–12.
4. Rudd MD. Suicide warning signs in clinical practice. Curr Psychiatry Rep. 2008;10:87–90.
5. World Health Organization. Epilepsy in the WHO eastern Mediterranean region: bridging the gap. Geneva: World Health Organization; 2010.
6. Mazza M, Bria P, Mazza S. Depression and suicide in epilepsy: a fact or artifact? J Neurol Sci. 2007;260:300–1.
7. Alsaadi T, Zamel K, Sameer A, Fathalla W, Koudier I. Depressive disorders in patients with epilepsy: why should neurologists care? Health. 2013;5(6A1):14–20.
8. Thompson AW, Miller JW, Katon W, Chayto N, Ciechanowski P. Sociodemographic and clinical factors associated with depression in epilepsy. Epilepsy Behav. 2009;14(4):655–60.
9. Meador KJ. Suicide in patients with epilepsy. Epilepsy Curr. 2008;8(2):40–2.
10. Pack AM. Epilepsy and suicidality: what's the relationship? Epilepsy Curr. 2016;16(4):236–8.

11. Jones JE, Hermann BP, Barry JJ, Gilliam FG, Kanner AM, Meador KJ. Rates and risk factors for suicide, suicidal ideation, and suicide attempts in chronic epilepsy. Epilepsy Behav. 2003;4:31–8.
12. Hamed SA, Elserogy YB, Abdou MA, Abdellah MM. Risks of suicidality in adult patients with epilepsy. World J Psychiatry. 2012;2(2):33–42.
13. Jallon P. Mortality in patients with epilepsy. Curr Opin Neurol. 2004;17:141–6.
14. Christensen J, Vestergaard M, Mortensen P, Sidenius P, Agerbo E. Epilepsy and risk of suicide: a population-based case–control study. Lancet Neurol. 2007;6:693–8.
15. Kanner AM. Suicidality and epilepsy: a complex relationship that remains misunderstood and underestimated. Curr Rev Clin Sci. 2009;9(3):63–6.
16. CDC. Suicide rate is 22% higher among people with epilepsy than the general population. Epilepsy Behav. 2016;61:210–7.
17. Kessler RC, Üstün TB. The world mental health (WMH) survey initiative version of the world health organization (WHO) composite international diagnostic interview (CIDI). Int J Methods Psychiatr Res. 2004;13(2):93–121.
18. Gelaye B, Williams MA, Lemma S, Deyessa N, Bahretibeb Y, Shibre T, Wondimagegn D, Lemenhe A, Fann JR, Vander Stoep A. Validity of the patient health questionnaire-9 for depression screening and diagnosis in East Africa. Psychiatry Res. 2013;210(2):653–61.
19. Bitew T, Hanlon C, Kebede E, Honikman S, Fekadu A. Antenatal depressive symptoms and perinatal complications: a prospective study in rural Ethiopia. BMC Psychiatry. 2017;17(1):301.
20. Meltzer H. Development of a common instrument for mental health. In: Nosikov A, Gudex C, editors. EUROHIS: developing common instruments for health surveys. Amsterdam: IOS Press Google Scholar; 2003.
21. Hecimovic H, Santos JM, Carter J, Attarian HP, Fessler AJ, Vahle V, Gilliam F. Depression but not seizure factors or quality of life predicts suicidality in epilepsy. Epilepsy Behav. 2012;24(4):426–9.
22. Andrijić NL, Alajbegović A, Zec SL, Loga S. Suicidal ideation and thoughts of death in epilepsy patients. Psychiatr Danub. 2014;26(1):52–5.
23. Stefanello S, Marín-Léon L, Fernandes PT, Li LM, Botega NJ. Psychiatric comorbidity and suicidal behavior in epilepsy: a community-based case–control study. Epilepsia. 2010;51(7):1120–5.
24. Espinosa AG, Machado RA, González SB, González ME, Montoto AP, Sotomayor GT. Wisconsin Card Sorting Test performance and impulsivity in patients with temporal lobe epilepsy: suicidal risk and suicide attempts. Epilepsy Behav. 2010;17:39–45.
25. Buljan R, Šantić AM. Suicide attempts in hospital-treated epilepsy patients. Acta Clin Croat. 2011;50(4):485–9.
26. Salgado PCB, Nogueira MH, Yasuda CL, Cendes F. Screening symptoms of depression and suicidal ideation in people with epilepsy using the beck depression inventory. J Epilepsy Clin Neurophysiol. 2012;18(3):85–91.
27. Seo JG, Lee JJ, Cho YW, Lee SJ, Kim JE, Moon HJ, Park SP. Suicidality and its risk factors in Korean people with epilepsy: a MEPSY study. J Clin Neurol. 2015;11(1):32–41.
28. Hara E, Akanuma N, Adachi N, Hara K, Koutroumanidis M. Suicide attempts in adult patients with idiopathic generalized epilepsy. Psychiatry Clin Neurosci. 2009;63:225–9.
29. Ajdacic-Gross V, Weiss MG, Ring M, Hepp U, Bopp M, Gutzwiller F, Rössler W. Methods of suicide: international suicide patterns derived from the WHO mortality database. Bull World Health Organ. 2008;86(9):726–32.
30. Tegegne MT, Mossie TB, Awoke AA, Assaye AM, Gebrie BT, Eshetu DA. Depression and anxiety disorder among epileptic people at Amanuel Specialized Mental Hospital, Addis Ababa, Ethiopia. BMC Psychiatry. 2015;15(210):210.
31. Tegegne MT, Awoke AA. Perception of stigma and associated factors in people with epilepsy at Amanuel Specialized Mental Hospital, Addis Ababa, Ethiopia. Int J Psychiatry Clin Pract. 2016;21(1):58–63.
32. World Health Organization. Suicide huge but preventable public health problem. Geneva: World Health Organization; 2004.
33. Christensen J, Vestergaard M, Mortensen PB, Sidenius P, Agerbo E. Epilepsy and risk of suicide: a population-based case–control study. Lancet Neurol. 2007;6(8):693–8.
34. Nilsson L, Ahlbom A, Farahmand BY, Asberg M, Tomson T. Risk factors for suicide in epilepsy: a case control study. Epilepsia. 2002;43(6):644–51.
35. Qin P, Agerbo E, Mortensen PB. Suicide risk in relation to family history of completed suicide and psychiatric disorders: a nested case–control study based on longitudinal registers. Lancet. 2002;360:1126–30.
36. Mainio A, Alamäki K, Karvonen K, Hakko H, Särkioja T, Räsänen P. Depression and suicide in epileptic victims: a population-based study of suicide victims during the years 1988–2002 in northern Finland. Epilepsy Behav. 2007;11:389–93.
37. Kanner AM. Depression in epilepsy: a neurobiologic perspective. Epilepsy Curr. 2005;5(1):21–7.
38. Hawton K, i Comabella CC, Haw C, Saunders K. Risk factors for suicide in individuals with depression: a systematic review. J Affect Disord. 2013;147(1):17–28.
39. Spina E, Trifirò G, Caputi AP. Pharmacovigilance in psychiatry: an introduction. In: Pharmacovigilance in psychiatry. Springer; 2016. p. 3–7.
40. Pompili M, Vanacore N, Macone S, Amore M, Perticoni G, Tonna M, Sasso E, Lester D, Innamorati M, Gazzella S, et al. Depression, hopelessness and suicide risk among patients suffering from epilepsy. Ann Ist super sAnItà 2007. 2007;43(4):425–9.

13

Cardiometabolic comorbidities, readmission, and costs in schizophrenia and bipolar disorder

Christoph U. Correll[1,2], Daisy S. Ng-Mak[3*], Dana Stafkey-Mailey[4], Eileen Farrelly[4], Krithika Rajagopalan[3] and Antony Loebel[5]

Abstract

Background: Serious mental illnesses are associated with increased risk of cardiometabolic comorbidities. The objective of this study was to evaluate the prevalence of cardiometabolic comorbidity and its association with hospitalization outcomes and costs among inpatients with schizophrenia or bipolar disorder.

Methods: This retrospective database analysis reviewed patients with an inpatient diagnosis of schizophrenia or bipolar disorder from the Premier Perspective® Database (4/1/2010–6/30/2012). Patients were categorized into 4 cohorts based on the number of ICD-9-CM cardiometabolic comorbidities (i.e., 0, 1, 2, or 3+). Outcomes included length of stay, mortality during the index hospitalization, healthcare costs, and 30-day all-cause readmission rates.

Results: Of 57,506 patients with schizophrenia, 66.1% had at least one cardiometabolic comorbidity; 39.3% had two or more comorbidities. Of 124,803 patients with bipolar disorder, 60.5% had at least one cardiometabolic comorbidity; 33.4% had two or more. Average length of stay was 8.5 (for patients with schizophrenia) and 5.2 (for patients with bipolar disorder) days. Each additional cardiometabolic comorbidity was associated with an increase in length of stay for patients with bipolar disorder ($p < .001$) but not for patients with schizophrenia. Mortality rates during the index hospitalization were 1.2% (schizophrenia) and .7% (bipolar disorder). Each additional cardiometabolic comorbidity was associated with a significant increase in mortality for patients with bipolar disorder (OR 1.218, $p < .001$), and a numerical increase in mortality for patients with schizophrenia (OR 1.014, $p = .727$). Patients with more cardiometabolic comorbidities were more likely to have a 30-day readmission (schizophrenia = 9–13%; bipolar disorder = 7–12%), and to incur higher costs (schizophrenia = $10,606–15,355; bipolar disorder = $7126–13,523) (all $p < .01$).

Conclusions: Over 60% of inpatients with schizophrenia or bipolar disorder had cardiometabolic comorbidities. Greater cardiometabolic comorbidity burden was associated with an increased likelihood of readmission and higher costs among patients with schizophrenia or bipolar disorder, and an increase in length of stay and mortality for patients with bipolar disorder.

Keywords: Schizophrenia, Bipolar disorder, Cardiometabolic comorbidity, Hospitalization, Healthcare costs

Background

Severe and persistent mental illnesses that are often debilitating to patients, such as schizophrenia and bipolar disorder, are associated with increased physical comorbidities and mortality [1–7]. Schizophrenia is characterized by psychosis, behavioral dysfunction, and cognitive impairment and has a prevalence of approximately 1% in the United States (US) [8]. Bipolar disorder is a mood disorder characterized by intermittent periods of mania and major depression that has an approximate lifetime prevalence of 4% among adults in the US [9]. The severe psychiatric symptoms and accompanying functional disability among patients that suffer from these

*Correspondence: daisy.ng-mak@sunovion.com
[3] Sunovion Pharmaceuticals Inc., 84 Waterford Dr., Marlborough, MA 01752, USA
Full list of author information is available at the end of the article

debilitating disorders often result in high rates of unemployment [10], incarceration [11], and suicide [12].

Compounding the psychiatric disability in schizophrenia and bipolar disorder, a growing literature suggests that physical comorbidities in this population reduce life expectancy by as much as 10–25 years and double the risk of premature mortality compared to the general population [7]. Patients with schizophrenia have 2.4 times the rate of metabolic syndrome and 2.0 times the rate of diabetes than the general population [1]. Similarly, patients with bipolar disorder have 2.0 times the rate of metabolic syndrome [2] and 1.7 times the rate of diabetes [3] than the general population. Furthermore, some evidence suggests that the prevalence of cardiometabolic risks is underestimated among patients with schizophrenia [4, 5] or bipolar disorder [9] due to under-diagnosis and under-treatment.

Complicating the inherent higher risk of cardiometabolic comorbidities in patients with schizophrenia or bipolar disorder, atypical antipsychotics, which are standard pharmacological treatment for schizophrenia and many patients with bipolar disorder, can exacerbate patients' risk of cardiometabolic disease [13]. For example, treatment with certain atypical antipsychotics is associated with an increasing risk of developing metabolic syndrome [14, 15], diabetes [16–19], and elevated low-density lipoprotein cholesterol levels [19–21].

Hospital readmissions within 30 days post-hospital discharges (i.e., 30-day readmissions) have become an important measure of health care quality due to the high 30-day readmission rates among US Medicare beneficiaries [22]. Evidence suggests that 30-day readmissions are a significant predictor of long-term mortality [23]. In order to reduce 30-day readmission rates, the Centers for Medicare and Medicaid Services implemented the Medicare Hospital Readmissions Reduction Program which, as a penalty, reduces Medicare payments to hospitals with excess 30-day readmissions relative to the mean national readmission rates in conditions such as acute myocardial infarction and heart failure [24]. In a statistical brief summarizing the readmission trend in 2013, schizophrenia, mood disorder, and diabetes were among the top 20 conditions with the highest all-cause 30-day readmission rates [25].

While the prevalence, outcomes, and costs of cardiometabolic comorbidities in patients with schizophrenia and bipolar disorder have been examined in some outpatient studies [1–3], these variables remain relatively unexplored in hospitalized patients. In addition, although there is extensive literature regarding 30-day readmissions attributed to particular illnesses such as mental (e.g., schizophrenia) or cardiometabolic conditions (e.g., diabetes), the incremental impact of cardiometabolic conditions on readmission among patients with schizophrenia or bipolar disorder remains unknown. Therefore, the objectives of this study were to determine the prevalence of cardiometabolic comorbidities among inpatients with schizophrenia and bipolar disorder and to assess the role of incremental cardiometabolic comorbidity burden on length of stay, mortality, and healthcare costs during the initial admission. Following discharge, the study also examined the role of incremental cardiometabolic comorbidity burden on the 30-day readmission rate.

Methods

Study design

This retrospective observational study used administrative hospital data from the Premier Perspective Database® (Premier, Inc., Charlotte, NC, USA) during the period from April 1, 2010 to June 30, 2012. The Premier database is the largest hospital administrative database in the US and provides detailed service information from over 700 geographically dispersed hospitals and over 50 million discharges since 2000. The database contained detailed service level information, diagnostic information, hospital characteristics, and patient demographic information. The database did not include any identifiable protected health information and, pursuant to the Health Insurance Portability and Accountability Act of 1996 [26], the study did not require institutional review board waiver or approval.

Patient selection

Patients with a primary, secondary, or admitting diagnosis of schizophrenia (International Classification of Diseases, 9th Revision, Clinical Modification [ICD-9-CM] code 295.xx) or bipolar disorder (ICD-9-CM codes 296.0, 296.1, 296.4–296.8, 301.11, or 301.13) coded during their hospitalization stays were identified between October 1, 2010 and May 31, 2012. The first such hospitalization record was designated as the patient's index hospitalization. Patients diagnosed with both schizophrenia and bipolar disorder, patients who were less than 18-year old, or patients who were transferred from another hospital or an unknown admission source were excluded from the analysis.

Variable definitions

Six cardiometabolic comorbidities were examined for both the patients with schizophrenia and bipolar disorder: cerebrovascular disease (ICD-9-CM 430–438.xx), coronary or ischemic heart disease (ICD-9-CM 410.xx–411.xx, 413.xx–414.xx), diabetes mellitus (ICD-9-CM 250.xx), hyperglycemia (ICD-9-CM 790.2), hyperlipidemia (ICD-9-CM 272.x), and hypertension (ICD-9-CM

401.x–405.x). Patients were categorized into 1 of 4 comorbidity cohorts based on the number of cardiometabolic comorbidity diagnoses recorded during their index hospitalization (i.e., 0, 1, 2, or 3+). In addition to examining these specific cardiometabolic comorbidities, the Charlson Comorbidity Index (CCI) was coded based on an algorithm developed for administrative data [27] using comorbidities reported during the index hospitalization as well as all inpatient or outpatient hospitalizations in the Premier database that occurred in 6 months prior to the index admission.

Outcome variables

Outcome variables during the index hospitalization included length of stay, mortality, and costs. Following discharge from the index hospitalization, 30-day all-cause readmission rates were also examined. Length of stay in days and mortality were obtained from the discharge record for the index hospitalization. The hospitals reported both the charges for each individual service based on their charge master and the costs the hospital reported incurring to deliver the services. This analysis focused on the costs to deliver services, which were split into pharmacy and medical costs with the medical costs representing all non-pharmacy costs. All costs were adjusted to 2014 US dollars using the medical care component of the Consumer Price Index from the US Bureau of Labor Statistics [28]. The 30-day all-cause readmission rates were defined as a subsequent readmission to the same hospital for any reason within 30 days of discharge.

Statistical analyses

Patient demographic and baseline characteristics were summarized using descriptive statistics. The relationship between cardiometabolic comorbidities and study outcomes were evaluated using multivariate statistical models controlling for the following baseline variables: age, gender, race, payer, CCI, hospital region (Midwest, Northeast, South, and West), hospital location (urban/rural), hospital type (teaching/non-teaching), and hospital bed count. For the dichotomous outcome variables, mortality and 30-day readmission, logistic regression models were used. Length of stay was treated as count data and a negative binomial regression was used. Finally, for the highly skewed cost variables, total costs, pharmacy costs, and medical costs, generalized linear models (GLMs) with a gamma distribution and log-link function were used. The statistical models were fit separately for the schizophrenia and bipolar samples. Statistical analyses were conducted using SAS version 9.4 (SAS Institute, Cary, NC, USA). All analyses were two-sided with alpha of .05.

Results

Patient selection

There were 118,065 patients with an inpatient hospitalization for schizophrenia. Of these, 51.3% (n = 60,559) were excluded for the following reasons: index hospitalization did not have the required 6-month prior observation or 1-month follow-up period; age younger than 18 years; transfer from another hospital or an unknown admission source; diagnoses of both schizophrenia and bipolar disorder. Among 229,974 patients with an inpatient hospitalization for bipolar disorder, 45.7% (n = 105,171) were excluded after applying the exclusion criteria as above. The final study sample included 57,506 and 124,803 inpatients with a diagnosis of schizophrenia and bipolar disorder, respectively.

Patient characteristics

Patient characteristics are described in Table 1. The average age of patients with schizophrenia and bipolar disorder was in the mid to late 40s. The most common cardiometabolic comorbidities were hypertension (52% bipolar disorder; 57% schizophrenia), hyperlipidemia (28% bipolar disorder; 30% schizophrenia), and diabetes (22% bipolar disorder; 28% schizophrenia), with each numerically higher for patients with schizophrenia than patients with bipolar disorder. Nearly two-thirds of patients with schizophrenia (66.1%) and bipolar disorder (60.5%) had at least one cardiometabolic comorbidity, and over one-third of patients with schizophrenia (39.3%) and bipolar disorder (33.4%) had 2 or more cardiometabolic comorbidities.

Outcomes

For the index hospitalization, the mean length of stay was 8.5 days for patients with schizophrenia and 5.2 days for patients with bipolar disorder. Multivariate analyses showed a negative association between cardiometabolic comorbidity burden with length of stay for schizophrenia ($p < .001$), but a positive association for bipolar disorder ($p < .001$) (see Fig. 1a).

The index hospitalization mortality rate was 1.2% for the patients with schizophrenia and .7% for the patients with bipolar disorder. For those with schizophrenia, the risk of death during the index hospitalization was not significantly associated with each additional cardiometabolic comorbidity (odds ratio [OR] 1.014; 95% confidence interval [CI] .937, 1.098, $p = .727$). Prior to correcting for baseline differences, a Chi square test showed that patients with schizophrenia who had one or more cardiometabolic comorbidities had a higher risk of mortality compared to those with no comorbidities (1.7 vs. .3%, $p < .001$). For those with bipolar disorder, the risk of death during the index hospitalization increased by 21.8% (OR

Table 1 Demographic, clinical, and hospital facility characteristics for patients with schizophrenia and bipolar disorder

Characteristic	Schizophrenia ($N = 57{,}506$)	Bipolar disorder ($N = 124{,}803$)
Demographics		
Age, years (mean)	49.8	45.4
Female (%)	43.0	63.0
Race (%)		
African American	29.0	10.0
Caucasian	51.0	73.0
Hispanic	2.0	1.0
Other	18.0	15.0
Region (%)		
Midwest	24.0	24.0
Northeast	23.0	20.0
South	36.0	41.0
West	17.0	15.0
Payer (%)		
Medicaid	30.0	25.0
Medicare	51.0	35.0
Commercial/private	9.0	24.0
Self-pay	6.0	9.0
Other	5.0	6.0
Comorbidities		
Charlson comorbidity index (mean)	1.1	1.0
Specific cardiometabolic comorbidities (%)		
Diabetes	28.0	22.0
Hyperglycemia	2.0	2.0
Hypertension	57.0	52.0
Hyperlipidemia	30.0	28.0
Ischemic heart disease	9.0	9.0
Cerebrovascular disease	4.0	3.0
Number of cardiometabolic comorbidities (%)		
0	33.9	39.5
1	26.7	27.1
2	19.9	16.6
3+	19.4	16.8
Hospital characteristics		
Bed size (mean)	436	409
Urban (%)	89.0	86.0
Teaching (%)	48.0	42.0

1.218; 95% CI 1.129, 1.314, $p < .001$) with each additional cardiometabolic comorbidity (Fig. 1c). Prior to correcting for baseline differences, a Chi square test showed that patients with bipolar disorder who had one or more cardiometabolic comorbidities had a higher risk of mortality compared to those with no comorbidities (1.45 vs. .10%, $p < .001$).

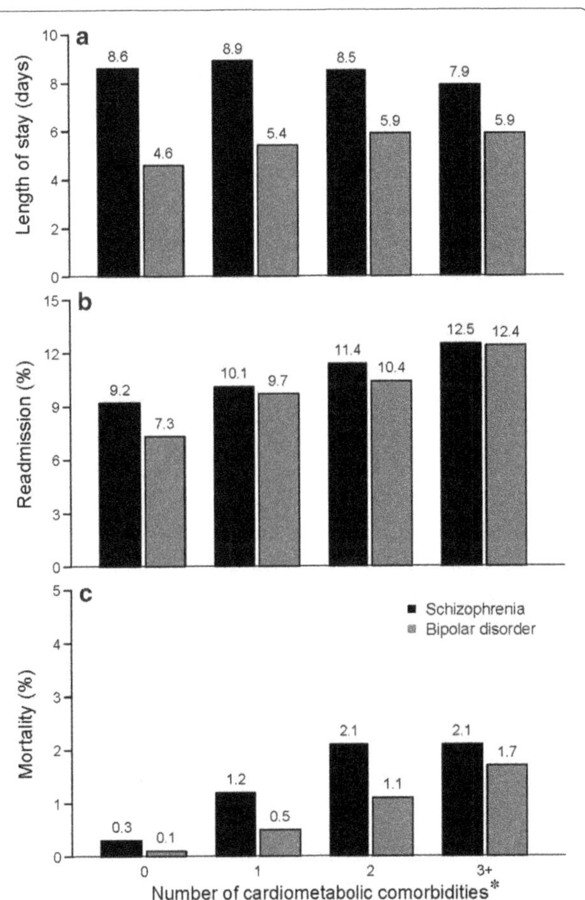

Fig. 1 Length of stay, 30-day all-cause readmission, and hospital mortality by number of cardiometabolic comorbidities. **a** The mean length of stay was 8.5 days for overall patients with schizophrenia and 5.2 days for patients with bipolar disorder. Negative binomial regressions showed a negative association between cardiometabolic comorbidity burden with length of stay for schizophrenia (−.015; 95% CI −.024, −.007, $p < .001$), but a positive association for bipolar disorder (.029; 95% CI .024, .034, $p < .001$). **b** Overall, 11.8% of the patients with schizophrenia and 9.3% of the patients with bipolar disorder were readmitted for any reason within 30 days of discharge from the index hospitalization. For each additional cardiometabolic comorbidity, logistic regressions showed the odds of readmission increased by 3.1% (OR 1.031; 95% CI 1.001, 1.061, $p = .042$) for schizophrenia and by 6.4% (OR 1.064; 95% CI 1.041, 1.087, $p < .001$) for bipolar disorder. **c** The index hospitalization mortality rate was 1.2% for overall patients with schizophrenia and .7% for patients with bipolar disorder. In schizophrenia, cardiometabolic comorbidity was not significantly associated with mortality (OR 1.014; 95% CI .937, 1.098, $p = .727$). A Chi square test showed that patients with schizophrenia who had one or more cardiometabolic comorbidities had a higher risk of mortality compared to those with no comorbidities (1.7 vs. .3%, $p < .001$). In bipolar disorder, each additional cardiometabolic comorbidity was associated with a 21.8% increase in mortality during the index hospitalization (OR 1.218; 95% CI 1.129, 1.314, $p < .001$). A Chi square test showed that patients with bipolar disorder who had one or more cardiometabolic comorbidities had a higher risk of mortality compared to those with no comorbidities (1.45 vs. .10%, $p < .001$). * The following covariates were included in all regression analyses: age, gender, race, payer, CCI, hospital region, hospital location (urban/rural), hospital type (teaching/non-teaching), and hospital bed count

Hospitalization costs increased as the number of cardiometabolic comorbidities increased (see Fig. 2). For patients with schizophrenia, the mean total cost for the index hospitalization was $12,781 per patient (medical and pharmacy costs of $11,771 and $1010 per patient, respectively). Medical costs increased by 6.8%, pharmacy costs by 25.9%, and total costs by 8.3% (all $p < .0001$) for each additional cardiometabolic comorbidity. For patients with bipolar disorder, the mean total cost for the index hospitalization was $9725 per patient (medical and pharmacy costs of $8878 and $847 per patient, respectively). Medical costs increased by 12.3%, pharmacy costs by 26.6%, and total costs by 13.4% (all $p < .0001$) for each additional cardiometabolic comorbidity.

Within 30-days of discharge from the index hospitalization, 11.8% of the patients with schizophrenia and 9.3% of the patients with bipolar disorder were readmitted for any reason. Odds of readmission increased by 3.1% (OR 1.031; 95% confidence interval [CI] 1.001, 1.061, $p = .042$) for patients with schizophrenia and by 6.4% (OR 1.064; 95% CI 1.041, 1.087, $p < .001$) for patients with bipolar disorder (see Fig. 1b) with each additional cardiometabolic comorbidity.

Discussion

In this large, nationally representative administrative database study of hospitalized patients with schizophrenia and bipolar disorder, cardiometabolic comorbidities were common. Over 60% of patients had ≥1 cardiometabolic comorbidity and over 30% had ≥2 cardiometabolic comorbidities. Increasing cardiometabolic comorbidity burden was associated with a significantly higher mortality rate (for bipolar disorder), and longer hospital stays (for bipolar disorder). Patients with schizophrenia appeared to have almost double the rates of mortality in comparison to patients with bipolar disorder. The average total all-cause hospitalization cost was $12,781 and $9725 per patient for schizophrenia and bipolar disorder, respectively. Each incremental cardiometabolic comorbidity was associated with an 8.3 and 13.4% increase in total hospital cost for patients with schizophrenia and bipolar disorder, respectively. While 1 in 10 schizophrenia or bipolar disorder patients had an all-cause readmission within 30-days after index hospitalization, the odds of 30-day readmission increased with each incremental cardiometabolic comorbidity.

The reported frequencies of cardiometabolic comorbidities in this study are generally consistent with those previously reported in the literature [1, 2, 15, 29, 30]. However, this study identified a higher prevalence of diabetes in patients with schizophrenia and bipolar disorder (28 and 22%, respectively) than previously reported (7–15%) [4, 6, 30–33]. This discrepancy in the reported prevalence of diabetes may be due to the study population; previous studies have typically been drawn from

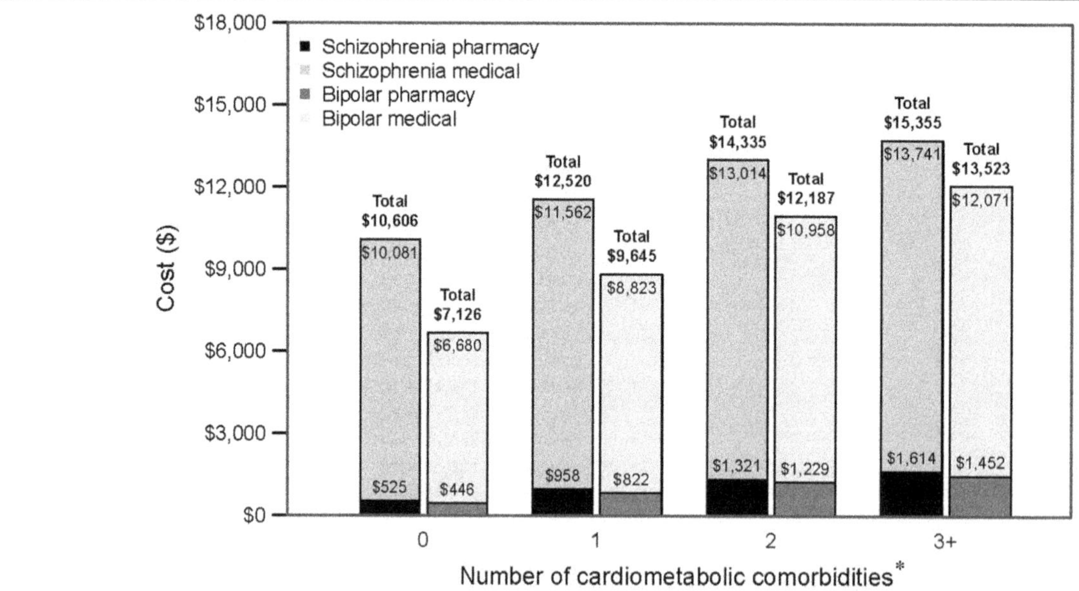

Fig. 2 Medical, pharmacy, and total costs by number of cardiometabolic comorbidities. *Dollar figures* reflect the costs to the hospital to deliver care in 2014 dollars. For both schizophrenia and bipolar disorder, increasing cardiometabolic comorbidity was associated with increased pharmacy, medical, and total index hospitalization costs (all $p < .001$). The following covariates were included in the gamma regression analyses with a log link: age, gender, race, payer, CCI, hospital region, hospital location (urban/rural), hospital type (teaching/non-teaching), and hospital bed count. * The data are presented by number of cardiometabolic comorbidities. Overall mean total cost for patients with schizophrenia was $12,781 per patient (medical and pharmacy costs of $11,771 and $1010 per patient, respectively). Overall mean total cost for patients with bipolar disorder was $9725 per patient (medical and pharmacy costs of $8878 and $847 per patient, respectively)

broader health system populations [30], clinical trial participants [4], or primary care settings [6]. Among the general population, nearly 20% of hospital stays in the US are associated with diabetes [34]. The prevalence of diabetes found among inpatients with schizophrenia (28%) or bipolar disorder (22%) in this study is therefore plausible, given that they are already considered a high-risk population for diabetes [33].

To the best of our knowledge, this is the first study to evaluate the risk of 30-day readmission among hospitalized patients with schizophrenia or bipolar disorder and its association with incremental cardiometabolic comorbidity burden. Our study showed that incremental cardiometabolic comorbidity burden was associated with a 3.1 and 6.4% increased risk of early readmission in patients with schizophrenia and bipolar disorder, respectively. A recent chart review study of 945 patients hospitalized in a psychiatric care facility found that psychiatric readmission in the following year was independently predicted by higher body mass index (BMI) [35]. The authors hypothesized that inflammation, which has been associated with both higher BMI and obesity as well as psychiatric disorders [36] may represent the link between the greater BMI and need for readmission, but research examining the mechanisms of early readmissions and cardiometabolic comorbidities is needed.

For patients with bipolar disorder, additional cardiometabolic comorbidity burden was associated with an increase in the length of stay (4.6 days for no comorbidities to 5.9 days for 3+ comorbidities). Surprisingly, increasing cardiometabolic comorbidity burden was associated with a small decrease in the length of stay among patients with schizophrenia (8.6 days for no comorbidities to 7.9 days for 3+ comorbidities). While the reasons for these differences in length of stay are not known, it is possible that bipolar disorder patients may have been more likely to receive medical assessment and/or intervention for comorbid conditions than were patients with schizophrenia in this study; alternatively it is possible that patients with schizophrenia were more likely to have medical comorbidities that were well established and known to treatment staff compared to patients with bipolar disorder.

Prior research has clearly established a link between cardiometabolic conditions and mortality in the general population [37]. The lack of statistical significance between the odds of mortality and cardiometabolic comorbidity burden in schizophrenia after correcting for demographic and hospital characteristics was unexpected; however, a univariate analysis showed a significant association with comorbidity burden and mortality. Given the small sample sizes and the rarity of mortality incidence in this dataset, it is also plausible that the potential association between mortality and cardiovascular comorbidity is underestimated. Cardiovascular disease, along with cancer and suicide, has also been established as one of the leading causes of death for patients with schizophrenia [38]. Although information about the cause of death was unavailable, confounding of the results by suicide is likely small, as all the patients were hospitalized at community hospitals and not psychiatric hospitals, indicating severity of a medical, rather than psychiatric condition at the time of admission.

Previous studies have reported increased outpatient or total costs for psychiatric patients with cardiometabolic comorbidities [39–41]. This study is unique in that it demonstrated the possible relationship between each additional cardiometabolic comorbidity and incremental costs per admission for patients with schizophrenia or bipolar disorder.

The results of this study highlight the importance of identifying optimal treatment regimens for patients with serious mental illness. Efforts should be taken to adequately monitor for and reduce the rates of cardiometabolic comorbidities in this vulnerable patient population, and perhaps consider antipsychotic therapeutic options with a limited liability for such comorbidities [13]. From a holistic approach of treating patients with serious mental illness, clinicians should coordinate care and consider a patients' medical profile when prescribing medications. Coordinated care can also improve quality of care and patient satisfaction [42], which may have a positive effect on reducing healthcare costs through shorter hospital stays and/or reduced early readmissions. Furthermore, improved physical health may also positively impact psychiatric health outcomes [35]. In 2013, four new measures of the Healthcare Effectiveness Data and Information Set were added to assess quality of care for patients with serious mental illness; two of these four measures focus on diabetes monitoring and cardiovascular monitoring, which highlights the importance of monitoring cardiometabolic risks among this susceptible patient population [43]. Monitoring patients' cardiometabolic profiles, consideration of these risk factors when selecting antipsychotic drug therapies, and striving to coordinate care delivery for both mental and physical symptoms may maximize patients' outcomes.

Limitations

The data used in this study were collected for administrative reasons rather than for research purposes. The study design precludes any determination of causal relationship between cardiometabolic comorbidities and the outcomes. The analysis was restricted to variables present in this particular database, and other factors that were not available in the database may have confounded the observed relationships. Information about the prior treatments for the mental and physical morbidities, prior hospitalizations, and reasons for death was unavailable. In particular, data on atypical antipsychotic utilization prior to hospitalization were not available, therefore it was not possible to assess the relationship between specific antipsychotic medications and cardiometabolic comorbidities, which have been previously described to vary substantially [2, 13, 20, 33].

The burden of cardiometabolic comorbidities in this study was measured using diagnostic ICD-9-CM codes of 6 disease entities. Studies that have used the more robust National Cholesterol Education Program's Adult Treatment Panel III report (ATP III) or International Diabetes Federation (IDF) definitions [15] have reported metabolic syndrome prevalence of approximately 33% for schizophrenia [15] and 37% for bipolar disorder [2]. The ICD-9-CM coding did not allow for the clear identification of bipolar II disorder (falls under "bipolar other"), precluding the assessment of differences in the number of cardiovascular comorbidities and outcomes between bipolar I and bipolar II subtypes. Moreover, there was no control group of inpatients without serious mental illness. The analysis of each patient was limited to a single index hospitalization and 30 days post-discharge, rather than attempting to determine hospital costs or outcomes over a longer duration of follow-up. Readmission rates in this study may be an underestimate, as these data only include admissions to the hospitals in the Premier network, and the likelihood of readmission to hospitals has been reported to be as high as 20% elsewhere [22].

Conclusions

In this large, retrospective, administrative database study, over 60% of patients with schizophrenia or bipolar disorder had at least one cardiometabolic comorbidity, and over 30% had two or more cardiometabolic comorbidities. For patients with schizophrenia, increasing cardiometabolic comorbidity burden had a significant impact on cost of index hospitalization, and 30-day readmission rates. For patients with bipolar disorder, increasing cardiometabolic comorbidity burden had a significant impact on length of stay, hospital mortality rates, cost of index hospitalization, and 30-day readmission rates. These results further underscore the need for improved detection and management of cardiometabolic risk factors in patients with schizophrenia or bipolar disorder across different clinical care settings. Further research is needed to better understand the long-term consequences of cardiometabolic comorbidity burden on patients with schizophrenia or bipolar disorder.

Abbreviations

ATP III: National Cholesterol Education Program's Adult Treatment Panel II; CCI: Charlson Comorbidity Index; GLMs: generalized linear models; ICD-9-CM: International Classification of Diseases, 9th Revision, Clinical Modification; IDF: International Diabetes Federation; US: United States.

Authors' contributions

Authors CUC, DSNM, DSM, EF, KR, and AL were involved in the study conception and design, drafting of the manuscript, data interpretation, and critical revision of the manuscript. Authors DSM and EF completed the data analysis in this study. All authors read and approved the final manuscript.

Author details

[1] Hofstra North Shore LIJ School of Medicine, Manhasset, NY, USA. [2] The Zucker Hillside Hospital, Glen Oaks, NY, USA. [3] Sunovion Pharmaceuticals Inc., 84 Waterford Dr., Marlborough, MA 01752, USA. [4] Xcenda, Palm Harbor, FL, USA. [5] Sunovion Pharmaceuticals Inc., Fort Lee, NJ, USA.

Acknowledgements

The authors acknowledge the contributions of Dr. Mariam Hassan and Dr. Chien-Chia Chuang who contributed to the design of this study and provided editorial support, respectively. Charles Meyer, who received support from Xcenda, and Dr. Michael Stensland of Agile Outcomes Research, Inc. both provided writing support.

Competing interests

Authors DSNM, KR, and AL are all employees of Sunovion Pharmaceuticals Inc. Other authors (DSM and EF) are employees of Xcenda LLC, which was compensated by Sunovion Pharmaceuticals Inc. All competing interests have been disclosed.

Funding

This research was funded by Sunovion Pharmaceuticals Inc., Marlborough, MA, USA. The authors who were employees of Sunovion Pharmaceuticals Inc. were involved in the final decision to publish study results and the sponsor reviewed the manuscript prior to submission, but publication of study results was not contingent on the sponsor's approval or censorship of the manuscript.

References

1. Vancampfort D, Wampers M, Mitchell AJ, et al. A meta-analysis of cardio-metabolic abnormalities in drug naïve, first-episode and multi-episode patients with schizophrenia versus general population controls. World Psychiatry. 2013;12(3):240–50.
2. Vancampfort D, Vansteelandt K, Correll CU, et al. Metabolic syndrome and metabolic abnormalities in bipolar disorder: a meta-analysis of prevalence rates and moderators. Am J Psychiatry. 2013;170(3):265–74.
3. Crump C, Sundquist K, Winkleby MA, Sundquist J. Comorbidities and mortality in bipolar disorder: a Swedish national cohort study. JAMA Psychiatry. 2013;70(9):931–9.
4. Nasrallah HA, Meyer JM, Goff DC, et al. Low rates of treatment for hypertension, dyslipidemia and diabetes in schizophrenia: data from the CATIE schizophrenia trial sample at baseline. Schizophr Res. 2006;86(1–3):15–22.
5. Correll CU, Robinson DG, Schooler NR, et al. Cardiometabolic risk in first episode schizophrenia-spectrum disorder patients: baseline results from the RAISE-ETP study. JAMA Psychiatry. 2014;71(12):1350–63.
6. Smith DJ, Martin D, McLean G, Langan J, Guthrie B, Mercer SW. Multimorbidity in bipolar disorder and undertreatment of cardiovascular disease: a cross sectional study. BMC Med. 2013;11:263.
7. Nordentoft M, Wahlbeck K, Hällgren J, et al. Excess mortality, causes of death and life expectancy in 270,770 patients with recent onset of mental disorders in Denmark, Finland and Sweden. PLoS ONE. 2013;8(1):e55176.
8. Narrow WE, Rae DS, Robins LN, Regier DA. Revised prevalence estimates of mental disorders in the United States: using a clinical significance criterion to reconcile 2 surveys' estimates. Arch Gen Psychiatry. 2002;59(2):115–23.
9. Merikangas KR, Akiskal HS, Angst J, et al. Lifetime and 12-month prevalence of bipolar spectrum disorder in the National Comorbidity Survey replication. Arch Gen Psychiatry. 2007;64(5):543–52.
10. Jääskeläinen E, Juola P, Hirvonen N, et al. A systematic review and meta-analysis of recovery in schizophrenia. Schizophr Bull. 2013;39(6):1296–306.

11. Thornicroft G, Tansella M, Becker T, et al. The personal impact of schizophrenia in Europe. Schizophr Res. 2004;69(2–3):125–32.
12. Olfson M, Gerhard T, Huang C, Crystal S, Stroup TS. Premature mortality among adults with schizophrenia in the United States. JAMA Psychiatry. 2015;72(12):1172–81.
13. De Hert M, Detraux J, van Winkel R, Yu W, Correll CU. Metabolic and cardiovascular adverse effects associated with antipsychotic drugs. Nat Rev Endocrinol. 2011;8(2):114–26.
14. Meyer JM, Davis VG, Goff DC, et al. Change in metabolic syndrome parameters with antipsychotic treatment in the CATIE Schizophrenia Trial: prospective data from phase 1. Schizophr Res. 2008;101(1–3):273–86.
15. Mitchell AJ, Vancampfort D, Sweers K, van Winkel R, Yu W, De Hert M. Prevalence of metabolic syndrome and metabolic abnormalities in schizophrenia and related disorders—a systematic review and meta-analysis. Schizophr Bull. 2013;39(2):306–18.
16. Smith M, Hopkins D, Peveler RC, Holt RI, Woodward M, Ismail K. First-v. second-generation antipsychotics and risk for diabetes in schizophrenia: systematic review and meta-analysis. Br J Psychiatry. 2008;192(6):406–11.
17. Nielsen J, Skadhede S, Correll CU. Antipsychotics associated with the development of type 2 diabetes in antipsychotic-naïve schizophrenia patients. Neuropsychopharmacology. 2010;35(9):1997–2004.
18. Ulcickas Yood M, Delorenze GN, Quesenberry CP Jr, et al. Association between second-generation antipsychotics and newly diagnosed treated diabetes mellitus: does the effect differ by dose? BMC Psychiatry. 2011;11:197.
19. American Diabetes Association, American Psychiatric Association, American Association of Clinical Endocrinologists, North American Association for the Study of obesity. Consensus development conference on antipsychotic drugs and obesity and diabetes. Diabetes Care. 2004;27(2):596–601.
20. Correll CU, Lencz T, Malhotra AK. Antipsychotic drugs and obesity. Trends Mol Med. 2011;17(2):97–107.
21. Rummel-Kluge C, Komossa K, Schwarz S, et al. Head-to-head comparisons of metabolic side effects of second generation antipsychotics in the treatment of schizophrenia: a systematic review and meta-analysis. Schizophr Res. 2010;123(2–3):225–33.
22. Jencks SF, Williams MV, Coleman EA. Rehospitalizations among patients in the Medicare fee-for-service program. N Engl J Med. 2009;360(14):1418–28.
23. Yian E, Zhou H, Schreiber A, et al. Early hospital readmission and mortality risk after surgical treatment of proximal humerus fractures in a community-based health care organization. Perm J. 2016;20(1):47–52.
24. Centers for Medicare & Medicaid Services: Readmissions Reduction Program. https://www.cms.gov/medicare/medicare-fee-for-service-payment/acuteinpatientpps/readmissions-reduction-program.html. Accessed 3 Aug 2016.
25. Fingar K, Washington R. Trends in hospital readmissions for four high-volume conditions, 2009–2013: Statistical Brief #196. Rockville: Agency for Healthcare Research and Quality. 2015. https://www.hcup-us.ahrq.gov/reports/statbriefs/sb196-Readmissions-Trends-High-Volume-Conditions.jsp. Accessed 3 Aug 2016.
26. United States Congress. Health Insurance Portability and Accountability Act of 1996. 1996. http://www.gpo.gov/fdsys/pkg/PLAW-104publ191/html/PLAW-104publ191.htm. Accessed 3 Aug 2016.
27. Deyo RA, Cherkin DC, Ciol MA. Adapting a clinical comorbidity index for use with ICD-9-CM administrative databases. J Clin Epidemiol. 1992;45(6):613–9.
28. U.S. Bureau of Labor Statistics. Measuring price change for medical care in the CPI. 2009. http://www.bls.gov/cpi/cpifact4.htm. Accessed 3 Aug 2016.
29. Kemp DE, Sylvia LG, Calabrese JR, et al, LiTMUS Study Group. General medical burden in bipolar disorder: findings from the LiTMUS comparative effectiveness trial. Acta Psychiatr Scand. 2014;129:24–34.
30. Bresee LC, Majumdar SR, Patten SB, Johnson JA. Prevalence of cardiovascular risk factors and disease in people with schizophrenia: a population-based study. Schizophr Res. 2010;117(1):75–82.
31. Cohen D, Stolk RP, Grobbee DE, Gispen-de Wied CC. Hyperglycemia and diabetes in patients with schizophrenia or schizoaffective disorders. Diabetes Care. 2006;29(4):786–91.
32. van Winkel R, De Hert M, Van Eyck D, et al. Prevalence of diabetes and the metabolic syndrome in a sample of patients with bipolar disorder. Bipolar Disord. 2008;10(2):342–8.
33. Vancampfort D, Correll CU, Galling B, et al. Diabetes mellitus in people with schizophrenia, bipolar disorder and major depressive disorder: a systematic review and large scale meta-analysis. World Psychiatry. 2016;15(2):166–74.
34. Fraze TK, Jiang HJ, Burgess J. Hospital stays for patients with diabetes, 2008. HCUP Statistical Brief #93. Rockville: Agency for Healthcare Research and Quality. 2010. http://www.hcup-us.ahrq.gov/reports/statbriefs/sb93.pdf. Accessed 3 Aug 2016.
35. Manu P, Khan S, Radhakrishan R, Russ MJ, Kane JM, Correll CU. Body mass index identified as an independent predictor of psychiatric readmission. J Clin Psychiatry. 2014;75(6):e573–7.
36. Manu P, Correll CU, Wampers M, et al. Markers of inflammation in schizophrenia: association vs. causation. World Psychiatry. 2014;13(2):189–92.
37. Casey DE, Haupt DW, Newcomer JW, Henderson DC, Sernyak MJ, Davidson M, Lindenmayer J-P, Manoukian SV, Banerji MA, Lebovitz HE, Hennekens CH. Antipsychotic-induced weight gain and metabolic abnormalities: implications for increased mortality in patients with schizophrenia. J Clin Psychiatry. 2004;65(S7):4–18.
38. Bushe CJ, Taylor M, Haukka J. Mortality in schizophrenia: a measurable clinical endpoint. J. Psychopharmacol. Oxf. Engl. 2010;24:17–25.
39. Chwastiak LA, Rosenheck RA, McEvoy JP, et al. The impact of obesity on the costs among persons with schizophrenia. Gen Hosp Psychiatry. 2009;31(1):1–7.
40. Jerrell JM, McIntyre RS, Tripathi A. Incidence and costs of cardiometabolic conditions in patients with schizophrenia treated with antipsychotic medications. Clin Schizophr Relat Psychoses. 2010;4(3):161–8.
41. Guo JJ, Keck PE, Li H, Patel NC. Treatment costs related to bipolar disorder and comorbid conditions among Medicaid patients with bipolar disorder. Psychiatr Serv. 2007;58(8):1073–8.
42. Horvitz-Lennon M, Kilbourne AM, Pincus HA. From silos to bridges: meeting the general health care needs of adults with severe mental illnesses. Health Aff (Millwood). 2006;25(3):659–69.
43. National Committee for Quality Assurance. HEDIS 2013: Technical Specifications for Health Plans. 2012. http://www.ncqa.org.

14

Suicidal ideation and suicide attempts among asthma

Jae Ho Chung[1], Sun- Hyun Kim[2*] and Yong Won Lee[1]

Abstract

Background: The present study aimed to investigate the mental health status in patients with asthma and assess the effects of asthma on suicidal ideation and attempts using a representative sample from Korea.

Methods: Individual-level data were obtained from 228,744 participants (6372 with asthma and 222,372 without asthma) of the 2013 Korean Community Health Survey. Demographic characteristics, socioeconomic status, physical health status, and mental health status were compared between patients with asthma and population without asthma. Multivariable logistic regression was performed to investigate the independent effects of the asthma on suicidal ideation and attempts.

Results: A depressed mood for 2 or more continuous weeks was reported by 12.0% of subjects with asthma and 5.7% of controls ($p < 0.001$). Suicidal thoughts were reported by 21.4% of patients with asthma and 9.8% of controls ($p < 0.001$). Suicidal attempts were reported by 1.0% of the patients with asthma and 0.4% of controls ($p < 0.001$). Following adjustment for age, sex, income, education, job, marital status, smoking, alcohol, exercise, and presence of diabetes mellitus, hypertension, stroke, arthritis, and depression, the ORs for suicidal ideation with asthma were 1.53 (95% CI 1.42–1.65) and that for suicidal attempts was 1.32 (95% CI 1.01–1.73).

Conclusions: We found that asthma increased the risk for suicidal ideation and attempts, even controlling for the effects of socioeconomic status, physical health status, comorbid chronic medical diseases, and depressive mood. Our finding suggests that asthma per se may be an independent risk factor for suicidality.

Keywords: Suicidal ideation, Suicidal attempt, Asthma

Background

Many chronic diseases are complicated by emotional and psychological disorders and yet the emotional dimensions of such chronic diseases are frequently overlooked when medical treatment is considered [1]. Several studies have found statistically significant correlates between asthma and suicide ideation and suicide attempts [2–6].

Suicide is the fourth leading cause of death in Korea [7]. Suicide rate was 33.3 per 100,000 persons in Korea in 2011, which ranked first among the Organization for Economic Co-operation and Development (OECD) countries (https://data.oecd.org/healthstat/suicide-rates.htm). Since asthma and suicide are important public health burdens, epidemiological study investigating the mental health status in asthma patients and its relationship with suicidal ideations and attempts would be required to assess the potential risk for suicide, and ultimately prevent suicidal completion in patients with asthma. However, very few studies about the relationship between asthma and suicide have been done in Asia especially South Korea. There are a number of epidemiological differences among the studies that have evaluated suicidal behavior, and an investigation of the various comorbidities and risk factors that lead to suicide in different ethnic groups is therefore necessary. As far as I know, this is the first study suicidal prevalence among asthma patients in Korea.

We aimed to compare the status of mental health including suicidal ideations and attempts between

*Correspondence: sunhyun@yahoo.com
[2] Department of Family Medicine, International St. Mary's Hospital, Catholic Kwandong University College of Medicine, Simgokro 100 Gil 25 Seo-gu, Incheon 22711, Republic of Korea
Full list of author information is available at the end of the article

patients with asthma and population without asthma using data from nationwide population-based health survey (The 2013 Korean Community Health Survey).

Methods

Study participants

For this study, we obtained data from the 2013 Korean Community Health Survey (KCHS, https://chs.cdc.go.kr/chs/index.do), which was carried out by the Korea Centers for Disease Control and Prevention (KCDC). The KCHS is a nationwide cross-sectional health interview survey, annually conducted since 2008, to investigate the patterns of disease prevalence and morbidity as well as personal lifestyle and health-related behaviors in adults aged 19 years or older. The sample size for the KCHS is 900 subjects in each of 253 community units, including 16 metropolitan cities and provinces. The KCHS expects a total of 227,700 survey participants per year, but the actual number of respondents approximates 230,000. The KCHS has a two-stage sampling process. The first stage involves selection of a sample area (tong/ban/ri) as a primary sample unit according to the number of households in the area using a probability proportional to size sampling technique. In the second stage, sample households are selected in each sample area (tong/ban/ri) using systematic sampling methods. This process ensures that the sample units can be representative of the entire population [8]. For the sample to be statistically representative of the population, the data from the survey are weighted based on the sample design. The KCHS employs interviewers who were trained in computer-assisted personal interviewing techniques to collect information.

The institutional review board at the Korea Centers for Disease Control and Prevention approved the study protocol (2013-06EXP-01-3C), and all participants gave written informed consents.

In total, 228,781 individuals participated in the 2013 survey. This study was based on 228,744 participants, excluding 37 with insufficient data to confirm a doctor's diagnosis with asthma. The final analysis identified 6372 asthma individuals who had been diagnosed by a doctor.

Baseline physical health

Physical health can affect an individual's mental health and future mortality risk [3]. Conditions comorbid that include hypertension, diabetes, stroke, and arthritis were investigated in this study. The number of comorbid conditions was also evaluated which were based on the answer "yes" to the question "Were you diagnosed with diseases by a physician?" to avoid bias generated by subjective assessment.

Socioeconomic status

Indicators of socioeconomic status are associated with suicidal thoughts [9], and the present study therefore evaluated education, occupation, and household income. Self-reported smoking, alcohol intake, and physical activity were estimated from questionnaire responses, and household income was categorized according to quartiles of total income for each member in the household. Marital status was categorized as married, single, or divorced/separated/widowed.

Suicide-related thoughts and behaviors are associated with health behaviors such as cigarette smoking [10], alcohol consumption [11], and exercise [12]. Thus, the present study assessed health behaviors such as smoking, drinking, and regular exercise using self-reported questionnaires. People who had smoked 100 cigarettes (5 packs) or more in their lifetime and currently smoked were classified as a 'smoker,' while everyone else belonged to the 'non-smoker' group. Risky drinking was defined as drinking more than five alcoholic beverages on one occasion, and individuals who had drunk more than 12 drinks on one occasion during the previous year were classified as risky drinkers [13]. Regular exercise was defined as routine walking at least five times per week for at least 30 min at a time or engaging during the survey period in regular moderate (at least five times per week for at least 30 min at a time) or strenuous (at least three times per week for at least 20 min at a time) exercise as defined by the American College of Sports Medicine Guidelines [14]. Self-rated health status was analyzed using a 5-point scale, with responses of 'very good,' 'good,' 'normal,' 'poor,' and 'very poor.'

Mental health measures

Psychosocial factors can affect the relationship between suicidal ideation and mortality, and suicidal ideation may also be considered as an indicator of psychosocial factors. Mental health surveys that included the same questions as those in the KCHS were provided to all participants. Three dimensions of mental health were determined within the domains of health status and mental health, namely stress, depression, and suicidal ideations and attempts. Participants reported their level of stress as none, mild, moderate, or severe. Depression was screened using the Korean version of the World Health Organization (WHO) Composite International Diagnostic Interview-Short Form (CIDI-SF), which was validated as a cost-effective screening instrument that could be easily integrated into health surveys [15]. The WHO CIDI-SF includes questions such as "In your lifetime, have you ever had 2 weeks or more when nearly every day you felt sad, blue, or depressed?" assess depression, subjects answered "yes" or "no" to a question of whether they had experienced a depressive mood for 2 or more continuous weeks during the previous year. Suicidal ideation was assessed by participants' positive answer to the question "In the last 12 months, did you think about committing suicide?" A "yes"' or "no" response was also used to determine whether the subjects had suicidal ideations; if the subject answered "yes," they were then asked about their suicide attempts, if any. This indicator is a well-documented predictor of suicide attempts that has been previously used in other surveys of adults [16].

Ethical issues

The institutional review board at the Korea Centers for Disease Control and Prevention approved the study protocol (2013-06EXP-01-3C), and all participants gave written informed consents.

Data analysis

Descriptive statistical methods were used to describe the basic characteristics of the study population; the numbers and percentages are reported for each variable. Student's t test and Chi-square test were used to compare variables between patients with asthma and population without asthma. Multivariable logistic regression analysis was conducted to calculate the adjusted odds ratios (ORs) for suicidal behavior among the asthma patients; we included age, sex, income, education, job, marital status, smoking, alcohol, exercise, presence of diabetes mellitus, hypertension, stroke, arthritis, and depression. Results were expressed with a 95% confidence interval (CI). All data were analyzed using the Statistical Package for Social Sciences (Version 20.0; IBM, Armonk, New York).

Results

The baseline characteristics of the study population ($n = 228{,}744$) are presented in Table 1. As compared to population without asthma ($n = 224{,}175$), patients with asthma ($n = 6372$) were older and had higher proportions of female, smoker, being alone (divorced/separated/widowed), hypertension, stroke, arthritis, and had lower level of education, lower level of income, lower proportions of alcohol drinking, regular exercise, and less having a job (all $p < 0.001$).

Differences in mental health status between asthma patients and population without asthma were presented in Table 2. Asthma patients reported more moderate to severe stress (33.4%) and depressive mood (12.0%) as compared to population without asthma (25.4%, $p < 0.001$; 5.7%, $p < 0.001$). The rate of asthma patients who had suicidal ideations (21.4%) was higher than twice the rate in population without asthma (9.8%, $p < 0.001$). The rate of asthma patients who had suicidal attempts (1.0%) was higher than three times the rate in population without asthma (0.4%, $p < 0.001$).

The ORs of suicidal ideation and attempts among the asthma patients in comparison to population without asthma was presented in Table 3. A multivariate analysis adjusting for age and sex (model 1) revealed that the ORs for suicidal ideations and attempts were 2.01 (95% CI 1.89–2.14) and 2.42 (95% CI 1.87–3.12), respectively. When additional adjustments were performed for socioeconomic factors (i.e., family income, education, job, and marital status; model 2), the ORs for suicidal ideations and attempts were 1.84 (95% CI 1.72–1.96) and 2.12 (95% CI 1.63–2.75), respectively. After additional adjustments for factors related to physical health (i.e., smoking, alcohol, exercise, diabetes, hypertension, stroke, and arthritis; model 3), the ORs for suicidal ideations and attempts were 1.71 (95% CI 1.59–1.82) and 1.79 (95% CI 1.37–2.33), respectively. In a final model adjusted for all of factors including depressive mood (model 4), the ORs for suicidal ideations and attempts were 1.53 (95% CI 1.42–1.65) and 1.32 (95% CI 1.01–1.73), respectively.

Discussion

Our study showed that asthma patients had more severe stress, depressive mood, suicidal ideations, and attempts than population without asthma. In addition, asthma was associated with an increase in the risk for suicidal ideations and attempts, even after adjusting for factors that are known to increase suicidality such as socioeconomic status, chronic medical diseases, and depressive symptoms.

Asthma is an important chronic condition that has previously been linked to a number of adverse outcomes including depression and risk-taking behavior. There is currently a body of research suggesting a link between suicidal behavior and asthma [2–6]. Clarke and colleagues [5] examined data on 5692 adults aged 18 and older participating in a United States nationwide health study showed that 12% of the participants had a history of asthma, 8.7% had experienced suicidal ideation, and 4.2% had suicidal attempts. Despite adjustments for smoking, concurrent mental conditions and demographic factors, a statistically significant association observed between asthma and suicide ideation and attempt. Goodwin and Eaton [2] reported a relationship between asthma and increased likelihood of suicidal ideation (OR 2.3; 95% CI 1.03–5.3) and suicidal attempts (OR 3.5; 95% CI 1.4–9.0). The same result was found in Puerto Rico [6]. An analysis of 6584 adults whose data were drawn from the Third National Health and Nutrition Examination Survey (NHANES III) also reported an association between current asthma and suicide ideation (Odds Ratio 1.77) and suicide attempt (OR 3.26), after

Table 1 Clinical characteristics of study populations

	No asthma ($n = 222,372$)	Asthma ($n = 6372$)	*P* value
Age (years)	51.8 ± 17.0	61.1 ± 17.8	<0.001
Sex (Male %)	100,089 (45.0)	2605 (40.9)	<0.001
Smoking status			<0.001
Smoker	81,882 (36.8)	2562 (40.2)	
Non-smoker	140,490 (63.2)	3810 (59.8)	
Alcohol drinking	59,896 (26.9)	1050 (16.5)	<0.001
Regular exercise	114,714 (51.6)	3047 (47.8)	<0.001
Marital status			<0.001
Married	152,061 (68.4)	3844 (60.4)	
Single	33,101 (14.9)	683 (10.7)	
Divorced/separated/widowed	37,072 (16.7)	1839 (28.9)	
Job	140,886 (63.4)	2914 (45.8)	<0.001
Family income			<0.001
Low	52,214 (24.3)	2705 (43.9)	
Moderate-low	43,285 (20.2)	1258 (20.6)	
Moderate-high	70,830 (33.0)	1303 (21.1)	
High	48,400 (22.5)	887 (14.4)	
Education			<0.001
≤Elementary	57,240 (25.8)	3067 (48.2)	
Middle school	25,346 (11.4)	811 (12.8)	
High school	64,235 (29.0)	1197 (18.8)	
≥College	75,165 (33.8)	1282 (20.2)	
DM	11,623 (5.2)	306 (4.8)	0.075
Hypertension	53,068 (23.9)	2523 (39.6)	<0.001
Stroke	4305 (1.9)	252 (4.0)	<0.001
Arthritis	29,761 (13.4)	1884 (29.6)	<0.001

Table 2 Mental health of asthma patients

	No asthma ($n = 222,372$)	Asthma ($n = 6372$)	*P* value
Stress			<0.001
Moderate to severe	56,507 (25.4)	2120 (33.4)	
None to mild	165,685 (74.6)	4236 (66.6)	
Perceived health status			<0.001
Very good	13,177 (5.9)	142 (2.2)	
Good	73,803 (33.2)	1016 (16.0)	
Moderate	89,422 (40.2)	2194 (34.5)	
Bad	35,534 (16.0)	2010 (31.6)	
Very bad	10,381 (4.7)	1006 (15.8)	
Experiences of depressive mood for 2 or more continuous weeks	12,602 (5.7)	764 (12.0)	<0.001
Suicidal thoughts during the previous year	21,804 (9.8)	1360 (21.4)	<0.001
Suicidal attempts during the previous year	929 (0.4)	64 (1.0)	<0.001

adjusting for confounding factors such as mood disorder, poverty, smoking, and demographics. Our study showed suicidal ideation (OR 1.53; 95% CI 1.42–1.65) and suicidal attempts (OR 1.32; 95% CI 1.01–1.73).

This present study cannot explain the mechanisms of the association between asthma and suicidal ideation and suicidal attempts. An association between asthma morbidity, risk-taking behavior, and depression has been

Table 3 Odds ratio (95% CI) suicidal ideation and suicidal attempts for asthma

	Suicidal ideation OR (95% CI)	Suicidal attempts OR (95% CI)
Model 1	2.01 (1.89–2.14)	2.42 (1.87–3.12)
Model 2	1.84 (1.72–1.96)	2.12 (1.63–2.75)
Model 3	1.71 (1.59–1.82)	1.79 (1.37–2.33)
Model 4	1.53 (1.42–1.65)	1.32 (1.01–1.73)

Adjusted for age, sex variable in model 1. Adjusted for age, sex, family income, education, job, marital status variables in model 2. Adjusted for age, sex, family income, education, job, marital status, smoking, alcohol, exercise, physician diagnosed diseases (diabetes, hypertension, arthritis, stroke) variables in model 3. Adjusted for age, sex, income, education, job, marital status, smoking, alcohol, exercise, physician diagnosed diseases, depression in model 4

presented in previous research, although the reasons and direction of this association are not clear [17]. Asthma may be associated with mood change, anxiety, and some difficulties in daily living which may themselves feel hopelessness and consequently increased suicide risk [18]. Another possible mechanism for this association concerns effects of hypoxia [19], and it has been suggested that an association between high altitude and suicide may be accounted for by metabolic stress associated with hypoxia in individuals who have mood disorders. Recent research reports that suicide rates are elevated in those living at higher altitudes [8, 20], smokers [21, 22] and asthma [6, 23]. A possible mechanism that was proposed is metabolic stress associated with hypoxia. Young SN propose that low brain serotonin synthesis due to hypoxia could be a factor in the high suicide rates seen in people living at altitude, smokers and patients with chronic obstructive pulmonary disease (COPD) and asthma [24]. As pulmonary function decreases, and as the disease progresses, the risk of alveolar hypoxia and consequent hypoxemia increases [25]. Another potential cause of depression in asthma sufferers is the use of particular medications, including corticosteroid or montelukast sodium, which, while reducing the symptoms of asthma, have also been linked to mood disturbances similar to the symptoms of major depression [26, 27].

The strength of our study is that data were obtained from a nationwide population-based survey with a large sample size ($n = 228{,}744$) and the sampling methods representative of the general population. Moreover, the survey provided information about a number of factors that might be related to suicidality, such as socioeconomic variables and physical health as well as mental health measures, which allows us to assess the independent effects of asthma on suicidality using multiple statistical adjustments.

Our study has some limitations that should be addressed. First, because this is a cross-sectional study, temporal relationship and causality between asthma and suicidality could not be determined. Second, all data in this survey are based on self-reported questionnaires; therefore, the recall bias leading to the possibility of over- or under-reporting cannot be excluded. In addition, our study sample might be biased toward mild asthma patients who could complete the questionnaires. Third, we could not obtain detailed information about severity of asthma.

Conclusion

In summary, we observed that asthma patients had more depressive mood and suicidal ideation and attempts than population without asthma using a large population-based survey. We also found that asthma increased the risk for suicidal ideation and attempts, independent of other factors that are known to be associated with suicidality, suggesting that asthma per se may be an independent risk factor for suicidality. Given that a previous suicidal attempt is among the strongest risk factors for future attempt [28], our findings may warrant the need for physicians to screen for suicidality and provide psychosocial support as well as interventions for preventing suicide in management of asthma patients. Hence any treatment modality for asthma, to minimize the possibility of suicide in patients with asthma, must incorporate. More research is required in the mental health field and asthma, but the indicators are clear that there is a significant association between asthma and suicide. Patients with asthma must be assessed not only for physical health but also for psychological morbidity.

Authors' contributions

JHC served as a principal investigator and had full access to all of the data in the study. YWL participated in its coordination and helped to draft the manuscript. SHK is responsible for the integrity and accuracy of the data. All authors read and approved the final manuscript.

Author details

[1] Department of Internal Medicine, International St. Mary's Hospital, Catholic Kwandong University College of Medicine, Incheon, Republic of Korea.
[2] Department of Family Medicine, International St. Mary's Hospital, Catholic Kwandong University College of Medicine, Simgokro 100 Gil 25 Seo-gu, Incheon 22711, Republic of Korea.

Acknowledgements

None.

Competing interests

The authors declare that they have no competing interests.

Funding

This work was supported by research fund of Catholic Kwandong University International St. Mary's Hospital (CKURF-201601560001). These funds were used for collection, analysis, and interpretation of data.

References

1. Turner J, Kelly B. Emotional dimensions of chronic disease. West J Med. 2000;172:124–8.
2. Goodwin RD, Eaton WW. Asthma, suicidal ideation, and suicide attempts: findings from the baltimore epidemiologic catchment area follow-up. Am J Public Health. 2005;95:717–22.
3. Druss B, Pincus H. Suicidal ideation and suicide attempts in general medical illnesses. Arch Intern Med. 2000;160:1522–6.
4. Farberow L, McKelligott JW, Cohen S, Darbonne A. Suicide among patients with cardiorespiratory illnesses. JAMA. 1966;195:422–8.
5. Clarke DE, Goodwin RD, Messias EL, Eaton WW. Asthma and suicidal ideation with and without suicide attempts among adults in the united states: What is the role of cigarette smoking and mental disorders? Ann Allergy Asthma Immunol. 2008;100:439–46.
6. Goodwin RD, Demmer RT, Galea S, Lemeshow AR, Ortega AN, Beautrais A. Asthma and suicide behaviors: results from the third national health and nutrition examination survey (NHANES III). J Psychiatry Res. 2012;46:1002–7.
7. 2010 annual report on the cause of death. Seoul, South Korea. 2011. https://kostat.go.kr/portal/korea/kor_nw/2/6/2/index.board?bmode=read&aSeq=250282.
8. Rim H, Kim H, Lee K, Chang S, Hovell MF, Kim YT, et al. Validity of self-reported healthcare utilization data in the community health survey in korea. J Korean Med Sci. 2011;26:1409–14.
9. Nock MK, Borges G, Bromet EJ, Alonso J, Angermeyer M, Beautrais A, et al. Cross-national prevalence and risk factors for suicidal ideation, plans and attempts. Br J Psychiatry. 2008;192:98–105.
10. Kessler RC, Borges G, Sampson N, Miller M, Nock MK. The association between smoking and subsequent suicide-related outcomes in the national comorbidity survey panel sample. Mol Psychiatry. 2009;14:1132–42.
11. Pfaff JJ, Almeida OP, Witte TK, Waesche MC, Joiner TE Jr. Relationship between quantity and frequency of alcohol use and indices of suicidal behavior in an elderly australian sample. Suicide Life Threat Behav. 2007;37:616–26.
12. Brown DR, Galuska DA, Zhang J, Eaton DK, Fulton JE, Lowry R, et al. Psychobiology and behavioral strategies. Physical activity, sport participation, and suicidal behavior: US High school students. Med Sci Sports Exerc. 2007;39:2248–57.
13. Coups EJ, Ostroff JS. A population-based estimate of the prevalence of behavioral risk factors among adult cancer survivors and noncancer controls. Prev Med. 2005;40:702–11.
14. Haskell WL, Lee IM, Pate RR, Powell KE, Blair SN, Franklin BA, et al. Physical activity and public health: updated recommendation for adults from the american college of sports medicine and the american heart association. Circulation. 2007;116:1081–93.
15. Gigantesco A, Morosini P. Development, reliability and factor analysis of a self-administered questionnaire which originates from the world health organization's composite international diagnostic interview—short form (cidi-sf) for assessing mental disorders. Clin Pract Epidemiol Ment Health. 2008;4:8.
16. Gaynes BN, West SL, Ford CA, Frame P, Klein J, Lohr KN, et al. Screening for suicide risk in adults: a summary of the evidence for the US Preventive services task force. Ann Intern Med. 2004;140:822–35.
17. Bender BG. Risk taking, depression, adherence, and symptom control in adolescents and young adults with asthma. Am J Respir Crit Care Med. 2006;173:953–7.
18. Wong KO, Hunter Rowe B, Douwes J, Senthilselvan A. Asthma and wheezing are associated with depression and anxiety in adults: an analysis from 54 countries. Pulm Med. 2013;2013:929028.
19. Kim N, Mickelson JB, Brenner BE, Haws CA, Yurgelun-Todd DA, Renshaw PF. Altitude, gun ownership, rural areas, and suicide. Am J Psychiatry. 2011;168:49–54.
20. Haws CA, Gray DD, Yurgelun-Todd DA, Moskos M, Meyer LJ, Renshaw PF. The possible effect of altitude on regional variation in suicide rates. Med Hypotheses. 2009;73:587–90.
21. Aubin HJ, Berlin I, Reynaud M. Current smoking, hypoxia, and suicide. Am J Psychiatry. 2011;168:326–7.
22. Li D, Yang X, Ge Z, Hao Y, Wang Q, Liu F, et al. Cigarette smoking and risk of completed suicide: a meta-analysis of prospective cohort studies. J Psychiatry Res. 2012;46:1257–66.
23. Goodwin RD. Asthma and suicide: current knowledge and future directions. Curr Psychiatry Rep. 2012;14:30–5.
24. Young SN. Elevated incidence of suicide in people living at altitude, smokers and patients with chronic obstructive pulmonary disease and asthma: possible role of hypoxia causing decreased serotonin synthesis. J Psychiatry Neurosci JPN. 2013;38:423–6.
25. Vestbo J, Hurd SS, Agusti AG, Jones PW, Vogelmeier C, Anzueto A, et al. Global strategy for the diagnosis, management, and prevention of chronic obstructive pulmonary disease: gold executive summary. Am J Respir Crit Care Med. 2013;187:347–65.
26. Patten SB, Neutel CI. Corticosteroid-induced adverse psychiatric effects: incidence, diagnosis and management. Drug Saf. 2000;22:111–22.
27. Philip G, Hustad C, Noonan G, Malice MP, Ezekowitz A, Reiss TF, et al. Reports of suicidality in clinical trials of montelukast. J Allergy Clin Immunol. 2009;124(691–696):e696.
28. Sokero TP, Melartin TK, Rytsala HJ, Leskela US, Lestela-Mielonen PS, Isometsa ET. Prospective study of risk factors for attempted suicide among patients with DSM-IV major depressive disorder. Br J Psychiatry. 2005;186:314–8.

15

Attempted suicide in Podgorica, Montenegro: higher rates in females and unemployed males

Lidija Injac Stevovic[1,2*] and Sanja Vodopic[3]

Abstract

Background: A change in suicide attempts is associated with comprehensive changes in mental and physical health and social environment. Attempted suicide and suicide are one of the biggest problems nowadays worldwide, not only in the field of mental health but also in the field of public health. The aim of the research was to determine the number of attempted suicides as well as the influence of clinical and demographic variables on the attempted suicide rate.

Methods: The data on the attempted suicide were analysed in the period 2012–2016 based on the data from the Emergency Ward of the Clinical Centre of Montenegro in Podgorica. The rate of attempted suicides as well as the unemployment rate was calculated. The statistical analysis included descriptive statistics of the raw data and relative numbers, Chi-squared test, Fisher's test and Spearman coefficient.

Results: The average age of males who attempted suicide was 38.35 ± 14.11, min 15 and max 88 years of age, and the age of women was 38.97 ± 16.81, min 16 and max 93 years of age. Women attempted suicide more frequently ($p < 0.05$). Female/male ratio during the investigation period slightly declined (1.93 in 2012 vs. 1.29 in 2016). The attempted suicide rates ranged from 103 per 100,000 residents in 2016 to 142 per 100,000 residents in 2015. Crude attempt rate was the highest in women in 2012 (102.42 per 100,000 residents) and for men in 2014 and 2015 (84.48 vs. 83.06 per 100,000 residents). Poisoning with psychotropic drugs was the dominant manner of attempt (93.2%), while the largest number of attempts was in the late spring and summer (May, June and July). Attempted suicide rate in man was associated with higher unemployment rate.

Conclusions: Although women make the majority of attempted suicide cases, there has been a decline in the value of the rate for women and a rise for men. The attempted suicide rates in Podgorica belong to lower rates compared to the WHO European multicentre study on parasuicide. Poisoning with psychotropic drugs was the predominant manner, while the highest number of attempted suicides was in the late spring and summer (May, June and July). Unemployment influences men to attempt suicide much more frequently.

Keywords: Attempted suicide, Montenegro, Rate, Risk factors, Unemployment

Background

Attempted suicide and suicide are one of the biggest problems nowadays worldwide, not only in the field of mental health but also in the field of public health. Little is known about attempted suicides in the world. It is estimated that in the countries of the WHO European Region, 150,000 people manage to commit suicide and 1,500,000 people attempt suicide annually [1].

According to the WHO data, the suicide rate in Montenegro in 2012 was 18.9/100,000 residents, which classified it in the tenth position in Europe [2].

Until 2009, Montenegro had official data on suicides which were published by the Statistical Office of Montenegro (MONSTAT) [3], while in 2010 this responsibility

*Correspondence: injacl19@gmail.com
[1] Clinical Department of Psychiatry, Clinical Centre of Montenegro, Podgorica, Montenegro
Full list of author information is available at the end of the article

was assumed by the Institute of Public Health, and since then there have been no official data on suicides or attempted suicides. Podgorica is the capital of Montenegro. The latest statistical data show that the population of Podgorica is 187,075, which represents 30% of the total population of Montenegro. Men make 49.39% and women 50.61% of the population [3]. A research of attempted suicide is extremely important, because we are a small country, so that this "disadvantage" of ours could be an advantage in monitoring and faster identification of such individuals.

Attempted suicide is the strongest predictor of suicide or parasuicide [4], so that those who attempted suicide are an important group for monitoring. Attempted suicides are more frequent than commited suicides and very often lead to hospitalization. The most important risk factors identified are younger age and female gender, single or divorced, unemployed, recent change in living situation, mental disorder and previous parasuicide incident [5].

Despite the current knowledge, it remains difficult to reliably establish the risk of attempted suicide among individuals and in the community. That is why the studies on attempted suicides list many challenges arising from the very nature of suicide. The aim of the research was to determine the number of attempted suicides as well as the influence of clinical and demographic variables on the attempted suicide rate.

Methods

The research was conducted in the Emergency Ward (EW) of the Clinical Centre of Montenegro (CCM) in Podgorica. We analysed the data on the attempted suicide in the period 2012–2016. The rate of attempted suicides and the unemployment rate were calculated. The data on population and the unemployment rate that we used were taken from the web site of the national Statistics Office MONSTAT [3]. CCM is the only hospital in Podgorica. The Emergency Ward operates 24 h a day within CCM. Each attempted suicide is registered on the basis of reports of patients or their families, as well as on the basis of the examinations carried out by psychiatrists and other specialists, including all relevant clinical and laboratory tests. All patients were accompanied by family members who provided additional information. All patients 18 years old and above, who attempted suicide in the period between 2012 and 2016, were included in the research. There were examined 608 patients in the Emergency Centre. The methodology will be used as a basis for the discussion on the situation with the population of Podgorica.

Statistics

The analysis included descriptive statistics of the raw data (absolute numbers) and relative numbers. Mortality rates were standardized to the 2011 Montenegro population census using the direct method. Rates are per 100,000 individuals per year. For the distribution of the method, Chi-squared test and Fisher's test were used. For the correlations of the unemployment rate and the attempted suicide, Spearman coefficient was used. The significance level was set at $p < 0.05$. Data analyses were performed in SPSS 16.0.

Results

In the period 2012–2016, 608 respondents attempted suicide. The largest number of attempted suicides was in 2015—142 attempts (23.40% of the sample) and the lowest number was in 2016—103 attempts (16.90%). Female/male ratio during the period of monitoring was on a slight decline (2012—1.93, and 2016—1.29) (Table 1). The average age of males who attempted suicide was 38.35 ± 14.11, and the average age of women was 38.97 ± 16.81.

Attempted suicides were mostly performed using psychotropic drugs in the total population (93.2%). This method of attempting suicide is statistically much more frequent in women than men (95.10% vs. 90.50%, $p = 0.043$). Hanging and drowning are statistically more frequent in men (2.90% vs. 0.30%, $p = 0.010$) (Table 2).

Table 1 Numbers of attempts concerning each sex in each year and the respective female-to-male ratio for absolute raw numbers

Year	Male		Female		Total	Female/male ratio
	Count	%	Count	%	Count	
2012	41	34.20	79	65.80	120	1.93
2013	41	37.60	68	62.40	109	1.66
2014	63	47.00	71	53.00	134	1.13
2015	69	48.60	73	51.40	142	1.06
2016	45	43.70	58	56.30	103	1.29

Table 2 Distribution of method of attempting suicide by gender

	Total		Male		Female		*p* value[†]
	N	%	*N*	%	*N*	%	
Medication	551	93.20	220	90.50	331	95.10	0.043
Hanging/drawing	8	1.40	7	2.90	1	0.30	0.010[‡]
Toxic	11	1.90	6	2.50	5	1.40	0.545
Blunt object	20	3.40	9	3.70	11	3.20	0.898
Firearms	1	0.20	1	0.4	0	0	0.410[‡]

[†] Male vs. female, Chi-squared test, [‡] Fisher's test

The highest frequency of attempted suicides was in May, June and July (10.50, 10.00 and 10.40%, respectively), i.e. during late spring and summer (Fig. 1). As for male patients, the highest frequency of attempted suicides was in May (12.00%), and when it comes to female respondents, the highest frequency was in June and July (11.20%).

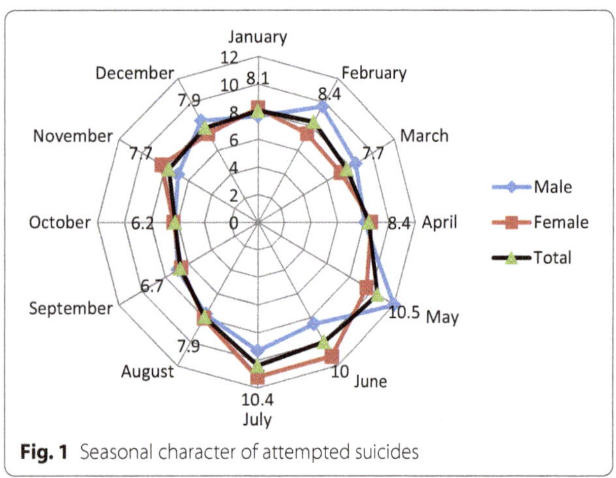

Fig. 1 Seasonal character of attempted suicides

Crude attempt rate was the highest in women in 2012—102.42 per 100,000 residents. As for male respondents, the peak of this rate was in 2014 and 2015 (84.48 and 83.06, respectively, per 100,000 residents) (Table 3).

Looking at the age-standardized attempt rate, we observe that during the monitoring period there is a balanced increase of the value of this rate in men, while there is a gradual decline of the value of age-standardized attempt rate among women for the same period. Age-standardized attempt rate for the whole population of the city of Podgorica follows the growth trend for the male population.

The highest correlation of the unemployment rate and the attempted suicide rate was observed in men ($\rho = -0.800$, and in the total population $\rho = -0.600$) (Table 4). While there is a negative correlation in men in the total population, there is a positive correlation

Table 3 Attempt rates (per 100,000 residents) for the period 2012–2016 (standard population: Montenegro census 2011)

	Year	Regional population (15+)	Number of attempts	Attempt rate (per 100,000 residents)	Age-standardized attempt rate	95% CI for standardized attempt rate
Male	2012	73,297	41	55.94	58.99	40.93–77.05
	2013	73,779	41	55.57	63.38	43.98–82.78
	2014	74,571	63	84.48	68.09	51.28–84.90
	2015	75,851	69	83.06	73.13	55.87–90.39
	2016	76,782	45	58.61	78.60	55.63–101.57
Female	2012	77,131	79	102.42	99.46	77.53–121.39
	2013	77,639	68	87.58	93.15	71.01–115.29
	2014	78,472	71	90.48	87.24	66.95–107.53
	2015	79,818	73	91.46	81.70	62.96–100.44
	2016	80,798	58	71.78	76.52	56.83–96.21
Total	2012	150,428	120	79.77	63.96	52.52–75.40
	2013	151,417	109	71.97	68.44	55.59–81.29
	2014	153,042	134	87.56	73.23	60.83–85.63
	2015	155,669	142	91.22	78.36	65.47–91.25
	2016	157,580	103	65.36	83.85	67.66–100.04

Table 4 Correlation of the unemployment rate and the attempted suicides

Indicator	Attempted suicide rate		
	Males	Females	Total
Unemployment rate			
P	−0.800	0.205	−0.600
p-value	0.145	0.741	0.285

p—Spearman coefficient, *p*-value < 0.05

($\rho = 0.205$) in women between these two indicators. The small number of observations makes any use of statistical significance problematic.

Discussion

This is the first study that has investigated attempted suicides in Podgorica, the capital of Montenegro. The paper deals with all the attempted suicides in the period of 5 years. During the observed period, 608 respondents attempted suicide, whereby the highest number was in 2015 and the lowest in 2016. The results show that the age of 38 in both sexes is the age of the highest risk for a suicide attempt. It has been observed that women attempted suicide more often than men, but in the monitoring period there was a slight decline of the attempted suicide in women compared to men (1.93/1.29). We could find similar data in similar Mediterranean countries such as Greece where the ratio is 2:1, which is a probable value for attempts, and 1:3.6 (more males) for committed suicides [6].

The largest number of attempts included poisoning with psychotropic drugs and statistically it occurs much more frequently in women, while, statistically, men rather use more lethal methods. These devastating results are in accordance with the studies conducted in England, Switzerland and Greece: over 75–95.93% attempted suicides were due to self-poisoning [6, 7]. It is worrying that overdosing is the most popular manner of attempt, while the others were used less frequently. It is a known fact that the availability of means leads to an increase of suicides. Control and distribution of psychoactive drugs in our country started only in mid-2016, which explains a lower rate of attempted suicides that year. Attempted suicides in men are more often linked with a strong suicidal intention and their attempts tend to be more lethal compared to women and more frequently point to a non-diagnosed mental disorder [8].

An epidemiological study in four European countries—Germany, Hungary, Ireland and Portugal—demonstrated that suicidal acts (fatal and non-fatal) were 3.4 times more lethal in men than in women and the proportion of serious suicide attempts among all non-fatal suicidal acts with known intentionality was significantly higher in men than in women [9]. In USA, males 1.6 times more likely than females use violent methods to attempt suicide [10].

The highest number of suicides took place during spring and summer. We identified three peaks: May, June and July. The increase in the number of suicides in May could be linked with the First May and the Independence Day holidays when alcohol is consumed and when man feel disappointed because of unemployment or return to work. June and July are the months when women have more expectations from holidays, which is followed by disappointment and dissatisfaction. Additionally, in Podgorica over the summer temperature is very high, about 40°, what has strong influence on the social life of the citizens.

In Greece, two peaks were identified for attempts—May and August (the border of summer) [6].

In Hungary, Seregi et al. [11] examined several environmental factors with periodic changes in intensity during the calendar year in order to explain the increase in suicide frequency during spring and summer. Their results strongly support the hypothesis that sunshine has a prompt, but very weak increasing effect on the risk of suicide (especially violent cases among males). The need to study the role of environmental factors in evoking suicidal behaviour is substantiated by the observation that suicide cases are unevenly distributed during the calendar year [12].

The attempted suicide rate in Podgorica ranged from 103 per 100,00 residents in 2016 to 142 per 100,000 residents in 2015, belonging to the group of the lowest rate compared to the WHO European multicentre study on parasuicide, where the male parasuicide rate varied from 45 to 314 per 100,000 and female parasuicide rate ranged from 69 to 462 per 100,000 of the population from the lowest to the highest level among the 13 participating countries [7].

As for age, standardized rates of attempts showed an increase in the value of rate for men, while for women there was a decline of the value, which shows that in Podgorica attempted suicide is not the behaviour that is characteristic not only for women but also for men. In Europe, the highest average male age-standardized rate of suicide attempts was found for Helsinki, Finland (314/100,000), and the lowest rate (45/100,000) was for Guipuzcoa, Spain. The highest average female age-standardized rate was found for Cergy-Pontoise, France (462/100,000), and the lowest (69/100,000) again for Guipuzcoa, Spain [7].

In Belgium, the rates are around 60–70 for males and 70–140 for females per 100,000 residents [13], and the same rates were recorded in Germany [14] and Sweden [14].

An increase of the rate of attempted suicides in men can be explained by the results of our research which point to a link of the unemployment rate and the attempted suicide rate, which means that unemployment represents a risk factor in men. Unemployment and low socioeconomic status represent important variables in the attempted suicides and committed suicides [13, 15, 16], while low education and unemployed young adult men and women had significantly higher rates of attempts [17].

For understanding the growth of the value of rates for men, it is of vital importance to bear in mind wider historical context and political changes in these areas, such as wars, the last one in the region in the 1990s, disintegration of Yugoslavia, NATO air-raids in 1999, political processes leading to the independence of Montenegro in 2006, the transition period and the World Economic Crisis in 2008. Education and the role of men who are expected to be strong and not to show emotions can have adverse effects in this social context. On the other hand, stigma and inadequate psychiatric services represent some of the reasons for not looking always for professional assistance.

Limitation of the study

We believe that the main limitation of the paper is that it only reflects the situation in the capital of Podgorica where one-third of the population of Montenegro lives. Among them, there are many who migrated from the North and the South of the country, so these data can also refer to them. However, one should bear in mind specific characteristics of the North and the South, cultural and other differences, as well as the factors such as isolation. Out of these reasons, we have started preparations to look into attempted suicides in other parts of the country.

Conclusions

This is the first study that has examined the attempted suicide rate in Podgorica. The results suggest that women attempt suicides most frequently and that in the observed period there was a decline of attempted suicides in females compared to males (1.93/1.29). Attempted suicide rates ranged from 103 per 100,000 residents in 2016 to 142 per 100,000 residents in 2015, and they belong to lower rates compared to the WHO European multicentre study on parasuicide.

Crude attempt rate was the highest in women in 2012—102.42/100,000 residents—and in men in 2014 and 2015—84.48 and 83.06, respectively, per 100,000 residents.

Poisoning with psychotropic drugs was a dominant method of attempts. The largest number of attempts was in late spring and summer (May, June and July). Unemployment influences men to attempt suicide much more frequently.

Abbreviations

EW: Emergency Ward of the Clinical Centre of Montenegro; CCM: Clinical Centre of Montenegro; WHO: World Health Organization; MONSTAT: Statistical Office of Montenegro; SPSS: Statistical Package for Social Sciences; SPSS Inc: statistical software.

Authors' contributions

With this, we want to confirm that LIS is the first and leading author of this publication. The authors participated in drafting the article and revising it critically for important intellectual content. They also made substantial contributions to conception and design, and acquisition of data, as well as data analysis and interpretation. They give their final approval of the version to be submitted. This article is an original work of the authors. We also want to confirm that this article is not previously published in any other journal, nor sent to revision of other journals. Study conception and design: LIS. Acquisition of data: LIS, SV. Analysis and interpretation of data: LIS, SV. Drafting of the manuscript: LIS. Critical revision: LIS, SV. Both authors read and approved the final manuscript.

Author details

[1] Clinical Department of Psychiatry, Clinical Centre of Montenegro, Podgorica, Montenegro. [2] Department of Psychiatry, School of Medicine, University of Montenegro, Dzona Dzeksona bb, Podgorica, Montenegro. [3] Clinical Department of Neurology, Clinical Centre of Montenegro, Dzona Dzeksona bb, Podgorica, Montenegro.

Acknowledgements

Not applicable.

Competing interests

The authors declare that they have no competing interests.

Consent for publication

Free, informed, written and unambiguousconsents were obtained from all participants for publication.

Funding

This research received no specific grant from any funding agency in the public, commercial or not-for-profit sectors.

References

1. World Health Organization—WHO Mental health—Suicide data. http://www.who.int/mental_health/prevention/suicide/suicideprevent/en/. Accessed 17 May 2017.
2. World Health Organization (WHO). Suicide data, 2016. http://www.who.int/gho/publications/world_health_statistics/2016/whs2016_AnnexA_Suicide.pdf?Ua=1&ua=1. Accessed 20 Feb 2017.
3. Zavod za statistiku Crne Gore (Statistical Office of Montenegro). http://www.monstat.org/cg/page.php?id=1001&pageid=1001#DSS. Accessed 7 Jan 2017.
4. Hawton K, Fagg J. Suicide, and other causes of death, following attempted suicide. Br J Psychiatry. 1988;152:359–66.
5. Welch SS. A review of the literature on the epidemiology of parasuicide in the general population. Psychiatr Serv. 2001;52(3):368–75.
6. Fountoulakis K, Savopoulos C, Apostolopoulo M, Dampali R, Zaggelidou E, Karlafti E, Fountoukidis I, Kountis P, Limenopoulos V, Plomaritis E, Theodorakis P, Hatzitolios A. Rate of suicide and suicide attempts and their relationship to unemployment in Thessaloniki Greece (2000–2012). J Affect Disord. 2015;174:131–6. doi:10.1016/j.jad.2014.11.047.
7. Schmidtke A, Bille-Brahe U, DeLeo D, Kerkhof A, Bjerke T, Crepet P, Haring C, Hawton K, Lönnqvist J, Michel K, Pommereau X, Querejeta I, Phillipe I, Salander-Renberg E, Temesvary B, Wasserman D, Fricke S, Weinacker B, Sampaio-Faria JG. Attempted suicide in Europe: rates, trends and sociodemographic characteristics of suicide attempters during the period 1989–1992. Results of the WHO/EURO Multicentre Study on Parasuicide. Acta Psychiatr Scand. 1996;93:327–38.

8. Hawton K, Houston K, Haw C, Townsend E, Harriss L. Comorbidity of axis I and axis II disorders in patients who attempted suicide. Am J Psychiatry. 2003;160:1494–500.
9. Mergl R, Koburger N, Heinrichs K, Székely A, Tóth MD, Coyne J, Quintão S, Arensman E, Coffey C, Maxwell M, Värnik A, van Audenhove C, McDaid D, Sarchiapone M, Schmidtke A, Genz A, Gusmão R, Hegerl U. What are reasons for the large gender differences in the lethality of suicidal acts? An epidemiological analysis in four European Countries. PLoS ONE. 2015;10(7):e0129062.
10. Canner J, Giuliano K, Selvarajah S, Hammond E, Schneider EB. Emergency department visits for attempted suicide and self harm in the USA 2006–2013. Epidemiol Psychiatr Sci. 2016;1–9. doi:10.1017/S2045796016000871.
11. Seregi B, Kapitány B, Maróti-Agóts A, Rihmer Z, Gonda X, Döme P. Weak associations between the daily number of suicide cases and amount of daily sunlight. Prog Neuropsychopharmacol Biol Psychiatry. 2017;73:41–8. doi:10.1016/j.pnpbp.2016.10.003.
12. Christodoulou C, Douzenis A, Papadopoulos FC, Papadopoulou A, Bouras G, Gournellis R, Lykouras L. Suicide and seasonality. Acta Psychiatr Scand. 2012;125(2):127–46.
13. Boffin N, Bossuyt N, Vanthomme K, Van Casteren V. Declining rates of suicidal behavior among general practice patients in Belgium: results from sentinel surveillance between 1993 and 2008. Arch Suicide Res. 2011;15:68–74.
14. Bogdanovica I, Jiang GX, Lohr C, Schmidtke A, Mittendorfer-Rutz E. Changes in rates, methods and characteristics of suicide attempters over a 15-year period: comparison between Stockholm, Sweden, and Wurzburg, Germany. Soc Psychiatry Psychiatr Epidemiol. 2011;46(11):1103–14.
15. O'Shea B. Self-harm and unemployment. Hosp Med. 2000;61:495–8.
16. Fountoulakis KN, Kawohl W, Theodorakis PN, Kerkhof AJ, Navickas A, Höschl C, Lecic-Tosevski D, Sorel E, Rancans E, Palova E, Juckel G, Isacsson G, Jagodic HK, Botezat-Antonescu I, Warnke I, Rybakowski J, Azorin JM, Cookson J, Waddington J, Pregelj P, Demyttenaere K, Hranov LG, Stevovic LI, Pezawas L, Adida M, Figuera ML, Pompili M, Jakovljević M, Vichi M, Perugi G, Andreassen O, Vukovic O, Mavrogiorgou P, Varnik P, Bech P, Dome P, Winkler P, Salokangas RK, From T, Danileviciute V, Gonda X, Rihmer Z, Benhalima JF, Grady A, Leadholm AK, Soendergaard S, Nordt C, Lopez-Ibor J. Relationship of suicide rates to economic variables in Europe: 2000–2011. Br J Psychiatry. 2014;205(6):486–96.
17. Kim JL, Kim JM, Choi Y, Lee TH, Park EC. Effect of Socioeconomic Status on the Linkage Between Suicidal Ideation and Suicide Attempts. Suicide Life Threat Behav. 2016;46(5):588–97.

16

Antidepressive response of inpatients with major depression to adjuvant occupational therapy

Marc-Andreas Edel[1*], Brian Blackwell[1], Markus Schaub[2], Barbara Emons[2], Tanja Fox[1], Friederike Tornau[2], Bernward Vieten[3], Patrik Roser[1], Ida Sibylle Haussleiter[1,2] and Georg Juckel[1,2]

Abstract

Background: Despite marked costs and limited evidence regarding effectiveness, occupational therapy (OT) is widely applied in psychiatric settings and financed by health insurance companies in European countries. This pilot study investigated the antidepressive effects of adjuvant OT for patients with major depression in a 6-week inpatient setting, stratified for females and males.

Methods: A total of 114 inpatients with major depression were assigned to either a standard OT group (using basic handcraft) or an active control group that played board games (2 h daily, 5 days a week). HAMD-21 scores were assessed as the primary outcome parameter after 3–6 weeks.

Results: The OT intervention was not superior to "board game" (BG) activities in reducing depressive symptoms. However, significant interaction effects were found in favor of the OT group regarding anxiety measures and other variables. Male participants displayed more significant interaction effects than female participants.

Conclusions: OT as an adjuvant short-term treatment for inpatients with major depression may be more efficacious than game interventions in terms of reducing anxiety and other symptoms, particularly in males.

Trial registration The study was registered in the EU Clinical Trials Register as a multicenter trial (EudraCT Number 2009-016463-10; https://www.clinicaltrialsregister.eu/ctr-search/trial/2009-016463-10/DE#A)

However, because of the elaborate setting requirements, the original study design with four centers was transformed into a solution with those two centers facilitating the pertinent resources. Furthermore, "mono-therapy with mirtazapine" was changed into "preferably mono-therapy with any antidepressant drug".

Keywords: Adjuvant occupational therapy, Major depression, Antidepressive effects

Background

Major depression is one of the most common and debilitating mental disorders. It causes enormous individual, social, and economic burden [18]. According to the German Information System of the Federal Health Monitoring, the diagnosis of a major depressive episode is the number one cause for inpatient treatment in German psychiatric hospitals based on consistent data collected in the years 2000–2010 [5].

In several European countries, occupational therapy (OT) is known as *Ergotherapie* (from the Greek *ergon* = work, exercise). In German-speaking countries, it is a traditional treatment that is most frequently applied in combination with other treatments, such as pharmacotherapy [14].

Occupational therapy is based on the positive relation between meaningful occupation and health, and views people as occupational beings [1]. "Occupational therapists should continue to be mindful of the humanistic

*Correspondence: marc-andreas.edel@rub.de
[1] Department of Psychiatry, Psychotherapy and Preventive Medicine, LWL University Hospital, Ruhr University Bochum, Alexandrinenstr. 1-3, 44791 Bochum, Germany
Full list of author information is available at the end of the article

ideals on which the profession was founded: the belief in the therapeutic value of meaningful occupation, the importance of the environment and of satisfactory interpersonal relationships, and balance in the daily routines of work, self-care and leisure" [13].

In Germany in particular, OT in inpatient psychiatric settings is mainly performed in group settings and is composed of four therapeutic facets. The first facet is the classical *Ergotherapie* that is the performance of various handcraft techniques with wood, stone, paper, and other materials. The second facet addresses the expression of inner states through drawing, painting, or modeling. The third facet focuses on the interactions and social skills of the group members while they are involved in common projects. The fourth facet concentrates on work performance and workplace reintegration aspects.

The extensive provision of OT for psychiatric patients in German-speaking countries causes marked costs, particularly in inpatient settings. According to Reuster [14], OT for inpatients in the Department of Psychiatry and Psychotherapy of the University of Dresden in 1998 was more expensive than pharmacotherapy for those patients. However, empirical data regarding the effectiveness and efficacy of OT in patients with mental disorders are lacking, and there are only few randomized controlled trials (RCTs) in this field.

Comparatively strong evidence exists for OT in community samples of people with dementia. Voigt-Radloff et al. [17] stated that the results of 5 of 7 RCTs suggested positive effects on activities of daily living (ADLs) or quality of life in persons with dementia or on their caregivers' skills, burden, and quality of life.

To date, OT for patients with schizophrenia has been investigated only in long-term RCTs [3, 4, 6].

Schene et al. [15] were the first to perform a long-term RCT on OT (vs. treatment as usual, TAU) in outpatients with major depressive disorder; however, in that study, the OT intervention was not superior to TAU with respect to depression outcome. In a subsequent similar RCT (TAU + OT vs. TAU) in sick-listed employees with major depression, the workgroup focused on *work participation* as the primary outcome parameter, but significant benefits of adjuvant OT pertaining to a quick return to work, improvement of work-related coping and self-efficacy were not demonstrated. However, the OT group showed greater improvement in depression symptoms and an increased probability of long-term symptom remission and long-term *return to work in good health* [9].

Reuster [14] was the first to conduct a short-term RCT in 216 inpatients with major depression ($n = 114$; $n_{+OT} = 63$, $n_{-OT} = 51$), mania ($n = 26$; $n_{+OT} = 16$, $n_{-OT} = 10$), and schizophrenia ($n = 76$; $n_{+OT} = 41$, $n_{-OT} = 35$). That author investigated the effects of daily add-on standard OT (performance and training of handcraft techniques using wood, stone, paper, and other materials) versus self-instructed unspecific activities on psychopathological variables over four weeks within a multimodal clinical setting. A significant reduction of symptomatology was only observed in the patients with major depression (43.9% decrease in the Bech Rafaelsen Melancholia Scale score vs. a 27.5% decrease in the activity group after 4 weeks). However, that study had multiple methodological problems; it lacked a primary outcome parameter, an assessment of functioning in ADL, and control for confounders, such as drug therapy, psychoeducative and psychotherapeutic sessions, and other covariates, such as exercise therapy.

Because the above-mentioned study by Reuster is the only investigation of short-term OT in inpatients with major depression to date, we felt inspired to study this topic further.

We planned and performed a pilot RCT in inpatients with moderate-to-severe major depression that compared a standard OT group program, i.e., everyday performance of handcraft activities, to a board game (BG) group as a semi-active control. In both groups, the interventions were in addition to basic antidepressant drug treatment and short daily supportive talks with staff members.

We avoided the major limitations of Reuster's study by defining the change in the total score of the Hamilton Depression Rating Scale (HAMD) from before to after the interventions as the primary outcome parameter. Moreover, we applied secondary assessments of psychopathological symptoms, such as anxiety, and we included a specific OT assessment (Ergo-Assess™) of functioning in ADLs, and we controlled for confounders (antidepressant drugs and psychiatric comorbidity).

We expected that the adjuvant OT intervention would result in significantly greater effects indicating decrease in depressive symptoms and secondary psychopathological characteristics. Furthermore, we hypothesized superiority of the OT over the BG intervention with respect to improvements in ADL and social functioning. Additionally, gender differences regarding effects indicating possible improvements were explored.

Methods

Participants

A total of 131 inpatients who experiences a moderate or severe major depressive episode diagnosed according to the DSM-IV criteria (moderate, 296.22, or severe episode without psychotic features, 296.23; recurrent major depressive disorder: moderate, 296.32, or severe episode without psychotic features, 296.33) were recruited from three similar inpatient units of two German psychiatric clinics and assessed for eligibility for participation in this study. All diagnoses were established using the Structured Clinical Interview for the DSM-IV (SCID I/II). Of the 131 patients who were screened, 14 did not meet the inclusion criteria and three refused to participate. Finally, 114 patients (55% female, mean age 45.7 ± 11.8 years) were randomly (by the block random method) assigned to either the experimental (OT) or the active comparison group (board game group, BG). During the first 3 weeks, 11 (19.3%) OT participants and 21 (36.8%) BG participants dropped out for motivational reasons. 46 OT participants and 36 BG participants participated in the study for at least three weeks ($n = 82$) and 29 OT participants and 22 BG participants completed the study (6 weeks, $n = 51$). The data were processed in per-protocol analyses.

No significant group differences emerged regarding sex, age, education, marital status, intelligence, axis-I or axis-II comorbidity, number of psychoactive drugs, or number of antidepressants. However, as the only particular difference between study groups, the female participants in the OT group took significantly more psychoactive drugs ($p = 0.020$) than the female participants in the BG group (Table 1). No overall gender differences were found between study groups concerning intelligence, axis-I or axis-II comorbidity, number of psychoactive drugs, or number of antidepressants.

Over 80% of the participants took at least one antidepressant drug before admission. Of these participants, only about 20% had only one antidepressant.

All participants gave written informed consent, and the Ethics Committee of the Medical Faculty of the Ruhr University Bochum approved the study (No. 3626-10FF).

Study design, interventions, and inclusion/exclusion criteria

The study was primarily designed as a 6-week pilot RCT with a block randomization. However, block size could not be fixed randomly in this study, but the trialists allocated blocks of three, four, or five participants to the groups alternately, according to the availability of eligible patients.

Table 1 Group comparisons (demographic and clinical data)

	Occupational therapy	Board game group	Chi square[a]/t[b]	df	p
Demographic data					
$N = 82$	$n = 46$	$n = 36$			
Sex (f:m)	26:20	18:18	0.38[a]	1	0.539
Age, years (SD)	46.8 (11.8)	44.8 (11.7)	0.84[b]	81.8	0.401
Age, females (SD)	45.7 (10.7)	45.4 (13.3)	0.11[b]	40.4	0.910
Age, males (SD)	48.2 (13.3)	44.1 (9.8)	1.18[b]	31.5	0.247
Age groups	6 groups ranging from 18 to 70 years of age		2.74[a]	5	0.740
Educational level	11 categories ranging from 'no degree' to 'university degree'		17.3[a]	10	0.068
Marital status	4 categories (single, married, divorced, widowed)		577[a]	3	0.124
Clinical data					
Intelligence, MWT-B, raw data (SD)	29.1 (14.8)	28.1 (4.8)	0.50[b]	71.2	0.617
Intelligence, females (SD)	30.3 (9.0)	27.7 (4.7)	0.77[b]	37.7	0.448
Intelligence, males (SD)	27.5 (4.8)	28.5 (5.0)	−0.70[b]	37	0.487
Axis-I disorders (SD)	1.7 (0.8)	1.5 (0.7)	0.18[b]	75	0.861
Axis-I disorders, females (SD)	1.8 (0.9)	1.4 (0.6)	1.62[b]	35.8	0.112
Axis-I disorders, males (SD)	1.3 (0.6)	1.7 (0.8)	−1.74[b]	36	0.090
Axis-II disorders (SD)	0.2 (0.4)	0.1 (0.3)	0.60[b]	75	0.550
Axis-II disorders, females (SD)	0.2 (0.4)	0.1 (0.3)	0.22[b]	39.7	0.827
Axis-II disorders, males (SD)	0.2 (0.4)	0.1 (0.3)	0.64[b]	36	0.524
Number of psychoactive drugs (SD)	2.6 (1.4)	2.4 (1.3)	0.63[b]	72	0.529
Number of psychoactive drugs, females (SD)	2.6 (1.3)	2.0 (0.8)	2.40[b]	42	0.020
Number of psychoactive drugs, males (SD)	2.4 (1.4)	2.9 (1.8)	−0.99[b]	36	0.331
Number of antidepressants (SD)	1.8 (1.0)	1.7 (0.8)	0.20[b]	77.8	0.848
Number of antidepressants, females (SD)	1.8 (0.8)	1.6 (0.8)	1.02[b]	38.7	0.311
Number of antidepressants, males (SD)	1.7 (1.2)	1.9 (0.72)	−0.64[b]	36	0.524

[a] relates to Pearson's Chi-square tests

[b] relates to *t* tests

Basic handcraft is the core OT activity in German-speaking countries. Therefore, the primary or experimental intervention comprised standardized performance of basic handcraft activities, such as painting and crafting with wood, stone, and other materials.

Board game activities were used for control condition. The resemblance of such activities with OT in a stricter sense should improve the acceptability of the control intervention, since many patients claim OT as an essential part of inpatient treatments.

Both interventions were conducted 2 h daily, 5 days a week. Only one handcraft activity (either crafting or painting) or board game (like Monopoly or cards, involving more than two persons, thus no chess or Scrabble) was performed in each 2-h session. Both interventions were provided for groups with 6–8 patients and conducted by professional occupational therapists. No cognitive or talk therapy was added to the interventions, but a basic antidepressant drug treatment and supportive or psychoeducative talks up to 20 min per day with staff members were allowed.

The inclusion criteria were the following: 18- to 65-year-old inpatients with moderate or severe major depression without psychotic or catatonic features (moderate, 296.22, or severe episode without psychotic features, 296.23; recurrent major depressive disorder: moderate, 296.32, or severe episode without psychotic features, 296.33) and a Hamilton Depression Rating Scale (HAMD-21) score ≥18. Any antidepressant medication was allowed, if possible as a mono-therapy. Z-drugs were permitted to treat sleep problems. In case of restlessness or agitation, promethazine (up to 75 mg per day), lorazepam (up to 3 × 1 mg per day) or quetiapine (up to 100 mg per day) could be prescribed.

The exclusion criteria were the following: contraindications for antidepressants; currently at risk of suicide; and a DSM-IV diagnosis of any of the following: dementia, schizophrenia spectrum disorders, cluster A and cluster B personality disorders, substance use disorders (abuse and dependence), eating disorders (anorexia and bulimia nervosa); acute, serious, or unstable medical conditions; and pregnancy in females.

Outcome measures

The primary outcome parameter was *decrease in depressivity* as measured by the Hamilton Depression Rating Scale, HAMD-21 [7]. The Beck Depression Inventory, BDI [2], was used as a secondary outcome measure. Compared to the (interviewer-rating) HAMD, the (self-rating) BDI assesses rather subjective depressivity, and reductions of BDI scores during therapy may depend on personality traits, particularly introversion and neuroticism, to a larger extent, than do changes in HAMD scores. Therefore, complementary performance of both instruments may be useful [16]. State anxiety was measured using the Hamilton Anxiety Rating Scale, HAMA [8]. Furthermore, the Personal and Social Performance Scale, PSP, an interviewer-rating instrument, was used to assess four features of social functioning (socially useful activities; personal and social relationships; self-care; and disturbing and aggressive behavior) over a one-month period [12, 11]. These scales were applied for screening and baseline ratings and for the follow-up assessments at 3–9 weeks after baseline. A physician and a psychologist from our work group carried out the assessments. The software package *Ergo-Assess*™ [10] was used to assess functioning in activities of daily living (ADL) in the six domains of the International Classification of Functioning, Disability and Health, ICF [19]: (1) activities of physical self-care, (2) activities of independent living, (3) neuropsychological functioning, (4) psychosocial functioning, (5) sensomotoric functions, and (6) basic work activities. In contrast to the other instruments, Ergo-Assess was used at 1–6 weeks, as opposed to 3–6 weeks, after baseline by a professional occupational therapist.

Data analysis

Statistical analyses were carried out using the Statistical package for the Social Sciences (SPSS™), version 20 for Mac, IBM Corp., Armonk, New York, United States. The one-sample Kolmogorov–Smirnov test was used to confirm that all interval-scaled variables were normally distributed. Group comparisons in respect to gender, age, education, depressive symptomatology, comorbidity, and medication were conducted using t tests and Pearson's Chi-square tests. A reduction of the HAMD-21 total score of ≥50% from baseline was defined as 'antidepressive response,' and a HAMD-21 total score of ≤7 was defined as *remission*. The groups were compared with respect to these HAMD factors by performing Pearson's Chi-square tests. Possible treatment effects were investigated using general linear models (GLM) with repeated measures analyses of variance. Age, IQ, axis-I and axis-II comorbidity, number of psychoactive drugs, and number of antidepressants were taken into account as covariates. Cohen's measure of sample effect size for comparing two samples means, i.e., pre- and post-means, was then used to assess possible treatment effects. Results with $p < 0.05$ were considered statistically significant.

Results

Antidepressive response and remission

No significant group differences were found in terms of antidepressive response or remission after three- and six-week treatment. Antidepressive response was found in 10 participants (21.7%) of the OT group ($n = 46$)

and 13 participants (36.1%) of the BG group ($n = 36$) after 3 weeks, and in 19 participants (65.5%) of the OT group ($n = 29$) and 12 participants (54.5%) of the BG group ($n = 22$) after 6 weeks. Remission was found in nine participants (19.6%) in the OT group vs. five participants (13.9%) in the BG group (Chi-square = 0.536, $df = 1$, $p = 0.464$) after 3 weeks, and in eight participants (27.6%) in the OT group vs. nine participants (40.9%) in the BG group after 6 weeks (Chi-square = 0.777, $df = 1$, $p = 0.378$).

Primary outcome parameter

The GLM analysis did not find any significant time-by-group interaction effects regarding the primary outcome parameter *HAMD total score* (after 3 weeks: $F = 0.141$, $p = 0.709$; after 6 weeks: $F = 0.177$, $p = 0.828$). This indicates that neither group reached antidepressive superiority.

Secondary outcome parameters

A significant time-by-group interaction effect regarding the HAMA total score in males after three weeks was observed which suggests superiority of the OT intervention over the BG intervention ($F = 5.226$, $p = 0.031$; $d = 1.23$ vs. 0.48) (Table 2). At 6 weeks, no significant interaction effect was found. No other significant interaction effects were observed regarding the other total scores (BDI, PSP and ErgoAssess).

Subscale parameters

Comparison after 3 weeks

The following significant time-by-group interactions were observed: *loss of interest* (BDI 12) in favor of the OT group ($F = 13.494$, $p = 0.001$; $d = 0.95$ vs. 0.00) in the male participants; *disturbed sleep pattern* (BDI 16) in favor of the BG group ($F = 4.983$, $p = 0.029$; $d = 0.92$ vs. 0.31) in both genders; *loss of sexual interest* (BDI 22) in favor of the OT group in the male participants ($F = 5.017$, $p = 0.034$; $d = 0.22$ vs. 0.00); *depressed mood* (HAMA 6) in favor of the OT group in both genders ($F = 4.190$, $p = 0.044$; $d = 1.20$ vs. 0.79); and *self-care* (PSP C) in favor of the BG group in the female participants ($F = 5.213$, $p = 0.029$; $d = 0.44$ vs. 0.00) (Table 2).

Comparison after 6 weeks

The following significant time-by-group interaction effects were found subscales of the various inventories assessed: *depersonalization and derealization* (HAMD 19) in favor of the BG group in all participants ($F = 4.321$, $p = 0.044$; $d = 0.71$ vs. 0.00) and in the subgroup of male participants ($F = 4.944$, $p = 0.039$; $d = 0.83$ vs. 0.00); *loss of energy* (BDI 15) in favor of the OT group in all participants ($F = 5.095$, $p = 0.030$; $d = 1.05$ vs. 0.46); *disturbed sleep pattern* (BDI 16) in favor of the OT group in the subgroup of female participants ($F = 6.415$, $p = 0.025$; $d = 0.92$ vs. 0.51); *loss of sexual interest* (BDI 22) in favor of the OT group in all participants ($F = 11.908$, $p = 0.001$; $d = 0.36$ vs. 0.00) and in the subgroup of male participants ($F = 6.642$, $p = 0.028$; $d = 0.57$ vs. 0.00); *anxious behavior during the interview* (HAMA 14) in favor of the OT group in the subgroup of male participants ($F = 6.301$, $p = 0.022$; $d = 1.26$ vs. 0.41); and *basic work skills* (ErgoAssess 3) in favor of the OT group in all participants ($F = 6.344$, $p = 0.017$; $d = 1.83$ vs. 0.16) (Table 3).

Discussion

Data on adjuvant occupational therapy (OT) in inpatient psychiatric settings is greatly lacking. In fact, there have only been two studies on this topic [6, 14] to date. Only one trial by Reuster evaluated the effects of short-term adjuvant OT; that study was on inpatients with schizophrenia, mania, and major depression. Unfortunately, that study has not been published in PubMed, and it is the only available work that is comparable to ours.

In this study, our purpose was to investigate the effects of short-term adjuvant OT in patients with a mental disorder of considerable epidemiologic and clinical relevance, i.e., major depression, in an inpatient (i.e., costly) setting. In German-speaking countries, OT is broadly applied and generally financed by health insurance companies. The main difficulty in designing this study was that a simple comparison of pharmacotherapy alone (preferably with a single drug) to pharmacotherapy plus OT was not possible because the standard psychiatric inpatient settings in German-speaking countries provide pharmacotherapy, psycho-education and psychotherapy in single and group settings and exercise therapy, different occupational therapies, and other treatments. Therefore, we attempted to merge the demands of patients and the requirements of health insurance companies into a study design that was as simple as possible and, most importantly, had the least possible number of confounders.

Our main finding was that the interventional OT group was not superior to the control board game (BG) group with respect to our primary outcome measures: The study did not show any reduction of depressivity and percentage of remissions as measured by the Hamilton Depression Scale (HAMD-21). However, some significant time-by-group effects indicated a superiority of the OT intervention over the BG intervention with respect to anxiety, i.e., reductions in anxiety in general (HAMA total score) in male participants after three weeks, depressed mood (HAMA subscale) in participants of both genders after three weeks, and anxious behavior

Table 2 Occupational therapy ($n = 46$) vs. board games ($n = 36$): general linear model (significant interaction effects at baseline and after 3 weeks)

Variable	Subgroup	GLM						Means, differences (pre-post) and effect sizes							
		Within-subject effects (time)		Between-subjects effects (group)		Interaction (time × group)		Occupational therapy				Board game group			
		F	*p*	F	*p*	F	*p*	M pre (SD)	M post (SD)	$\Delta_{Mpre\text{-}Mpost}$	ES	M pre (SD)	M post (SD)	$\Delta_{Mpre\text{-}Mpost}$	ES
BDI 12	Total	0.429	0.515	4.579	0.036	1.001	0.298	1.21 (0.87)	0.83 (0.74)	0.38	0.47	0.83 (0.75)	0.65 (0.65)	0.18	0.26
	m	0.010	0.922	1.237	0.276	13.494	0.001	1.25 (0.90)	0.53 (0.61)	0.72	0.95	0.53 (0.70)	0.81 (0.75)	–	–
	f	0.000	0.992	2.445	0.128	2.559	0.119	1.18 (0.86)	1.04 (0.76)	0.14	0.16	1.10 (0.70)	0.50 (0.51)	0.60	0.98
BDI 16	Total	0.003	0.954	0.769	0.376	4.983	0.029	1.63 (1.09)	1.30 (1.07)	0.33	0.31	1.90 (1.01)	1.06 (0.81)	0.84	0.92
	m	0.000	0.991	3.057	0.092	1.047	0.315	1.50 (1.02)	1.16 (1.07)	0.34	0.32	2.00 (1.08)	1.13 (0.72)	0.87	0.97
	f	0.006	0.937	0.006	0.938	1.607	0.214	1.75 (1.14)	1.41 (1.08)	0.34	0.31	1.82 (0.96)	1.00 (0.91)	0.82	0.87
BDI 22	Total	0.481	0.490	0.000	0.993	3.094	0.083	1.52 (1.16)	1.33 (1.12)	0.19	0.17	1.37 (1.20)	1.47 (1.16)	–	–
	m	2.190	0.150	0.493	0.489	5.017	0.034	1.54 (1.06)	1.00 (1.00)	0.54	0.52	1.30 (1.13)	1.55 (1.13)	–	–
	f	0.022	0.883	0.271	0.606	0.150	0.702	1.50 (1.26)	1.56 (1.16)	–	–	1.43 (1.29)	1.55 (1.29)	–	–
HAMA total	Total	0.635	0.428	5.715	0.020	1.291	0.260	20.07 (7.06)	12.86 (6.73)	7.21	1.04	20.95 (6.75)	16.60 (8.78)	4.35	0.56
	m	0.023	0.882	4.511	0.044	5.226	0.031	19.38 (7.56)	10.94 (5.07)	8.52	1.23	19.11 (5.61)	16.35 (5.78)	2.76	0.48
	f	0.108	0.744	2.060	0.160	0.120	0.731	20.58 (6.75)	14.12 (7.45)	6.46	0.91	22.55 (7.34)	16.83 (11.07)	5.72	0.62
HAMA 6	Total	0.230	0.633	3.001	0.088	4.190	0.044	2.81 (0.64)	1.84 (0.97)	0.97	1.20	2.83 (0.71)	2.23 (0.81)	0.60	0.79
	m	0.023	0.880	0.305	0.586	3.669	0.067	2.88 (0.45)	1.88 (0.86)	1.00	1.52	2.74 (0.56)	2.24 (0.66)	0.50	0.82
	f	0.010	0.919	2.156	0.151	0.189	0.666	2.76 (0.75)	1.81 (1.06)	0.95	1.04	2.91 (0.87)	2.22 (0.94)	0.69	0.77
PSP C	Total	0.000	0.991	1.309	0.256	1.908	0.171	1.20 (0.56)	1.16 (0.42)	0.04	0.08	1.36 (0.62)	1.17 (0.51)	0.19	0.33
	m	0.835	0.368	0.283	0.599	0.013	0.911	1.33 (0.76)	1.21 (0.54)	0.12	0.18	1.35 (0.59)	1.22 (0.55)	0.13	0.36
	f	1.400	0.245	3.341	0.076	5.213	0.029	1.10 (0.30)	1.12 (0.33)	–	–	1.36 (0.66)	1.11 (0.47)	0.25	0.44

BDI 12: loss of interest

BDI 16: disturbed sleep pattern

BDI 22: loss of sexual interest

$HAMA_{total}$: total score

HAMA 6: depressed mood

PSP C: self-care

GLM general linear model (controlled for age, IQ, axis-I/II comorbidity, number of psychoactive drugs and number of antidepressants), stratified for gender (*m* males, *f* females); *M pre/post* mean pre/post, *SD* standard deviation, $\Delta_{Mpre\text{-}Mpost}$ difference between re- and post-mean, *ES* effect size (Cohen's d). *BDI* Beck Depression Inventory, *HAMA* Hamilton Anxiety Scale, *PSP* Personal and Social Performance Scale

Table 3 Occupational therapy ($n = 29$) vs. board games ($n = 22$): general linear model (significant interaction effects at baseline and after 6 weeks)

Variable	Sub-group	GLM						Means, differences (pre-post) and effect sizes							
		Within-subject effects (time)		Between-subjects effects (group)		Interaction (time × group)		Occupational therapy				Board game group			
		F	p	F	p	F	p	M pre (SD)	M post (SD)	$\Delta_{Mpre-Mpost}$	ES	M pre (SD)	M post (SD)	$\Delta_{Mpre-Mpost}$	ES
HAMD 19	Total	3.682	0.062	2.500	0.121	4.321	0.044	0.02 (0.13)	0.03 (0.19)	–	–	0.12 (0.33)	0.00 (0.00)	0.12	0.71
	m	1.814	0.194	3.291	0.085	4.944	0.039	0.00 (0.00)	0.06 (0.25)	–	–	0.10 (0.31)	0.00 (0.00)	0.10	0.63
	f	1.003	0.331	2.509	0.132	2.509	0.132	0.03 (0.17)	0.00 (0.00)	0.03	0.33	0.14 (0.35)	0.00 (0.00)	0.14	0.78
BDI 15	Total	0.290	0.594	0.060	0.808	5.095	0.030	1.88 (0.70)	1.11 (0.75)	0.77	1.05	1.67 (0.85)	1.25 (0.97)	0.42	0.46
	m	1.452	0.245	0.202	0.659	0.928	0.349	1.88 (0.68)	1.06 (0.77)	0.82	1.12	1.65 (0.75)	1.11 (0.93)	0.56	0.67
	f	0.025	0.877	0.850	0.373	0.757	0.400	1.89 (0.74)	1.18 (0.75)	0.71	0.95	1.68 (0.95)	1.36 (1.03)	0.32	0.32
BDI 16	Total	0.008	0.930	7.164	0.011	0.555	0.461	1.63 (1.09)	0.81 (0.74)	0.82	0.89	1.90 (1.01)	1.43 (1.17)	0.47	0.43
	m	1.205	0.287	7.065	0.016	0.075	0.787	1.50 (1.02)	0.81 (0.66)	0.69	0.82	2.00 (1.08)	1.60 (1.17)	0.40	0.35
	f	6.150	0.028	0.002	0.970	6.415	0.025	1.75 (1.14)	0.82 (0.87)	0.93	0.92	1.82 (0.96)	1.27 (1.19)	0.55	0.51
BDI 22	Total	0.002	0.960	0.156	0.695	11.908	0.001	1.52 (1.16)	1.11 (1.12)	0.41	0.36	1.37 (1.20)	1.55 (1.18)	–	–
	m	0.023	0.882	0.313	0.583	5.642	0.028	1.54 (1.06)	0.94 (0.93)	0.60	0.57	1.30 (1.13)	1.55 (1.13)	–	–
	f	0.526	0.481	0.775	0.395	0.114	0.741	1.50 (1.26)	1.36 (1.36)	0.14	0.11	1.43 (1.29)	1.55 (1.29)	–	–
HAMA 14	Total	0.131	0.720	0.779	0.283	2.412	0.128	1.19 (0.93)	0.38 (0.62)	0.81	1.04	1.07 (0.69)	1.55 (4.64)	–	–
	m	2.839	0.109	0.489	0.493	6.301	0.022	1.29 (1.12)	0.38 (0.62)	0.91	1.26	0.95 (0.71)	0.64 (0.81)	0.31	0.41
	f	0.101	0.755	1.332	0.265	1.424	0.250	1.12 (0.78)	0.38 (0.65)	0.74	1.03	1.18 (0.66)	2.45 (6.53)	–	–
Ergo-Asses 3	Total	1.753	0.195	0.172	0.681	6.344	0.017	13.90 (3.51)	10.96 (3.59)	2.94	0.83	12.72 (5.12)	11.90 (5.03)	0.82	0.16
	m	1.036	0.329	3.697	0.079	2.245	0.160	14.45 (4.12)	11.92 (4.38)	2.53	0.60	11.94 (5.49)	9.70 (3.53)	2.24	0.50
	f	0.667	0.429	3.089	0.102	2.210	0.161	13.50 (3.01)	9.91 (2.21)	3.59	1.38	13.38 (4.81)	14.10 (5.49)	–	–

HAMD 19: depersonalization and derealization

BDI 15: loss of energy

BDI 16: disturbed sleep pattern

BDI 22: loss of sexual interest

HAMA 14: anxious behavior during interview

Ergo-Assess 3: basic work skills

GLM general linear model (controlled for age, IQ, axis-I/II comorbidity, number of psychoactive drugs and number of antidepressants), stratified for gender (*m* males, *f* females), *M pre/post* mean pre/post, *SD* standard deviation, $\Delta_{Mpre-Mpost}$ difference between pre- and post-mean, *ES* effect size (Cohen's d). *HAMD* Hamilton Depression Scale, *BDI* Beck Depression Inventory, *HAMA* Hamilton Anxiety Scale, *Ergo-Assess*™ German Occupational Therapy Assessment

during the interview (HAMA subscale) in male participants after six weeks.

Moreover, significant interaction effects in regards to some subscales of the Beck Depression Inventory (BDI) indicated the superiority of OT over BG, including loss of general interest and loss of sexual interest in males after 3 weeks, loss of energy in all participants after six weeks, disturbed sleep pattern in females after 6 weeks, and loss of sexual interest in both genders after 6 weeks. However, a significant interaction effect with respect to disturbed sleep pattern in participants of both genders after 3 weeks suggested a superiority of BG over OT. Other measures in favor of BT included self-care (from the Personal and Social Performance Scale) after 3 weeks in the female participants and depersonalization and derealization (from the HAMD) after 6 weeks in participants of both genders.

Finally, basic work skills (assessed with Ergo-Assess™) improved significantly more in the OT participants of both genders after 6 weeks. Effect sizes with respect to the superior group, i.e., predominantly the OT group, were mainly in the high range ($d > 0.8$).

There were several limitations to this study: We faced difficulties concerning the comparability of the two groups; for example, patients found the OT intervention much more pleasant and effective than the BG activities, which was reflected by a far greater dropout rate during the first 3 weeks in the BG group, 36.8%, compared to the OT group, 19.3%.

The ("semi-active") BG group was not a true control group, such as a placebo or waitlist group; thus, we can only discuss 'effects' but not 'efficacy' of the OT intervention in comparison to the BG activities.

For comparability reasons, each group intervention was completely structured and standardized as to content and procedure, which entailed limited performance of individually meaningful activities and accomplishment of personal goals. Thus, the OT intervention was limitedly representative of standard OT group interventions for inpatients. Moreover, our "OT" intervention is by no means representative of occupational therapy in general.

We were not able to explain why BDI but not HAMD scores decreased during the intervention. Changes in BDI scores rather than HAMD scores emerged to be associated with personality features like introversion and neuroticism [16]; however, this study lacked assessment of personality traits.

Insufficient qualitative and process-related assessment of pharmacotherapy represents a major shortcoming of this study. However, the numbers of psychoactive and antidepressant drugs were considered as covariates, and 80% of the participants were known to enter the study taking at least one antidepressant.

Finally, the study was underpowered, as it had an even smaller study sample size than that of Reuster's investigation (82 participants in our study vs. 114 participants in Reuster's study). Thus, this study has to be regarded as a pilot project.

Conclusions

In conclusion, the OT group in our study showed more significant effects indicating improvement with respect to features of anxiety, loss of energy, sexual and general interest, and work skills than the BG group. Moreover, the results of this study suggest a greater benefit of the OT intervention in males than in females.

Together, our results suggest that adjuvant standard occupational treatment may be superior to mere board game activities and may be a feasible adjunct therapy to pharmacotherapy (and possibly other treatments) in a psychiatric short-term setting for inpatients with major depression.

Abbreviations

ADL: activities of daily living; BDI: Beck Depression Inventory; BG (group): board game (group); DSM-IV: Fourth edition of the Diagnostic and Statistical Manual of the American Psychiatric Association; Ergo-Assess™: instrument for the assessment of occupational therapy outcome; GLM: general linear model; HAMA: Hamilton Anxiety Rating Scale; HAMD (-21): Hamilton Depression Rating Scale (with 21 items); ICF: International Classification of Functioning, Disability and Health; OT (group): occupational therapy (group); PSP: scale personal and social performance scale; RCT: randomized controlled trial; SCID: Structured Clinical Interview for the DSM-IV; SPSS: statistical package for the social sciences; TAU: treatment as usual; WHO: World Health Organization.

Authors' contributions

All of us authors made substantial contributions to the conception and design or analysis and interpretation of data. Furthermore, all of us were involved substantially in drafting or revising the article for important and novel content, and gave approval of the final version to be submitted. Particularly, MAE, BV, PR, ISH and GJ were substantially involved in the planning of the study design, providing treatment facilities, supervising occupational therapists, evaluating study results, and writing of the paper. BB, MS, BE, and FT coordinated the allocation of participants and took care of the assessment, evaluation, analysis, and presentation of data; moreover, the colleagues were involved in drafting and revising the manuscript. TF was part of our study team. As the leading occupational therapist, she was involved in the conceptualization of the study, moreover in active performance and supervising colleagues concerning occupational therapy and "game therapy" in the study groups, and in the final presentation of results. All authors have read and approved the final manuscript.

Author details

[1] Department of Psychiatry, Psychotherapy and Preventive Medicine, LWL University Hospital, Ruhr University Bochum, Alexandrinenstr. 1-3, 44791 Bochum, Germany. [2] Institute of Mental Health, LWL University Hospital Bochum, Bochum, Germany. [3] LWL Hospital Paderborn, Paderborn, Germany.

Acknowledgements

We thank Birgit Zander, Petra Nengelken, and Bettina Finger for acquisition of the literature we have used and referred to in our paper, and for drafting the manuscript. Moreover, many thanks to the colleagues of our inpatient occupational therapy unit for therapeutic activities and support, and to all patients who participated in the study.

Competing interests

The authors declare that they have no competing interests.

Funding
The study was financed by the participating hospitals without any external sponsorship.

References

1. American Occupational Therapy Association. Occupational therapy practice framework: domain and process. Am J Occup Ther. 2008;62:625–83.
2. Beck AT, Ward CH, Mendelson M, Mock J, Erbaugh J. An inventory for measuring depression. Arch Gen Psychiatry. 1961;4:561–71.
3. Buchain PC, Vizzotto AD, Henna Neto J, Elkis H. Randomized controlled trial of occupational therapy in patients with treatment-resistant schizophrenia. Rev Bras Psiquiatr. 2003;25:26–30.
4. Cook S, Chambers E, Coleman JH. Occupational therapy for people with psychotic conditions in community settings: a pilot randomized controlled trial. Clin Rehabil. 2009. doi:10.1177/0269215508098898.
5. Die Gesundheitsberichterstattung des Bundes [Transl.: The German Information System of the Federal Health Monitoring]. Wiesbaden: Statistisches Bundesamt; 2006. http://www.gbe-bund.de. Accessed 5 Aug 2016.
6. Foruzandeh N, Parvin N. Occupational therapy for inpatients with chronic schizophrenia: a pilot randomized controlled trial. Jpn J Nurs Sci. 2013. doi:10.1111/j.1742-7924.2012.00211.x.
7. Hamilton M. A rating scale for depression. J Neurol Neurosurg Psychiatry. 1960;23:56–62.
8. Hamilton M. The assessment of anxiety states by rating. Br J Med Psychol. 1959;32:50–5.
9. Hees HL, de Vries G, Koeter MW, Schene AH. Adjuvant occupational therapy improves long-term depression recovery and return-to-work in good health in sick-listed employees with major depression: results of a randomised controlled trial. Occup Environ Med. 2013;70:252–60.
10. Heiss HW, Voigt-Radloff S, Schochat T. Occupational Therapy Assessment (OTA): validity and reliability for adults of various ages. Eur J Ger. 2003;5:23–9.
11. Juckel G, Schaub D, Fuchs N, Naumann U, Uhl I, Witthaus H, Hargarter L, Bierhoff HW, Brüne M. Validation of the Personal and Social Performance (PSP) Scale in a German sample of acutely ill patients with schizophrenia. Schizophr Res. 2008. doi:10.1016/j.schres.2008.04.037.
12. Morosini PL, Magliano L, Brambilla L, Ugolini S, Pioli R. Development, reliability and acceptability of a new version of the DSM-IV Social and Occupational Functioning Assessment Scale (SOFAS) to assess routine social functioning. Acta Psychiatr Scand. 2000;101:323–9.
13. Paterson CF. History of occupational therapy in mental health. In: Bryant W, Fieldhouse J, Bannigan K, editors. Creek's Occupational Therapy and Mental Health. 5th ed. London: Churchill/Livingstone (Elsevier); 2014.
14. Reuster T. Effektivität der Ergotherapie im psychiatrischen Krankenhaus [Transl.: Effectiveness of occupational therapy in the psychiatric hospital]. Vol. 112. Darmstadt; 2006.
15. Schene AH, Koeter MW, Kikkert MJ, Swinkels JA, McCrone P. Adjuvant occupational therapy for work-related major depression works: randomized trial including economic evaluation. Psychol Med. 2007;37:351–62.
16. Schneibel R, Brakemeier EL, Wilbertz G, Dykierek P, Zobel I, Schramm E. Sensitivity to detect change and the correlation of clinical factors with the Hamilton Depression Rating Scale and the Beck Depression Inventory in depressed inpatients. Psychiatry Res. 2012;198:62–7.
17. Voigt-Radloff S, Ruf G, Vogel A, van Nes F, Hüll M. Occupational therapy for elderly: evidence mapping of randomised controlled trials from 2004 to 2012. Z Gerontol Geriatr. 2015;48:52–72.
18. World Health Organization. Depression, a global public health concern. Geneva: World Health Organization; 2012.
19. World Health Organization. International Classification of Functioning, Disability and Health. Geneva: World Health Organization; 2001.

17

Strength-based assessment for future violence risk: a retrospective validation study of the Structured Assessment of PROtective Factors for violence risk (SAPROF) Japanese version in forensic psychiatric inpatients

Hiroko Kashiwagi[1*], Akiko Kikuchi[2], Mayuko Koyama[1], Daisuke Saito[1] and Naotsugu Hirabayashi[1]

Abstract

Background: The Structured Assessment of PROtective Factors for violence risk (SAPROF) was recently developed as a strength-based addition to the risk assessment of future violent behavior. We examined the interrater reliability and predictive accuracy of the SAPROF for violence in forensic mental health inpatient units in Japan.

Methods: This retrospective record study provides an initial validation of the SAPROF in a Japanese sample of 95 forensic psychiatric inpatients from a complete 2008–2013 cohort. Violent outcomes were assessed 6 and 12 months after hospitalization.

Results: We observed moderate-to-good interrater reliability for the SAPROF total score and the internal factors, motivational factors, external factors, and the Final Protection Judgment scores. According to a receiver operating characteristic analysis, the SAPROF total score and all subscale scores predicted violence at both 6 and 12 months after hospitalization with high accuracy. Furthermore, the predictive validity of a combination of the SAPROF with the Historical Clinical Risk Management-20 (HCR-20) outperformed that of the HCR-20 alone.

Conclusions: The results provide evidence of the value of considering protective factors in the assessment of future violence risk among Japanese forensic psychiatric inpatients. The SAPROF might allow for a more balanced assessment of future violence risk in places where the population rates of violent crime are low, such as Japan, but a validation study in a different setting should confirm this. Moreover, future studies should examine the effectiveness of treatment and promoting community re-integration on motivating patients and treatment staff.

Keywords: Protective factor, SAPROF, Violence, Risk assessment, Forensic inpatients

Background

Over the last few decades, our knowledge of violence risk assessment and the risk factors for violence have increased markedly. Risk-focused assessment tools, such as the Historical Clinical Risk Management-20 (HCR-20) [1], are widely used in forensic settings worldwide. However, very little attention has been paid to the factors that might compensate for these risk factors and thereby reduce the risk of violence recidivism, namely protective factors.

According to the manual of the Structured Assessment of PROtective Factors for violence risk (SAPROF), protective factors refer to any characteristic of a person, his/her environment, or his/her situation that reduces the risk of future violent behavior [2, 3]. The identification of specific protective factors is a major challenge for

*Correspondence: hkashiwagi@ncnp.go.jp
[1] Department of Forensic Psychiatry, National Center Hospital of Neurology and Psychiatry, 4-1-1, Ogawahigashicho, Kodaira, Tokyo 187-8553, Japan
Full list of author information is available at the end of the article

the future [4–6]. A balanced risk assessment involves the evaluation of both risk and protective factors. In other words, when these protective factors are not considered, risk assessment becomes unbalanced, thereby leading to inaccurate predictions [5]. Further, this might lead to pessimism among both offenders, who are often stigmatized, and therapists, which might lead to the long-term detention of forensic psychiatric patients. Protective factors might explain the reason for the lack of recidivism in some high-risk individuals [7], such as individuals with severe psychopathy. As the reduction of violent re-offenses is a major goal of treatment, interventions should not focus on merely curtailing risk factors, but also on strengthening protective factors [8, 9]. Moreover, insight into the presence or absence of protective factors might offer a complete view of the individual in their context and provide guidelines for treatment and risk management. The standardized assessment of protective factors might also have a positive and motivating effect on both patients and treatment staff [2, 3]. Therefore, such a strength-based approach might be particularly effective when integrated into psychosocial treatment, such as that which uses a problem-solving approach and seeks empowerment (e.g., the Good Lives Model) [10, 11].

Inspired by past research and reinforced by the desire of clinicians to focus more on the changeable positive factors in risk assessment, de Vogel and colleagues [2, 3] developed the SAPROF, a positive, dynamic addition to the collection of structured risk assessment tools. The SAPROF is a checklist of 17 protective factors identified in a literature review on the protective and contextual factors of future violence [12], contextual factors related to violent recidivism, and the clinical experience of the mental health professionals and researchers at the Van der Hoeven clinic in the Netherlands [2, 3]. Two of the factors are considered static and 15 dynamic, and its overall aim is to inform clinicians of potential goals for treatment intervention. The SAPROF might offer valuable guidance in narrowing the gap between risk assessment and violence prevention [13]. The SAPROF validation study further revealed that it has a good interrater reliability and good predictive validity for forensic inpatients and outpatients [2, 3, 13].

In Japan, there are no widely used structured risk assessment tools for violence. In accordance with a new mental health act (the Medical Treatment and Supervision Act [MTSA], 2005), the Ministry of Health, Labour and Welfare developed and introduced 17 specific risk assessment items (Kyoutu Hyouka Koumoku in Japanese) for common points of view among various professionals. These items share many commonalities with the items of the HCR-20 [1]. Of course, in addition to the focus on problem extraction and evaluation from a negative perspective, there have been voices pointing out the importance of positive evaluations that focus on protective factors. Consequently, from the initial implementation of the MTSA, the necessity of attending to this positive perspective of future violence assessment, on which the SAPROF is based, and treatment through a recovery model has been recognized. Still, evaluation tools based on this perspective do not currently exist, which has necessitated the development of the SAPROF Japanese Version.

In this study, a Japanese translation of the SAPROF was completed, and its back translation was subsequently certificated by the original authors. We then sought to validate the measure in Japanese forensic settings by examining its predictive accuracy for violent incidents among forensic psychiatric inpatients in Japan.

Methods

We conducted a retrospective record study of a complete cohort of patients admitted to the National Center Hospital of Neurology and Psychiatry, which has 66 beds dedicated to forensic psychiatric patients.

Participants

In Japan, individuals who have committed serious harm to others while in a state of insanity or diminished responsibility because of a mental disorder receive a court order for hospitalization that is pursuant to the MTSA. Forensic psychiatric wards are dedicated to the containment and treatment of such individuals. In this study, we included all such patients admitted to the forensic psychiatric wards of the National Center Hospital of Neurology and Psychiatry between April 2008 and November 2012, and followed them up through November 2013. Patients who were hospitalized for less than 1 year were excluded because we used two observation periods for the occurrence of violence: 6 and 12 months.

Diagnosis

Participants were diagnosed by a consulting psychiatrist according to the International Classification of Diseases, Tenth Edition (ICD-10) criteria [14]. The classification was based on single-digit ICD-10 codes (F0 to F9), and when a participant had multiple psychiatric diagnoses, we included only the primary diagnosis, consistent with the previous validation study on the HCR-20 in Japanese forensic inpatients [15]. We determined which diagnosis was considered primary based on which diagnosis was directly connected to the offense for which the patient was hospitalized.

Assessment

SAPROF

The SAPROF is a checklist of protective factors that is intended for use in conjunction with structured professional judgment risk assessment tools, such as the HCR-20. The SAPROF comprises 17 protective factors (see Table 1), all of which are rated on a three-point scale (0 = the protective factor is clearly absent or there is no evidence that the protective factor is present, 1 = the protective factor may be present or is present to some extent, 2 = the protective factor is clearly present) reflecting the extent to which they are present for a given patient in a specific situation. After rating all the protective factors, a Final Protection Judgment score, which reflects the degree of protection against relapse into violence, is rated on a five-point scale (low, low–moderate, moderate, moderate–high, high). The SAPROF items are organized into three scales: internal factors, motivational factors, and external factors. Items 1 and 2 (internal factors) are considered static, whereas the other 15 factors are dynamic and, therefore, changeable during treatment. Items 3–14 are expected to improve during treatment because higher scores on these factors indicate greater balance in internal and social functioning and increased motivation. Items 15–17, by contrast, are expected to decrease during treatment because they relate to the protection offered by external professional care, which is expected to be reduced as much as possible by the end of treatment. A total SAPROF protection score is the sum of the scores of the 17 items. The total SAPROF internal, motivational, and external scores are the sums of the five (items 1–5), seven (items 6–12), and five (items 13–17) item scores in these factors, respectively. The total SAPROF protection score ranges from 0 to 34.

Table 1 The SAPROF-17 factors and expected changes during treatment

	Expected changes during treatment
Internal factors	
1. Intelligence	Static
2. Secure attachment in childhood	Static
3. Empathy	Improving
4. Coping	Improving
5. Self-control	Improving
Motivational factors	
6. Work	Improving
7. Leisure activities	Improving
8. Financial management	Improving
9. Motivation for treatment	Improving
10. Attitudes toward authority	Improving
11. Life goals	Improving
12. Medication	Improving
External factors	
13. Social network	Improving
14. Intimate relationship	Improving
15. Professional care	Decreasing
16. Living circumstances	Decreasing
17. External control	Decreasing

The procedure for translating the SAPROF into Japanese was as follows. First, the original English version was translated into Japanese by the first author (HK), the second author (AK), the last author (NH), and five others. Second, back translation was done by a native English speaker, whose second language was Japanese. Finally, the back-translated version of the SAPROF was confirmed and approved by the researchers who had originally developed the SAPROF in the Netherlands.

The SAPROF was completed based on a psychiatric evaluation report recorded by a psychiatrist, a life and environmental report recorded by a probation officer, and clinical records of multi-disciplinary professionals within the first 2 weeks following hospitalization. The SAPROF was scored by the first author (HK), who is a forensic psychiatrist and had attended English and Japanese training sessions for scoring the SAPROF. To establish interrater reliability, 30 randomly selected cases were coded independently by two different raters, HK and MK (the latter of whom is a clinical psychologist and was trained to score the SAPROF).

HCR-20

The HCR-20 is a commonly used risk-focused, structured professional judgment assessment tool for future violence. We used the HCR-20 version 2, Japanese Edition [15]. The HCR-20 comprises 20 items across the following subscales: historical (10 items), clinical (five items), and risk management (5 items). Each item is scored on a three-point scale as 0 (absent), 1 (possibly present or present only to a limited extent), or 2 (present). The risk management items are scored separately for the likelihood of institutional (In) and community (Out) violence. In the current study, we included only the scores for the risk of institutional violence because all the participants were inpatients. Psychopathy was omitted from the scale following the Japanese HCR-20 version 2 validation study [15] because there is evidence that it adds little to this assessment, and guidelines warn against the use of this item unless psychopathy is rated using the Hare Psychopathy Checklist-Revised (PCL-R) [16]. There is no validation study on the PCL-R Japanese version. Furthermore, high-psychopathic inpatients are very rare in the MTSA wards in Japan because these individuals tend to be sentenced to prison, as they are regarded to assume full responsibility for their offense. Consequently, the HCR-20 total score ranges from 0 to 38.

As described above, designated evaluation items (Kyoutu Hyouka Koumoku) are typically used in Japanese forensic units, whereas HCR-20 scores are recorded only for research and are not intended for clinical practice in Japan. The HCR-20 version 2, Japanese Edition was administered by trained psychiatrists at admission, 3, 6 months, and 1 year after hospitalization, as well as at discharge. In our study, only HCR-20 admission scores were used because we also administered the SAPROF at admission. We obtained these data for the HCR-20 from original validation study conducted by Arai et al. [15].

We also calculated an overall total risk and protection score by subtracting the SAPROF total score from the HCR-20 total score: this HCR-20–SAPROF total score ranges from − 34 to 38.

Violent outcomes

Data on the incidents of violence in forensic psychiatric wards were obtained from the patients' electronic medical records. We searched these records for the following: (1) records with tags related to interpersonal violence; (2) records with tags related to loss of impulse control; (3) records associated with advanced observation level; and (4) records related to administration of restraint or seclusion. This search protocol yielded almost all incidents of violence during hospitalization. In their introduction to the HCR-20, Webster et al. [1] defined violence as actual, attempted, or threatened harm to another individual. Thus, any behavior directed at a typical person that would make that person experience fear can be regarded as violence. More specifically, we used the following definition of violence based on the validation study of the HCR-20 (version 2) Japanese Edition [15]:

1. An act attempting to harm another person physically (e.g., striking, kicking, biting, or throwing something at another person);
2. Intentional destruction of property in front of others (e.g., breaking glass or slamming a table to the floor);
3. Sexual offenses/harassment.

Although threats of harm are regarded as "verbal violence," they are not always documented in medical records [17]. Therefore, they were excluded from the present study.

Violent incidents were measured at 6 and 12 months after hospitalization. Violent incidents that occurred within 6 months of hospitalization were included in both the 6- and 12-month analyses. The data on violence were collected independently from the HCR-20 and SAPROF data by different researchers, each blind to others' ratings.

Data analysis

The interrater reliability of the SAPROF was examined via the intraclass correlation coefficient (ICC) using a two-way random-effect variance model that assesses the consistency of agreement [18]. The critical values for single-measure ICCs are as follows: ICC $\geq$ 0.75 = excellent; 0.60 $\leq$ ICC < 0.75 = good; and 0.40 $\leq$ ICC < 0.60 = moderate [19].

The predictive validity of the SAPROF and HCR-20 and the combined score of both measures were examined at 6 and 12 months using receiver operating characteristic (ROC) analyses. The ROC curve is created by plotting the sensitivity against the specificity at various cut-off points. The predictive ability of the measure is determined by the area under the curve (AUC), with 0.5 representing a prediction no better than chance and 1 representing a perfect positive prediction. An AUC greater than 0.71 is regarded as a large effect size [20]. Note that values on the SAPROF (total score, subscale scores, and Final Protection Judgment) do not reflect the risk of violent incidents but, rather, their absence. Conversely, values on the HCR-20 and the HCR-20–SAPROF are considered to reflect risk of violent incidents.

Results

Background characteristics and occurrence of violence

During the study period, 128 patients were admitted. Eight patients were excluded because of insufficient data, and 25 patients were excluded because they were discharged within 1 year. Thus, a total of 95 patients were included in analyses.

Table 2 shows the demographic characteristics of the participants. All the participants were Asians and Japanese-speaking adults ($\geq$ 20 years old). Most of them had been diagnosed with a schizophrenic disorder, while the second most frequent diagnosis involved mental and behavioral disorders resulting from psychoactive substance use. No participant had a primary diagnosis of a personality disorder. The index offense of most participants involved interpersonal violence.

Diagnostic categories are based on ICD-10 codes as follows: F00–09: organic, including symptomatic, mental disorders; F10–19: mental and behavioral disorders because of psychoactive substance use; F20–29: schizophrenia, schizotypal, and delusional disorders; F30–39: mood [affective] disorders; F60–69: disorders of adult personality and behavior; F80–89: disorders of psychological development.

Scores on the SAPROF, HCR-20, and HCR-20–SAPROF, as well as incidents of violence following hospitalization, are shown in Table 3. Electronic medical records showed that at 6 and 12 months, 11 (11.6%) and 17

Table 2 Participant demographic characteristics

	n = 95	
Age		
	Mean age (SD)	45.73 (14.12)
	20–29	12 (12.6%)
	30–39	28 (29.4%)
	40–49	21 (22.1%)
	50–59	17 (17.9%)
	60–69	10 (10.5%)
	70–79	6 (6.3%)
	80–89	1 (1.1%)
Sex		
	Male	83 (87.4%)
	Female	12 (12.6%)
Diagnosis		
	F00-09	2 (2.1%)
	F10-19	14 (15.8%)
	F20-29	70 (73.7%)
	F30-39	6 (6.3%)
	F60-69	1 (1.1%)
	F80-89	1 (1.1%)
Index offence		
	Murder	35 (36.8%)
	Bodily injury	33 (34.7%)
	Arson	18 (18.9%)
	Sexual offence	3 (3.2%)
	Robbery	6 (6.3%)

(17.9%) of the patients, respectively, had committed at least one violent act.

Reliability

Cronbach's alpha of the whole SAPROF was 0.81 (data available for 93 participants). The interrater reliability analyses of the randomly selected 30 cases are shown in Table 4. They revealed single-measure ICCs for the total SAPROF score, the internal score, the motivational score, the external score, the Final Protection Judgment score, and for the individual items in the SAPROF. The professional care, living circumstances, and external control items (all external factors) were scored 2 for all participants because all the participants were hospitalized, treated, and under observation according to a court order.

Predictive accuracy of the SAPROF for violence

Table 5 shows the results of the ROC analysis of the predictive accuracy of the SAPROF, HCR-20 and HCR-20–SAPROF at 6 and 12 months. Six months after hospitalization, the AUCs for the total SAPROF score and for the internal factors, motivational factors, external factors, Final Protection Judgment, HCR-20, and HCR-20–SAPROF scores were all > 0.71. Twelve months after admission, all scores were > 0.71, except for that of the HCR-20 (AUC = 0.67). Notably, the predictive validity of the combined HCR-20–SAPROF outperformed the predictive validity of the HCR-20 alone at both 6 and 12 months after admission.

Table 3 SAPROF, HCR-20, and HCR-20-SAPROF scores and the occurrence of violence

	6 months	12 months
Number	95	95
Interpersonal violence	9	13
Property destruction	2	4
Sexual violence	0	0

	6 months			12 months		
Violence	Yes	No	*P*	Yes	No	*P*
Number	11	84[a]		17	78[a]	
SAPROF total (SD)	12.1 (1.9)	17.4 (4.1)	< 0.001	12.7 (2.3)	17.6 (4.1)	< 0.001
Internal (SD)	2.0 (0.9)	4.0 (1.8)	< 0.001	2.1 (1.0)	4.1 (1.8)	< 0.001
Motivational (SD)	3.8 (1.8)	6.4 (2.2)	< 0.001	4.2 (1.6)	6.5 (2.2)	< 0.001
External (SD)	6.3 (0.5)	7.0 (0.9)	0.015	6.4 (0.5)	7.0 (0.9)	0.006
Final judgment (SD)	1.8 (0.8)	2.9 (0.9)	< 0.001	1.9 (0.7)	3.0 (0.9)	< 0.001
HCR-20 (SD)	24.7 (4.3)	18.6 (6.4)	0.003	22.2 (5.4)	18.7 (6.5)	0.045
HCR-20-SAPROF (SD)	12.6 (3.9)	1.3 (9.1)	< 0.001	9.5 (6.1)	1.1 (9.3)	< 0.001

T tests were calculated to compare group means

[a] One participant's intelligence could not be evaluated because of the patient's refusal to take an IQ test, and one participant did not take any medications, so the number of participants contributing to the mean SAPROF internal and motivational scores in the nonviolent group was 83 at 6 months and 77 at 12 months, while that contributing to the mean SAPROF total score in the nonviolent group was 82 at 6 months and 76 at 12 months

Table 4 Interrater reliability of the SAPROF

Scale	ICC	P
SAPROF total	0.70	< 0.001
Internal	0.78	< 0.001
Motivational	0.57	< 0.001
External	0.76	< 0.001
Final judgment	0.60	< 0.001
Items		
Intelligence	0.96	< 0.001
Secure attachment in childhood	0.71	< 0.001
Empathy	0.71	< 0.001
Coping	0.32	0.042
Self-control	0.44	0.007
Work	0.46	0.004
Leisure activity	0.32	0.041
Financial management	0.36	0.024
Motivation for treatment	0.043	0.410
Attitude toward authority	0.50	0.002
Life goals	0.53	0.001
Medication	0.51	0.002
Social network	0.72	< 0.001
Intimate relationship	0.81	< 0.001

The critical values for single-measure ICCs are as follows: ICC $\geq$ 0.75 = excellent; 0.60 $\leq$ ICC < 0.75 = good; and 0.40 $\leq$ ICC < 0.60 = moderate. The professional care, living circumstances, and external control items (all external factors) were excluded because they were scored 2 for all participants

Table 5 ROC analysis of the predictive accuracy of the SAPROF, HCR-20, and HCR-20–SAPROF for violence

Observation period	Scale	Area under the curve	95% confidence interval
6 months	SAPROF total	0.87	0.79–0.95
	Internal	0.83	0.73–0.93
	Motivational	0.82	0.70–0.94
	External	0.74	0.60–0.89
	Final judgment	0.82	0.69–0.95
	HCR-20	0.79	0.69–0.90
	HCR-20–SAPROF	0.87	0.79–0.94
12 months	SAPROF total	0.85	0.77–0.94
	Internal	0.83	0.74–0.92
	Motivational	0.8	0.70–0.91
	External	0.72	0.59–0.85
	Final judgment	0.82	0.72–0.92
	HCR-20	0.67	0.54–0.80
	HCR-20–SAPROF	0.78	0.67–0.88

The values on the SAPROF (total score, subscale scores, and Final Protection Judgment) do not reflect risk of violent incidents but, rather, their absence. Conversely, values on the HCR-20 and the HCR-20–SAPROF reflect risk of violent incidents

Discussion

This is the first study to examine the predictive ability of the SAPROF for future violence (i.e., the absence of violence) in a sample of forensic psychiatric inpatients in Japan. The interrater reliability analysis indicated that there was moderate-to-good reliability for the total SAPROF score, as well as the scores on the three subscales (internal, motivational, and external factors) and the Final Protection Judgment score. Furthermore, according to the ROC analysis, the total SAPROF score, as well as the scores on the three subscales and the Final Protection Judgment score, predicted the absence of violence at 6 and 12 months with high accuracy.

The fact that the SAPROF Japanese version had predictive validity is consistent with a previous study conducted among a Dutch sample of inpatients [21]. In this Dutch inpatient study, most of the patients (89%) had been diagnosed with at least one personality disorder (particularly Cluster B disorders), while 53% of the patients had been diagnosed with a major mental illness (primarily psychotic disorders, such as schizophrenia) [21]. The duration of observation for violence was 12 months after the initial assessment. While they included verbal aggression as well as physical aggression (e.g., hitting, pushing) among the incidents of violence, the overall observed violent incident rate was 11%. In the present study, most participants (73.7%) had been diagnosed with a schizophrenic disorder, suggesting that the diagnostic characteristics are different from the Dutch sample; nevertheless, the observation duration and violent incident rate were similar to that sample. One possible reason for this might be that differences in the treatment environment and management skills affected the violence rate. Abidin et al. [22], in a prospective study conducted in Ireland, reported that the total score on the SAPROF predicted the absence of violence (AUC = 0.847) in forensic inpatients at 6 months after admission, with a violent incident rate of 13.3%. In that study, most participants (85%) had a primary diagnosis of either schizophrenia or schizoaffective disorder [22].

The predictive validity results are not, however, entirely consistent with a Swiss retrospective cross-validation study [23], which showed that the total SAPROF score had an AUC of 0.70, while the total HCR-20 score had an AUC of 0.85 for violent and sexual incidents 3 years after release. In that study, almost half the participants were sex offenders, 58.8% had been diagnosed with a personality disorder, and 27% had mental retardation, whereas only 5.9% had exhibited psychosis. In addition, about 30% of the offenders were reconvicted within 3 years of their release.

Singh et al. [24] reported that the rates of violence in persons identified as high risk by structured risk assessment instruments showed substantial variation. In addition, they suggested that the rates were elevated when the population rates of violence were higher, when a structured professional judgment instrument was used, and when there was a lower population of men in a study. Given that population rates of violent crime in Japan are low in comparison with other countries (as reported by the Ministry of Justice) [25], we can infer that using only risk-focused assessment tools might increase the rates of false positives. Thus, the HCR-20 might not be sufficient if used alone. Assessing protective factors alongside risk factors might thus help in providing more accurate and balanced predictions of future violence in Japan. Our findings encourage clinicians working in forensic psychiatric settings to take these protective factors into account when assessing violence risk. Additionally, focusing on strengths or protective factors might be useful for psychosocial treatment, particularly by motivating both clinicians and patients. Future studies on the effectiveness of assessing protective factors using the SAPROF or other strength-based assessment tools for treatment and promoting re-integration into society among forensic psychiatric patients are warranted.

Limitations

This study has some limitations. First, while both the HCR-20 and SAPROF were mainly based on a psychiatric evaluation report recorded by a psychiatrist, a life and environmental report recorded by a probation officer, and clinical records of multi-disciplinary professionals within the first 2 weeks following hospitalization, the HCR-20 was assessed by the psychiatrist in charge so that the psychiatrists could begin seeing the patients. Second, the study design, along with the short observation period for the initial assessment (i.e., within 2 weeks of hospitalization) on the clinical records, might have negatively impacted interrater reliability, as the ICCs of coping, leisure activities, financial management, and motivation for treatment were all < 0.4. Third, the data on the occurrence of violence were limited to incidents reported in the electronic clinical records. Fourth, the sample size was insufficient to allow sub-group analyses. Therefore, we cannot determine the predictive validity of the SAPROF for men and women separately and in different diagnostic categories. Finally, the applicability of our results is limited to forensic psychiatric inpatients admitted under the MTSA in Japan. The predictive accuracy of the SAPROF among forensic outpatients, general psychiatric patients, or individuals in other forensic settings in Japan is unknown.

Conclusion

The SAPROF Japanese version, a structured professional judgment tool focused on the protective factors against violence, is an effective tool as a significant predictor of desistance from violent behavior among Japanese forensic psychiatric inpatients. The SAPROF might allow for a more balanced assessment of future violence risk in places where the population rates of violent crime are low, such as Japan, but a validation study in a different setting is needed to confirm this.

Abbreviations

AUC: area under the curve; HCR-20: Historical Clinical Risk Management-20; ICC: intraclass correlation coefficient; ICD-10: International Classification of Diseases, Tenth Edition; MTSA: Medical Treatment and Supervision Act; ROC: receiver operating characteristic; SAPROF: Structured Assessment of PROtective Factors.

Authors' contributions

HK contributed to scoring the SAPROF, drafting the manuscript, and statistical analyses. AK contributed to the predictive validation analyses. MK assessed the SAPROF for interrater reliability and investigated the occurrence of violence among participants to whom she did not administer the SAPROF. DS investigated the occurrence of violence. HK, AK, MK, DS, and NH all contributed to the design and management of the study. All authors read and approved the final manuscript.

Author details

[1] Department of Forensic Psychiatry, National Center Hospital of Neurology and Psychiatry, 4-1-1, Ogawahigashicho, Kodaira, Tokyo 187-8553, Japan.
[2] Department of Forensic Psychiatry, National Institute of Mental Health, National Center of Neurology and Psychiatry, Kodaira, Tokyo, Japan.

Acknowledgements

We thank all the participants and staff who were involved in the study. We are profoundly grateful to the authors of the original SAPROF for permitting us to develop a Japanese version of this instrument. We sincerely thank Kaoru Arai, Department of Psychiatry, Kagoshima University Graduate School of Medical and Dental Sciences, for sharing the dataset of the HCR-20 (version 2).

Competing interests

The authors declare that they have no competing interests.

Consent for publication

Informed consent was obtained in the form of opt-out on the website.

Funding

This study was supported by a Grant-in-Aid for Young Scientists (B) to HK from the Japan Society for the Promotion of Science (JSPS) (KAKENHI No. 16K19793).

References

1. Webster CD, Douglas KS, Eaves D, Hart SD. HCR-20. Assessing the risk of violence. Version 2. Burnaby: Mental Health, Law, and Policy Institute, Simon Fraser University; 1997.
2. de Vogel V, de Ruiter C, Bouman Y, de Vries Robbé M, de Handleiding bij, SAPROF. Structured assessment of protective factors for violence risk. Versie1. Utrecht: Forum Educatief; 2007 **(in Dutch)**.
3. de Vogel V, de Ruiter C, Bouman Y, de Vries Robbé. SAPROF. Guidelines for the assessment of protective factors for violence risk. English version. Utrecht: Forum Educatief; 2009.
4. Farrington DP. Key results from the first forty years of the Cambridge Study in delinquent development. In: Thornberry TP, Krohn MD, editors. Taking stock of delinquency: an overview of findings from contemporary longitudinal studies. New York: Kluwer/Plenum; 2003. p. 137–84.

5. Rogers R. The uncritical acceptance of risk assessment in forensic practice. Law Hum Behav. 2000;24:595–605.
6. Salekin RT, Lochman JE. Child and adolescent psychopathy. The search for protective factors. Crim Justice Behav. 2008;35:159–72.
7. DeMatteo D, Heilbrun K, Marczyk G. Psychopathy, risk of violence, and protective factors in a noninstitutionalized and noncriminal sample. Int J Forensic Ment Health. 2005;4:147–57.
8. Blum RW, Ireland M. Reducing risk, increasing protective factors: findings from the Caribbean Youth Health Survey. J Adolesc Health. 2004;35:493–500.
9. Resnick MD, Ireland M, Borowsky I. Youth violence perpetration: What protects? What predicts? Findings from the National Longitudinal Study of Adolescent Health. J Adolesc Health. 2004;35:424.
10. Ward T, Brown M. The good lives model and conceptual issues in offender rehabilitation. Psychol Crime Law. 2004;10:243–57.
11. Ward T, Mann RE, Gannon TA. The good lives model of offender rehabilitation: clinical implications. Aggress Viol Behav. 2007;12:87–107.
12. de Carvalho CCJ. Innovatie in risicotaxatie: Protectieve factoren voor het plegen van geweld in de toekomst. Amsterdam: University of Amsterdam; 2002 **(in Dutch)**.
13. de Vries Robbé M, de Vogel V, de Spa E. Protective factors for violence risk in forensic psychiatric patients: a retrospective validation study of the SAPROF. Int J Forensic Ment Health. 2011;10(3):178–86.
14. World Health Organization. The ICD-10 classification of mental and behavioural disorders. Geneva: World Health Organization; 1992.
15. Arai K, Takano A, Nagata T, Hirabayashi N. Predictive accuracy of the Historical-Clinical-Risk Management-20 for violence in forensic psychiatric wards in Japan. Crim Behav Ment Health. 2016. https://doi.org/10.1002/cbm.2007.
16. Hare RD. Manual for the psychopathy checklist-revised. 2nd ed. Toronto: Multi-Health Systems; 2003.
17. Speroni KG, Fitch T, Dawson E, Dugan L, Atherton M. Incidence and cost of nurse workplace violence perpetrated by hospital patients or patient visitors. J Emerg Nurs. 2014;40:218–28. https://doi.org/10.1016/j.jen.2013.05.014.
18. McGraw KO, Wong SP. Forming inferences about some intraclass correlation coefficients. Psychol Methods. 1996;1:46.
19. Fleiss JL. The design and analysis of clinical experiments. New York: Wiley; 1986.
20. Rice ME, Harris GT. Comparing effect sizes in follow-up studies: ROC area, Cohen's d, and r. Law. Hum Behav. 2005;29:615–20.
21. de Vries Robbé M, de Vogel V, Wever EC, Douglas KS, Nijman HLI. Risk and protective factors for inpatient aggression. Crim Justice Behav. 2016;43(10):1364–85.
22. Abidin Z, Davoren M, Naughton L, Gibbons O, Nulty A, Kennedy HG. Susceptibility (risk and protective) factors for in-patient violence and self-harm: prospective study of structured professional judgement instruments START and SAPROF, DUNDRUM-3 and DUNDRUM-4 in forensic mental health services. BMC Psychiatry. 2013;13:197. https://doi.org/10.1186/1471-244X-13-197.
23. Abbiati M, Azzola A, Palix J, Gasser J, Moulin V. Validity and predictive accuracy of the structured assessment of protective factors for violence risk in criminal forensic evaluations. A Swiss cross-validation retrospective study. Crim Justice Behav. 2017;44(4):493–510.
24. Singh JP, Fazel S, Gueorguieva R, Buchanan A. Rates of violence in patients classified as high risk by structured risk assessment instruments. Br J Psychiatry. 2014;204(3):180–7. https://doi.org/10.1192/bjp.bp.113.131938.
25. The Ministry of Justice. White paper on crime. 2016. http://hakusyo1.moj.go.jp/jp/63/nfm/mokuji.html. Accessed 22 Dec 2017.

18

Suicidal ideation and attempts among people with severe mental disorder, Addis Ababa, Ethiopia

Bereket Duko[1*] and Getinet Ayano[2]

Abstract

Background: People with severe mental disorders are associated with increased risk of suicide and suicide attempts compared to the general population. In low and middle-income countries, research concerning suicide attempts and completed suicide among people living with severe mental disorder is limited. The objective of this study was to assess suicide and attempts in people with severe mental disorder at Amanuel Mental Specialized Hospital, Addis Ababa, Ethiopia.

Methods: Institution-based cross-sectional study was conducted in August–September 2016. Patients with schizophrenia and bipolar disorder were selected using systematic random-sampling technique. The composite international diagnostic interview was used to assess suicide that was administered by psychiatry professionals. Substance use disorder was assessed through face-to-face interviews using structured clinical interview of DSM-IV.

Results: A total of 542 (272 schizophrenia + 270 bipolar disorder) patients were included in the study. One hundred nineteen (43.75%) of schizophrenic participants and 128 (47.1%) of bipolar participants have suicidal ideation. Fifty-six (20.7%) of schizophrenic participants and 58 (21.3%) of bipolar participants have suicidal attempt. Among the schizophrenic and bipolar patients who had suicidal ideation, 31.8 and 32.60% had co-morbid substance use disorder, respectively.

Conclusion: In this study, which was performed in Ethiopia, suicidal ideation and attempt were shown to be common problems in people with schizophrenia and bipolar disorder. Co-morbid substance use disorder was a more frequent phenomenon among patients with suicidal ideation and attempt. Attention should be given to screen and assess suicidal ideation and attempt in persons with schizophrenia and bipolar disorder.

Keywords: Suicidal ideation, Suicidal attempt, Schizophrenia, Bipolar disorder

Background

Suicide is a huge but largely preventable health problem causing almost half of all violent deaths and resulting in one million fatalities each year, as well as economic costs in billions of dollars. Estimates suggest that suicide could rise to 1.5 million by 2020. Globally, suicide represents 1.4% of the global burden of diseases [1]. Suicide is usually a cause of great distress to victim, family, friends, and community and largely to the nation [2, 3].

According to different studies among all suicides over 90% of are explained by mental disorders [4–9] mostly mood disorders, alcohol and substance use disorders [9–12].

A recent review of the literatures estimated that up to 50% of schizophrenic patients attempt suicide and up to 13% of all deaths due to suicide are attributable to

*Correspondence: berkole.dad@gmail.com
[1] Faculty of Health Sciences, College of Medicine and Health Sciences, Hawassa University, P. O. Box 1560 Hawassa, Ethiopia
Full list of author information is available at the end of the article

schizophrenia [13]. Compared to the general population (suicide prevalence about 1%), people with schizophrenia have a more than eightfold increased risk of suicide [14]. Suicide is the major cause of premature death among individuals with schizophrenia. Evidences indicated that up to 10% of patients with schizophrenia die by suicide [15–17]. Being young, male, and in the early years of the illness and having a history of multiple previous episodes or previous suicide attempts are the common risk factors for suicide in schizophrenia [18–21]. A substantial percentage of patients with schizophrenia also attempt suicide, with estimates of lifetime occurrence ranging from 18 to 55% [8].

Evidences indicated that persons with bipolar disorder are 30 times more likely to make a suicide attempt during their lifetime compared to those with no psychiatric disorder [22]. Close to one-third of persons with bipolar disorder attempt suicide [23, 24]. Researchers estimate that in the general population 29% of bipolar patients made at least one suicide attempt during their lives. In clinical samples, 25–56% of the patients with BD report at least one suicide attempt during their lives and 10–19% die by suicide [22–24]. A number of factors have been reported to be associated with the occurrence of suicide attempts in bipolar disorder and co-morbid substance use disorders (SUDs) [23, 25–27] is among those factors.

In persons with severe mental disorders co-morbid substance use disorders (SUD) are very common throughout the course of illness, with an estimated prevalence of 50–60% [28–31]. Nicotine and alcohol use disorders are particularly common among persons with severe mental disorders [8, 9]. Substance use disorder co-morbidity is eventually associated with worse outcome and higher suicidal risk [29, 30].

Evidences have shown that people with severe mental disorders (SMD) are at higher risk of suicide. However, in low- and middle-income countries (LMIC), including Ethiopia there is limited research concerning suicide attempts and suicide ideations in people with severe mental disorders (SMDs). The objective of this study was to assess suicide and suicide attempts in people with schizophrenia and bipolar disorder.

Methods

Study setting and population

Institution-based cross-sectional study was conducted in August 2016 at Amanuel Mental Specialized Hospital, Addis Ababa, Ethiopia. Amanuel Mental specialized hospital is the only hospital in Ethiopia giving services for mental health for long time. A total of 542 patients; 272 patients with the diagnosis of schizophrenia and 270 with bipolar disorder were included in the study. Study participants were included using systematic random-sampling technique.

Inclusion and exclusion criteria

All patients with established DSM-IV diagnoses of schizophrenia and bipolar disorder who had treatment follow-up assessment were included in this study. Suicidal gesture or attempt was defined as a self-inflicted act associated with intent to die or use of a method with potential for lethality.

Data collection instruments

Demographic variables were collected using semi-structured questionnaire. Data were collected by trained psychiatry professionals. The composite international diagnostic interview (CIDI) was administered by psychiatry professionals and used to assess suicide. Substance use disorder was assessed through face-to-face interviews using structured clinical interview of DSM-IV (SCID).

Data processing and analyses

The statistical program for social science (SPSS version 20) was used for data analyses. Socio-demographic (age, sex, marital status, areas of residence, religion, education) and clinical factors (diagnosis, history of alcohol, cannabis, nicotine and khat abuse or dependence) was analyzed and reported using words, tables and charts.

Results

Socio-economic and demographic characteristics

A total of 572 patients; 270 patients with the diagnosis of schizophrenia and 272 with bipolar disorder were included in the study. The mean age of the respondents was 32.62 ($\pm$SD = 9.43) and 33.71 ($\pm$SD = 9.35) years for bipolar and schizophrenic participants, respectively. Among the total participants (bipolar and schizophrenia), 107 (39.3%) and 105 (38.8%) of participants had completed secondary educational level, respectively. Regarding income, the average monthly family income was 1450 ($\pm$SD = 648.50) and 1463 ($\pm$SD = 647.93) Ethiopian birr with respect to bipolar and schizophrenic participants (Table 1).

Suicidal ideation and attempt in patients with severe mental disorders

One hundred nineteen (43.75%) of schizophrenic participants and 128 (47.1%) of bipolar patients had suicidal ideation. In addition to this, 56 (20.7%) of schizophrenic

Table 1 Sociodemographic characteristics of people with severe mental disorders (schizophrenia, $n=270$ and bipolar disorder, $n=272$) Amanuel Hospital, Addis Ababa, Ethiopia, August, 2016

Characteristics	Schizophrenia		Bipolar disorder	
	Frequency	%	Frequency	%
Sex				
Male	186	68.8	196	72.1
Female	84	31.1	76	28.9
Age in years				
20–27	105	38.8	101	37.2
28–38	96	35.6	98	36
39–53	69	25.6	73	26.8
Marital status				
Single	157	58.2	159	58.5
Married	73	27	79	29
Separated	14	5.2	14	5.1
Divorce	26	9.6	20	7.4
Place of residence				
Urban	186	68.9	182	66.9
Rural	84	31.1	90	33.1
Religion				
Orthodox	168	62.3	166	61
Muslim	73	27	81	29.8
Protestant	24	8.8	19	7
Catholic	5	1.9	6	2.2
Educational level				
No school	30	11.1	27	9.9
Primary	78	28.9	86	31.6
Secondary	105	38.9	105	38.6
Higher education	57	21.1	54	19.9
Occupation				
Government employee	23	8.5	28	10.2
Private employee	89	33	87	32
Merchant	56	20.6	57	21
Unemployed	23	8.5	22	8.1
Student	59	21.9	53	19.5
Others	20	7.5	25	9.2
Monthly income				
300–1000	106	39.2	107	39.3
1001–1900	92	34.2	91	33.5
1901–3000	72	26.6	74	27.2
Ethnicity				
Amhara	63	23.3	58	21.3
Tigray	40	14.8	38	14
Oromo	102	37.8	100	36.8
Gurage	55	20.4	64	23.5
Others	10	3.7	12	4.4

Table 2 Distribution of patients with severe mental disorders by suicidal ideation and attempt (schizophrenia, $n=270$ and bipolar disorder, $n=272$) Amanuel Mental Specialized Hospital, Addis Ababa, Ethiopia, August, 2016

Suicidal behavior	Schizophrenia		Bipolar disorder	
	Yes	No	Yes	No
Suicidal ideation	119 (43.75%)	151 (56.25%)	128 (47.1%)	144 (52.9%)
Suicidal attempt	56 (20.7%)	214 (79.3%)	58 (21.3%)	214 (78.7%)

participants and 58 (21.3%) of bipolar participants have suicidal attempt, respectively (Table 2).

Substance use disorders in patients with schizophrenia and bipolar disorders

Regarding khat, 137 (50.3%) of bipolar and 125 (36.6%) of schizophrenic patients had used in their life time. Concerning alcohol, 107 (39.1%) of bipolar and 99 (36.6%) schizophrenic patients had used in their life time. From schizophrenic patients, 130 (48.1%) and bipolar patients 86 (31.6%) had poly substance use disorder (Table 3).

Discussion

This study revealed that the magnitude of suicidal ideation and suicide attempts in patients with schizophrenia and bipolar disorder was comparable with study conducted in high-income country settings [13, 14, 22, 24]. In the current study, 119 (44.1%) of schizophrenic participants and 128 (47.1%) of bipolar participants have suicidal ideation and, 56 (20.58%) of schizophrenic participants and 58 (21.32%) of bipolar participants have suicidal attempt. This finding is in agreement with other studies [13, 22, 24].

In this study, both suicidal ideation and attempt were more commonly seen in people with bipolar disorder compared to those with schizophrenia. This finding is in agreement with other studies that reported significantly higher rates of suicide ideation and attempt among patients with bipolar disorder [13, 14, 22, 24].

Suicidal ideation and attempt are common among patients with schizophrenia and bipolar disorder as compared to evidences suicidal ideation and attempt in general population. These findings are in line with other studies that revealed significantly higher suicidal ideation and attempt in patients with severe mental disorder than general population [9, 11, 12, 14].

Our study revealed that patients with severe mental disorders are using different substances. This finding is in line with other studies [20] but higher than [31] and lower than [32, 33]. The possible reasons for this difference might be due to the difference in data collection

Table 3 Distribution of patients with Schizophrenia and Bipolar disorder by their substance use disorders (schizophrenia, *n* = 270 and bipolar disorder, *n* = 272) Amanuel Mental Specialized Hospital, Addis Ababa, Ethiopia, August, 2016

Substance use	Schizophrenia		Bipolar disorder	
Disorders	Current use disorder	Life time use (ever had used) disorder	Current use disorder	Life time use (ever had used) disorder
Alcohol use disorder	71 (27.3%)	99 (36.6%)	74 (28.4%)	107 (39.1%)
Khat/chat use disorder	123 (47.3%)	125 (46.3%)	130 (49.8%)	137 (50.3%)
Nicotine use disorder	34 (13.1%)	34 (13.1%)	33 (12.6%)	34 (13%)
Cannabis use disorder	4 (1.5%)	4 (1.5%)	4 (1.5%)	4 (1.5%)
Any substance use disorder	160 (61.5%)	165 (63.5%)	167 (64%)	172 (65.9%)
Poly substance use disorders	95 (36.5%)	130 (48.1%)	71 (27.2%)	86 (31.6%)

instrument, socio-demographics and culture. Unlike other studies [32–35], 132 (50.6%) (bipolar patients) and 125 (48.1%) (schizophrenic patients), had used khat in their life time. The possible reasons for this difference might be due to differences in socio-demographics and culture.

Conclusion

Suicidal ideation and attempt were more commonly seen in people with bipolar disorder compared to those with schizophrenia. Co-morbid substance use disorder was a more frequent phenomenon among patients with suicidal ideation and attempt than those without suicidal ideation and attempt was identified in the current study that majority of those who have history of suicidal ideation and attempt have co-occurring substance use disorders as compared to those who have no suicidal ideation and attempt. Co-morbid substance use disorders are common in person with suicidal ideation and attempt. As a result, this indicates the need for further screening and attention of co-morbidity in persons with suicide. Further studies concerning effects and specific relationships between suicide and co-morbid substance use disorders and exploring other factors are recommended.

Limitation of study

This study only assessed the descriptive part. It will be better to asses factors associated with suicidal ideation and attempt.

Authors' contributions

Both authors conceived the study and were involved in the study design, reviewed the article, analysis, report writing and drafted the manuscript. Both authors read and approved the final manuscript.

Author details

[1] Faculty of Health Sciences, College of Medicine and Health Sciences, Hawassa University, P. O. Box 1560 Hawassa, Ethiopia. [2] Research and Training Directorate, Amanuel Mental Specialized Hospital, Addis Ababa, Ethiopia.

Acknowledgements

The authors acknowledge Amanuel Mental Specialized Hospital, Ethiopia for funding the study. The authors appreciate the study participants for their cooperation in providing the necessary information.

Competing interests

The authors declare that they have no competing interests.

Consent for publication

Not applicable.

Funding

Amanuel Mental Specialized Hospital, Addis Ababa, Ethiopia partially funded the research work.

References

1. World Health Organization. Suicide huge but preventable public health problem. Geneva: WHO; 2004.
2. Gelden M, Gath D, Mayou R. Concise oxford text book of psychiatry. 9th ed. Oxford: Oxford University Press; 1993. p. 255–61.
3. Jacobsson L, Renberg ES. On suicide and suicide prevention as a public health issue. Med Arh. 1999;53(3):175–7.
4. Cavanagh JT, Carson AJ, Sharpe M, Lawrie SM. Psychological autopsy studies of suicide: a systematic review. Psychol Med. 2003;33(3):395–405.
5. Hawton K, Appleby L, Platt S, Foster T, Cooper J, Malmberg A, Simkin S. The psychological autopsy approach to studying suicide: a review of methodological issues. J Affect Disord. 1998;50(2–3):269–76.
6. APA. Practice guideline for the assessment and treatment of patients with suicidal behaviors. Am J Psychiatry. 2003;160(Supp. 11):1–6.
7. CDC. Web-based injury statistics query and reporting system (WISQARSTM). National center injury prevention and control: center for disease control; 2009.
8. Uwakwe R, Gureje O. The relationship of comorbidity of mental and substance use disorders with suicidal behaviors in the Nigerian survey of mental health and wellbeing. Soc Psychiatry Psychiatr Epidemiol. 2011;46(3):173–80.
9. WHO. Suicide prevention (SUPRE). Geneva: WHO; 2012.
10. Joe S, Stein DJ, Seedat S, Herman A, Williams DR. Prevalence and correlates of non-fatal suicidal behaviour among South Africans. Br J Psychiatry. 2008;192(4):310–1.
11. Cassidy F. Risk factors of attempted suicide in bipolar disorder. Suicide Life Threat Behav. 2011;41(1):6–11.
12. Posada-Villa J, Camacho JC, Valenzuela JI, Arguello A, Cendales JG, Fajardo R. Prevalence of suicide risk factors and suicide-related outcomes in the national mental health study, Colombia. Suicide Life Threat Behav. 2009;39(4):408–24.

13. Caldwell CB, Gottesman II. Schizophrenia—a high-risk factor for suicide: clues to risk reduction. Suicide Life Threat Behav. 1992;22:47–493.
14. Caldwell CB, Gottesman II. Schizophrenics kill themselves too: a review of risk factors for suicide. Schizophr Bull. 1990;16:571–89.
15. Miles CP. Conditions predisposing to suicide: a review. J Nerv Ment Dis. 1977;164:231–46.
16. Roy A. Suicide in schizophrenia. In: Roy A, editor. Suicide. Baltimore: Williams & Wilkins; 1986. p. 97–109.
17. Drake RE, Gates C, Whitaker A, Cotton PG. Suicide among schizophrenics: a review. Compr Psychiatry. 1985;26:90–100.
18. Johns CA, Stanley M, Stanley B. Suicide in schizophrenia. In: Mann JJ, Stanley M, editors. Psychobiology of suicidal behavior. New York: New York Academy of Sciences; 1986. p. 294–300.
19. Caldwell CB, Gottesman II. Schizophrenia—a high-risk factor for suicide: clues to risk reduction. Suicide Life Threat Behav. 1992;22:479–93.
20. Haas GL. Suicidal behavior in schizophrenia. In: Maris RW, Silverman NM, Canetto SS, editors. Review of suicidology, 1997. New York: Guilford Press; 1997. p. 202–36.
21. Chen YW, Dilsaver SC. Lifetime rates of suicide attempts among subjects with bipolar and unipolar disorders relative to subjects with other Axis I disorders. Biol Psychiatry. 1996;39:896–9.
22. Goodwin FK, Jamison KR. Maniac-depressive illness: bipolar disorders and recurrent depression. 2nd ed. New York: Oxford University Press; 2007.
23. Harris EC, Barraclough B. Suicide as an outcome for mental disorders: a meta-analysis. Br J Psychiatry. 1997;170:205–28.
24. Dunner DL, Gershon ES, Goodwin FK. Heritable factors in the severity of affective illness. Biol Psychiatry. 1976;11:31–42.
25. Endicott J, Nee J, Andeasen N, Clayton P, Keller M, Coryell W. Combine or keep separate? J Affect Disord. 1985;8(1):17–28.
26. Vieta E, Benabarre A, Colom F, Gasto C, Nieto E, Otero A, Vallejo J. Suicidal behavior in bipolar I and bipolar II disorder. J Nerv Ment Disord. 1997;185(6):407–9.
27. American Psychiatric Association. Diagnostic and statistical manual of mental disorders. 4th ed. Washington, D.C.: American Psychiatric Press; 1994.
28. Center for Substance Abuse Treatment. Substance abuse treatment for persons with co-occurring disorders. Treatment improvement protocol (TIP) Ser., No. 42. DHHS Publ. No. (SMA) 05-3992. Rockville: Substance Abuse and Mental Health Services Administration and Center for Mental Health Services; 2005.
29. Center for Substance Abuse Treatment. Definitions and terms relating to co-occurring disorders. COCE overview paper. DHHS Publ. No. (SMA) 07-4163. Rockville: Substance Abuse and Mental Health Services Administration and Center for Mental Health Services; 2007.
30. Center for Substance Abuse Treatment. The epidemiology of co-occurring substance use and mental disorders. COCE overview paper 8. DHHS Publ. No. (SMA) 07-4308. Rockville: Substance Abuse and Mental Health Services Administration and Center for Mental Health Services; 2007.
31. Ashton K, Streem D. Nicotine dependence: disease management project. Lyndhurst: Centre for Continuing Education. Cleveland Clinic; 2006.
32. Cassidy F, Ahearn EP, Carroll BJ. Substance abuse in bipolar disorder. Bipolar Disord. 2001;3:e120–88.
33. Tohen M, Greenfield SF, Weiss RD, Zarate CA Jr, Vagge LM. The effect of comorbid substance use disorders on the course of bipolar disorder: a review. Harv Rev Psychiatry. 1998;6:133–41.
34. Dalton EJ, Cate-Carter TD, Mundo E, Parikh SV, Kennedy JL. Suicide risk in bipolar patients: the role of co-morbid substance use disorders. Bipolar Disord. 2003;5:58–61.
35. Regier DA, Farmer ME, Rae DS, Locke BZ, Keith SJ, et al. Comorbidity of mental disorders with alcohol and other drug abuse. Results from the epidemiologic catchment area (ECA) study. JAMA. 1990;264:2511–8.

19

Exploring PTSD in emergency operators of a major University Hospital in Italy: a preliminary report on the role of gender, age, and education

Claudia Carmassi[1*], Camilla Gesi[1], Martina Corsi[1], Ivan M. Cremone[1], Carlo A. Bertelloni[1], Enrico Massimetti[1], Maria Cristina Olivieri[2], Ciro Conversano[1], Massimo Santini[2] and Liliana Dell'Osso[1]

Abstract

Background: Emergency services personnel face frequent exposure to potentially traumatic events, with the potential for chronic symptomatic distress. The DSM-5 recently recognized a particular risk for post-traumatic stress disorder (PTSD) among first responders (criterion A4) but data are still scarce on prevalence rates and correlates.

Objective: The aim of the present study was to explore the possible role of age, gender, and education training in a sample of emergency personnel diagnosed with DSM-5 PTSD.

Methods: The Trauma and Loss Spectrum-Self-Report (TALS-SR) and the Work and Social Adjustment Scale (WSAS) were administered to 42 between nurses and health care assistants, employed at the emergency room of a major University Hospital (Pisa) in Italy.

Results: 21.4% of the sample reported DSM-5 PTSD with significantly higher scores in the TALS-SR domain exploring the acute reaction to trauma and losses among health care assistants, older, and non-graduated subjects. A significant correlation between the number of the TALS-SR symptoms endorsed, corresponding to DSM-5 PTSD diagnostic criteria emerged in health care assistants.

Conclusions: Despite further studies are needed in larger samples, our data suggest a high risk for PTSD and post-traumatic stress spectrum symptoms in nurses and health care workers operating in an emergency department, particularly among health care assistants, women, older, and non-graduated operators.

Keywords: Post-traumatic stress disorder (PTSD), Emergency personnel, Nurses, Health care assistants, Work and social functioning/adjustment, Age, Gender, Education

Background

The DSM-5 encoded important changes for what concern post-traumatic stress conditions, particularly post-traumatic stress disorder (PTSD). Besides changes in the symptomatological diagnostic criteria, the actual edition of the manual better specified Criterion A about the trauma eliminating the need of person's response to the event involving *intense fear, helplessness, or horror* (criterion A2) and better clarifying the characteristics of the potentially traumatic experiences including, for the first time, *a repeated or extreme indirect exposure to aversive details of the event(s), usually in the course of professional duties (e.g., first responders, collecting body parts; professionals repeatedly exposed to details of child abuse)* (criterion A4).

Psychological distress in health care workers may vary across different specialties but increasing evidence highlights that staff operating in emergency planning, such

*Correspondence: ccarmassi@gmail.com
[1] Section of Psychiatry, Department of Clinical and Experimental Medicine, University of Pisa, Via Roma 67, 56100 Pisa, Italy
Full list of author information is available at the end of the article

as doctors, nurses, and paramedics, to be at high risk for PTSD [1]. Emergency departments, in fact, may be challenging because of frequent unpredictability of daily work cases, coping with the acute phase of most disorders, including traumatic incident exposure, frequently facing patients' and their families' expectations in unexpected and acute critical cases/situations. This induced researchers to investigate work-related psychological disorders, such as Burnout Syndrome, an occupational health concept of emotional and physical exhaustion, depersonalization and decreased personal accomplishment [2] and, most recently, PTSD [3, 4].

The prevalence of PTSD in the general population has been reported to be approximately 6.8% [5] with lower rates in Italy [6, 7], but studies on emergency services personnel have reported higher rates showing an increased risk in such populations. PTSD prevalence rates ranging between 10 and 17% have in fact been reported among emergency unit operators [4, 8–10], with even higher percentages (18–44%) being reported among nurses [3, 11]. In a study investigating the relationship between exposure to critical incidents and mental health problems among emergency medical care personnel, Ward et al. [12] found that symptoms of anxiety, depression, or PTSD intensified when exposure to critical incidents increased. However, the rate at which symptoms increased eventually slowed over time, suggesting that there may be a time-dependent desensitization to the effects of repeated work-related traumatic exposures [12]. Mealer et al. [3] investigated 332 University hospital nurses operating in the University of Colorado Hospital (USA), reporting a PTSD diagnosis in 18% of the sample, with 22% of it showing PTSD symptoms. An extensive systematic review of all empirical articles regarding emergency medical responders and conceptual literature on the constructs of interest in other related populations, reported exposure to traumatic events to be between 80 and 100%, and rates of PTSD higher than 20%. In this same review, a modification of the stress process model is suggested to explain the relationships among occupational stress exposure, PTSD, and high risk of alcohol and other drug use [13]. More recently, Fjeldheim et al. [14] reported 94% of 131 South African university paramedic trainees to have directly experienced trauma, with 16% meeting PTSD criteria and 7% chronic perceived stress, suggesting the need for efficient, ongoing screening of PTSD symptomatology in trauma-exposed high-risk groups. Emergency care workers trainees, in fact, have been suggested to be at an even higher risk of developing PTSD due to exposure to a novel environment, age, inexperience in the field, and the added pressure of academic evaluation [15]. Resilient coping strategies with mitigation of common maladaptive psychological symptoms may be in fact developed during the course of professional career as seen in some nurses [11].

Little data are yet available on DSM-5 PTSD rates among operators of the emergency units in Europe, particularly in Italy [16, 17]. Slight differences in PTSD symptomatological rates have been reported on subjects exposed to mass trauma and assessed according to either the DSM-IV or the DSM-5 PTSD criteria, suggesting the need for further investigation on the possible rates detected by means of the new criteria. The aim of the present study was to assess PTSD symptoms among nurses and health care working in the Emergency Unit of a major University Hospital in Italy.

Methods

Study design

A total sample of 42 subjects employed, at the time of enrollment, at the emergency room of the Azienda Ospedaliero-Universitaria Pisana (AOUP) was included in this study. According to the study protocol, the whole medical staff employed at the emergency room of the AOUP was asked to participate in the study with the only exception of the doctors. According to the Italian health care system, we thus included nurses and health care assistants. Medical doctors were excluded as, upon the organization of the services of the AOUP, they rotate between two different services, that are the emergency room and the emergency medicine, aim of the present study was to assess post-traumatic stress symptoms in the former department in order to have a more selected sample operating the first health care interventions.

The subjects were asked to fulfill the self-report instruments immediately before or after their work schedule.

The study was conducted in accordance to Helsinki Declaration and received the approval of the Ethics Committee of Area Vasta Nord Ovest Toscana.

Instruments and assessment

All subjects were assessed by means of the Trauma and Loss Spectrum-Self-Report (TALS-SR) [18, 19], for post-traumatic stress spectrum symptoms developed after exposure to trauma in the work place according to PTSD criterion A4 of the DSM-5 and the Work and Social Adjustment Scale (WSAS) [21] for work and social functioning.

The TALS-SR was developed by the authors, who comprise an international (Italian–American) collaboration research project named Spectrum Project (http://www.spectrum-project.org/), established to develop and test assessment instruments for assessment of the spectrum of clinical features associated with the current version of the DSM psychiatric disorders. In particular, the TALS-SR includes 116 items exploring the lifetime experience of a range of losses and/or traumatic events and lifetime symptoms, behaviors, and personal characteristics that might represent manifestations and/or risk factors for the development of a stress response syndrome. The instrument is organized into nine domains including loss events (I); grief reactions (II); potentially traumatic events (III); reactions to losses or upsetting events (IV); re-experiencing (V); avoidance and numbing (VI); maladaptive coping (VII); arousal (VIII); and personal characteristics/risk factors (IX). The responses to the items are coded in a dichotomous way (yes/no) and domain scores are obtained by counting the number of positive answers. In the Italian version, test–retest/inter-rater reliability was excellent, with infraclass correlation coefficient values exceeding .90 for each of the domains [18, 19].

The Work and Social Adjustment Scale is a test used to evaluate and measure the work and social adjustment. It includes five items that assess the individual's ability to perform the activities of everyday life and how these are affected, in the week prior to the assessment. The first item investigates the work ability of the subject. The second item assesses the ability to cope with household chores, such as cleaning the house, looking after the children and shopping. The third item assesses private recreational activities carried out by the patient, such as reading, going to cinema and museum. The fourth and fifth items investigate the family interaction and relationship: in particular, the fourth item investigates the social activities carried out exclusively with people who are not part of the family, and includes activities such as parties, tours of pleasure, go clubbing or show up to sentimental appointments. The fifth item analyzes only the relations with family members with whom the person lives, and if any problem of the subject under examination has interfered with this type of relationship. Each of the 5 item is rated on a nine-point scale ranging from 0 (not at all) to 8 (severe interference), so that the total scores are between 0 and 40 reliability [20].

In accordance with the aims of the study, all participants were asked to report symptoms related to work-related trauma exposure, referring to their work activity at the emergency room of the Azienda Ospedaliero-Universitaria Pisana (AOUP). Due to the sample characteristics, the criterion A was considered satisfied. According to previous studies [21–29], symptomatological PTSD prevalence rates according to either the DSM-IV-TR and the DSM-5 criteria were assessed by means of a matching between the TALS-SR and the DSM PTSD symptoms. In particular, in the present study a symptomatological DSM-5 diagnosis of PTSD was assessed by using the following matching between DSM-5 symptoms criteria and TALS-SR items, a scheme already used in 2014 to assess gender differences in PTSD scores on a sample of 512 survivors to the L'Aquila earthquake [23]:

> Criterion B ($B1=80$; $B2=77$; $B3=79$; $B4=78$; $B5=81$);
> Criterion C ($C1=86$; $C2=87$ and/or 88 and/or 89);
> Criterion D ($D1=90$; $D2=95$; $D3=85$; $D4=96$; $D5=91$; $D6=93$; $D7=92$); and
> Criterion E ($E1=108$; $E2=99$ and/or 100 and/or 102 and/or 103 and/or 104; $E3=106$; $E4=107$; $E5=105$; $E6=109$).

Statistical analysis

In order to compare the rates of PTSD in the groups examined, we adopted exact Fisher test. As considered variables are not normally distributed, we adopted non-parametric Mann–Whitney test to compare groups. In particular, the study protocol provided for a total sample of 120 subjects in order to ensure an 80% statistical power when comparing groups for the total WSAS scores, considering an effect of clinical relevance a difference of at least two points related to an expected standard deviation within groups equal to 5.

All the processing statistics were conducted using the Statistical Package for Social Science (SPSS Inc.), version 22.

Results

A total sample of 42 subjects was included in the study: 32 (76.2%) nurses and 10 (23.8%) health care assistants. Among the whole sample, 13 (31.0%) subjects of the total sample were males, 22 (52.4%) aged below 40 years old, 25 (59.5%) graduated (this included only younger nurses that according to new Italian laws require a University Degree).

With regard to the presence of PTSD, nine subjects (21.4%) met DSM-5 criteria for the diagnosis of the disorder with higher, despite not significantly, rates among health care assistants, females, older, and non-graduated subjects (see Table 1).

When comparing the TALS-SR symptomatological domain IV, that explores the acute reactions to losses or traumatic events, between subsamples, we found statistically significant higher scores in health care assistants, older, and non-graduated subjects (see Table 2).

Discussion

The low percentages of response to self-assessment questionnaires are largely attributable to the fact that the design of the study provided that the questionnaires were fulfilled immediately before or after operators work schedule and many subjects declined and complained.

Table 1 Prevalence of PTSD and comparison of WSAS total mean scores among study groups

	Total sample *n* (%)	PTSD		Total WSAS	
		Rates *n* (%)	(Fisher) *p*	Mean ± SD, (mean rank)	(Mann–Whitney) *p*
Occupation					
Nurses	32 (76.2)	6 (18.8)	.660	7.06 ± 6.94, (21.61)	.919
Health care assistants	10 (23.8)	3 (30.0)		8.10 ± 9.78, (21.15)	
Gender					
Males	13 (31.0)	2 (15.4)	.695	5.15 ± 7.42, (16.88)	.103
Females	29 (69.0)	7 (24.1)		8.28 ± 7.59, (23.57)	
Age					
≤ 40 years old	22 (52.4)	4 (18.2)	.714	6.91 ± 7.63, (20.70)	.658
> 40 years old	20 (47.6)	5 (25.0)		7.75 ± 7.72, (22.38)	
Education					
Graduated	25 (59.5)	5 (20.0)	1.00	6.80 ± 7.59, (20.30)	.440
Non-graduated	17 (40.5)	4 (23.5)		8.06 ± 7.75, (23.26)	
Total	42 (100)	9 (21.4)			

Table 2 TALS-SR domain IV (reactions to losses or upsetting events) scores comparisons between subgroups

Groups	Reaction to losses or traumatic upsetting events Mean ± SD	*p*
Occupation		
Nurses (*n* = 32)	4.50 ± 2.93	.028
Health care assistants (*n* = 10)	7.00 ± 3.33	
Age		
≤ 40 years old (*n* = 22)	4.09 ± 2.82	.030
> 40 years old (*n* = 20)	6.20 ± 3.24	
Education		
Non-graduated (*n* = 17)	6.65 ± 3.16	.007
Graduated (*n* = 25)	4.04 ± 2.78	

Nevertheless, the results of the present study corroborate increasing literature highlighting the fact that emergency services personnel face frequent exposure to potentially traumatic events with the potential for chronic symptomatic distress, such as PTSD and post-traumatic stress spectrum symptoms [14, 30–32].

According to previous literature [1, 3, 11, 16] we reported PTSD rates among health professionals operating in the emergency in Italy higher than those reported, despite with different methodological approaches, in the general population [6, 33]. The rates we found are in the range of prior works developed worldwide [3, 14, 34, 35], but appear to be in the higher range of prior works on nurses and health care workers operating in the emergency services across Europe, where PTSD prevalence rates ranging between 10 and 21% have been reported [8, 16, 34, 36]. Clohessy and Ehlers [8], in fact, exploring a sample of paramedics and emergency medical technicians in the UK, showed that 21% of enrolled subjects was affected by PTSD, diagnosed by both DSM-III and DSM-IV. Maia and Ribeiro [16], reported high exposure to events as evaluated as traumatic but low prevalence of PTSD (3.4%) among 59 between nurses and medical staff from the National Institute of Medical Emergency in the north of Portugal. Bennet and colleagues [36], exploring the psychological reactions in a sample of emergency ambulance personnel in a combination of rural and urban setting in the UK, found a 22% overall rate of PTSD. Further, Johnson and colleagues [34] showed a prevalence of post-traumatic stress disorder around 15% among Swedish ambulance personnel.

Our results also seem to be in line with the current literature which recognizes female gender as a risk factor for PTSD [37, 38]. However it is important to notice that studies exploring the possible confounding role of other risk factors for PTSD, including work-related training and education, reported gender difference may be lowered when a specific professional training has been performed, as reported among nurses [11], police officers, and fire workers [12, 39].

It is also noteworthy to underline as higher PTSD rates, as well as higher scores in all the symptomatological TALS-SR domains, were found among health care assistants with respect to nurses, as well as non-graduated with respect to graduated subjects. Some authors highlighted a possible relationship between education level and PTSD [13, 40]; accordingly, epidemiological data from the ESEMeD study in Italy reported significantly higher PTSD rates in subjects with lower instruction levels [6]. Despite conflicting results have been reported in the possible relationship between education level and PTSD [35, 39], the strongest evidence seem to suggest lower levels of education to render subjects at higher risk for PTSD. Health care assistants represent a professional category in Italy that perform basic care and administrative duties in a doctor's office, clinic or hospital, and their specific roles vary by health care specialty, but common duties include gathering patient information, checking vital signs, taking notes during a physician's visit. Upon Italian legislation, no bachelor's degree is required for this role. For what concern nurses, Italian legislation changed since 1994, when a specific bachelor's degree became a compulsory requirement to be hired by public and private health services. Thus, younger nurses all acquired a higher education level with respect to older ones. We may thus argue that our results suggest a preventive role of professional education on the risk to develop PTSD according to previous data [13, 16, 40]. In fact, Mealer and colleagues [11] highlight the possible development of resilient coping strategies among nurses during the course of their professional career. These considerations corroborate the importance of education and training as an important prevention factor in the developing of PTSD.

Our results show older subjects reporting higher rates of PTSD with respect to younger ones and we speculate that most likely older subjects reported the lower education levels, adding evidence to the previous findings. In addiction, some authors correlate the time spent in the same working place with an increased risk for PTSD and a more severe symptomatology [4, 41]. Specifically Berger and colleagues [4] reported higher incidence of PTSD in specific occupational groups of rescue workers including those with a longer job experience.

Interestingly, we reported statistically significant higher post-traumatic stress spectrum scores in the TALS-SR domain exploring symptoms of acute reaction to trauma. Prior studies documented the relationship between acute distress reaction and the risk of PTSD highlighting the fact PTSD represents the ideal candidate for secondary prevention programs [42, 43]. In this regards, Maia and Ribeiro [16] found peri-traumatic dissociation and distress symptoms to be the only predictor of PTSD symptoms among a group of health emergency operators.

The finding regarding the severity of impairment in work and social-related adjustment in the randomized groups strengthens the consideration that women with a lower educational level are more at risk to develop work trauma-related PTSD symptomatology.

Interpretation of our results should keep in mind some important limitations of the study. As already mentioned, the most important is related to the limited sample size and the lack of a control group of health worker not employed in the Emergency Department that could affect the methodological strength of our study and consequently the generalizability of our results; nevertheless, this is a pilot study with preliminary data on a topic ignored in Italy in the actual literature which shed light on the need to better explore post-traumatic stress symptomatology on emergency health workers. Second limitation is the use of a self-report instrument to detect PTSD symptoms and even the diagnosis. We opted for an accurate self-report since the only comparable international validated instrument for PTSD is the Clinician-Administered PTSD Scale (CAPS) which is a semi-structured interview and we dreaded for high percentages of drop out and risk of bias of untruthful answers as we were on the workplace of the subjects recruited. A further limitation of the study is the lack of information on the presence of Axis I psychiatric comorbidities that may have an impact on some of the variables explored, particularly the work and social functioning levels.

Conclusions

Despite the limitations mentioned above, this report suggests emergency health professionals, in particular older subjects and women, to be a category at high risk of post-traumatic stress spectrum. Further research is thus needed to advance scientific understanding on the real impact of trauma on this population in order to better clarify which are the categories at higher risk and develop specific education and training interventions for prevention programs.

Authors' contributions

CC, MCO, LD, and MS participated to the conception and design of the study. CC, CAB, MC, CG and LD participated to the interpretation of the data, the draft, and critical revision of this article. CG, CC, EM, and IMC participated to the critical revision of the manuscript. All authors agreed to be cited as co-authors, accepting the order of authorship, and approved the final version of manuscript and the manuscript submission to Annals of General Psychiatry. All authors read and approved the final manuscript.

Author details

[1] Section of Psychiatry, Department of Clinical and Experimental Medicine, University of Pisa, Via Roma 67, 56100 Pisa, Italy. [2] Emergency Medicine and Emergency Room Unit, AOUP, Pisa, Italy.

Acknowledgements

None.

Competing interests

The authors do not have an affiliation with or financial interest in any organization that might pose a competing interests.

Consent for publication

Not applicable.

Funding
None.

References

1. Papathanasiou IV, Damigos D, Mavreas V. Higher levels of psychiatric symptomatology reported by health professionals working in medical settings in Greece. Ann Gen Psychiatry. 2011;10(1):28.
2. Embriaco N, Papazian L, Kentish-Barnes N, Pochard F, Azoulay E. Burnout syndrome among critical care healthcare workers. Curr Opin Crit Care. 2007;13(5):482–8.
3. Mealer M, Burnham EL, Goode CJ, Rothbaum B, Moss M. The prevalence and impact of post traumatic stress disorder and burnout syndrome in nurses. Depress Anxiety. 2009;26(12):1118–26.
4. Berger W, Coutinho ES, Figueira I, Marques-Portella C, Luz MP, Neylan TC, Marmar CR, Mendlowicz MV. Rescuers at risk: a systematic review and meta-regression analysis of the worldwide current prevalence and correlates of PTSD in rescue workers. Soc Psychiatry Psychiatr Epidemiol. 2012;47(6):1001–11.
5. Kessler RC, Chiu WT, Demler O, Merikangas KR, Walters EE. Prevalence, severity, and comorbidity of 12-month DSM-IV disorders in the National Comorbidity Survey Replication. Arch Gen Psychiatry. 2005;62(6):617–27.
6. Carmassi C, Dell'Osso L, Manni C, Candini V, Dagani J, Iozzino L, Koenen KC, de Girolamo G. Frequency of trauma exposure and post-traumatic stress disorder in Italy: analysis from the World Mental Health Survey Initiative. J Psychiatr Res. 2014;59:77–84.
7. Helzer JE, Robins LN, McEvoy L. Post-traumatic stress disorder in the general population. Findings of the epidemiologic catchment area survey. N Engl J Med. 1987;317(26):1630–4.
8. Clohessy S, Ehlers A. PTSD symptoms, response to intrusive memories and coping in ambulance service workers. Br J Clin Psychol. 1999;38(Pt 3):251–65.
9. Grevin F. Posttraumatic stress disorder, ego defense mechanisms, and empathy among urban paramedics. Psychol Rep. 1996;79(2):483–95.
10. Hegg-Deloye S, Brassard P, Jauvin N, Prairie J, Larouche D, Poirier P, Tremblay A, Corbeil P. Current state of knowledge of post-traumatic stress, sleeping problems, obesity and cardiovascular disease in paramedics. Emerg Med J. 2014;31(3):242–7.
11. Mealer M, Conrad D, Evans J, Jooste K, Solyntjes J, Rothbaum B, Moss M. Feasibility and acceptability of a resilience training program for intensive care unit nurses. Am J Crit Care. 2014;23(6):e97–105.
12. Ward CL, Lombard CJ, Gwebushe N. Critical incident exposure in South African emergency services personnel: prevalence and associated mental health issues. Emerg Med J. 2006;23(3):226–31.
13. Donnelly E, Siebert D. Occupational risk factors in the emergency medical services. Prehosp Disaster Med. 2009;24(5):422–9.
14. Fjeldheim CB, Nothling J, Pretorius K, Basson M, Ganasen K, Heneke R, Cloete KJ, Seedat S. Trauma exposure, posttraumatic stress disorder and the effect of explanatory variables in paramedic trainees. BMC Emerg Med. 2014;14:11.
15. Lowery K, Stokes MA. Role of peer support and emotional expression on posttraumatic stress disorder in student paramedics. J Trauma Stress. 2005;18(2):171–9.
16. Maia AC, Ribeiro E. The psychological impact of motor vehicle accidents on emergency service workers. Eur J Emerg Med. 2010;17(5):296–301.
17. Jonsson A, Segesten K. Daily stress and concept of self in Swedish ambulance personnel. Prehosp Disaster Med. 2004;19(3):226–34.
18. Dell'Osso L, Carmassi C, Rucci P, Conversano C, Shear MK, Calugi S, Maser JD, Endicott J, Fagiolini A, Cassano GB. A multidimensional spectrum approach to post-traumatic stress disorder: comparison between the Structured Clinical Interview for Trauma and Loss Spectrum (SCI-TALS) and the Self-Report instrument (TALS-SR). Compr Psychiatry. 2009;50(5):485–90.
19. Dell'Osso L, Shear MK, Carmassi C, Rucci P, Maser JD, Frank E, Endicott J, Lorettu L, Altamura CA, Carpiniello B, et al. Validity and reliability of the Structured Clinical Interview for the Trauma and Loss Spectrum (SCI-TALS). Clin Pract Epidemiol Ment Health. 2008;4:2.
20. Mundt JC, Marks IM, Shear MK, Greist JH. The Work and Social Adjustment Scale: a simple measure of impairment in functioning. Br J Psychiatry 2002;180:461–64.
21. Carmassi C, Stratta P, Massimetti G, Bertelloni CA, Conversano C, Cremone IM, Miccoli M, Baggiani A, Rossi A, Dell'Osso L. New DSM-5 maladaptive symptoms in PTSD: gender differences and correlations with mood spectrum symptoms in a sample of high school students following survival of an earthquake. Ann Gen Psychiatry. 2014;13:28.
22. Carmassi C, Antonio Bertelloni C, Massimetti G, Miniati M, Stratta P, Rossi A, Dell'Osso L. Impact of DSM-5 PTSD and gender on impaired eating behaviors in 512 Italian earthquake survivors. Psychiatry Res. 2015;225(1–2):64–9.
23. Carmassi C, Akiskal HS, Bessonov D, Massimetti G, Calderani E, Stratta P, Rossi A, Dell'Osso L. Gender differences in DSM-5 versus DSM-IV-TR PTSD prevalence and criteria comparison among 512 survivors to the L'Aquila earthquake. J Affect Disord. 2014;160:55–61.
24. Dell'Osso L, Stratta P, Conversano C, Massimetti E, Akiskal KK, Akiskal HS, Rossi A, Carmassi C. Lifetime mania is related to post-traumatic stress symptoms in high school students exposed to the 2009 L'Aquila earthquake. Compr Psychiatry. 2014;55(2):357–62.
25. Carmassi C, Akiskal HS, Yong SS, Stratta P, Calderani E, Massimetti E, Akiskal KK, Rossi A, Dell'Osso L. Post-traumatic stress disorder in DSM-5: estimates of prevalence and criteria comparison versus DSM-IV-TR in a non-clinical sample of earthquake survivors. J Affect Disord. 2013;151(3):843–8.
26. Dell'Osso L, Carmassi C, Stratta P, Massimetti G, Akiskal KK, Akiskal HS, Maremmani I, Rossi A. Gender differences in the relationship between maladaptive behaviors and post-traumatic stress disorder. A study on 900 L'Aquila 2009 earthquake survivors. Front Psychiatry. 2009;2012(3):111.
27. Dell'Osso L, Carmassi C, Massimetti G, Stratta P, Riccardi I, Capanna C, Akiskal KK, Akiskal HS, Rossi A. Age, gender and epicenter proximity effects on post-traumatic stress symptoms in L'Aquila 2009 earthquake survivors. J Affect Disord. 2013;146(2):174–80.
28. Dell'Osso L, Carmassi C, Massimetti G, Conversano C, Daneluzzo E, Riccardi I, Stratta P, Rossi A. Impact of traumatic loss on post-traumatic spectrum symptoms in high school students after the L'Aquila 2009 earthquake in Italy. J Affect Disord. 2011;134(1–3):59–64.
29. Dell'Osso L, Carmassi C, Massimetti G, Daneluzzo E, Di Tommaso S, Rossi A. Full and partial PTSD among young adult survivors 10 months after the L'Aquila 2009 earthquake: gender differences. J Affect Disord. 2011;131(1–3):79–83.
30. Beaton R, Murphy S, Johnson C, Pike K, Corneil W. Coping responses and posttraumatic stress symptomatology in urban fire service personnel. J Trauma Stress. 1999;12(2):293–308.
31. Berger W, Figueira I, Maurat AM, Bucassio EP, Vieira I, Jardim SR, Coutinho ES, Mari JJ, Mendlowicz MV. Partial and full PTSD in Brazilian ambulance workers: prevalence and impact on health and on quality of life. J Trauma Stress. 2007;20(4):637–42.
32. Corneil W, Beaton R, Murphy S, Johnson C, Pike K. Exposure to traumatic incidents and prevalence of posttraumatic stress symptomatology in urban firefighters in two countries. J Occup Health Psychol. 1999;4(2):131–41.
33. de Girolamo G, Polidori G, Morosini P, Scarpino V, Reda V, Serra G, Mazzi F, Alonso J, Vilagut G, Visona G, et al. Prevalence of common mental disorders in Italy: results from the European Study of the Epidemiology of Mental Disorders (ESEMeD). Soc Psychiatry Psychiatr Epidemiol. 2006;41(11):853–61.
34. Jonsson A, Segesten K, Mattsson B. Post-traumatic stress among Swedish ambulance personnel. Emerg Med J. 2003;20(1):79–84.
35. Perrin MA, DiGrande L, Wheeler K, Thorpe L, Farfel M, Brackbill R. Differences in PTSD prevalence and associated risk factors among World Trade Center disaster rescue and recovery workers. Am J Psychiatry. 2007;164(9):1385–94.
36. Bennett P, Williams Y, Page N, Hood K, Woollard M. Levels of mental health problems among UK emergency ambulance workers. Emerg Med J. 2004;21(2):235–6.
37. Christiansen DM, Elklit A. Risk factors predict post-traumatic stress disorder differently in men and women. Ann Gen Psychiatry. 2008;7:24.
38. Ditlevsen DN, Elklit A. Gender, trauma type, and PTSD prevalence: a re-analysis of 18 nordic convenience samples. Ann Gen Psychiatry. 2012;11(1):26.

39. Pole N, Best SR, Weiss DS, Metzler T, Liberman AM, Fagan J, Marmar CR. Effects of gender and ethnicity on duty-related posttraumatic stress symptoms among urban police officers. J Nerv Ment Dis. 2001;189(7):442–8.
40. Engel CC, Litz B, Magruder KM, Harper E, Gore K, Stein N, Yeager D, Liu X, Coe TR. Delivery of self training and education for stressful situations (DESTRESS-PC): a randomized trial of nurse assisted online self-management for PTSD in primary care. Gen Hosp Psychiatry. 2015;37(4):323–8.
41. Wagner D, Heinrichs M, Ehlert U. Prevalence of symptoms of posttraumatic stress disorder in German professional firefighters. Am J Psychiatry. 1998;155(12):1727–32.
42. Zohar J, Juven-Wetzler A, Sonnino R, Cwikel-Hamzany S, Balaban E, Cohen H. New insights into secondary prevention in post-traumatic stress disorder. Dialogues Clin Neurosci. 2011;13(3):301–9.
43. Zohar J, Sonnino R, Juven-Wetzler A, Cohen H. Can posttraumatic stress disorder be prevented? CNS Spectr. 2009;14(1 Suppl 1):44–51.

Prevalence of postpartum depression and interventions utilized for its management

Reindolf Anokye[1*], Enoch Acheampong[1], Amy Budu-Ainooson[2], Edmund Isaac Obeng[3] and Adjei Gyimah Akwasi[1]

Abstract

Introduction: Postpartum depression is a mood disorder that affects approximately 10–15% of adult mothers yearly. This study sought to determine the prevalence of postpartum depression and interventions utilized for its management in a Health facility in Ghana.

Methods: A descriptive cross-sectional study design using a quantitative approach was used for the study. The study population included mothers and healthcare workers. Simple random sampling technique was used to select 257 mothers, while a convenience sampling technique was used to select 56 health workers for the study. A Patient Health Questionnaire was used to screen for depression and a structured questionnaire comprising closed-ended questions was used to collect primary data on the interventions for the management of postpartum depression. Data were analyzed using statistical software SPSS version 16.0.

Results: Postpartum depression was prevalent among 7% of all mothers selected. The severity ranged from minimal depression to severe depression. Psychosocial support proved to be the most effective intervention ($p = 0.001$) that has been used by the healthcare workers to reduce depressive symptoms.

Conclusion: Postpartum depression is prevalent among mothers although at a lower rate and psychosocial support has been the most effective intervention in its management. Postpartum depression may affect socialization behaviors in children and the mother, and it may lead to thoughts of failure leading to deeper depression. Frequent screening exercises for postpartum depression should be organized by authorities of the hospitals in conjunction with the Ministry of Health.

Keywords: Prevalence, Psychosocial and psychological intervention, Postpartum depression, Ghana

Introduction

Postpartum depression (PPD) is a mood disorder that affects approximately 10–15% of adult mothers yearly with depressive symptoms lasting more than 6 months among 25–50% of those affected [1]. Postpartum depression often occurs within a few months to a year after birth. However, some studies have reported the occurrence of postpartum depression 4 years after birth [2]. Causes of PPD may be physiological, situational, or multifactorial [3].

Major predisposing factors for developing PPD are social in nature usually stressful life events, childcare stress, and prenatal anxiety appears to have predictive value for PPD. In addition, a history of the previous episode of PPD [4], marital conflict, and single parenthood are also predictive [5]. It was believed for a long time that only women from western societies suffered from PPD and that postnatal mood disorders were defined by culture [6]. However, conditions with similar symptoms have also been identified in other countries [7]. Some studies have found the same prevalence of PPD in different societies [8]; however, European and Australian women appear to have lower levels of PPD than women in the United States of America (USA). Women from Asia and South Africa have been identified as being most at risk

*Correspondence: reindolfanokye@yahoo.com
[1] Centre for Disability and Rehabilitation Studies, Department of Community Health, Kwame Nkrumah University of Science and Technology, Kumasi, Ghana
Full list of author information is available at the end of the article

[9]. The symptoms are similar to symptoms of depression at other times of life, but in addition to low mood, sleep disturbance, change in appetite, diurnal variation in mood, poor concentration, and irritability, women with PPD also experience guilt about their inability to look after their new baby [10]. For most women, symptoms are transient and relatively mild known as postpartum blues; however, 10–15% of women experience a more disabling and persistent form of mood disturbance [11].

More recent evidence suggests that postpartum psychiatric illness is virtually indistinguishable from psychiatric disorders that occur at other times during a woman's life [12]. Interventions for PPD include pharmacologic interventions, supportive interpersonal and cognitive therapy, psychosocial support through support groups, and complementary therapies. Electroconvulsant therapy has proven effective for mothers with severe PPD [5]. In severe cases of postpartum depression, especially in mothers who are at risk of suicide, inpatient hospitalization may be required [13].

Psychosocial interventions such as support groups have been reported as effective [1, 13]. Beck [1] states that support group attendance can give mothers a sense of hope through the realization that they are not alone. Support groups for couples can teach coping strategies and offer encouragement. They also give couples an opportunity to express needs and fears in a nonjudgmental environment [3].

Interpersonal psychotherapy conceptualizes depression as having three components symptom formation, social functioning, and personal contributions. Emphasis is placed on interpersonal relationships relating to role changes that accompany parenthood rather than on the depression itself. Interpersonal psychotherapy can also be initiated during pregnancy for women who are considered at high risk [13]. Recent research has found that women receiving IPT were significantly more likely to have a reduction in symptoms and recover from PPD than women who did not receive IPT treatment [25].

A study from the United Kingdom found that three brief home-based visits using counseling techniques were effective at accelerating the recovery rate for women suffering from PPD [23].

Prevalence of PPD has been difficult to determine because of the difference in criteria for the time of onset used by the DSM-IV and that used by most epidemiological studies. Prevalence has also been difficult to establish because of underreporting by mothers themselves [2]. It has been estimated that only 20% of women who experience symptoms of PPD report those symptoms to their healthcare providers. Symptoms of PPD are often minimized by both mothers and care providers as normal, natural consequences of childbirth [13]. Evidence has been presented that mothers may also be reluctant to disclose their feelings of depression for fear of stigmatization and fear that their depressive symptoms might be determined as evidence of being a "bad mother". Cooper et al. [23] reported that "almost half of those independently identified as depressed were not detected as such by their health visitor.

Despite the growing recognition as a global childbirth-related problem, the importance of detecting and treating it has until recently been largely overlooked in practice and it seems that knowledge about this problem is not very high [14]. PPD is a serious social issue due to its consequences, including an increased risk of suicide and infanticide. PPD is often under-diagnosed and untreated; therefore, efforts are needed to improve perinatal mental healthcare [15].

This research was carried out to determine the Prevalence of postpartum depression and interventions utilized by healthcare workers for its management in a Health facility in Ghana.

Methods

The study was conducted at Komfo Anokye Teaching Hospital in Ghana. The selected hospital is a primary government-owned health facility having several units such as Maternity unit, Reproductive and family planning services, Medical unit, Surgical unit, Adolescent unit, Child Welfare clinic, Outpatient Department, Radiology unit, Accounts, Administration, Medical records, Security, Health insurance unit among others and offer psychiatric services to patients. In this study, a cross-sectional study design with a quantitative approach was used. In cross-sectional studies, investigators do not follow individuals over time. Instead, they look at the prevalence of disease and/or exposure at one moment in time [16]. These studies take a "snapshot" of the proportion of individuals in the population that are, for example, diseased and nondiseased at one point in time. Descriptive cross-sectional studies simply characterize the prevalence of a health outcome in a specified population [16]. This study design was deemed appropriate for this study. The study population included mothers who were within 12 months after delivery because postpartum depression usually affects women within 12 months after giving birth and health workers who were recruited for this study to provide information on the psychosocial and psychological interventions that has been used in the management of postpartum depression at the hospital. The study was conducted within a period of 2 months.

Simple random sampling technique was used to select the mothers. This method selected by chance or none zero mothers for the study and data was collected within a period of 1 month using 5 research assistants. In selecting the respondents for the study, random numbers from a prepared random number table was assigned to names of mothers who were present each day data was collected. The numbers were randomly picked and whichever name that was assigned to the selected numbers that were picked was selected to take part in the study. The Yamane formula for determining samples was used to determine the appropriate sample for the study. A 95% confidence level [The value of $(1-\alpha)$ in standard normal distribution z-table, which is 1.96 for 95%] and a Precision level/sampling error or margin of error of 0.05 or 5% which is the generally acceptable margin of error for social researches [17] were used to calculate for the sample using the equation;

$$n = \frac{N}{1+N(e)^2}$$

n represents the sample size to be determined; N represents the estimated total population size, and e represents the level of precision/sampling error or margin of error. The population of the mothers who had given birth and were within 12 months after delivery at Komfo Anokye Teaching Hospital was estimated to be 451 for the month data was collected.

Therefore;

$$N = 451$$

$$1+N(e)^2 = 1+451(.05)^2$$

$$n = \frac{451}{1+451(.05)^2}$$

$$n = 212$$

Assuming that 20% will not respond to the questionnaire due to the sensitive nature of the study, 45 (rounded from 42.4) were added to 212. and therefore the total sample size selected amounted to 257 mothers. A convenience sampling technique was also used to select 56 health workers for the study. They were recruited based on their availability and willingness to be part of the study. By the time the investigators completed data collection 56 health workers had availed themselves to be part of the study. The 56 health workers were recruited for this study to provide information on the psychosocial and psychological interventions that have been used in the management of postpartum depression at the hospital.

A Patient Health Questionnaire (PHQ-9) was used to screen for depression at the selected hospital. The PHQ-9 is a 9-question instrument given to patients in a primary care setting to screen for the presence and severity of depression. The PHQ-9 has been validated against in-depth mental health interviews [18, 19] and is reported to be specific (> 86% at scores of > 10) for identification of people with major depressive disorders (MDD) [18, 19].

A structured questionnaire with closed-ended questions was used. The questionnaire was deemed an appropriate instrument for data collection in this study to reap its advantages of cost efficiency, easy administration, and easy quantitative analysis. The questionnaire comprised of four (4) subsections which included questions on the demographic characteristics of respondents; interventions as well as the duration of intervention and influence of interventions on reduction of depressive symptomatology.

Data were analyzed using both descriptive and inferential statistical tools incorporated in statistical software SPSS version 16.0. To ensure validity and reliability of instruments, the questionnaire was pretested at the Animwaa Hospital, and conflicting issues were resolved before the final data collection (Fig. 1).

Results

Demographic characteristics of respondents

The mean age was 27 years while more than half (54%) were married and the majority were Akan's. Also, more than half (66%) of the respondents had completed JHS/SHS whiles majority (83%) were working in the informal sector as shown in Table 1.

Prevalence of postpartum depression

Figure 2 illustrates the prevalence of postpartum depression among 212 respondents. Out of this total number of respondents, the majority (93%) did not have any

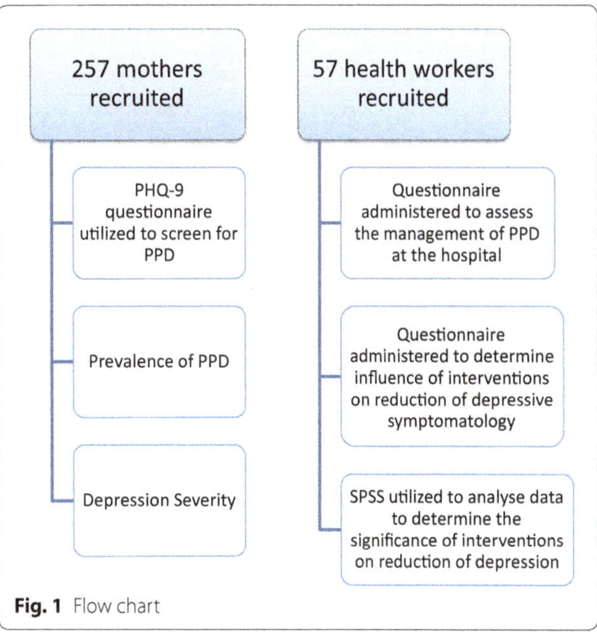

Fig. 1 Flow chart

Table 1 The demographic characteristics of respondents *Source* Field survey, 2017

Variables	Characteristics	Frequency ($N=313$)	Percentage (%)	
Age	18–21 years	48	15	
	22–30 years	69	22	
	31–40 years	79	25	
	41–50 years	69	22	Mean = 27.3
	51 years and above	48	15	SD = 8.31
Marital status	Married	115	37	
	Single	74	24	
	Widowed	43	14	
	Divorced	39	12	
	Separated	42	13	
Ethnicity	Akan	155	49	
	Ga/Adagme	56	18	
	Ewe	53	17	
	Gonja	49	16	
Education	No formal education	13	4	
	JHS/SHS	139	44	
	Certificate/diploma	124	40	
	Bachelors	35	11	
	Masters	2	1	
Occupation	Unemployed	22	7	
	Formal	60	19	
	Informal	175	56	
	Midwife	47	15	
	Psychologist	5	2	
	Psychiatrist	4	1	

indications of postpartum depression (PPD), while 7% had postpartum depression (PPD).

Depression severity

The severity of depression among respondents in the study was further examined and the outcomes are represented in Fig. 3 which shows that 39% out of the total number of respondents had minimal depression; 22% had moderate depression and mild depression, respectively; 6% had moderately severe depression with 11% of the respondents had severe depression.

Interventions utilized by healthcare workers for the management of postpartum depression

Figure 4 indicates the interventions used in the management of postpartum depression among respondents. The most common interventions used in the management of postpartum depression among respondents were psychosocial support (34%), professionally based postpartum home visits (28%), interpersonal psychotherapy (20%), and cognitive therapy (18%).

Duration of intervention

Table 2 shows the durations of interventions utilized by healthcare workers for the management of postpartum depression. From the table, it is observed that all the interventions were applied up to 6 months.

Influence of interventions on reduction of depressive symptomatology (positive outcome)

From Table 3, cognitive therapy ($p=0.14$), interpersonal psychotherapy ($p=0.356$), and professionally based

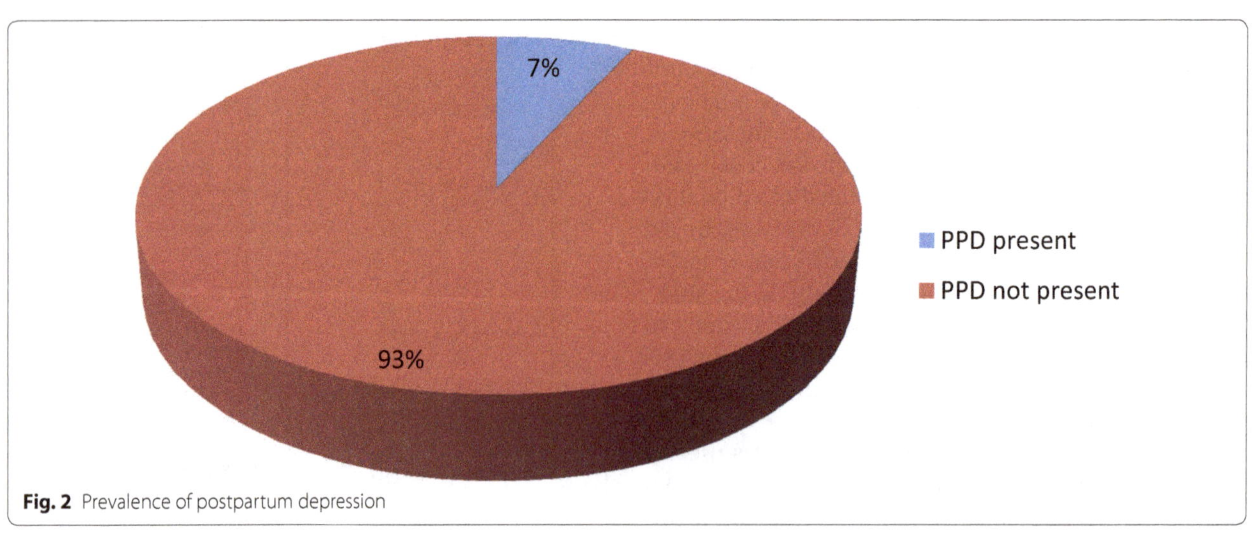

Fig. 2 Prevalence of postpartum depression

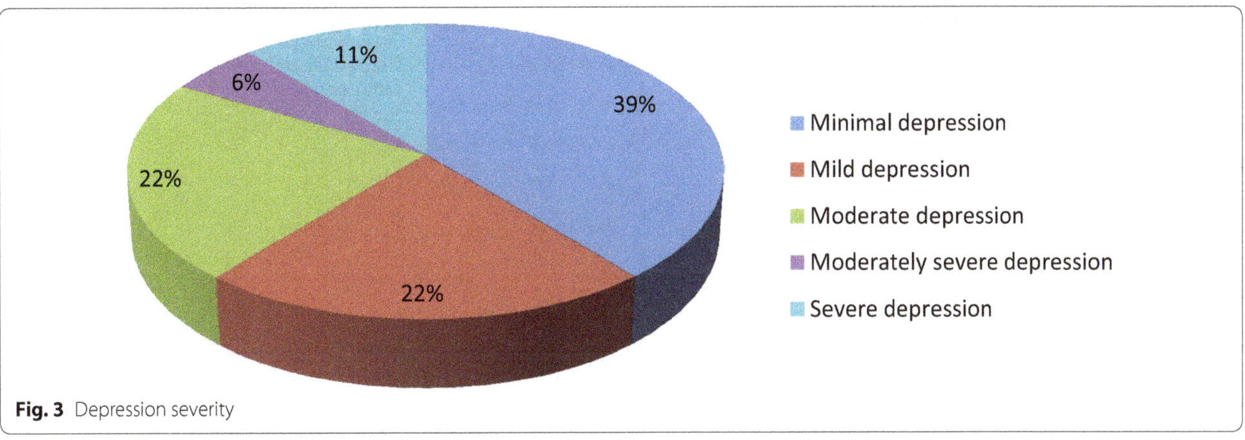

Fig. 3 Depression severity

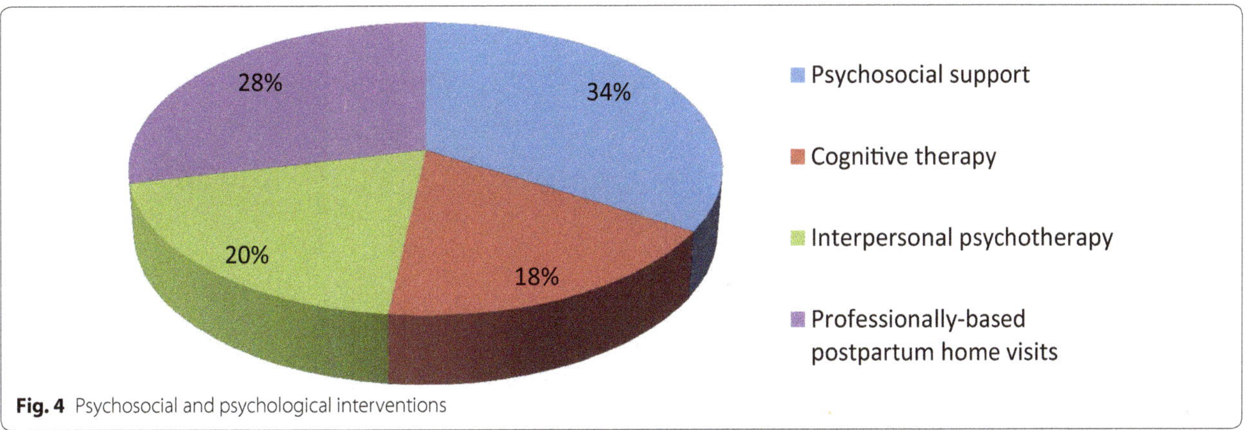

Fig. 4 Psychosocial and psychological interventions

Table 2 Durations of interventions *Source* field survey, 2017

Interventions ($n=53$)	Less than a month	1–3 months	4–6 months	SD
Psychosocial support	7	10	6	2.08
Cognitive therapy	3	6	3	1.73
Interpersonal psychotherapy	8	3	2	3.21
Professionally based postpartum home visits	1	3	1	1.15

postpartum home visits ($p=0.121$) had no significant impact on depressive symptomatology reduction, and only psychosocial support ($p=0.001$) was found to significantly impact on depressive symptomatology reduction.

Association between demographic characteristics and depressive symptoms

Table 4 summarizes the result of the univariate and multivariate analysis of the association between demographic characteristics and the presence of depressive symptoms. In both the univariate analysis and the multivariate analysis, ethnicity and occupation had an association with depressive symptoms. Respondents who were Gonja's were 8.46 times more likely to develop Depressive Symptoms than those in another ethnicity: adjusted Odds Ratio (AOR) = 8.46 [95% confidence interval (CI) 1.57–65.2]. Respondents who were employed were 4.7 times more likely to develop depressive symptoms: adjusted Odds Ratio (AOR) = 4.72 [95% confidence interval (CI) 1.021–14.01].

Discussion

Findings from this study showed a lower prevalence (7%) of postpartum depression among respondents compared to those found in similar African countries [20–22]. This may be attributed to the instruments used as the PHQ-9 instrument used for this study is different from the other instruments used in the other studies. Respondent's

Table 3 Influence of interventions on reduction of depressive symptomatology *Source* field survey, 2017

Interventions (*n* = 53)	Applied	Not applied	Depressive symptomatology reduction	*p* value*
Psychosocial support	23	28	7	0.001
Cognitive therapy	12	39	0	0.14
Interpersonal psychotherapy	13	38	0	0.356
Professionally based postpartum home visits	5	46	1	0.121

Table 4 Odds ratio with 95% confidence interval for the association between demographic characteristics and depressive symptoms

Variables	Depressive symptoms		Univariate		Multivariate*	
	Present (*n* = 18)	Not present (*n* = 239)	OR (95% CI)	*p* value	AOR (95% CI)	*p* value
Age						
< 40	10	109	1.10 (0.48–2.48)	0.797	0.85 (0.19–3.09)	0.698
> 40	8	130	1.00		1.00	
Marital status						
Married	7	135	1.02 (0.44–2.35)	0.838	1.62 (0.41–5.66)	0.529
Not married	11	104	1.00		1.00	
Ethnicity						
Akan	2	130	1.00		1.00	
Ga/Adagme	1	46	2.01	0.139	1.21 (0.28–6.27)	0.706
Ewe	1	16	1.00			
Gonja	4	47	12.5 (3.54–45.49)	< 0.001	8.46 (1.57–65.2)	0.014
Education						
No formal education	3	10	1.00		1.00	
JHS/SHS	6	109	0.89 (0.41–3.02)	0.797	1.29 (0.35–4.81)	0.122
Certificate/diploma	6	101	2.86 (1.13–20.28)	0.121	1.31 (0.04–2.19)	0.211
Bachelors	3	19	1.00		1.00	
Masters	0	0	1.00		1.00	
Occupation						
Employed	12	223	8.21 (3.12–20.18)	< 0.001	4.72 (1.021–14.01)	0.044
Unemployed	6	16	1.00		1.00	

OR odds ratio, *CI* confidence interval, *AOR* Adjusted Odds Ratio

* Mutually adjusted

depressive symptoms varied from being minimal, moderate, mild, moderately severe depression and severe depression. A similar finding was found in South Africa study where prevalence rates of various depressive symptoms were found [23]. The most common interventions used in the management of postpartum depression among respondents were psychosocial support, professionally based postpartum home visits, interpersonal psychotherapy, and cognitive therapy. However, among these interventions the one which had a significant influence on the reduction of depressive symptomatology (positive outcome) was the psychosocial support while the others had minimal influence. Psychosocial interventions are unstructured and nonmanualized and include nondirective counseling and peer support. Psychosocial interventions such as support groups have been reported as effective [1, 13]. The effectiveness of this intervention in the management of postpartum depression (PPD) has been established by Holden [24] in his study 50 women with PPD were randomized to 8 weekly nondirective counseling sessions with a health visitor or routine primary care and it was found that the rate of recovery from PPD for counseling was significantly greater (69%) than that of the control group (38%). From this study, interpersonal psychotherapy intervention and cognitive therapy did not significantly influence the reduction of depressive symptoms. This implies that interpersonal psychotherapy cannot be relied on as an intervention for PPD in the study area. However, the effectiveness of interpersonal psychotherapy in postpartum depression management was confirmed in several studies, including a large randomized trial with a control group [25]. O'Hara et al. randomized 120 women with postpartum depression to receive 12 weekly 60-min individual sessions of manualized interpersonal psychotherapy by a trained therapist versus control condition of a waitlist [25]. The women who received interpersonal psychotherapy had a significant decrease in their depressive symptomatology (measured by Hamilton Depression Rating Scale and Beck Depression Inventory) compared to the waitlist group, as well as significant improvement in social adjustment scores. In another study by Clark et al. [26], 35 women with postpartum depression were assigned to individual interpersonal psychotherapy (12 sessions) versus mother–infant group therapy versus a waitlist condition. Both interpersonal psychotherapy and mother–infant group therapy were associated with greater reduction in depressive symptoms compared to the waitlist conditions. Both studies support the effectiveness of interpersonal psychotherapy as a treatment for PPD, though there is not enough data to suggest a specific benefit to interpersonal psychotherapy compared with other therapeutic modalities. It could, therefore, serve as the first-line treatment, especially for breastfeeding mothers [27].

The study was limited by a smaller sample size, the use of one screening tool for depression among other tools. The study, therefore, missed out on the many other mothers who were not present at the hospital at the time of the study. Moreover, the study failed to determine the prevalence of PPD based on the tools used in other epidemiological studies. However, the Patient Health Questionnaire (PHQ-9) is a multipurpose instrument for screening, diagnosing, monitoring, and measuring the severity of depression. The PHQ-9 incorporates DSM-IV depression diagnostic criteria with other leading major depressive symptoms into a brief self-report tool. While there may be limitations inherent in the study design and methods used, these limitations by no means, compromise the results reported.

Conclusion

Prevalence of PPD has been difficult to determine because of several factors. The interventions for PPD include pharmacologic interventions, supportive interpersonal and cognitive therapy, psychosocial support through support groups, and complementary therapies. This study found that postpartum depression was prevalent among mothers who were within 12 months after delivery though at a lower rate. Some of the respondents had minimal depression, moderate depression, and mild depression, as well as moderately severe depression, and extremely severe depression. The major predisposing factors for developing PPD are stressful life events, childcare stress, and prenatal anxiety, as well as the history of the previous episode of PPD.

The most-common psychosocial and psychological interventions utilized in the management of postpartum depression were psychosocial support, professionally based postpartum home visits, interpersonal psychotherapy, and cognitive therapy. However, among these interventions, psychosocial support proved to be the most effective intervention as it was reported to have influenced the reduction of depressive symptoms.

Postpartum depression may affect socialization behavior in children and the mother, and it may lead to thoughts of failure leading to deeper depression.

Recommendations

Frequent screening exercises for postpartum depression should be organized by authorities of the Komfo Anokye Teaching Hospital in conjunction with the Ministry of Health, Ghana Health Service and Nongovernmental Organizations.

The Ministry of Health and Ghana Health Service should collaborate with the National Commission on Civic Education to embark on public education on the effective use of psychosocial support as an intervention for postpartum depression at the various health facilities in Ghana.

Abbreviations

KATH: Komfo Anokye Teaching Hospital; CBT: cognitive therapy; MDD: major depressive disorders; PHQ-9: Patient Health Questionnaire; ECN: early childhood nurses; PPD: postpartum depression.

Authors' contributions

The collection of data was done by the fifth and fourth authors (EIO and AGA). The secondary data compilation, data analysis, and interpretation were done by the first author (RA). The second and third authors (EA and AB) revised the manuscript thoroughly with their individual expertise. In the analysis of data, all authors played a significant part as well as in designing and preparing the manuscript. Proofreading and the final approval process was also shared accordingly among all authors, and all authors have agreed for its submission for publication. All authors read and approved the final manuscript.

Author details

[1] Centre for Disability and Rehabilitation Studies, Department of Community Health, Kwame Nkrumah University of Science and Technology, Kumasi, Ghana. [2] School of Public Health, Department of Health Education and Promotion, Kwame Nkrumah University of Science and Technology, Kumasi, Ghana. [3] Methodist University College, Accra, Ghana.

Acknowledgements
Our gratitude goes out to the management and staff of the Komfo Anokye Teaching Hospital, Kumasi as well as all mothers who participated in this study. Further thanks to all whose works on postpartum depression helped in putting this work together.

Competing interests
The authors declare that they have no competing interests.

Consent to publish
Not applicable.

Funding
No external funding was received for the purpose of this study. All cost related to this research was covered by the researchers themselves.

References
1. Beck CT, Records K, Rice M. Further development of the postpartum depression predictors inventory-revised. J Obstet Gynecol Neonatal Nurs. 2006;35(6):735–45.
2. Mauthner NS. Re-assessing the importance and role of the marital relationship in postnatal depression: Methodological and theoretical implications. Journal of Reprod Infant Psychol. 1998;16(2–3):157–75.
3. Fishel AH. Mental health disorders and substance abuse. Maternity & women's health care; 2004:960–82.
4. Leopold KA, Zoschnick LB. Women's primary health grand rounds at the University of Michigan: postpartum depression. Female Patient Total Health Care Women 1997;22:12–30.
5. Andrews-Fike C. A review of postpartum depression. Primary Care Companion J Clin Psychiatry. 1999;1(1):9.
6. Bina R. The impact of cultural factors on postpartum depression: a literature review. Health Care Women Int. 2008;29(6):568–92.
7. Cox JL, Holden JM, Sagovsky R. Detection of postnatal depression: development of the 10-item Edinburgh Postnatal Depression Scale. Br J Psychiatry. 1987;150(6):782–6.
8. Huang YC, Mathers N. Postnatal depression–biological or cultural? A comparative study of postnatal women in the UK and Taiwan. J Adv Nurs. 2001;33(3):279–87.
9. Affonso DD, De AK, Horowitz JA, Mayberry LJ. An international study exploring levels of postpartum depressive symptomatology. J Psychosom Res. 2000;49(3):207–16.
10. Keller MC, Nesse RM. The evolutionary significance of depressive symptoms: different adverse situations lead to different depressive symptom patterns. J Pers Soc Psychol. 2006;91(2):316.
11. Craske MG. Origins of phobias and anxiety disorders: why more women than men?. New York: Elsevier; 2003. p. 13.
12. Buist A, Bilszta J, Milgrom J, Barnett B, Hayes B, Austin MP. Health professional's knowledge and awareness of perinatal depression: results of a national survey. Women Birth. 2006;19(1):11–6.
13. Nonacs R, Cohen LS. Postpartum mood disorders: diagnosis and treatment guidelines. J Clin Psychiatry. 1998;59:34–40.
14. McCue Horwitz S, Briggs-Gowan MJ, Storfer-Isser A, Carter AS. Prevalence, correlates, and persistence of maternal depression. J Women's Health. 2007;16(5):678–91.
15. Drozdowicz LB, Bostwick JM. Psychiatric adverse effects of pediatric corticosteroid use. In: Mayo clinic Proceedings 2014 Jun 1, vol. 89, no 6. New York: Elsevier. p. 817–834.
16. Lorraine KA, Lopes B, Ricchetti-Masterson K, Yeatts KB. ERIC notebook. Chapel Hill: The University of North Carolina at Chapel Hill, Department of Epidemiology Courses: Epidemiology; 2013. p. 710.
17. Barlett JE, Kotrlik JW, Higgins CC. Organizational research: Determining appropriate sample size in survey research. Inf Technol Learn Perform J. 2001;19(1):43.
18. Gilbody S, Richards D, Brealey S, Hewitt C. Screening for depression in medical settings with the Patient Health Questionnaire (PHQ): a diagnostic meta-analysis. J Gen Intern Med. 2007;22(11):1596–602.
19. Kroenke K, Spitzer RL, Williams JB. The phq 9. J Gen Intern Med. 2001;16(9):606–13.
20. Chinawa JM, Odetunde OI, Ndu IK, Ezugwu EC, Aniwada EC, Chinawa AT, Ezenyirioha U. Postpartum depression among mothers as seen in hospitals in Enugu, South-East Nigeria: an undocumented issue. Pan Afr Med J. 2016;23(1):180.
21. Nakku JN, Nakasi G, Mirembe F. Postpartum major depression at six weeks in primary health care: prevalence and associated factors. Afr Health Sci. 2006;6(4):207–14.
22. Sawyer A, Ayers S, Smith H. Pre-and postnatal psychological wellbeing in Africa: a systematic review. J Affec Disord. 2010;123(1):17–29.
23. Cooper PJ, Tomlinson M, Swartz L, Woolgar M, Murray L, Molteno C. Postpartum depression and the mother-infant relationship in a South African peri-urban settlement. Br J Psychiatry. 1999;175(6):554–8.
24. Holden JM, Sagovsky R, Cox JL. Counselling in a general practice setting: controlled study of health visitor intervention in treatment of postnatal depression. BMJ. 1989;298(6668):223–6.
25. O'Hara MW, Stuart S, Gorman LL, Wenzel A. Efficacy of interpersonal psychotherapy for postpartum depression. Arch Gen Psychiatry. 2000;57(11):1039–45.
26. Clark R, Tluczek A, Wenzel A. Psychotherapy for postpartum depression: a preliminary report. Am J Orthopsychiatry. 2003;73(4):441.
27. O'Hara MW, Stuart S, Watson D, Dietz PM, Farr SL, D'Angelo D. Brief scales to detect postpartum depression and anxiety symptoms. J Women's Health. 2012;21(12):1237–43.

21

The frequency of *DRD2* rs1076560 and *OPRM1* rs1799971 in substance use disorder patients from the United Arab Emirates

Hiba Alblooshi[1,2], Gary Hulse[2,3], Wael Osman[4], Ahmed El Kashef[5], Mansour Shawky[5], Hamad Al Ghaferi[5], Habiba Al Safar[4,6] and Guan K. Tay[2,3,4,6*]

Abstract

Background: Dopaminergic and opioid systems are involved in mediating drug reward and reinforcement of various types of substances including psychoactive compounds. Genes of both systems have been candidate for investigation for associations with substance use disorder (SUD) in various populations. This study is the first study to determine the allele frequency and the genetic association of the *DRD2* rs1076560 SNP and *OPRM1* rs1799971 SNP variants in clinically diagnosed patients with SUD from the United Arab Emirates (UAE).

Methods: A cross-sectional case–control cohort that consisted of 512 male subjects was studied. Two hundred and fifty patients with SUD receiving treatment at the UAE National Rehabilitation Center were compared to 262 controls with no prior history of mental health and SUD. DNA from each subject was extracted and genotyped using the TaqMan® SNP genotyping assay.

Results: There were no significant associations observed for *DRD2* rs1076560 SNP, *OPRM1* rs1799971 SNP, and combined genotypes of both SNPs in the SUD group.

Conclusion: Further research is required with refinements to the criteria of the clinical phenotypes. Genetic studies have to be expanded to include other variants of the gene, the interaction with other genes, and possible epigenetic relationships.

Keywords: Substance use disorder, *DRD2* gene, *OPRM1* gene, rs1076560, rs1799971, UAE

Background

The dopaminergic and opioid systems are part of a network involved in rewarding response following the consumption of opioids and other psychoactive substances [1, 2]. The dopamine system has been central to theories in reward of substance use disorder (SUD) that has been debated for several decades [3]. The consumption of addictive substances stimulates the release of dopamine into nucleus accumbens (NAc) elevating the dopamine level to above basal levels [4]. There are different mechanisms of action and target molecules in the dopamine system for the variety of substances that are commonly consumed. This dopaminergic system comprises an array of dopamine receptors, transporters, and substance-metabolising enzymes. Members of the family of the dopamine receptor genes, *DRD1, DRD2, DRD3, DRD4,* and *DRD5,* have been widely studied as risk factors for SUD [2]. The dopamine D2 receptor is a part of G protein-coupled receptors (GPCRs) that is encoded by the *DRD2* gene. It is located on chromosome 11q23, spanning a region of 65.56 kilobases and comprises 8 exons separated by 7 introns. During the splicing process of the *DRD2* mRNA precursor, two alternative subtypes of the D2 receptors are formed: a 443 amino acid D2L or a 414 amino acid D2S form. The longer D2L form is more common [5]. This 29 amino acid difference between the two isoforms does not appear to affect the pharmacological

*Correspondence: guan.tay@ku.ac.ae
[4] Center of Biotechnology, Khalifa University of Science, Technology and Research, PO Box 127788, Abu Dhabi, United Arab Emirates
Full list of author information is available at the end of the article

properties of the dopamine D2 receptor. The D2L/S variation changes the localization of the third intracellular loop of the receptor that interacts with the G coupled protein; hence, it affects the intracellular signalling mechanism. The mechanisms of dopamine receptor signal transduction and regulation are not only mediated via G protein signalling, but also involve G protein independent signalling events [6].

Understanding the reward and the treatment responses highlight the necessity of reviewing the relation between the genetic variants of these dopaminergic genes and SUD [7]. Patriquin et al. [7] reviewed the correlation of dopaminergic genes to SUD. The genetic variants of *DRD2* have been a focus of intense research to determine their link to SUD. Two single-nucleotide polymorphisms (SNPs) of the *DRD2* loci; rs2283265 in intron 5 and rs1076560 in intron 6 have been reported to be associated with cocaine use [8]. A *DRD2* variant (rs1076560) has also been studied in various populations. Clark et al. [9] reported the association between rs1076560 and opioid use in African Americans (AA) ($p = 0.03$) and European Americans (EA) ($p = 0.02$). These findings introduced insights into the possible roles of these dopaminergic variants on SUD. However, the extent of genetic variations acting as a risk factor for SUD is still not understood.

The opioid receptor gene family has been extensively studied to identify if there are any associations with SUD. There three subtypes are μ, κ, and δ, encoded by the *OPRM1*, *OPRK1*, and *OPRD1* genes, respectively. The product of the *OPRM1* gene plays a role in facilitating the analgesia and euphoria effects of opioids. The G protein-coupled mu opioid receptor encoded by the *OPRM1* gene is a multiple trans-membrane protein that has a high affinity for endogenous and exogenous opioids [10]. The *OPRM1* gene consists of 9 exons which encode over 100 variants that produce between 19 and 39 splice forms of the protein [11]. The rs1799971 (A118G) site is an SNP that is located in exon 1 of the *OPRM1* gene. This variant encodes a missense change in *OPRM1* at position 40 resulting in a change from an asparagine to an aspartate (Asn40Asp) in the extracellular domain of the receptor. This substitution eliminates an *N*-glycosylation site in the extracellular domain, which affects endogenous opioid binding and receptor activity [12]. The role of the rs1799971 in SUD remains in dispute [13, 14]. The effect of the variants of rs1799971 on different classes of substance has been extensively studied in various populations [10, 11, 13, 15–20]. However, only two studies [21, 22] have looked into rs1799971 variants in the Arab population. Several studies have reported associations between A118G with different substances of use in patients from different ethnic groups [10, 11, 13, 15–20], with others not finding significant associations with SUD [23, 24].

This study is the first study to report on the allele frequency for the rs1076560 SNP of *DRD2* and the rs1799971 SNP of *OPRM1* in individuals with SUD from the United Arab Emirates (UAE). This case–control study investigated the genetic association between the *DRD2* rs1076560 SNP and *OPRM1* rs1799971 SNP and SUD in the UAE population. The allele frequencies of *DRD2* rs1076560 SNP in the UAE population were compared to other global populations. The allele frequencies of the *OPRM1* rs1799971 SNP in this UAE study were compared with SUD cohorts in other Arab populations.

Methods

Subject information

A total of 250 male nationals of the UAE were recruited from the National Rehabilitation Center (NRC) based on the nation's capital of Abu Dhabi. All participants were previously diagnosed with SUD based on the DSM-5 criteria. Saliva samples were collected from each patient who had agreed to participate in this study, using the DNA Oragene saliva kit (DNA Genotek, Ottawa, Ontario, Canada). In addition, 262 male nationals of the UAE with no prior history of SUD or mental illness were recruited as controls. These individuals were part of an ongoing population study towards the establishment of the Emirates Family Registry (EFR) [25]. The characteristics of the cohort are summarised in Alblooshi et al. [26] which includes socio-demographic data as well as the combination and types of substances that were used. The study was conducted in accordance with standards set by the World Medical Association of Helsinki [27]. Specifically, approval to study human subjects was obtained from the NRC in Abu Dhabi. In addition, reciprocal approval was obtained from the human ethic committee at the University of Western Australia (RA/4/1/6715).

Genotyping of single-nucleotide polymorphism (SNP)

Genomic DNA was isolated from the cells in human saliva samples using the laboratory protocol for manual extraction of DNA as recommended by Genoteck (Ottawa, Ontario, Canada). SNP genotyping was preformed using a TaqMan® SNP genotyping assay on the viiA™7 (Applied Biosystems Inc. (ABI); Foster City, CA, USA). For quality control (QC) purposes, 10% of samples that were studied were randomly selected. These QC samples were genotyped at least twice. There was 100% concordance between the genotypes recorded for replicates from the same individual. The Hardy–Weinberg equilibrium (HWE) was calculated for both the cases and controls. No significant deviation from HWE was observed.

Identification and inclusion criteria of relevant studies for comparison purposes

Life science journal articles containing information related to genotyping studies of the two SNPs of interest: *DRD2* rs1076560 and *OPRM1* rs1799971 were retrieved from a search of electronic publication databases. Specifically, articles in PubMed/MEDLINE (US National Library of Medicine), EMBASE (Elsevier B.V., Amsterdam, The Netherlands), and ISI Web of Science (Thomson Reuters, New York, NY, USA) that were published to 15 March 2017 were retrieved. The search process was set up to specifically identify case–control studies that examined associations between each SNP (*DRD2* rs1076560 and *OPRM1* rs1799971) with different types of SUD in different populations or ethnic groups. Data that were specifically extracted from these published studies for comparison included: (1) the number of cases and controls; (2) the ethnicity of the study population; (3) the genotyping method used; (4) allele and genotype frequency data; (5) information related to Hardy–Weinberg equilibrium; and (6) the significance of the levels of associations identified (p values and statistical tests).

Statistical analysis

Allele and genotype frequencies in the cases and controls from this study were calculated using the GenAlex package (Peakall and Smouse 2006, 2012) and association was determined using the STATA statistical software (College Station, TX, USA).

Results

The allele frequencies of the *DRD2* rs1076560 SNP in the patient and control groups were compared. The Minor Allele Frequency (MAF) for *DRD2* rs1076560 was the "A" allele, with a frequency of 11.80% in the substance use group compared with 13.20% in the controls. Correspondingly, the "C" allele was 88.20% in cases and 86.80% in controls (Table 1). The χ^2 allelic association between the *DRD2* rs1076560 SNP and substance use was not significant in the UAE population that was studied [$p=0.52$, odds ratio (OR) = 0.88].

The results of this UAE study were compared with published data that included association studies between the *DRD2* rs1076560 SNP and the use of different substances (e.g., alcohol, cocaine, opioids, and poly-substances) in a number of different populations (e.g., Caucasians, African Americans, Asians, and Jordanian Arabs) (Table 1). Six relevant publications matched the selection criteria described in the "Methods" section. All the studies identified were case versus control studies. Clark et al. [9] studied a relatively large population of EA and AA (999 EA cases versus 656 EA controls and 278 AA cases versus 750 AA controls) and showed that the *DRD2* rs1076560 SNP was significantly associated with opioid use in both

Table 1 Summary of the meta-analysis of the *DRD2* rs1076560 in association with SUD in different populations

Population	Substance	Phenotype	Number	Allele's frequency (%)		p	OR (95% CI)	References
				C	A			
Caucasians	Alcohol	Case	171	79.00	21.00	0.14	1.34 (0.90–1.98)	[30]
		Control	160	83.00	17.00			
African Americans	Opioid	Case	278	88.00	12.00	*0.03*	1.43 (1.04–1.97)	[9]
		Control	750	91.00	9.00			
European Americans		Case	999	83.00	17.00	*0.02*	1.27 (1.04–1.54)	
		Control	656	86.00	14.00			
African Americans	Cocaine	Case	45	94.00	6.00	0.53	0.66 (0.18–2.40)	[27]
		Control	31	92.00	8.00			
Caucasians		Case	74	76.00	24.00	*0.003*	2.74 (1.38–5.45)	
		Control	63	90.00	10.00			
Japanese	Alcohol	Case	297	59.90	40.10	*0.03*	1.30 (1.02–1.66)	[29]
		Control	425	66.00	34.00			
Jordanian Arabs	Poly-substance	Case	220	84.30	15.70	*0.03*	1.53 (0.90–2.68)	[30]
		Control	240	89.20	10.80			
UAE Cohort	Mixed[a]	Case	250	88.20	11.80	0.52**	0.88 (0.61–1.28)	This study
		Control	262	86.80	13.20			

CI confidence intervals, *OR* odds ratio

** p value of Armitage test using the status of mixed opioids ($n=250$) versus no addiction ($n=262$)

[a] Mixed: include single substance and poly-substance users

populations with p values of 0.02 and 0.03, respectively. The MAF of the *DRD2* rs1076560 SNP was higher in EA case group (17.0%) when compared to EA control group (14.0%) as well as in AA cases (12.0%) versus AA controls (9.0%) [9]. Moyer et al. [28] studied cocaine users in the same two ethnic groups (EA and AA) and showed that the *DRD2* rs1076560 SNP was associated with cocaine use in EA ($p=0.003$, OR = 2.74), but not in AA ($p=0.53$, OR = 0.66). A polish study of European alcohol users reported results that were not significant ($p=0.14$, OR = 1.34). In a study of Japanese patients, the risk allele "A" of the *DRD2* rs1076560 SNP was associated with alcohol use ($p=0.03$, OR = 1.30) [29]. To date, there has only been one other study of patients of Middle Eastern descent. Al-Eitan et al. [30] found the *DRD2* rs1076560 SNP to be associated with poly-substance use in a Jordanian Arab population ($p=0.03$, OR = 1.53).

The *OPRM1* rs1799971 SNP genotype frequencies studied in two case–control studies of SUD in populations of Arab descent are summarised in Table 2. In this study, the MAF "G allele" was 15.4% in cases and 18.9% in controls. Overall, the association of the *OPRM1* rs1799971 SNP was not significant in the UAE patients with SUD ($p=0.12$, OR = 0.78). In comparison with an Egyptian Arab population, no significant association was reported between the *OPRM1* rs1799971 SNP and Tramadol use ($p=0.54$, OR = 0.73) with MAF "G allele" of 5.2% in cases and 7.0% in controls. Simple combinations in both populations indicate significant association between the MAF "G allele" with SUD ($p=0.04$, OR = 0.73). This enhanced the odd ratio value with no heterogeneity observed. The combined data were adjusted using Cochran–Mantel–Haenszel test that was close to the UAE cohort.

The combined genotype frequencies for the *DRD2* rs1076560 SNP and *OPRM1* rs1799971 SNP are summarised in Table 3. There were no significant associations between the combined genotypes of both SNPs in cases ($p=0.88$) and controls ($p=0.23$). The combined genotype CC/AA was the highest in cases (55.6%) and controls (50.8%). This was followed by the combined genotype CC/AG with similar representation in cases (22.0%) and controls (22.9%). The combined genotype of the AC/GG was not observed in any individuals in the case group. Whereas, this combined genotype was observed in 1.2% of the control group. There were no cases or controls subjects with the combined genotype, AA/GG.

Discussion

In the UAE cohort represented in this study, there was no significant genetic association between the *DRD2* rs1076560 SNP ($p=0.52$) and SUD. The MAF of the *DRD2* rs1076560 SNP was higher in the controls (13.2%) when compared to the substance users (11.8%). This was similar to the observations made in an AA population studied by Moyer et al. [28], where the MAF in cocaine

Table 2 Distribution of the allele frequency of rs1799971 among Arab population

Cohort	Case					Control					p*	OR (95% CI)	p-hetero**
	AA	AG	GG	Sum	MAF (%)	AA	AG	GG	Sum	MAF (%)			
UAE	175	73	2	250	15.4	171	83	8	262	18.9	0.12	0.78 (0.56–1.08)	
Egypt-Arabs	69	8	0	77	5.2	43	7	0	50	7.0	0.54	0.73 (0.26–2.07)	
Simple combination	244	81	2	327	13.0	214	90	8	312	17.0	*0.04*	0.73 (0.51–0.99)	
M-H adjusted[a]												0.78 (0.57–1.06)	0.75

CI confidence intervals, *MAF* minor allele frequency, *OR* odds ratio

* p value of Cochran–Armitage test using allelic model

** p-hetero: p value of heterogeneity of Breslow–Day of homogeneity test

[a] Cochran–Mantel–Haenszel test (CMH) is a test used in the analysis of stratified or matched categorical data

Table 3 *DRD2* rs1075650 and *OPRM1* rs1799971 genotype combination among case–control of this cohort

SNPs	*OPRM1* rs1799971 Genotype							
	Case			p	Control			p
	AA	AG	GG		AA	AG	GG	
DRD2 rs1076560 genotype								
CC	55.60	22.00	0.80	0.88	50.76	22.90	1.91	0.23
AC	13.20	6.40	0.00		12.60	8.78	1.15	
AA	1.20	0.80	0.00		1.91	0.00	0.00	

users (6.0%) was lower than in the control group at 8.0%. In general, Moyer et al. [28] reported an association between the *DRD2* rs1076560 SNP and cocaine use, in EA but not the AA. The overall odds ratio of 1.94 in population ($n = 214$) was attributed to an artefact arising from the small sample size that was studied [9]. In a more recent study, Clark et al. [9] replicated the Moyer et al. [28] study by increasing sample size. The *DRD2* rs1076560 SNP was found to be associated with opioid use disorder in the two populations examined in this subsequent study (EA: $p = 0.02$, AA: $p = 0.03$), but not cocaine use (EA: $p = 0.23$, AA: $p = 0.19$). The MAF of the *DRD2* rs1076560 SNP, the "A allele", was found to be higher in the cases when compared to controls in both populations: EA at 17.0% versus 14.0%, respectively, and in AA at 12.0% versus 9.0%, respectively [9].

The different association outcomes between the studies may account for the differences in the substance of use or the pattern of use in the cohorts that were studied. Table 1 summarises the type of substances in each study, which included alcohol, opioid, cocaine, and poly-substance use. Stratifying these studies based on the type or pattern of substance used is important to identify more specific genetic risk variants [31]. Iacono et al. [32] suggested that specific substances influenced the nature of the genes that are involved in the pharmacodynamics and pharmacokinetics of that substance [31, 32]. However, it is a challenge to stratify patients according to substance of use, as often there is no single substance that is used by patients and there are overlaps between the substances are used. Clark et al. [9] investigated associations with a single substance. However, their study was plagued with difficulties related to overlap between different types of the used substances [9]. In addition, the differences in the genetic architecture between populations could dictate whether a variant is associated or not (Table 1). For example, the association between *DRD2* rs1076560 SNP and alcohol use was statistically significant ($p = 0.03$, $OR = 1.30$) in a Japanese population [29]. However, the same SNP was not statistically significant in the Polish patients with alcohol use disorder ($p = 0.14$, $OR = 1.30$) [33]. Even though the findings of Malecka et al. [33] were not significant, the MAF "A allele" in the group of alcohol users was higher in the cases (21.0%) than in the controls (17.0%). In contrast, the MAF "A allele" in this UAE study and the AA group in Moyer et al. [28] were opposite, where the MAF "A allele" was higher in controls than in cases (Table 1).

This study found no significant genetic association between the *OPRM1* rs1799971 SNP ($p = 0.12$) with SUD among patients from the UAE population. The association between the *OPRM1* rs1799971 SNP and various phenotypes of SUD has been studied and includes being a risk factor to different types of substances of use including tobacco consumption [34], alcohol use and sensitivity [13, 19, 34, 35], and opioid use [16, 36]. Other studies looked into inducing clinical symptoms or mediating responses to therapeutic treatment [11, 17, 37, 38]. The association between the *OPRM1* rs1799971 SNP and SUD failed to reach statistical significance in our study ($p = 0.12$) and in a previous study by Enabah et al. [22] ($p = 0.54$). In addition, the MAF of the *OPRM1* rs1799971 SNP or "G allele" in our study (case = 15.4%, control = 18.9%) was distributed in a similar pattern to Enabah et al. [22] (case = 5.2%, control = 7.0%), where the MAF "G allele" was lower in cases than in the controls. However, by combining the two cohorts, as shown in Table 3, the increase in numbers resulted in a significant association between the *OPRM1* rs1799971 SNP and substance use. This suggests that a larger population size in future studies is required. The *OPRM1* rs1799971 SNP association varies and appears to depend on the study population and the nature of the substance of use. For example, Chen et al. [35] examined the association between the *OPRM1* rs1799971 SNP and alcohol use disorder in two different populations (Asian and Caucasian) in a meta-analysis study. They reported an association with the *OPRM1* rs1799971 SNP in Asians ($p \leq 0.001$) but not in Caucasian ($p = 0.76$). Other studies have reported a lack of association with alcohol use [24] and with heroin and/or cocaine use [16, 23]. Since the *OPRM1* rs1799971 SNP has been widely studied in different populations, we focused on compiling data based on the Arab studies (Table 2). Another Arab study by Al-Eitan et al. [21] investigated the role of *OPRM1* variants including the rs1799971 SNP on the outcomes of therapeutic treatment for opioids. This association between *OPRM1* rs1799971 SNP and the possibility of an increased chance of relapse in patients undergoing Naltrexone treatment for opioid use disorder in Jordanian patients was not significant ($p = 0.55$). The variability of the findings from the range of studies conducted to date highlights some contribution by the *OPRM1* rs1799971 SNP. However, the variability in associations found to date requires further study to understand the contribution of this SNP.

This study is the first to examine if there is any association between combined genotypes of two genes (*DRD2* rs1076560 SNP and *OPRM1* rs1799971 SNP) and the susceptibility to SUD in patients of Arabian ancestry. There was no significant association found between the combined genotype frequencies of the two SNPs and disease in this case–control study (cases $p = 0.88$ and controls $p = 0.23$). Although some studies support the combined effect of variants of these two genes (*DRD2* and *OPRM1*), the exact mechanism remains elusive. This may suggest the involvement of other genetic variants within or in the vicinity of the *DRD2* and *OPRM1* genes. For example, Zhang et al. [10] examined 13 SNPs in the *OPRM1* gene using haplotype analysis in an association study involving substance use patients from two populations: European and Russian ancestries [10]. They reported the involvement of the intronic variants of *OPRM1* (rs511435, rs534731, rs3823010, rs2075572, and rs609148) in increasing risk to SUD. Some of these SNPs were located in linkage disequilibrium (LD) with *OPRM1* rs1799971 SNP and others have been postulated to be involved in transcription regulation or alternative gene splicing. The findings in Zhang et al. [10] highlighted the limitation of selecting a single SNP of a candidate gene to examine the genetic association with SUD.

Interaction between the *DRD2* and *OPRM1* genes with other genes has been examined across different substances of use. For instance, Lechner et al. [39] examined the combined effect of the *OPRM1* rs1799971 SNP and the *DRD4* exon 3 VNTR variants on cigarette craving after alcohol consumption. The study reported that the presence of the G allele is associated with an increase in cigarette craving after alcohol consumption. However, no significant association between to the exon 3 VNTR variants of the *DRD4* were found with the condition [39]. In addition, Sullivan et al. [40] reported a gene–gene interaction between the dopamine receptors gene (*DRD2*) and the dopamine transporter gene (*DAT*) in cocaine users. The interaction between the regulatory variant of *DRD2* (rs2283265) and dopamine transporters gene altered *DAT* protein activity, supporting the possibility that variants being a risk factors for cocaine use [40].

Conclusion

This study provides insights into two major genes that are thought to be risk factors of substance use. Specifically, the *DRD2* rs1076560 SNP and the *OPRM1* rs1799971 SNP were studied in substance use patients from the UAE population. No significant association between the *DRD2* rs1076560 SNP, the *OPRM1* rs1799971 SNP, and the combined genotype of the two SNPs and SUD was identified in this cohort. Nevertheless, future studies must consider stratification of the disease phenotype to assess possible association with *DRD2* and *OPRM1*. In addition, the findings of this study might suggest the involvement of other variants or genes in the mechanism of the disorder. Haplotype analyses for *DRD2* and *OPRM1* variants can be considered in future studies to evaluate the interaction of variants on each gene. Alternatively, genome-wide association study (GWAS) could be more objective strategy, since it does not rely on any previous conclusions from other populations.

Abbreviations

SUD: substance use disorder; UAE: United Arab Emirates; NRC: National Rehabilitation Center; EFR: Emirates Family Registry; DSM-5: Diagnostic and Statistical Manual_5; SNP: single nucleotide polymorphism; QC: quality control; HWE: Hardy Weinberg equilibrium; AA: African American; EA: European American; VNTR: variable number of tandem repeats.

Authors' contributions

HA contributed to the design of the study, processing the samples, analysing the data, and preparing the manuscript. The NRC team, comprising of AEK, MS, and HAG, was involved in recruiting patients and accessing data for patients. WO provided further assistance with statistical analysis. GH, HAS, and GT are supervisors of HA, who is a doctoral student at the University of Western Australia. They contributed on all elements of the study. All authors read and approved the final manuscript.

Author details

[1] School of Human Sciences, The University of Western Australia, Crawley, WA, Australia. [2] School of Psychiatry and Clinical Neurosciences, The University of Western Australia, Crawley, WA, Australia. [3] School of Medical and Health Sciences, Edith Cowan University, Perth, WA, Australia. [4] Center of Biotechnology, Khalifa University of Science, Technology and Research, PO Box 1227788, Abu Dhabi, United Arab Emirates. [5] United Arab Emirates National Rehabilitation Center, Abu Dhabi, United Arab Emirates. [6] Faculty of Biomedical Engineering, Khalifa University of Science, Technology and Research, Abu Dhabi, United Arab Emirates.

Acknowledgements

We acknowledge the support of staff at Center of Biotechnology at Khalifa University of Science and Technology in Abu Dhabi, UAE. We also thank the nursing and clinical staff of the UAE National Rehabilitation Center (NRC) in Abu Dhabi for their assistance in recruiting substance use patients to this study. Miss Alblooshi would like to acknowledge scholarship support from UAE Higher Ministry of Education and Scientific Research that funded her candidature as a Ph.D. student at the University of Western Australia.

Competing interests

The authors declare that they have no competing interests.

Consent for publication

All participants provided their consent for their de-identified data to be published.

Funding

This research was funded by the UAE National Rehabilitation Center (NRC), Abu Dhabi, UAE.

References

1. Contet C, Kieffer BL, Befort K. Mu opioid receptor: a gateway to drug addiction. Curr Opin Neurobiol. 2004;14(3):370–8.
2. Gorwood P, Le Strat Y, Ramoz N, Dubertret C, Moalic JM, Simonneau M. Genetics of dopamine receptors and drug addiction. Hum Genet. 2012;131(6):803–22.
3. Nutt DJ, Lingford-Hughes A, Erritzoe D, Stokes PRA. The dopamine theory of addiction: 40 years of highs and lows. Nat Rev Neurosci. 2015;16(5):305–12.
4. Volkow ND, Wang GJ, Fowler JS, Tomasi D, Telang F. Addiction: beyond dopamine reward circuitry. Proc Natl Acad Sci USA. 2011;108(37):15037–42.
5. Vallone D, Picetti R, Borrelli E. Structure and function of dopamine receptors. Neurosci Biobehav Rev. 2000;24(1):125–32.
6. Beaulieu JM, Gainetdinov RR. The physiology, signaling, and pharmacology of dopamine receptors. Pharmacol Rev. 2011;63(1):182–217.

7. Patriquin MA, Bauer IE, Soares JC, Graham DP, Nielsen DA. Addiction pharmacogenetics: a systematic review of the genetic variation of the dopaminergic system. Psychiatr Genet. 2015;25(5):181–93.
8. Zhang Y, Bertolino A, Fazio L, Blasi G, Rampino A, Romano R, et al. Polymorphisms in human dopamine D2 receptor gene affect gene expression, splicing, and neuronal activity during working memory. Proc Natl Acad Sci USA. 2007;104(51):20552–7.
9. Clarke T-K, Weiss TN, Weiss T, Ferarro K, Kampman C, Dackis H, et al. The dopamine receptor D2 (DRD2) SNP rs1076560 is associated with opioid addiction. Ann Hum Genet. 2014;78(1):33–9.
10. Zhang H, Luo X, Kranzler HR, Lappalainen J, Yang B-Z, Krupitsky E, et al. Association between two μ-opioid receptor gene (OPRM1) haplotype blocks and drug or alcohol dependence. Hum Mol Genet. 2006;15(6):807–19.
11. Manini AF, Jacobs MM, Vlahov D, Hurd YL. Opioid receptor polymorphism A118G associated with clinical severity in a drug overdose population. J Med Toxicol. 2013;9(2):148–54.
12. Oertel BG, Kettner M, Scholich K, Renne C, Roskam B, Geisslinger G, et al. A common human micro-opioid receptor genetic variant diminishes the receptor signaling efficacy in brain regions processing the sensory information of pain. J Biol Chem. 2009;284(10):6530–5.
13. Koller G, Zill P, Rujescu D, Ridinger M, Pogarell O, Fehr C, et al. Possible association between OPRM1 genetic variance at the 118 locus and alcohol dependence in a large treatment sample: relationship to alcohol dependence symptoms. Alcohol Clin Exp Res. 2012;36(7):1230–6.
14. Levran O, Awolesi O, Linzy S, Adelson M, Kreek MJ. Haplotype block structure of the genomic region of the mu opioid receptor gene. J Hum Genet. 2011;56(2):147–55.
15. Arias A, Feinn R, Kranzler HR. Association of an Asn40Asp (A118G) polymorphism in the μ-opioid receptor gene with substance dependence: a meta-analysis. Drug Alcohol Depend. 2006;83(3):262–8.
16. Clarke T-K, Crist RC, Kampman KM, Dackis CA, Pettinati HM, O'Brien CP, et al. Low frequency genetic variants in the μ-opioid receptor (OPRM1) affect risk for addiction to heroin and cocaine. Neurosci Lett. 2013;542:71–5.
17. Dlugos AM, Hamidovic A, Hodgkinson C, Shen PH, Goldman D, Palmer AA, et al. OPRM1 gene variants modulate amphetamine-induced euphoria in humans. Genes Brain Behav. 2011;10(2):199–209.
18. Gelernter J, Gueorguieva R, Kranzler HR, Zhang H, Cramer J, Rosenheck R, et al. Opioid receptor gene (OPRM1, OPRK1, and OPRD1) variants and response to naltrexone treatment for alcohol dependence: results from the VA cooperative study. Alcohol Clin Exp Res. 2007;31(4):555–63.
19. Hendershot CS, Claus ED, Ramchandani VA. Associations of OPRM1 A118G and alcohol sensitivity with intravenous alcohol self-administration in young adults. Addict Biol. 2016;21:125–35.
20. Miranda R, Ray L, Justus A, Meyerson LA, Knopik VS, McGeary J, et al. Initial evidence of an association between OPRM1 and adolescent alcohol misuse. Alcohol Clin Exp Res. 2010;34(1):112–22.
21. Al-Eitan LN, Jaradat SA, Su SY, Tay GK, Hulse GK. Mu opioid receptor (OPRM1) as a predictor of treatment outcome in opiate-dependent individuals of Arab descent. Pharmacogenomics Pers Med. 2012;5:99–111.
22. Enabah D, El Baz H, Moselhy H. Higher frequency of C.3435 of the ABCB1 gene in patients with tramadol dependence disorder. Am J Drug Alcohol Abuse. 2014;40(4):317–20.
23. Nikolov MA, Beltcheva O, Galabova A, Ljubenova A, Jankova E, Gergov G, et al. No evidence of association between 118A>G OPRM1 polymorphism and heroin dependence in a large Bulgarian case–control sample. Drug Alcohol Depend. 2011;117(1):62–5.
24. Rouvinen-Lagerström N, Lahti J, Alho H, Kovanen L, Aalto M, Partonen T, et al. μ-Opioid receptor gene (OPRM1) polymorphism A118G: lack of association in Finnish populations with alcohol dependence or alcohol consumption. Alcohol Alcohol. 2013;48:519–25.
25. Alsafar H, Jama-Alol K, Hassoun AK, Tay G. The prevalence of type 2 diabetes mellitus in the United Arab Emirates: justification for the establishment of the Emirates Family Registry. Int J Diab Dev Ctries. 2012;32(1):25–32.
26. Alblooshi H, Hulse GK, El Kashef A, Al Hashmi H, Shawky M, Al Ghaferi H, et al. The pattern of substance use disorder in the United Arab Emirates in 2015: results of a National Rehabilitation Centre cohort study. Subst Abuse Treat Prev Policy. 2016;11(1):19.
27. World medical association declaration of helsinki. Recommendations guiding physicians in biomedical research involving human subjects. JAMA. 1997;277(11):925–6.
28. Moyer RA, Wang D, Papp AC, Smith RM, Duque L, Mash DC, et al. Intronic polymorphisms affecting alternative splicing of human dopamine D2 receptor are associated with cocaine abuse. Neuropsychopharmacology. 2011;36(4):753–62.
29. Sasabe T, Furukawa A, Matsusita S, Higuchi S, Ishiura S. Association analysis of the dopamine receptor D2 (DRD2) SNP rs1076560 in alcoholic patients. Neurosci Lett. 2007;412(2):139–42.
30. Al-Eitan LN, Jaradat SA, Hulse GK, Tay GK. Custom genotyping for substance addiction susceptibility genes in Jordanians of Arab descent. BMC Res Notes. 2012;5:497.
31. Gizer IR, Ehlers CL. Genome-wide association studies of substance use: considerations regarding populations and phenotypes. Biol Psychiat. 2015;77(5):423–4.
32. Iacono WG, Malone SM, McGue M. Behavioral disinhibition and the development of early-onset addiction: common and specific influences. Annu Rev Clin Psychol. 2008;4:325–48.
33. Malecka I, Jasiewicz A, Suchanecka A, Samochowiec J, Grzywacz A. Association and family studies of DRD2 gene polymorphisms in alcohol dependence syndrome. Postepy higieny i medycyny doswiadczalnej. 2014;68:1257–63.
34. Francés F, Portolés O, Castelló A, Costa JA, Verdú F. Association between opioid receptor mu 1 (OPRM1) gene polymorphisms and tobacco and alcohol consumption in a Spanish population. Bos J Basic Med Sci. 2015;15(2):31–6.
35. Chen D, Liu L, Xiao Y, Peng Y, Yang C, Wang Z. Ethnic-specific meta-analyses of association between the OPRM1 A118G polymorphism and alcohol dependence among Asians and Caucasians. Drug Alcohol Depend. 2012;123(1–3):1–6.
36. Woodcock EA, Lundahl LH, Burmeister M, Greenwald MK. Functional mu opioid receptor polymorphism [OPRM1 A(118) G] associated with heroin use outcomes in Caucasian males: a pilot study. Am J Addict. 2015;24(4):329–35.
37. Ziauddeen H, Nestor LJ, Subramaniam N, Dodds C, Nathan PJ, Miller SR, et al. Opioid antagonists and the A118G polymorphism in the mu-opioid receptor gene: effects of GSK1521498 and naltrexone in healthy drinkers stratified by OPRM1 genotype. Neuropsychopharmacology. 2016;41:2647–57.
38. Schwantes-An TH, Zhang J, Chen LS, Hartz SM, Culverhouse RC, Chen X, et al. Association of the OPRM1 variant rs1799971 (A118G) with non-specific liability to substance dependence in a collaborative de novo meta-analysis of European-ancestry cohorts. Behav Genet. 2016;46(2):151–69.
39. Lechner WV, Knopik VS, McGeary JE, Spillane NS, Tidey JW, McKee SA, et al. Influence of the A118G polymorphism of the OPRM1 gene and exon 3 VNTR polymorphism of the DRD4 gene on cigarette craving after alcohol administration. Nicotine Tob Res. 2016;18(5):632–6.
40. Sullivan D, Pinsonneault JK, Papp AC, Zhu H, Lemeshow S, Mash DC, et al. Dopamine transporter DAT and receptor DRD2 variants affect risk of lethal cocaine abuse: a gene–gene–environment interaction. Transl Psychiatry. 2013;3:e222.

22

EFFORT-D study process evaluation: challenges in conducting a trial into the effects of running therapy in patients with major depressive disorder

Frank Kruisdijk[1,2*], Ingrid Hendriksen[2,3], Erwin Tak[2,3], Aart-Jan Beekman[4] and Marijke Hopman-Rock[2,3,5]

Abstract

Background: Exercise is currently seen as an effective treatment for major depressive disorder (MDD). However, existing studies have focused mainly on mild-to-moderate depression. The moderate positive effect of exercise found in meta-analyses concerning these studies differs, however, from the harsh daily clinical practice, when trying to implement exercise as an adjunctive treatment. We aimed to evaluate the feasibility of aerobic exercise in MDD and identify future problems for implementation.

Methods: The EFFect Of Running Therapy on Depression (EFFORT-D) study was a randomized clinical trial examining the effectiveness of running therapy or Nordic walking in inpatients and outpatients with MDD. We conducted a process evaluation based on the method of Linnan and Steckler. Participant inclusion, dropout and no show were registered qualitatively and quantitatively.

Results: The inclusion and delivered dose of the exercise interventions were limited (60 and 75%, respectively), leading to 80% less inclusion than foreseen. Motivational doubts were the main reason not to participate in the study. The unexpected high dropout rates (40% after 3 months and 80% after 12 months) were frequently related to lack of motivation due to disease characteristics and severity. The duration of the intervention, longer than 3 months was another underlying factor for poor adherence.

Conclusions: Depression severity appeared to be the key factor determining dropout, followed by the duration of exercise intervention, expressed by a pre- and post-inclusion lack of motivation. Both running therapy and Nordic walking were apparently unsuitable for most patients with MDD in the current format. Emphasis on motivational issues is necessary from the early start of the intervention in these patients with MDD. Also a tailored and stepped-care approach is advised for future implementation.

Trial registration The randomized controlled trial protocol of EFFORT-D was approved by the Medical Ethical Committee for Mental Health (Metigg Kamer Noord), CCMO (Central Committee on Research Involving Human Subjects) Protocol Number: NL.26169.097.08. Registration in the Netherlands Trial Register (NTR): NTR1894 on July 2, 2009

Background

Major depressive disorder (MDD) has huge effects on wellbeing and daily personal and professional functioning. It is the second leading cause of disease burden based on years lived with disability [1], and the loss of daily-adjusted life years is considerable [2]. Depressive symptoms are common in various populations [3]. Recurrence of symptoms of MDD occurs in an unfavourable but fluctuating course in 44% of the patients and a severe chronic course in 12–32% of the patients [4, 5]. Pharmacotherapy and psychotherapy, i.e. cognitive behaviour therapy and interpersonal therapy, are the mainstays of treatment [6,

*Correspondence: f.kruisdijk@planet.nl
[1] Department Innova, GGz Centraal Innova, Amersfoort, The Netherlands
Full list of author information is available at the end of the article

7]. Effective use of antidepressant medication is often compromised by side effects, while both the availability of trained therapists and lack of motivation on the part of patients may limit the utility of antidepressant psychotherapy [8]. Although for instance cognitive therapy treatment has a positive effect, about 50% of the patients relapse after 2 years with an estimated 80% relapse after 5 years [9]. Meta-analysis of standard MDD treatment showed a clinically and statistically heterogeneous outcome of treatment as usual: about 30% of the patients remitted from depression, but depressive symptoms also worsened in 12% [10].

Exercise is currently seen as a promising alternative to pharmacotherapy and psychotherapy, because it has low costs and few side effects, and is also considered safe for most patients. Previous research showed that a low level of physical activity is highly prevalent in individuals with depression [11] and that exercise has a positive effect on physical health in such a population [12–14]. Physical activity also has additional advantages in the large group of patients that suffer from a combination of mental and physical problems, such as depression and diabetes, in which prevention of metabolic syndrome by enhancing physical activity is vital [15, 16].

Using exercise therapy as (part of the) regular treatment for MDD seems, therefore, a logical consequence. However, studies focussing on exercise therapy as (part of the) treatment for depression usually involved patients with mild to moderate depression. These patients were mostly recruited through public announcements, and attracted participants who are different from the population with MDD that is hospitalised in recognised mental health care institutions. Of the 28 studies selected by Mead et al. [17] in their Cochrane review on exercise and depression, only two were randomized controlled trials (RCTs) that included adult inpatients [18, 19]. In a follow-up Cochrane review of Cooney et al. [20], only seven of 39 studies recruited participants from clinical populations, i.e. hospital inpatients or outpatients referred by a general practitioner (GP). The studies included in the latter review, that reported positive effects on quality of life and symptom severity in severely depressed inpatients, were all short-term studies.

One of the few studies into severe MDD inpatients, which was not included in the aforementioned Cochrane reviews, had an add-on design with, besides exercise, treatment as usual consisting of pharmacotherapy and/or electroconvulsive therapy [20]. Although this study lasted only 2 weeks, it showed a significant effect on depressive symptoms as well as physical and psychological domains of quality of life; however, 50% of the eligible patients were not motivated to participate. The eight trials with a longer follow-up in the Cochrane review of Cooney et al. [21] using an intervention time between 10 and 16 weeks and follow-up measurements with a maximum of 10 months, showed only a moderate effect on depression with a pooled standardised mean difference (SMD) of – 0.33. This is in line with the review of Krogh et al. [22] studying RCTs in adults with a clinical depression. This review showed a significant SMD of – 0.40 in 13 trials, with an inverse relationship between duration of the intervention and the magnitude of the association between exercise and depression. Also, a pooled analysis of five trials with a long-term follow-up (9–26 months), suggested no long-term benefit (SMD – 0,01). Consequently, when implementing exercise in for instance a guideline for treatment of MDD, a diminishing effect of exercise in the long run should be considered.

Limited evidence is found that short-term interventions are as effective as long-term interventions in MDD [23]. The latest review in this field advised moderate exercise to be suitable as part of a multidimensional approach [24]. A limitation of existing studies is that bias must be considered regarding inadequate blinding of participants and observers. When studies with adequate allocation concealment, intention-to-treat-analysis and blinded outcome assessment were analysed, the pooled SMD (– 0.18) for the primary outcome of depression scores was small and no longer significant [17, 21, 25].

An important aspect of MDD is the unpredictable duration of a depressive period. In an epidemiological cohort study, half of those with MDD and a minor depressive episode recovered within 6 months with standard treatment, wherein only a short period without treatment seemed, however, defensible. Treatment was urgently advised for those with greatest need, a lower functioning at onset and experiencing comorbidity [5]. However, it is unknown how long an intervention should take. The abovementioned controversy between moderate positive results from meta-analyses and treatment of severe (inpatient) MDD in the harsh clinical daily practice still exists, leaving clinicians and patients uncertain about the optimal use of exercise as a part of their treatment. As a result, more high-quality research into the relationship between MDD and exercise as a (add-on) treatment was needed.

The EFFect Of Running Therapy on Depression (EFFORT-D) study, which has been described in a previous publication, was both aimed at severe (inpatient) MDD and a long-term exercise intervention in an add-on RCT design [26]. During the EFFORT-D study, which was carried out between 2012 and 2015, both an effect evaluation (results to be published) and a process evaluation were conducted. The process evaluation enabled us to determine influencing factors to the outcome results in different phases and identify topics for future research, such as implementation strategies in clinical practice and advices for depressive patients. To our knowledge, only few process evaluation studies in this field have been published [27–29]. The importance of a process evaluation has been demonstrated by Linnan and Steckler [30]. Although their examples focused on preventive population interventions, their framework can also be applied to our study focusing on curative interventions for patients. Therefore, the aim of this process evaluation was to gain insight into the context, reach and dose of the exercise intervention of the EFFORT-D study.

Methods

EFFORT-D study

Aim

The main objective of the EFFORT-D study was to assess the effectiveness of exercise therapy [running therapy (RT) or Nordic walking (NW)], in addition to usual care, on MDD in adult (in) patients. We hypothesised that adding exercise therapy to usual care would result in a larger reduction in depressive symptoms [as measured with the Hamilton Rating Scale of Depression (HAM-D_{17})], during a 6-month treatment programme as well as at 6 months follow-up, compared to usual care without exercise therapy.

Design

EFFect Of Running on Depression was an observer-blinded randomised controlled parallel trial conducted in three Dutch mental health care hospitals between December 2012 and January 2015. Participants were randomly assigned to 6 months of RT or NW twice a week in addition to their treatment as usual. Both groups were followed during 1 year with measurements at inclusion (T0), 3 months (T3), 6 months (T6) and a final after 12 months (T12).

It was expected that patients in the usual care group (control group) would respond with a mean reduction in HAM-D_{17} of six points, because they were all following the standard MDD treatment protocol. Adding exercise to usual care (intervention group) was expected to result in a decline of at least eight points on the HAM-D_{17} score. To detect this difference, with an α (two-tailed) of 5% and a power $(1 - \beta)$ of 80%, using two equal groups and a standard deviation of 5 points, 100 patients were needed in each group. Taking 30% dropout into account, 140 patients had to be included in each group.

Because EFFORT-D focussed on patients with MDD, an add-on design with exercise was indicated due to ethical considerations: no active treatment at all versus exercise was no option due to the nature, type and severity of the participant's MDD.

Participants

The study was performed in three regions of a large specialised mental health care institution. Included patients were either inpatients, day-hospital patients or outpatients referred by specialised mental health care such as emergency services (in- and day-hospital patients) and Dutch general practitioners (GPs) for outpatients.

The study population of EFFORT-D consisted of patients with MDD with a Hamilton depression scale (HAM-D_{17}) score $\geq$ 14, indicating at least a moderate depression at the time of inclusion. Because the GPs already had started with the depression protocol several months before the start of this study, the depressive symptoms of these outpatients were usually in partial remission.

Measurements and procedure

The control group received treatment as usual, which consisted of pharmacotherapy, supportive psychotherapy and daily activation for the hospitalized participants or those in-day treatment, and pharmacotherapy and cognitive therapy for the outpatients. The experimental group received an exercise intervention in addition to treatment as usual. This consisted of a group-based Running Therapy (RT) or Nordic Walking (NW) session of 1 h, twice a week for the duration of 6 months, with increasing intensity following a training protocol with the possibility for individual adaptations. The control group was only allowed to practice low-intensity, non-aerobic exercises. Participants were monitored closely: no shows and dropouts were registered including the arguments of the participant. Participants were followed up using the Hamilton Depression Scale (HAM-D_{17}) scores, the Åstrand submaximal cycling test and questionnaires at 3, 6 and 12 months (T3, T6 and T12, respectively). All participants gave their informed consent for participation in the study.

Methodological framework of this process evaluation

In their model, Linnan and Steckler mentioned several factors that are important in a process evaluation [30]. In the current process evaluation, we used the factors context, reach and dose from their model, because these were assumed to be the most suitable to evaluate our intervention study:

- Context refers to aspects of the larger social, political and economic environment that may influence the intervention.
- Reach describes the proportion of the intended population that participates in the intervention or study.

- Dose, which consists of dose delivered and dose received, measures the intended intervention and the extent to which participants adhere to it.

Furthermore, the exercise trainers and the research assistant were asked by a questionnaire to answer nine open questions for evaluation purposes. These questions were based on the context, reach and dose factors as defined by Linnan and Steckler, along with two general evaluative questions. Answers were received by email and summarised by the first author.

Results

Context

Much less than the required 200 subjects (100 in both the intervention and control group) was included. The financial crisis and the associated changes in the Dutch mental healthcare system had a major—and unexpected—impact on the social, political and economic environment in which this study took place. As a result, the recruitment of patients was restrained. Regarding the inclusion sites, 17% of the participants were initially assigned to a locked emergency ward. After stabilization and reduction of suicide risk, they continued their stay voluntarily in an open crisis ward. They were invited to participate in the study after a clinician indicated that they could give informed consent; they often continued their treatment in a day hospital followed by an outpatient programme. The other inclusion sites were day hospitals as a start of the treatment and outpatient clinics. Finally, 45% of the included participants were treated MDD inpatients or were day-hospitalized.

Reach

Due to the abovementioned developments at the start of the study, the reach was severely reduced. An important contextual reason for reduced inclusion was the exclusion of three of the original five study locations. Budgetary cuts and strategic decisions about the affective disorders programme were underling arguments. The previously estimated reach in the population was approximately 3500 patients in a programme for depressive disorders and about 500 patients from emergency wards. With the loss of three locations, the reach was reduced to approximately 1200 patients in a programme and about 200 patients from emergency wards, which caused a decrease of approximately 60% potentially to reach. Table 1 shows the demographic characteristics of the included participants.

Table 1 Baseline demographic characteristics of the participants

	N = 48
Age, years (SD)	41.6 (9.1)
Female, %	62.5
Education, %	PS: 5; SecS: 30; LVE/MVE: 28; HS/HVE/acad: 37
Country of origin, %	Netherlands: 79 Turkey/Morocco: 8 Other[a]: 13
Civil status, %	M: 55; S: 35; D: 10

PS primary school, *SecS* secondary school, *LVE* lower vocational, *MVE* medium vocational, *HS/HVE/acad* high school/higher vocational/academic, *M* married, *S* single, *D* divorced

[a] Include Surinam, Aruba, Curacao and Iraq

Dose-related findings

In total, 183 patients were screened for eligibility to participate within the 2-year time-frame of the EFFORT-D study. Ultimately only 48 participants could be included in the study, with 25 participants in the intervention arm, instead of the required 100 participants in each group. The relatively high number of eligible participants that were excluded ($n = 135$) was due to several causes. First, 20% of the patients referred by a GP were admitted to the affective disorder programmes after completing the intake procedure, but by the time they were rated on the HAM-D_{17}, their cut-off score was below 14, which made them ineligible to participate. Their HAM-D_{17} score was probably higher before referral to specialist care, but standard treatment was already initiated before the research assistant could make a screening appointment to measure the HAM-D_{17}. Other causes for exclusion were other health problems during screening (14%), already exercising twice a week for at least 30 min (14%) and a contraindication for the intervention given by the primary treating psychiatrist (12%). The largest barrier to inclusion, however, resulted from the large proportion of patients (40%) who expected that they were not able to organise their daily life in such a way that they could participate in the exercise intervention twice a week. The programme was too time consuming, they were too tired and, in their own opinion, were unable to invest in exercise and commitment to the study. These reasons were assumed to be associated with MDD symptoms as fatigue, loss of energy and initiative. The planned dose of exercise was finally delivered to 25 participants in the intervention group, of which 45% were inpatients of an emergency ward or were being treated in a day hospital. As expected, due to the severity of their depression, the average HAM-D_{17} score at inclusion for inpatient or day hospital participants (25.7) was higher than for outpatients (20.5). The patient flow during all measurements (T0, T3, T6 and T12) is presented in Fig. 1.

Between allocation to the intervention group (T0) and the first follow-up measurement (T3), already 10

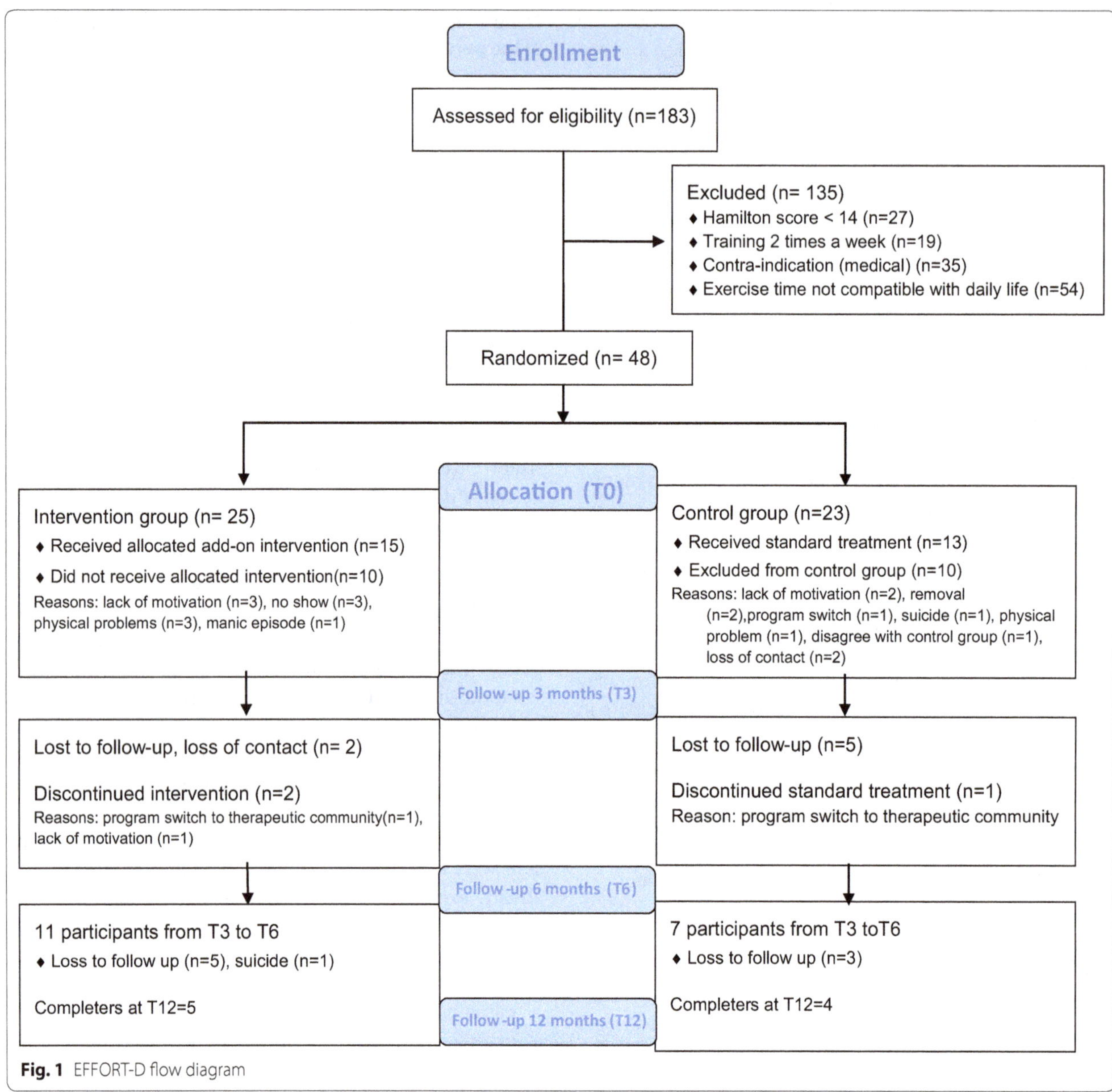

Fig. 1 EFFORT-D flow diagram

of the 25 participants (40%) dropped out. This dropout increased to 56% at T6 and 80% at T12. In the non-intervention arm the same pattern was seen. For the drop-out reasons see Fig. 1.

Evaluation of the nine-item questionnaire

We decided not to contact the participants at the end of the study for the process evaluation. Participants who dropped out could not easily be contacted by the research assistant, and the small proportion of participants who reached the T12 evaluation (20%) in the intervention arm could cause bias in favour of the RT and NW activities. The answers to nine open questions showed that the trainers ($n = 2$) and the research assistant had positive attitudes about their role in the study.

However, they all reported that it was unexpectedly difficult to motivate the participants. The expectation of a positive effect of the RT and NW was still present, but trainers and research assistant developed a more realistic view on the feasibility of implementing RT and NW in these depressive patients. The many dropouts at every stage of the study compelled them to be cautious for any positive expectations. According to the exercise trainers (see questions described in Table 2), the 'ideal patient' who can benefit from RT or NW is a female patient

Table 2 Evaluation questionnaire for exercise trainers and the research assistant

Context-related questions	What aspects went well during the study? What would have been the ideal environment for the study?
Reach-related questions	Did the participation in the study meet your expectations? Describe the profile of a patient suffering from depression who improves with exercise Describe the profile of a patient for whom exercise will have little effect
Dose-related questions	Estimate the percentage of participants in the intervention arm that completed the intervention Did the participation in the study meet your expectations?
General questions about context, reach and dose	What needs improvement? What advice can you give to other researchers studying exercise in depressive patients in the future? Did your opinion about the importance of exercise in depressive patients change?

between 30 and 50 years old, who is native Dutch and has previous positive exercise experiences with running.

This positive exercise experience could have been a long time ago, but could be reactivated during the RT and/or NW intervention. For depressed inpatients who are not native Dutch, middle aged, male and with no exercise experience, a very modest form of walking without training goals was reported to be most feasible. According to the exercise trainers, the inpatients were serious about participating, but training two times a week according to the protocol was ultimately too difficult for these patients to maintain. Even when the programme was adapted, without violating the protocol, whereby patients were coached individually and started with gradual walking exercises, the participants could not keep up participation. For outpatients, who had to travel to the intervention site, the intervention often was too time consuming. At the time the patients started the first series of training, their motivation to complete the intervention was considered high by the trainers and the research assistant, so during the intervention it appeared difficult to maintain their motivation. When asked to suggest improvements for the study, the trainers and research assistant referred to a shorter intervention period, with a suggested maximum of 3 months. The trainers indicated that this could have a positive effect on the inclusion because it will be easier to motivate the patients with a time horizon of 3 months, and at the same time the costs for trainers could be reduced. In addition, they suggested that a shorter travel distance to the intervention site could have a positive effect.

Another constraint of this research, according to the trainers, was the winter weather in the Netherlands. To complete the exercise intervention, dry weather and moderate temperatures were seen as ideal. Indoor training was not preferred, because the ideal training environment for RT or NW is in the woods or at the countryside, but indoor facilities are necessary for the continuity of the activities. In this study enduring wintry conditions caused too much discontinuity in the trainings scheme. When asked to estimate the percentage of participants that would complete the intervention, provided that the first sessions were finished, the trainers indicated 70%, while the research assistant indicated only 30%. To prevent potential demotivation of the research assistant, he was intensively coached by the project leader during the rest of the study. Furthermore, the trainers and research assistant both indicated that communication between them was lacking at several times during the intervention period. The fact that one exercise site was in another region as the research centre was an important causal factor.

Discussion

This process evaluation showed that economic conditions had an important negative influence on the implementation of the EFFORT-D study. A severely reduced reach, combined with a large loss of dose delivered was shown. Once included in the intervention group, it turned out to be very difficult to motivate patients with MDD to participate in the aerobic exercise therapy and the long-term measurements. The duration of the intervention seemed to be too long according to the evaluative questionnaire. During this study, the research team faced substantial challenges in several areas. An unexpected high proportion (almost three quarters) of the eligible participants was excluded before randomization. As a result, only about one-fifth of the intended number of patients could be included in this study. Also, contextual difficulties, due to an organisational merger and an economic-driven reorganisation, reduced the reach and the number of available patients in the research population. Forty percent of the eligible participants reported that they were unable to incorporate the exercise programme in their daily lives. They argued that they were too tired and the required investment in time was too high. This can be interpreted as a lack of motivation and it seems to form a structural problem for implementation of exercise in MDD. This motivational issue was also found to be a perceived barrier to exercise in another qualitative study

[27]. Patients in that study were screened for preferences of exercise as a treatment for depression. They reported mood problems, tiredness and lack of motivation as the biggest barriers for exercise in both men and women. In another systematic review on motivating factors and barriers towards exercise, mood problems and stress were also identified as major barriers for engaging in exercise during severe mental illness [31]. Comparable trials in MDD inpatients or severe depressed outpatients who were referred by GPs or psychiatrists also show 25–50% of the eligible participants that refuse to participate. This may be an indication that severity of depression might be the underlying factor for refusal [20, 32]. However, severity of depression seemed not to be an important factor of non-adherence to exercise in a pooled analysis from two clinical trials [33]. This result could be explained by the fact that a population with mild to moderate depression was included in these trials. Finally, in 20% of the outpatients referred by a GP in our study, depressive symptoms fell below the required threshold for inclusion during the intake procedure. This was possibly due to the mechanism of spontaneous recovery [34] or was a result of treatment that was already started by the GP. The fact that the dropout rate in both arms of our study was comparable could indicate that the intervention itself was not the main cause of the high dropout. It might also mean that strain of the follow-up testing was too high for these severely depressed participants. This was, however, not confirmed by the evaluative questions answered by the exercise leaders and research assistant. The follow-up arguments for quitting the study showed that participating in the early stages of the intervention did not provide enough incentive to remain on board. These kinds of motivational problems are also described in patients with affective disorders such as MDD, bipolar disorder [35] and with schizophrenia [36].

The concept of 'autonomous motivation' to exercise, meaning an intrinsic motivation and an identification with the benefits of a healthy lifestyle, seems to play a vital role in maintaining involvement in the exercise programme. Somewhat hopeful here is the fact that 14% of our eligible participants were excluded because they already trained twice a week for 30 min. Possibly, the use of a depression guideline of the GPs explains this effect, because it recommends prescribing exercise for mild to moderate depression. It seems that the EFFORT-D intervention and study design in its current form does not seem to be feasible in these MDD patients, certainly not for hospitalised inpatients. So, regarding implementation of exercise programmes in the treatment of MDD, motivational themes need a lot of attention throughout the programme. This is very important, because people with severe psychiatric disorders, such as MDD, are at higher risk for chronic physical conditions [37–39] and tend to be very sedentary [40]. It might seem more adequate to treat MDD patients using the activation principles of patients with other severe mental illnesses such as schizophrenia or bipolar disorder. As described in recent publications, aiming the exercise intervention on improvement of quality of life and cardiorespiratory fitness, besides the improvement of depression, is indicated [11, 38, 41]. A broader multidisciplinary lifestyle intervention, incorporating light-to-moderate physical activity in daily life, in addition to lifestyle interventions aimed at smoking and eating habits, seems effective. A disadvantage of such a multidimensional approach is that it will be difficult to determine the effect of the physical exercise separately, but an advantage is a probably broader health gain. An alternative approach might be indoor training, as used in other studies of depressed patients [32, 42] and in studies of patients with schizophrenia [43]. This could also prevent training absences during wintry conditions with icy running tracks. However, a combination of indoor and outdoor exercise is preferred due to indications that a green environment contributes to wellbeing [44, 45]. Another option is to launch a pre-study training, in which participants are given the opportunity to personalise their programme with help from a physical therapist with the aim of increasing their fitness level and preventing injuries. This is in line with recommendations based on a qualitative study of patients' viewpoints in general practice involving 33 participants [28]. Once participants have a sufficient fitness level, they can participate in the group intervention. An advantage of this personalised approach is that the form of exercise can be adapted to the patients' preferences and possibilities, for instance cycling in the case of joint problems. In addition, also E-learning environments, supporting technical tools such as electronic devices for self-registration of activity and smartphone applications (including WhatsApp and social media) can be considered. These can potentially encourage participants in daily life and promote more adherence to exercise [46].

Prevention of early dropouts needs more attention in future research. It is a paradox, however, that the estimated length of an optimal exercise study is 3–4 months, whereas the preferred length of an exercise programme is longer. A single study, with a long follow-up of 10 months, showed that it is worthwhile to invest in long-term motivation to persist in exercising because of maintenance of the therapeutic effect and prevention of a relapse [47]. The latest results of the Dutch NEMISIS-study show that the median time for a depressive episode was 6 months in MDD and 3 months for a minor depressive episode with a full remission of 75% after 1 year for both [5]. This means that exercise as an adjunctive treatment probably can contribute to remission in the first 6 months, after this period it is probably meaningful to prevent a relapse.

This process evaluation had several limitations. First, evaluative questioning of participants was not appropriate, because the expected bias in favour of exercise was estimated to be high: practically only the very small group of completers of the intervention at T12 were able to give feedback. This diminished potential informative and qualitative suggestions for future research from a patient perspective. In particular, evaluation of the larger group of dropouts could have given more detailed information about blockades for exercise or suggestions to solve these, but that was not feasible. Second, the questions directed at the trainers and research assistant for this process evaluation were sent by e-mail. Instead, a (semi)-structured interview would have led to more in-depth information. At last the numbers of included patients were small so the conclusion that this type of exercise in these particular patients does not fit MDD patients cannot be generalised easily. Nevertheless, this process evaluation of an exercise intervention in patients with MDD is one of the few delivered and may be of value for both researchers as well as clinicians in the field. Researchers can profit from the described pitfalls, whereas the clinicians may recognise their own patients and prevent obstacles when planning an (add-on) exercise intervention.

Conclusions

Our process evaluation showed that both the intervention as well as the study design of EFFORT-D were not feasible for patients with MDD in terms of motivation and compliance. In future interventions, applying electronic self-registration devices is advised, which not only can motivate the participant through direct feedback, but they also enable researchers to objectively measure the intensity and time spent on physical activity. Besides, social media use could enhance more adequate communication (for instance forming an easy accessible WhatsApp or Facebook group). Further research is needed to define the optimal duration of an exercise intervention in MDD. Finally, a tailored and stepped-care intervention method is advised in case of aerobic exercise training such as running therapy or Nordic walking, starting with a pre-study phase in which a physical therapist can prepare the potential participant. Flexibility in aerobic activity fitting the individual participant, and combining in- and outdoor facilities, may also help to retain the participants and enhance motivation for exercise, making it part of their lifestyle.

Abbreviations

MDD: major depressive disorder; RCT: randomized controlled trial; GP: general practitioner; SMD: standard mean difference; EFFORT-D study: EFFect Of Running on Depression study; RT: running therapy; NW: Nordic walking; HAM-D_{17}: 17-item Hamilton Depression Rating Scale; T0, T3, T6, T12: measurements at inclusion, 3, 6 and 12 months.

Authors' contributions

FK: study design, collection and analysis of data, drafting and revising the manuscript, IH: study design and revising the manuscript, ET: study design and revising the manuscript, AJB: revising the manuscript, MH: study design, supporting data analysis and revising the manuscript. All authors contributed to the manuscript. All authors read and approved the final manuscript.

Author details

[1] Department Innova, GGz Centraal Innova, Amersfoort, The Netherlands. [2] Body@Work, TNO-VU University Medical Center, Amsterdam, The Netherlands. [3] The Netherlands Organisation for Applied Scientific Research TNO, Leiden, The Netherlands. [4] Department of Psychiatry, VU University Medical Center, Amsterdam, The Netherlands. [5] Department of Public and Occupational Health, EMGO Institute for Health and Care Research, VU University Medical Center, Amsterdam, The Netherlands.

Acknowledgements

The authors would like to thank all patients and mental healthcare professionals of GGz Centraal who have made efforts to collect all the data, which formed the basis for this publication. Prof. Dr. Erik Knorth for his valuable explanation of the systematic approach of research process evaluations.

Competing interests

AJB received honorarium as a speaker from Lundbeck (no connection with this study). Other authors: no competing interests.

Consent for publication

Not applicable.

Funding

Grant support (unrestricted gift) was received from the former "Open Ankh Foundation" (since March 2008 "Zorgcoöperatie Nederland").

References

1. Vos T, Flaxman AD, Naghavi M, Lozano R, Michaud C, Ezzati M, Shibuya K, Salomon JA, Abdalla S, Aboyans V, et al. Years lived with disability (YLDs) for 1160 sequelae of 289 diseases and injuries 1990–2010: a systematic analysis for the Global Burden of Disease Study 2010. Lancet. 2012;380:2163–96.
2. Murray CJL, Lopez AD. Measuring the global burden of disease. N Engl J Med. 2013;369(5):448–57.
3. Salomon JA, Wang H, Freeman MK, Vos T, Flaxman AD, Lopez AD, Murray CJ. Healthy life expectancy for 187 countries, 1990–2010: a systematic analysis for the Global Burden Disease Study 2010. Lancet. 2012;380:2144–62.
4. Beekman AF, Geerlings SW, Deeg DH, et al. The natural history of late-life depression: a 6-year prospective study in the community. Arch Gen Psychiatry. 2002;59:605–11.
5. Ten Have M, Penninx B, Tuithof M, van Dorsselaer S, Kleinjan M, Spijker J, de Graaf R. Duration of major and minor depressive episodes and associated risk indicators in a psychiatric epidemiological cohort study of the general population. Acta Psychiatr Scand. 2017;136:300–12.
6. Cuijpers P, Donker T, Weissman MM, Ravitz P, Cristea IA. Interpersonal psychotherapy for mental health problems: a comprehensive meta-analysis. Am J Psychiatry. 2016;173:680–7.

7. Cuijpers P, Cristea IA, Karyotaki E, Reijnders M, Huibers MJ. How effective are cognitive behavior therapies for major depression and anxiety disorders? A meta-analytic update of the evidence. World Psychiatry. 2016;15:245–58.
8. Hollon SD, Munoz RF, Barlow DH, Beardslee WR, Bell CC, Bernal G, Clarke GN, Franciosi LP, Kazdin AE, Kohn L, et al. Psychosocial intervention development for the prevention and treatment of depression: promoting innovation and increasing access. Biol Psychiatry. 2002;52:610–30.
9. Vittengl JR, Clark LA, Dunn TW, Jarrett RB. Reducing relapse and recurrence in unipolar depression: a comparative meta-analysis of cognitive-behavioral therapy's effects. J Consult Clin Psychol. 2007;75:475–88.
10. Kolovos S, van Tulder MW, Cuijpers P, Prigent A, Chevreul K, Riper H, Bosmans JE. The effect of treatment as usual on major depressive disorder: a meta-analysis. J Affect Disord. 2017;210:72–81.
11. Stubbs B, Koyanagi A, Schuch FB, Firth J, Rosenbaum S, Veronese N, Solmi M, Mugisha J, Vancampfort D. Physical activity and depression: a large cross-sectional, population-based study across 36 low- and middle-income countries. Acta Psychiatr Scand. 2016;134:546–56.
12. Blumenthal JA. Effects of exercise and stress management training on markers of cardiovascular risk in patients with ischemic heart disease: a randomized controlled trial. JAMA J Am Med Assoc. 2005;293:1626–34.
13. Bridle C, Spanjers K, Patel S, Atherton NM, Lamb SE. Effect of exercise on depression severity in older people: systematic review and meta-analysis of randomised controlled trials. Br J Psychiatry. 2012;201:180–5.
14. Stubbs B, Rosenbaum S, Vancampfort D, Ward PB, Schuch FB. Exercise improves cardiorespiratory fitness in people with depression: a meta-analysis of randomized control trials. J Affect Disord. 2016;190:249–53.
15. Mezuk B, Eaton WW, Albrecht S, Golden SH. Depression and type 2 diabetes over the lifespan: a meta-analysis. Diabetes Care. 2008;31:2383–90.
16. Vancampfort D, Stubbs B. Physical activity and metabolic disease among people with affective disorders: prevention, management and implementation. J Affect Disord. 2016;224:87–94.
17. Mead G, Morley W, Campbell P, Greig C, Murdo MM, Lawlor D. Exercise for depression. Cochrane Database Syst Rev. 2009;(3):CD004366. https://doi.org/10.1002/14651858.CD004366.pub4.
18. Knubben K, Reischies FM, Adli M, Schlattmann P, Bauer M, Dimeo F. A randomised, controlled study on the effects of a short-term endurance training programme in patients with major depression. Br J Sports Med. 2007;41:29–33.
19. Martinsen E, Medhus A, Sandvik L. Effects of aerobic exercise on depression: a controlled study. BMJ. 1985;291(6488):109.
20. Schuch FB, Vasconcelos-Moreno MP, Borowsky C, Zimmermann AB, Rocha NS, Fleck MP. Exercise and severe major depression: effect on symptom severity and quality of life at discharge in an inpatient cohort. J Psychiatr Res. 2015;61:25–32.
21. Cooney G, Dwan K, Greig CA, Lawlor DA, Rimer J, Waugh FR, McMurdo M, Mead GE. Exercise for depression. Cochrane Database Syst Rev. 2013;(9):CD004366. https://doi.org/10.1002/14651858.CD004366.pub6.
22. Krogh J, Nordentoft M, Sterne JA, Lawlor DA. The effect of exercise in clinically depressed adults: systematic review and meta-analysis of randomized controlled trials. J Clin Psychiatry. 2011;72:529–38.
23. Excellence NIfHaC. Depression: the treatment and management of depression in adults. London: National Institute for Health and Clinical Excellence; 2009.
24. Ledochowski L, Stark R, Ruedl G, Kopp M. Physical activity as therapeutic intervention for depression. Nervenarzt. 2017;88:765–78.
25. Spedding S. Exercise for depression: Cochrane systematic reviews are rigorous, but how subjective are the assessment of bias and the practice implications? Adv Integr Med. 2015;2:63–5.
26. Kruisdijk FR, Hendriksen IJM, Tak ECPM, Beekman ATF, Hopman-Rock M. Effect of running therapy on depression (EFFORT-D). Design of a randomised controlled trial in adult patients. BMC Public Health. 2012;12:50.
27. Busch AM, Ciccolo JT, Puspitasari AJ, Nosrat S, Whitworth JW, Stults-Kolehmainen M. Preferences for exercise as a treatment for depression. Mental Health Phys Act. 2016;10:68–72.
28. Searle A, Calnan M, Lewis G, Campbell J, Taylor A, Turner K. Patients' views of physical activity as treatment for depression: a qualitative study. Br J Gen Pract. 2011;61:149–56.
29. Pickett K, Kendrick T, Yardley L. "A forward movement into life": a qualitative study of how, why and when physical activity may benefit depression. Mental Health Phys Act. 2017;12:100–9.
30. Linnan L, Steckler A, editors. Process evaluation for public health, interventions and research. San Francisco: Jossey-Bass; 2002.
31. Firth J, Rosenbaum S, Stubbs B, Gorczynski P, Yung AR, Vancampfort D. Motivating factors and barriers towards exercise in severe mental illness: a systematic review and meta-analysis. Psychol Med. 2016;46:2869–81.
32. Krogh J, Saltin B, Gluud C, Nordentoft M. The DEMO trial: a randomized, parallel-group, observer-blinded clinical trial of strength versus aerobic versus relaxation training for patients with mild to moderate depression. J Clin Psychiatry. 2009;70:790–800.
33. Krogh J, Lorentzen AK, Subhi Y, Nordentoft M. Predictors of adherence to exercise interventions in patients with clinical depression—a pooled analysis from two clinical trials. Mental Health Phys Act. 2014;7(1):50–4.
34. Posternak MA, Miller I. Untreated short-term course of major depression: a meta-analysis of outcomes from studies using wait-list control groups. J Affect Disord. 2001;66:139–46.
35. Vancampfort D, Madou T, Moens H, De Backer T, Vanhalst P, Helon C, Naert P, Rosenbaum S, Stubbs B, Probst M. Could autonomous motivation hold the key to successfully implementing lifestyle changes in affective disorders? A multicentre cross sectional study. Psychiatry Res. 2015;228:100–6.
36. Firth J, Carney R, Pownall M, French P, Elliott R, Cotter J, Yung AR. Challenges in implementing an exercise intervention within residential psychiatric care: a mixed methods study. Mental Health Phys Act. 2017;12:141–6.
37. Fleischhacker WW, Cetkovich-Bakmas M, De Hert M, Hennekens CH, Lambert M, Leucht S, Maj M, McIntyre RS, Naber D, Newcomer JW, et al. Comorbid somatic illnesses in patients with severe mental disorders: clinical, policy, and research challenges. J Clin Psychiatry. 2008;69:514–9.
38. Vancampfort D, Rosenbaum S, Schuch F, Ward PB, Richards J, Mugisha J, Probst M, Stubbs B. Cardiorespiratory fitness in severe mental illness: a systematic review and meta-analysis. Sports Med. 2017;47(2):343–52.
39. Correll CU, Solmi M, Veronese N, Bortolato B, Rosson S, Santonastaso P, Thapa-Chhetri N, Fornaro M, Gallicchio D, Collantoni E, et al. Prevalence, incidence and mortality from cardiovascular disease in patients with pooled and specific severe mental illness: a large-scale meta-analysis of 3,211,768 patients and 113,383,368 controls. World Psychiatry. 2017;16:163–80.
40. Kruisdijk F, Deenik J, Tenback D, Tak E, Beekman AJ, van Harten P, Hopman-Rock M, Hendriksen I. Accelerometer-measured sedentary behaviour and physical activity of inpatients with severe mental illness. Psychiatry Res. 2017;254:67–74.
41. Schuch FB, Vancampfort D, Rosenbaum S, Richards J, Ward PB, Stubbs B. Exercise improves physical and psychological quality of life in people with depression: a meta-analysis including the evaluation of control group response. Psychiatry Res. 2016;241:47–54.
42. Krogh J, Videbech P, Thomsen C, Gluud C, Nordentoft M. DEMO-II trial. Aerobic exercise versus stretching exercise in patients with major depression—a randomised clinical trial. PLoS ONE. 2012;7:e48316.
43. Pajonk FG, Wobrock T, Gruber O, Scherk H, Berner D, Kaizl I, Kierer A, Muller S, Oest M, Meyer T, et al. Hippocampal plasticity in response to exercise in schizophrenia. Arch Gen Psychiatry. 2010;67:133–43.
44. Lovell R, Wheeler BW, Higgins SL, Irvine KN, Depledge MH. A systematic review of the health and well-being benefits of biodiverse environments. J Toxicol Environ Health B Crit Rev. 2014;17:1–20.
45. Fruhauf A, Niedermeier M, Elliott LR, Ledochowski L, Marksteiner J, Kopp M. Acute effects of outdoor physical activity on affect and psychological well-being in depressed patients—a preliminary study. Mental Health Phys Act. 2016;10:4–9.
46. Naslund JA, Aschbrenner KA, Bartels SJ. Wearable devices and smartphones for activity tracking among people with serious mental illness. Mental Health Phys Act. 2016;10:10–7.
47. Babyak M, Blumenthal JA, Herman S, Khatri P, Doraiswamy M, Moore K, Craighead WE, Baldewicz TT, Krishnan KR. Exercise treatment for major depression: maintenance of therapeutic benefit at 10 months. Psychosom Med. 2000;62:633–8.

23

Personality traits and health-related quality of life: the mediator role of coping strategies and psychological distress

Angela J. Pereira-Morales[1], Ana Adan[2,3], Sandra Lopez-Leon[4*] and Diego A. Forero[1*]

Abstract

Background: The study of health-related quality of life (HRQOL) is an important topic in mental health around the globe. However, there is the need for more evidence about the cumulative influence of psychological variables on HRQOL. The main aim of the study was to evaluate how specific personality traits might explain scores in HRQOL and to explore how this relationship might be mediated by coping styles and psychological distress.

Methods: Young Colombian subjects (*N* = 274) were included (mean age: 21.3; SD = 3.8). The Short-Form Health Survey was used to measure HRQOL. For assessment of psychological variables, the Hospital Anxiety and Depression Scale, the Zung Self-Rating Anxiety Scale, The Coping Inventory for Stressful Situations and the short version of Big Five Inventory were used.

Results: The personality trait that was the best predictor of HRQOL was openness to experience, forming an explanatory model for HRQOL, along with emotional coping style and depressive and anxious symptoms. Emotional coping style and psychological distress were significant mediators of the relationship between openness and HRQOL.

Conclusions: Our findings provide additional data about the cumulative influence of specific psychological variables on HRQOL, in a mostly young female Latin American sample.

Keywords: Five-factor personality model, Coping, Health-related quality of life, Latin America, Mental health

Background

Health-related quality of life (HRQOL) has been defined by the World Health Organization as: "An individual's perception of their position in life, in the context of the culture and values in which they live and in relation to their goals, expectations, standards, and concerns" [1]. In developing countries, a low HRQOL has been associated with lower socioeconomic status (SES) [2]. Research has shown that a lower SES is associated with a poor mental health in young adults; this relationship can be explained by several risk factors, such as disadvantageous work characteristics, reduced social support and risky health behaviors [3–6].

In general, young people in South American countries are exposed to many vulnerabilities, such as inadequate access to education and social and health services, high rates of violence and a relatively easy access to drugs [7]. These susceptibilities might have important impacts on mental health [8], given the fact that psychosocial vulnerabilities during youth have been shown to have short- and long-term implications for the individuals and the society [8].

In terms of adaptation and coping, the emotional and cognitive evaluations of life satisfaction are important factors for understanding HRQOL [9]. Coping typically includes cognitive and behavioral strategies that are used to overcome or to resolve problematic life circumstances (e.g., problem solving) [10]. In addition, coping strategies are used to manage the emotional consequences

*Correspondence: sandra.lopez@novartis.com; diego.forero@uan.edu.co
[1] Laboratory of Neuropsychiatric Genetics, Biomedical Sciences Research Group, School of Medicine, Universidad Antonio Nariño, Bogotá 110231, Colombia
[4] Novartis Pharmaceuticals Corporation, One Health Plaza, East Hanover, NJ 07936-1080, USA
Full list of author information is available at the end of the article

of stressful situations [10]. In accordance with previous works [11], coping can be understood through three main dimensions or styles: task oriented, emotional, and avoidant, which represents self-reported responses to stressful circumstances. The task-oriented style is represented by subjects who generally take a problem-solving approach to stressful situations. In contrast, those who habitually engage in maladaptive behaviors, such as ruminating activities or becoming emotional in response to stress, have a predominantly emotional style. On the other hand, individuals who typically employ behaviors aimed at circumventing the stressful situation have a predominantly avoidant style [12]. Although there is evidence for stability in coping styles over time, they can change across the life span and across different stressful situations and the effect of the coping strategies depends on the specific situations [10, 13].

Personality is an important factor for the perception of stressful events and is considered as fundamental for having the required resources to cope in an unexpected situation [14]. Several studies have established evidence of associations between coping styles and personality [15], showing that the neurotic trait is positively correlated with the avoidant coping strategies and negatively correlated with the task-oriented coping style, while openness has been associated with active coping strategies, such as seeking social support [16–23].

The study of HRQOL is an important topic in mental health worldwide, taking into account its relationship with subjective well-being and other health outcomes [9]. Although HRQOL is influenced by life circumstances and demographic characteristics (such as socioeconomic status), more evidence is needed about the cumulative effect of multiple psychological variables on physical and mental health-related quality of life. The main aim of the current study was to test, in a sample of young Colombian subjects, the hypothesis that specific personality traits might explain scores in HRQOL and that this relationship might be mediated by coping styles and psychological distress.

Materials and methods

Participants

Two hundred seventy-four young Colombian healthy subjects were included in this study. Recruitment of the participants started with an invitation in two universities in Bogotá, Colombia. The aims and procedures of the study were explained to the interested subjects and they were invited for the application of the psychosocial evaluations. The mean of age was 21.3 years (standard deviation, SD = 3.8), 75.1% were females and 24.9% were males. The participants did not have a personal history of neuropsychiatric disorders, according to self-report. The study followed the ethical standards of the Helsinki Declaration and all subjects signed a written informed consent, with prior approval of the study by the Institutional Ethics Committee of the Antonio Nariño University.

Psychological scales and instruments

HRQOL was assessed with the 12-Item Short-Form Health Survey (SF-12). The SF-12 is a self-report scale that provides a reliable measure of the perception of physical (PCS) and mental (MCS) health. PCS dimension includes the physical functioning, physical health problems, general health and bodily pain domains. Meanwhile, MCS dimension includes the social functioning, emotional problems, mental health and vitality domains [24]. The scores are standardized to population norms (based on a European normative sample), with the mean score set at 50 (SD = 10); scores above 50 indicate better perception of health status [25]. The method used to compute values for the two main dimensions (PCS and MCS) was based on the algorithm provided by Andersen et al. [26], which was based on the procedure described in the SF-12 manual. The SF-12 has been validated in Spanish and in Colombia, with adequate reliability and psychometric properties [27]. In the current study, the Cronbach's alphas were 0.74 and 0.72 for PCS and MCS, respectively.

Psychological distress was assessed using the Hospital Anxiety and Depression Scale (HADS) and the Zung Self-Rating Anxiety Scale (ZSAS). We used two scales for the assessment of anxiety symptomatology since ZSAS includes somatic aspects of anxiety that HADS-A does not evaluate. In addition, HADS-A assesses generalized anxiety symptoms, such as tension, worry, panic, difficulties in relaxing, and restlessness. The *HADS* is a self-report screening instrument created to indicate the possible presence of anxiety and depression states. It includes two sub-factors: Depression (HADS-D) and Anxiety (HADS-A), each one with 7 items. It has demonstrated excellent reliability and validity in English and Spanish languages, including Colombia [28]. The cutoff points are ≥ 6 for depression, ≥ 8 for anxiety and ≥ 13 for the total test. The Cronbach's alpha for the current study was 0.83 for the total HADS score, 0.77 for the anxiety subscale and 0.65 for the depression subscale. The ZSAS is an instrument that provides a self-report of symptoms, based on the characteristic signs of anxiety. It has shown excellent reliability and validity in Spanish and in Colombia [29]. The Cronbach's α for the ZSAS was 0.85 in this sample.

Coping was measured with the Coping Inventory for Stressful Situations (CISS-SF), in the short form version with 21 items [30]. This inventory assesses three different dimensions or coping styles (task-oriented, emotional, and avoidant). CISS items exemplify different ways of coping in a particular stressful situation. Good internal consistency has been found for its subscales in the English language and it has been previously used in the Spanish language [30]. In the current study, the internal consistency of the emotional coping style was $\alpha = 0.84$, of 0.80 for task-oriented style and of 0.65 for the avoidant style.

To assess personality dimensions, the Big Five Inventory (BFI-S; 15-items) was used [31]. The Big Five personality trait model is one of the most established and used approaches to measure individual differences in personality. This self-report inventory measures five dimensions of personality: N (Neuroticism), E (Extraversion), O (Openness to experience), C (Conscientiousness) and A (Agreeableness) on a 7-point Likert scale. It has been validated in the English language by Lang et al. [31] and it has been widely used in several countries, such as Spain [32]. In the current study, the Cronbach's alpha was 0.61 for Extraversion, 0.73 for Openness, 0.42 for Consciousness, 0.47 for Agreeableness and 0.62 for Neuroticism. The instruments selected for this work (SF-12, HADS, ZSAS, CISS-SF and BFI-S) are reliable and efficient tools for psychosocial measurement, which are broadly used and have been validated in Spanish.

Statistical analysis

Normal distributions of the scores for the used scales were explored with previously described methods, including analyses of skewness and kurtosis [33]. The psychometric properties of the instruments used were evaluated using Cronbach's alpha and exploratory factorial analysis.

The association of the HRQOL (total SF-12 scores and PCS/MCS dimensions) and predictor variables (psychological distress, coping and personality traits) was examined using Pearson correlations and multiple regression models, controlling for age and gender. Collinearity was examined with the variance inflation factor (VIF) and independence assumption on the residuals was evaluated with the Durbin–Watson test. For a better characterization of HRQOL and its predictors, two models of multiple regression analyses were conducted: (1) one for SF-12/Physical Component Score and (2) one for SF-12/Mental Component Score.

The Statistical Package for the Social Sciences V. 18 (SPSS Inc., Chicago, Illinois, United States) was used for all the statistical analyses. The Bonferroni correction for multiple testing [34] was included. For the current study, the Bonferroni corrected p value for the regression models 1 and 2 was 0.012.

Mediation analysis was performed to evaluate the mediator role of coping styles and psychological distress in the relationship between HRQOL and personality traits. Only significant predictors for HRQOL in the regression model were included in mediation analysis. Following the procedures recommended by Hayes [35], mediation-in-serial models using multiple regressions with three mediators were carried out. Direct effects, indirect effects, and total effects were calculated using specification model 6 with three mediators in the PROCESS plugin (V.2014) [35] in SPSS (V.18).

Openness was inserted as an independent variable, HRQOL was included as an outcome variable and emotional coping style, task-oriented coping style and psychological distress (depressive and anxious symptoms) were inserted as the mediator variables. To assess the magnitude of the indirect effects, we report *partially standardized indirect effects* of the independent variable on the outcome variable. According to Preacher et al. [36], this index is interpreted as the number of standard deviations by which the outcome variable is expected to increase or decrease per each change in independent variable indirectly via the mediator variables.

Results

Descriptive data and Associations between variables

The majority of the participants were from low and medium SES (33.5 and 44.5%, respectively). The most common education level and marital status of the subjects were secondary (78.8%) and single (93%), respectively. Sixteen and thirteen percent of the subjects showed lower scores of PCS and MCS, respectively. The mean scores for the psychological distress scales were 13.9 (SD = 5.4) for HADS scale and 38.5 (SD = 9.4) for ZSAS. The preferred coping style was task oriented (mean = 22.7; SD = 5.0), followed by emotional (mean = 19.9; SD = 6.0) and avoidant (mean = 17.6; SD = 5.1). In terms of the personality traits, Factor O showed the highest mean value (5.4; SD = 1.0), followed by factor C (mean = 4.9; SD = 1.0). Neuroticism was the personality trait with the lowest average value (4.1; SD = 1.2).

Pearson's correlations are summarized in Table S1. HRQOL/PCS was negatively correlated with task-oriented coping style, openness and conscientiousness ($r = -0.171$, $r = -0.175$, $r = -0.136$, $p < 0.01$, respectively) and positively correlated with emotional coping style and neuroticism ($r = 0.194$, $r = 0.169$, $p < 0.01$). HRQOL/MCS was negatively correlated with psychological distress (measured with HADS and ZSAS) and with emotional coping style and neuroticism ($r = -0.568$, $r = -0.547$, $r = -0.533$, $r = -0.442$, $p < 0.01$, respectively) and correlated positively with task-oriented coping style, openness, conscientiousness, extraversion and agreeableness ($r=0.254$, $r=0.205$, $r=0.139$, $r=0.211$, $r=0.187$, $p<0.01$, respectively).

Task-oriented coping style was negatively correlated with psychological distress (measured with HADS and ZSAS), emotional coping style and neuroticism ($r=-0.303$, $r=-0.328$, $r=-0.133$, $r=-0.228$, $p<0.01$, respectively) and it was positively correlated with openness, conscientiousness and agreeableness ($r=0.310$, $r=0.291$, 0.312, $p<0.01$, respectively). Finally, emotional coping style positively correlated with psychological distress (measured with HADS and ZSAS) and with neuroticism ($r=0.509$, 0.576, 0.486, $p<0.01$, respectively) and avoidance coping style correlated with extraversion ($r=0.222$, $p<0.01$).

Multivariate analyses

Model 1

The best regression model for HRQOL/PCS was composed by emotional coping style ($\beta=0.28$, $p=0.0001$), openness ($\beta=-0.14$, $p=0.018$), anxiety symptoms (measured with ZSAS, $\beta=-0.19$, $p=0.008$) and task-oriented coping style ($\beta=-0.15$, $p=0.017$) (Table 1).

Model 2

For HRQOL/MCS, the best regression model found was composed by psychological distress (measured with HADS total score, $\beta=-0.27$, $p=0.00003$), ZSAS ($\beta=-0.17$, $p=0.010$), emotional coping style ($\beta=-0.28$, $p=1.4508E^{-06}$) and openness ($\beta=0.10$, $p=0.025$) (Table 2).

In this sample of young adults, anxiety symptoms, emotional coping style, task-oriented coping style and openness explained 8% of the variance on HRQOL in its physical dimension; while psychological distress (anxiety and depressive symptoms), emotional coping style and openness explained 42% of the variance on HRQOL in its mental dimension.

Direct and indirect effects of openness on HRQOL Physical Component Score via coping styles and anxious symptoms

The first mediation model (Fig. 1) tested the relationship of openness to experience with HRQOL/PCS, via the effects of task-oriented coping style, emotional-focused coping, and ZSAS. Openness affected HRQOL/PCS directly (coefficient: -1.228, SE$=0.42$, $p=0.0040$) (Fig. 1), as well as indirectly through emotional coping style, task-oriented coping style and anxiety symptoms measured with ZSAS (coefficient: -1.0257, SE$=0.43$, $p=0.0183$). The total indirect effect of openness on HRQOL/PCS, via emotional coping style, task-oriented coping style, and anxiety symptoms was not significant (coefficient: -0.203, 95% CI -0.622 to 0.170) (Table 2).

Direct and indirect effects of openness on HRQOL Mental Component Score via emotional coping style and psychological distress

The second mediation model (Fig. 2) tested the relationship of openness to experience with HRQOL/MCS, via emotional-focused coping, total HADS score, and ZSAS. Openness affected HRQOL (SF-12 MCS) directly (coefficient: 3.402, SE$=0.99$, $p=0.0007$), as well as indirectly via emotional coping style and psychological distress (coefficient: 1.777, SE$=0.79$, $p=0.0257$) (Table 2). The total indirect effect of openness on HRQOL/MCS

Table 1 Stepwise multiple regression models for HRQOL and associated psychological factors

Variable	Model 1 HRQOL (SF-12 PCS)[a]			Model 2 HRQOL (SF-12 MCS)[b]		
	β	SE	R^2	β	SE	R^2
Emotional coping style	0.19**	7.1	0.03			
Emotional coping style × openness	0.18** × − 0.16**	7.0	0.05			
Emotional coping style × openness × ZSAS	0.27** × − 0.18** × − 0.14*	6.9	0.07			
Emotional coping style × Openness × ZSAS × Task-oriented coping style	0.28** × − 0.14* × − 0.19** × − 0.15*	6.9	0.08			
HADS				− 0.58**	14.0	0.32
HADS × emotional coping style				− 0.40** × − 0.33**	13.2	0.39
HADS × emotional coping style × ZSAS				− 0.30** × − 0.27** × − 0.18**	13.0	0.41
HADS × emotional coping style × ZSAS × openness				− 0.27** × − 0.28** × − 0.17** × 0.10*	12.9	0.42

ZSAS Zung Self-Rating Anxiety Scale, *HADS* Hospital Anxiety and Depression Scale, *SE* standard error

* Significant at $p<0.05$

** Significant after Bonferroni correction for multiple testing

[a] Model 1: Outcome variable measured with 12-Item Short-Form Health Survey-Physical Component Score

[b] Model 2: Outcome variable measured with 12-Item Short-Form Health Survey-Mental Component Score

Table 2 Multiple mediation effect for HRQOL (SF-12 PCS) and HRQOL (SF-12 MCS)

		Coefficient	CI lower	CI upper	Effect size (95% CI)
Mediation model 1: HRQOL (SF-12 PCS)	Indirect effect via M1[a]	0.204	0.030	0.507	0.028 (0.003–0.068)
	Indirect effect via M1 and M2[b]	− 0.169	− 0.401	− 0.039	− 0.023 (− 0.054 to − 0.005)
	Indirect effect via M1 and M3[c]	− 0.051	− 0.159	− 0.004	− 0.007 (− 0.022 to − 0.0006)
	Indirect effect via M2 and M3[d]	− 0.003	− 0.039	0.003	− 0.0005 (− 0.005–0.0004)
	Indirect effect via M1, M2 and M3[e]	0.006	− 0.003	0.035	0.0008 (− 0.0005–0.0049)
	Total indirect effect	− 0.203	− 0.622	0.170	− 0.028 (− 0.084–0.023)
Mediation model 2: HRQOL (SF-12 MCS)	Indirect effect via M1	0.126	− 0.004	0.351	0.025 (0.0001–0.0696)
	Indirect effect via M1 and M2	0.406	0.082	0.944	0.023 (0.004–0.053)
	Indirect effect via M1 and M3	0.377	0.075	0.970	0.022 (0.004–0.052)
	Indirect effect via M2 and M3	− 0.041	− 0.206	0.270	− 0.002 (− 0.011–0.0016)
	Indirect effect via M1, M2 and M3	0.071	0.014	0.256	0.004 (0.0009–0.0136)
	Total indirect effect	1624	0.323	3.019	0.095 (0.017–0.175)

Model 1: M1 = mediator 1 (anxiety symptoms measure with ZSAS); M2: mediator 2 (emotional coping style); M3: mediator 3 (task-oriented coping style). Model 2: M1 = mediator 1 (anxiety symptoms measure with ZSAS); M2: mediator 2 (emotional coping style); M3: mediator 3 (psychological distress measure with HADS)

CI confidence interval

[a] The indirect effect of the openness on health-related quality of life via anxiety symptoms measure with ZSAS

[b] The indirect effect of the Openness on Health-related Quality of Life via anxiety symptoms measure with ZSAS and emotional coping style

[c] The indirect effect of the openness on health-related quality of life via anxiety symptoms measure with ZSAS and task-oriented coping style

[d] The indirect effect of the openness on health-related quality of life via emotional coping style and task-oriented coping style

[e] The indirect effect of the openness on health-related quality of life via anxiety symptoms measure with ZSAS, Emotional coping style and Task-oriented coping style

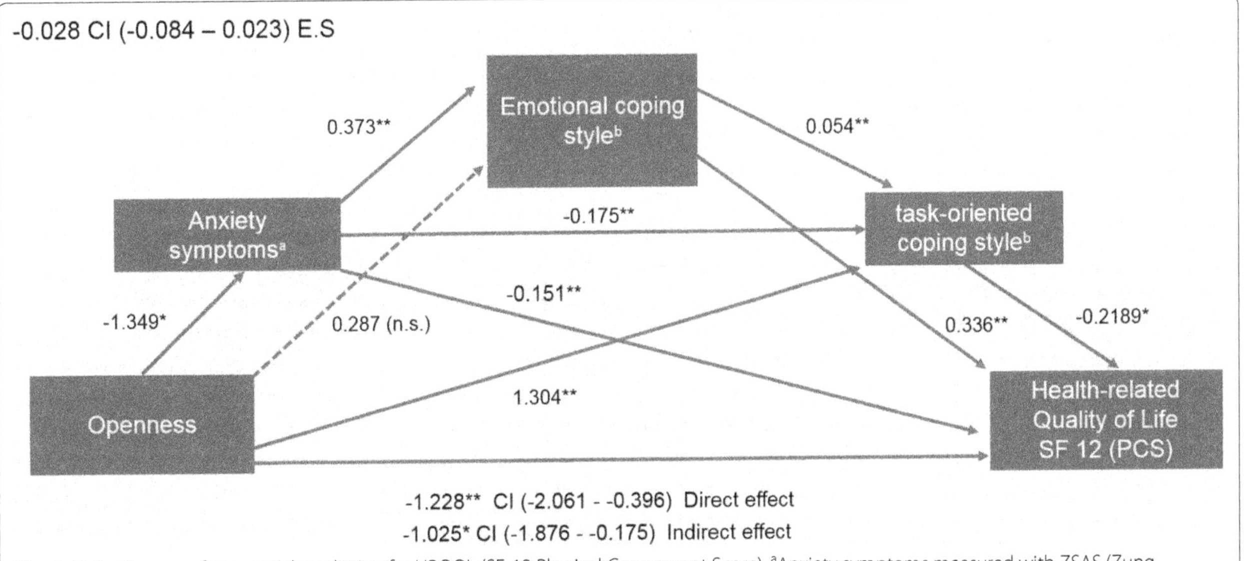

Fig. 1 Path diagram of sequential mediation for HRQOL (SF-12 Physical Component Score). [a]Anxiety symptoms measured with ZSAS (Zung Self-Rating Anxiety Scale). [b]Coping styles measured with the Coping Inventory for Stressful Situations (CISS-SF). *E.S* effect size of total indirect effect for the mediation model, *CI* confidence interval, *n.s.* no significant. $^{*}p<0.05$; $^{**}p<0.001$

through emotional coping style and psychological distress (measured with HADS and ZSAS) was significant (coefficient: 1.624, 95% CI 0.323–3.019) (Table 2).

The partially standardized indirect effect for openness on subjective well-being (SF-MCS) via emotional coping style and psychological distress (measured with ZSAS and HADS) was 0.095 (95% CI 0.017–0.175). It implies that HRQOL/MCS is expected to increase by 0.095 standard deviations for every increase in one unit in openness, indirectly through emotional coping style and psychological distress. Other significant effect sizes for the indirect effects were found (Table 2).

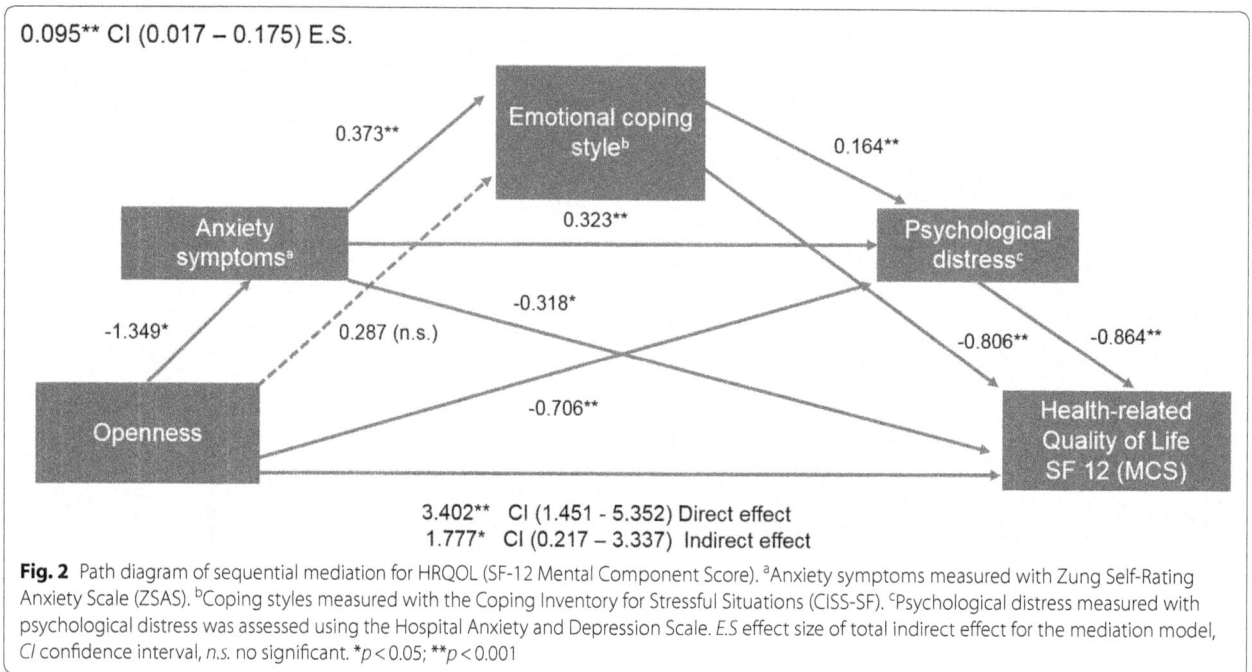

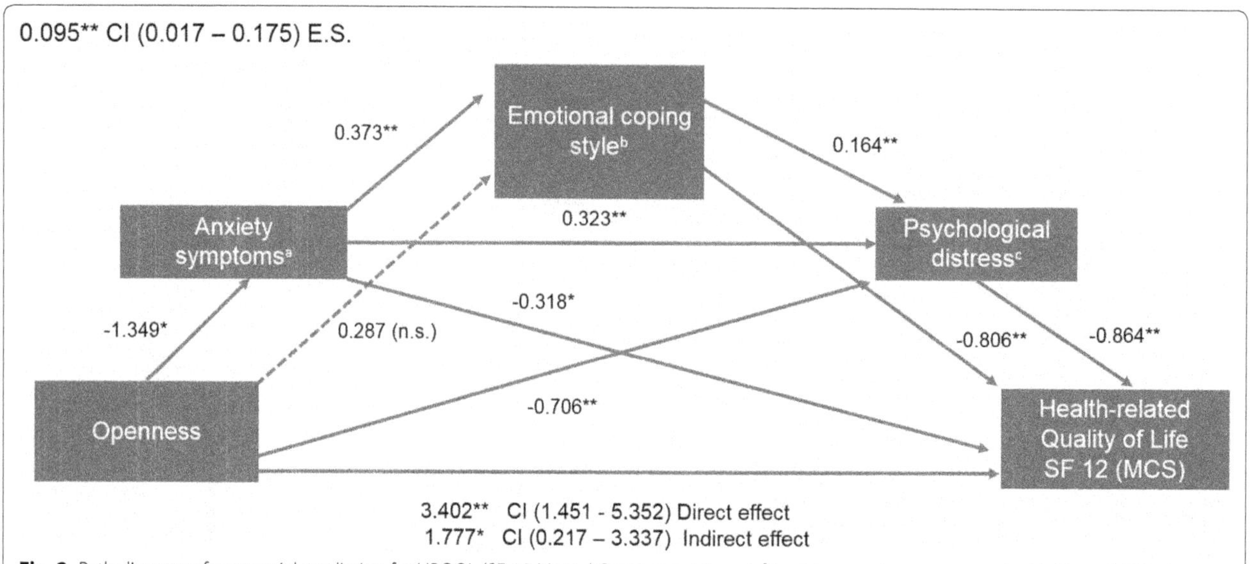

Fig. 2 Path diagram of sequential mediation for HRQOL (SF-12 Mental Component Score). [a]Anxiety symptoms measured with Zung Self-Rating Anxiety Scale (ZSAS). [b]Coping styles measured with the Coping Inventory for Stressful Situations (CISS-SF). [c]Psychological distress measured with psychological distress was assessed using the Hospital Anxiety and Depression Scale. *E.S* effect size of total indirect effect for the mediation model, *CI* confidence interval, *n.s.* no significant. *$p < 0.05$; **$p < 0.001$

Discussion

In this work, in a sample of young Colombian subjects, we tested the hypothesis that specific personality traits might explain scores in HRQOL and that this relationship might be mediated by coping styles and psychological distress. We found that the personality trait that best predicted HRQOL was openness, forming an explanatory model for HRQOL, along with emotional coping style and depressive and anxious symptoms. We also found that emotional coping style and psychological distress were significant mediators of the relationship between openness and HRQOL.

Over the past three decades, there has been considerable progress on research on health-related quality of life [37]. Previous studies have indicated that HRQOL is influenced by both personality and coping [38]. However, there is the need for inclusion of other relevant psychological variables, in addition to personality and coping, in the analytical models and studies [39]. This is important taking into account that HRQOL is a multidimensional construct that has been under-investigated for a long time in young populations in developing countries [9]. The results for HRQL in the current sample are similar to findings in other studies [23]. Our results provide a multidimensional model for HRQOL, which includes personality, coping and emotional variables and that explains a considerable percentage of HRQOL variance, in a Colombian sample of young adults.

The relationship between personality traits and HRQOL has been reported in previous studies, finding that personality is one of the strongest and most consistent predictors for HRQOL in the general population [40]. Specifically, it has been suggested that neuroticism has an interactive effect on HRQOL, as well that agreeableness, conscientiousness, and extraversion have been also predictors of self-rated health [41]. Openness to experience has the fewest documented links to health; nevertheless, recent studies have found higher levels of openness as protective against earlier mortality [42].

It has been proposed that personality may affect the selection of coping strategies directly or indirectly, facilitating the use of specific approaches [16]. Some investigations have found that certain personality traits are related to specific coping styles. Neurotic subjects (characterized by high reactivity to stress) generally show emotional or avoidant coping strategies [17]. On the other hand, individuals who have low-stress reactivity, such as subjects with high scores in consciousness and openness personality traits, have been shown to prefer task-oriented coping strategies [43].

Previous studies have shown a positive association between openness and approach coping strategies [15] and other reports found an association between approach coping strategies and increased distress and non-productive worry [15]. These previous results are consistent with our findings of psychological distress as a mediator of the relationship between openness and HRQOL. Moreover, both emotional coping style and psychological distress were explanatory factors (negatively correlated) for HRQOL (physical and mental dimensions). In addition, task-oriented coping style was a significant factor for the HRQOL physical dimension. Although the effect of the coping strategies depends on the specific situations, these patterns of relationships might indicate that individuals with high scores in openness can experience a recovery from the initial emotional reaction to a stressful event and move on to deal with the source of the stress more quickly and effectively than neurotic individuals do, who generally prefer emotional coping strategies and show low scores in HRQOL. This is supported in part by a previous study [44] and by another report that has shown that openness reflects a more flexible, imaginative, and intellectually curious approach to problem solving [45]. On the other hand, in our second model of mediation, when emotional coping style and with psychological distress were included, the relationship between openness and HRQOL mental dimension was diminished. This finding can be explained in terms of the evidence that has shown that passive coping strategies, such as emotional coping style, involve avoidance and withdrawal behaviors, instead of a rational approach in dealing with difficulties, which is more characteristic of subjects with higher scores in openness experience [46]. In turn, it is well known that healthy adaptive strategies are positively associated with active coping behaviors and with a better perception of quality of life [47]; and are inversely associated with maladaptive strategies, such as emotional-focused styles, and with lower levels of openness experience [48, 49].

Nonetheless, in some cases, emotional coping strategies may also be a protective factor. For example, some emotional coping style strategies, such as acceptance or religion, can help to reduce depressive symptoms and contribute to HRQOL [50], particularly if a problem is unlikely to be resolved. However, other avoidant coping attitudes, such as denial and substance use, are often less useful and have been associated with impulsivity and anxious symptoms [51].

A considerable amount of previous studies have documented the impact of neuroticism and conscientiousness on objective measures of health and its perception [52], but few previous studies have shown evidence that higher levels of openness are also a significant factor for perception of HRQOL. Future studies would help to confirm the role of personality and coping in HRQOL processes, which might help to keep people healthy as they move across the decades of adulthood [52].

In the context of coping strategies, personality traits are considered an important factor for having the required resources to cope in stressful situations [14] as well as in the perception of stressful events and on HRQOL. In our sample, openness, conscientiousness, and agreeableness were significantly correlated with the task-oriented coping style. In our study, openness, task-oriented coping style, anxiety symptoms and emotional coping style formed an associative model for HRQOL in its physical dimension. This is relevant because the task-oriented coping style is a strategy employed usually more frequent in subjects who generally take an active problem-solving approach to stressful situations [11]. A task-oriented coping style, in conjunction with conscientiousness, agreeableness and openness, may be an important protective factor for affective disorders [53].

In our mediation analyses, the relationship between HRQOL-MCS and openness (with emotional coping style and psychological distress as mediators) showed a significant effect size. This may suggest that these factors are more important variables for HRQOL-MCS, in comparison with HRQOL-PCS. Openness was significant (direct effect) in the mediation model for HRQOR-MCS after a Bonferroni correction for multiple testing. This is relevant because an openness to experience involves the tendency to be creative, curious, flexible, and inclined toward new activities and ideas [54]. These tendencies may facilitate engagement in coping strategies that require considering new perspectives, such as cognitive restructuring and problem solving [15].

This study has some limitations: the effect sizes found were small and these findings should be treated with caution, because mediation analysis is employed for testing casual relationships in experimental designs where is possible to conclude that causality has occurred. When using this method in behavioral studies, we should consider that the relationships in such contexts might be reciprocal, as it is possible that the independent variable affects the mediator and that the mediator might influence the independent variable as well [55]. In addition, the nature of our sample, composed mainly by females and educated participants, does not allow the generalization of the results to the general population (Additional file 1).

In future studies, it will be important to carry out an analysis of the genetic and epigenetic factors involved in HRQOL, as well as the possible interaction of these factors with environmental influences on HRQOL and perceived mental health.

Conclusion

In this study, we tested the hypothesis that specific personality traits might explain scores in HRQOL and that this relationship might be mediated by coping styles and psychological distress. Our study provides novel mediational models that may help to understand the association between personality and coping in the context of HRQOL, in both their physical and mental dimensions. In addition, our findings provide additional data about

the cumulative influence of specific psychological variables on health-related quality of life in a Latin American sample, composed mainly by young females.

Authors' contributions

AJP participated in study design, acquisition and analysis of psychological data and drafting and critical revision of the manuscript. AA participated in analysis of psychological data and drafting and critical revision of the manuscript. SL-L participated in analysis of data and drafting and critical revision of the manuscript. DAF participated in study design, analysis of psychological data, drafting and critical revision of the manuscript. All authors read and approved the final manuscript.

Author details

[1] Laboratory of Neuropsychiatric Genetics, Biomedical Sciences Research Group, School of Medicine, Universidad Antonio Nariño, Bogotá 110231, Colombia. [2] Department of Clinical Psychology and Psychobiology, School of Psychology, University of Barcelona, Barcelona, Spain. [3] Institute of Neurosciences, University of Barcelona, Barcelona, Spain. [4] Novartis Pharmaceuticals Corporation, One Health Plaza, East Hanover, NJ 07936-1080, USA.

Acknowledgements

The authors thank to Andres Camargo, who assisted with recruitment and evaluations of subjects.

Competing interests

The authors declare that they have no competing interests.

Consent for publication

Not applicable.

Funding

This study was supported by a research grant from Colciencias (Grant # 823-2015). AA was supported by a grant from the Spanish Ministry of Economy, Industry and Competitiveness (#PSI2015-65026; MINECO/FEDER/UE).

References

1. Thoma A, Kaur MN, Ignacy TA, Levis C, Martin S, Duku E, Haines T. Psychometric properties of health-related quality of life instruments in patients undergoing palmar fasciectomy for dupuytren's disease: a prospective study. Hand (N Y). 2014;9:166–74.
2. Savadogo G, Souares A, Sie A, Parmar D, Bibeau G, Sauerborn R. Using a community-based definition of poverty for targeting poor households for premium subsidies in the context of a community health insurance in Burkina Faso. BMC Public Health. 2015;15:84.
3. Von Rueden U, Gosch A, Rajmil L, Bisegger C, Ravens-Sieberer U. Socioeconomic determinants of health related quality of life in childhood and adolescence: results from a European study. J Epidemiol Community Health. 2006;60:130–5.
4. Barriuso-Lapresa L, Hernando-Arizaleta L, Rajmil L. Social inequalities in mental health and health-related quality of life in children in Spain. Pediatrics. 2012;130:e528–35.
5. Meyer OL, Castro-Schilo L, Aguilar-Gaxiola S. Determinants of mental health and self-rated health: a model of socioeconomic status, neighborhood safety, and physical activity. Am J Public Health. 2014;104:1734–41.
6. Callan MJ, Kim H, Matthews WJ. Predicting self-rated mental and physical health: the contributions of subjective socioeconomic status and personal relative deprivation. Front Psychol. 2015;6:1415.
7. Mokdad AH, Forouzanfar MH, Daoud F, Mokdad AA, El Bcheraoui C, Moradi-Lakeh M, Kyu HH, Barber RM, Wagner J, Cercy K, et al. Global burden of diseases, injuries, and risk factors for young people's health during 1990-2013: a systematic analysis for the Global Burden of Disease Study 2013. Lancet. 2016;387:2383–401.
8. Blum RW, Nelson-Mmari K. The health of young people in a global context. J Adolesc Health. 2004;35:402–18.
9. Ed D, Suh EM, Lucas RE, Smith HL. Subjective well-being: three decades of progress. Psychol Bull. 1999;125:276–302.
10. Compas BE, Connor-Smith JK, Saltzman H, Thomsen AH, Wadsworth ME. Coping with stress during childhood and adolescence: problems, progress, and potential in theory and research. Psychol Bull. 2001;127:87–127.
11. Endler NS, Parker JD. Assessment of multidimensional coping: task, emotion, and avoidance strategies. Psychol Assess. 1994;6:50.
12. Lin HS, Probst JC, Hsu YC. Depression among female psychiatric nurses in southern Taiwan: main and moderating effects of job stress, coping behaviour and social support. J Clin Nurs. 2010;19:2342–54.
13. Diehl M, Chui H, Hay EL, Lumley MA, Gruhn D, Labouvie-Vief G. Change in coping and defense mechanisms across adulthood: longitudinal findings in a European American sample. Dev Psychol. 2014;50:634–48.
14. Dumitru VM, Cozman D. The relationship between stress and personality factors. Hum Vet Med. 2012;4:34–9.
15. Carver CS, Connor-Smith J. Personality and coping. Annu Rev Psychol. 2010;61:679–704.
16. Bolger N, Zuckerman A. A framework for studying personality in the stress process. J Pers Soc Psychol. 1995;69:890–902.
17. Amirkhan JH, Risinger RT, Swickert RJ. Extraversion: a "hidden" personality factor in coping? J Pers. 1995;63:189–212.
18. Afshar H, Roohafza HR, Keshteli AH, Mazaheri M, Feizi A, Adibi P. The association of personality traits and coping styles according to stress level. J Res Med Sci. 2015;20:353–8.
19. Fornes-Vives J, Garcia-Banda G, Frias-Navarro D, Rosales-Viladrich G. Coping, stress, and personality in Spanish nursing students: a longitudinal study. Nurse Educ Today. 2016;36:318–23.
20. Montero J, Gomez-Polo C. Association between personality traits and oral health-related quality of life: a cross-sectional study. Int J Prosthodont. 2017;30:429–36.
21. Lin F, Ye Y, Ye S, Wang L, Du W, Yao L, Guo J. Effect of personality on oral health-related quality of life in undergraduates. Angle Orthod. 2018;88:215–20.
22. Hasanoglu Erbasar GN, Alpaslan C. Influence of coping strategies on oral health-related quality of life in patients with myalgia. Cranio. 2017. https://doi.org/10.1080/08869634.2017.1398300.
23. Husson O, Zebrack B, Block R, Embry L, Aguilar C, Hayes-Lattin B, Cole S. Personality traits and health-related quality of life among adolescent and young adult cancer patients: the role of psychological distress. J Adolesc Young Adult Oncol. 2017;6:358–62.
24. Islam N, Khan IH, Ferdous N, Rasker JJ. Translation, cultural adaptation and validation of the English "Short form SF 12v2" into Bengali in rheumatoid arthritis patients. Health Qual Life Outcomes. 2017;15:109.
25. Karatzias T, Yan E, Jowett S. Adverse life events and health: a population study in Hong Kong. J Psychosom Res. 2015;78:173–7.
26. Andersen HH, Mühlbacher A, Nübling M, Schupp J, Wagner GG. Computation of standard values for physical and mental health scale scores using the SOEP version of SF-12v2. Schmollers Jahrbuch. 2007;127:171–82.
27. Ramirez-Velez R, Agredo-Zuniga RA, Jerez-Valderrama AM. The reliability of preliminary normative values from the short form health survey (SF-12) questionnaire regarding Colombian adults. Rev Salud Publica (Bogota). 2010;12:807–19.
28. Hinz A, Finck C, Gomez Y, Daig I, Glaesmer H, Singer S. Anxiety and depression in the general population in Colombia: reference values of the Hospital Anxiety and Depression Scale (HADS). Soc Psychiatry Psychiatr Epidemiol. 2014;49:41–9.
29. De La Ossa S, Martinez Y, Herazo E, Campo A. Study of internal consistency and factor structure of three versions of the Zung's rating instrument for anxiety disorders. Colombia Méd. 2009;40:71–7.
30. Inostroza C, Cova F, Bustos C, Quijada Y. Desesperanza y afrontamiento centrado en la tarea median la relación entre sintomatologia depresiva y conducta suicida no letal en pacientes de salud mental. Rev Chil Neuro-psiquiatr. 2015;53:231–40.

31. Lang FR, John D, Ludtke O, Schupp J, Wagner GG. Short assessment of the Big Five: robust across survey methods except telephone interviewing. Behav Res Methods. 2011;43:548–67.
32. Chamorro-Premuzic T, Gomà-i-Freixanet M, Furnham A, Muro A. Personality, self-estimated intelligence, and uses of music: a Spanish replication and extension using structural equation modeling. Psychol Aesthet Creat Arts. 2009;3:149.
33. Kim HY. Statistical notes for clinical researchers: assessing normal distribution (2) using skewness and kurtosis. Restor Dent Endod. 2013;38:52–4.
34. Streiner DL, Norman GR. Correction for multiple testing: is there a resolution? Chest. 2011;140:16–8.
35. Hayes AF. Introduction to mediation, moderation, and conditional process analysis: a regression-based approach. New York: Guilford Press; 2013.
36. Preacher KJ, Kelley K. Effect size measures for mediation models: quantitative strategies for communicating indirect effects. Psychol Methods. 2011;16:93–115.
37. Diener E. New findings and future directions for subjective well-being research. Am Psychol. 2012;67:590–7.
38. van Straten A, Cuijpers P, van Zuuren FJ, Smits N, Donker M. Personality traits and health-related quality of life in patients with mood and anxiety disorders. Qual Life Res. 2007;16:1–8.
39. Pocnet C, Antonietti JP, Strippoli MF, Glaus J, Preisig M, Rossier J. Individuals' quality of life linked to major life events, perceived social support, and personality traits. Qual Life Res. 2016;25:2897–908.
40. Sprangers MA, Schwartz CE. Integrating response shift into health-related quality of life research: a theoretical model. Soc Sci Med. 1999;48:1507–15.
41. Smith TW, Williams PG. Personality and health: advantages and limitations of the five-factor model. J Pers. 1992;60:395–425.
42. Hampson SE, Friedman HS. Personality and health: a lifespan perspective. In: John OP, Robins RW, Pervin LA, editors. Handbook of personality: theory and research. New York: Guilford Press; 2008. p. 770–94.
43. Connor-Smith JK, Flachsbart C. Relations between personality and coping: a meta-analysis. J Pers Soc Psychol. 2007;93:1080–107.
44. Gohm CL, Clore GL. Four latent traits of emotional experience and their involvement in well-being, coping, and attributional style. Cogn Emot. 2002;16:495–518.
45. Watson D, Hubbard B. Adaptational style and dispositional structure: coping in the context of the five-factor model. J Pers. 1996;64:737–74.
46. Jia H, Uphold CR, Wu S, Reid K, Findley K, Duncan PW. Health-related quality of life among men with HIV infection: effects of social support, coping, and depression. AIDS Patient Care STDS. 2004;18:594–603.
47. Folkman S, Lazarus RS, Gruen RJ, DeLongis A. Appraisal, coping, health status, and psychological symptoms. J Pers Soc Psychol. 1986;50:571–9.
48. DeLongis A, Holtzman S. Coping in context: the role of stress, social support, and personality in coping. J Pers. 2005;73:1633–56.
49. Schaller M, Murray DR. Pathogens, personality, and culture: disease prevalence predicts worldwide variability in sociosexuality, extraversion, and openness to experience. J Pers Soc Psychol. 2008;95:212–21.
50. Evans LD, Kouros C, Frankel SA, McCauley E, Diamond GS, Schloredt KA, Garber J. Longitudinal relations between stress and depressive symptoms in youth: coping as a mediator. J Abnorm Child Psychol. 2015;43:355–68.
51. Lightsey OR Jr, Hulsey CD. Impulsivity, coping, stress, and problem gambling among university students. J Couns Psychol. 2002;49:202.
52. Turiano NA, Pitzer L, Armour C, Karlamangla A, Ryff CD, Mroczek DK. Personality trait level and change as predictors of health outcomes: findings from a national study of Americans (MIDUS). J Gerontol B Psychol Sci Soc Sci. 2012;67:4–12.
53. Chioqueta AP, Stiles TC. Personality traits and the development of depression, hopelessness, and suicide ideation. Personal Individ Differ. 2005;38:1283–91.
54. McCrae RR, John OP. An introduction to the five-factor model and its applications. J Pers. 1992;60:175–215.
55. Preacher KJ, Hayes AF. Asymptotic and resampling strategies for assessing and comparing indirect effects in multiple mediator models. Behav Res Methods. 2008;40:879–91.

An open-label, flexible dose adaptive study evaluating the efficacy of vortioxetine in subjects with panic disorder

Anish Shah[1*] and Joanne Northcutt[2]

Abstract

Background: Despite the current treatments available for panic disorder (PD), as many as one-third of patients have persistent and treatment-resistant panic attacks. Vortioxetine is an approved medicine for major depressive disorder and has been shown to have anxiolytic properties. The purpose of this study was to evaluate its efficacy and safety in an adult population with a diagnosis of PD.

Methods: The study design was open label with flexible dose strategies (5, 10, or 20 mg) with a treatment period of 10 weeks. 27 male and female subjects aged between 18 and 60 years, who met DSM-IV criteria for PD with or without agoraphobia, or who had a Panic Disorder Severity Scale (PDSS) score > 8 at baseline were enrolled. Statistical significance was established by the Student's *T* test.

Results: A statistically significant decrease in the occurrence of panic attacks was measured with the PDSS with vortioxetine. In addition, a moderate improvement in the quality of life and no significant side effects were observed using the Quality-of-Life Scale and Monitoring of Side Effects Scale, respectively.

Conclusions: These results provide some support for the use of vortioxetine in the management of panic disorder.

Trial registration ClinicalTrials.gov ID#: NCT02395510. Registered March 23, 2015, https://clinicaltrials.gov/ct2/show/NCT02395510

Keywords: Panic disorder, Vortioxetine, Anxiety, Agoraphobia, Depression

Background

Panic disorder (PD) is a common anxiety disorder affecting up to 5% of the population at a given time [1, 2]. It is characterized by one or more unexpected panic attacks followed by anticipatory worry about additional attacks, including a morbid fear of death. PD has been strongly linked to age, female gender, smoking, and depleted financial resources [3]. It can be severely disabling and can greatly worsen quality of life when associated with agoraphobia [2, 4]. PD has a strong co-morbidity with other anxiety disorders, especially social phobia and obsessive–compulsive disorder [5].

There are multiple neurobiological theories posited with regard to the genesis of PD. Three chemicals seem to be of particular importance: serotonin (5-HT), noradrenaline, and gamma-aminobutyric acid (GABA) [6]. While there are also other neurobiological mechanisms involving corticotrophic releasing factor (CRF), dysfunction of the hypothalamic–pituitary–adrenal gland, and disrupted GABA and glutamate activity, the following are the proposed mechanisms of action controlling panic attacks:

(1) Whereas 5-HT neurons located at the dorsal raphe nucleus are involved in the regulation of both inhibitory avoidance and escape, those of the median raphe nucleus are primarily implicated in panic attacks.

*Correspondence: ashah@siyanclinical.com
[1] Siyan Clinical Corporation, 480 Tesconi Dr., Santa Rosa, CA 95401, USA
Full list of author information is available at the end of the article

(2) Facilitation of 5-HT1A- and 5-HT2A-mediated neurotransmission in the dorsal periaqueductal gray (dPAG) is likely to mediate a panicolytic drug action.
(3) Stimulation of 5-HT2C receptors in the basolateral amygdala increases anxiety and is implicated in the anxiogenesis caused by short-term administration of antidepressant drugs.
4) 5-HT1A and the μ-opioid receptors work together in the dPAG to modulate escape or panic attacks.

In one meta-analysis of PD treatments, medications (especially serotonin–noradrenaline reuptake inhibitors) were found to be more effective based on calculated effect sizes, compared to psychotherapies and other therapies [7]. PD is generally treated very effectively with benzodiazepines, but these medications have a high risk for addiction, physical weakness, and cognitive impairment [8, 9] indicating the need for more effective long-term treatment. There are multiple drugs within the selective serotonin reuptake inhibitor (SSRI) and serotonin and norepinephrine reuptake inhibitor (SNRI) class that have proven efficacy in treating patients with PD [10–16]. Studies of treatment with paroxetine, venlafaxine, and escitalopram indicate positive results in the treatment of PD. The following antidepressants are significantly superior to placebo for PD patients, listed in increasing order of effectiveness: escitalopram, sertraline, paroxetine, fluoxetine, and venlafaxine for panic symptoms; paroxetine, fluoxetine, fluvoxamine, venlafaxine, and mirtazapine for overall anxiety symptoms [10–16].

Vortioxetine is an atypical antidepressant that has been approved for the treatment of the major depressive disorder [17]. The primary aim of this study was to evaluate the efficacy of vortioxetine in an adult patient population of PD with or without agoraphobia. Although the unique, multimodal mechanism of action of vortioxetine is not fully understood, it is thought to be related to enhancement of serotonergic activity in the CNS through inhibition of the reuptake of serotonin (5-HT) [18]. It also has several other functions, including 5-HT3 receptor antagonism and 5-HT1A receptor agonism. In vitro studies have shown it to be a 5HT1D and 5HT7 receptor antagonist and 5HT1B receptor partial agonist [19, 20].

In mouse models of anxiety and depression-like behavior, the antidepressant and anxiolytic effects produced by vortioxetine were greater than those produced by fluoxetine and comparable (in the open-field test) with those produced by diazepam [21]. In humans, a double-blind, randomized, fixed-dose (15 or 20 mg), placebo-controlled study showed that scores on the Hamilton Anxiety Rating Scale (HAM-A) decreased significantly from baseline with regular doses of vortioxetine [22]. No statistically significant gender differences have been observed in its action [23].

Based upon the evidence for the multimodal action of the drug and recent published data, the authors believe that vortioxetine may have clinical relevance in the treatment of PD, and our primary aim was to provide support for this hypothesis. The secondary aim of this study was to monitor the quality of life of subjects with PD when treated with vortioxetine.

Methods

Study design and patient recruitment

We designed an open-label 10 week-long study with fixed doses (5, 10, or 20 mg) to evaluate the safety, tolerability, and efficacy of vortioxetine for the treatment of PD, see Fig. 1 for the transparent reporting of evaluations with nonrandomized design (TREND) flowchart. 27 male and female subjects aged between 18 and 60 years, who met DSM-IV criteria for PD with or without agoraphobia, or who had a Panic Disorder Severity Scale (PDSS) score > 8 at baseline were screened. Institutional Review Board (IRB) approval for this study was obtained from the Schulman Associates IRB (Approval #: 201500056) and this study was conducted according to the World Medical Association Declaration of Helsinki. Only patients with active ongoing panic disorder were selected (as diagnosed by the Investigator as per the Diagnostic and Statistical Manual of Mental Disorders-Fourth Edition [DSM-IV] criteria using the MINI International Neuropsychiatric Interview 6.0); the previous treatment had not succeeded in eliminating their symptoms. Five patients were excluded for not meeting inclusion criteria, or not wishing to participate. After providing written informed consent, 22 subjects underwent a 7–14 day washout period of their current SSRI or SNRI medications. In the case of a subject taking a medication with a long half-life such as fluoxetine, a 5-week washout period prior to Baseline was allowed. There was no washout requirement for subjects using benzodiazepines or hypnotics prior to study enrollment. Subjects were allowed to continue concomitant treatment with these medications during the study; however, treatment was not initiated with benzodiazepines or hypnotics for any of the enrolled subjects, which allowed for a better overall assessment in the efficacy of vortioxetine for panic disorder. All subjects who participated in the study met the designated inclusion criteria and none of the exclusion criteria. Four patients discontinued the study, suffering from diarrhea, nausea, akathisia, dry skin, and itchiness. All patients with adverse events were monitored, serious, or otherwise. One patient suffered a serious adverse event (SAE) of a pulmonary embolus after completing the study; this event was not deemed as related to the study treatment.

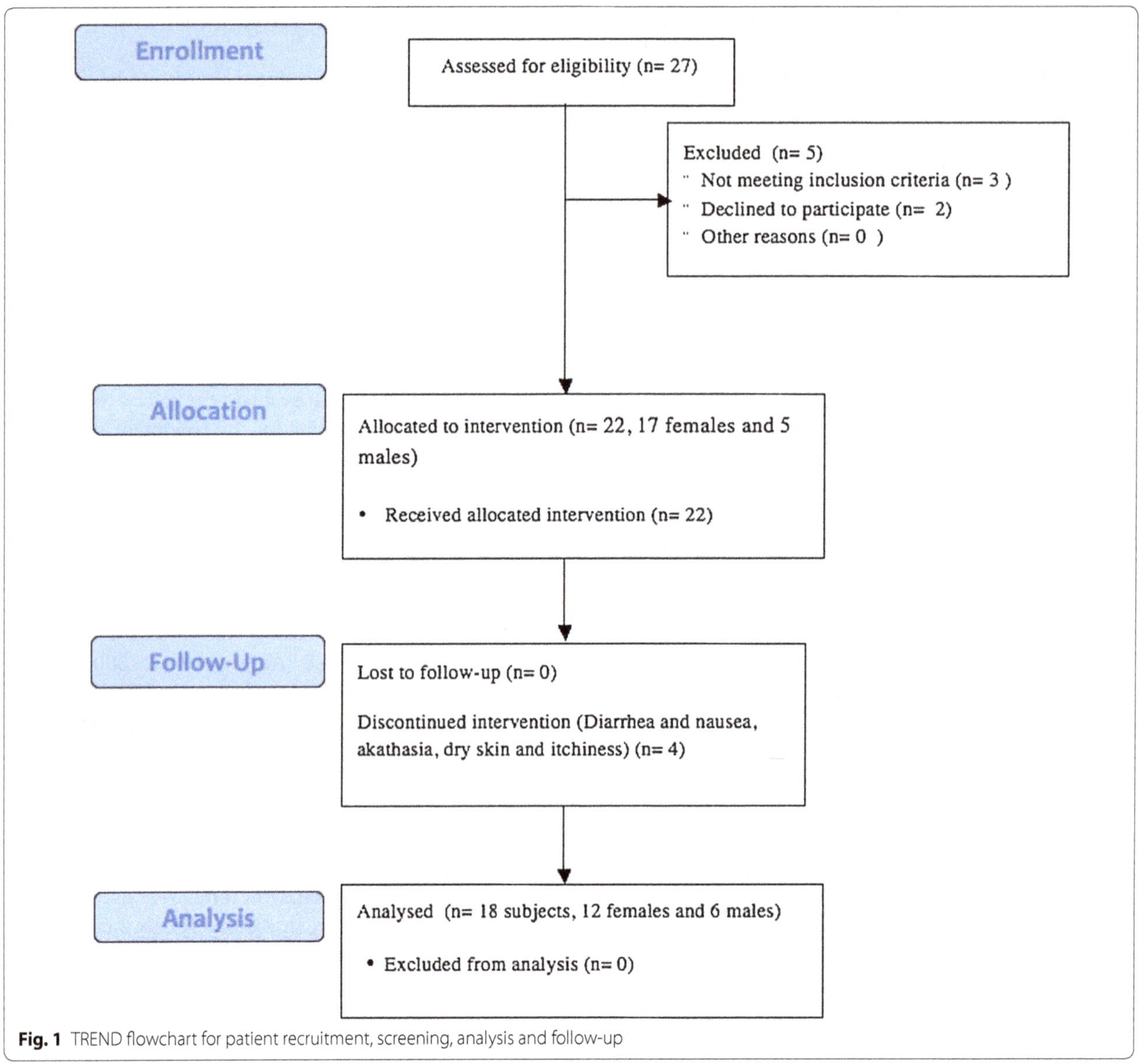

Fig. 1 TREND flowchart for patient recruitment, screening, analysis and follow-up

Dosing

Subjects received 5 mg of vortioxetine and were instructed to take one capsule orally, once daily in the morning, starting at the baseline visit (visit 1). Subjects were then seen bi-weekly following the baseline visit for a period of 10 weeks. The study medication was given on a flexible titration schedule until an optimal dose or response (in the opinion of the investigator) had been achieved for each subject. This design allowed the investigator to focus on the most effective dose for each subject with the total daily dose of vortioxetine not exceeding 20 mg.

Assessments

Two efficacy and two safety assessments were used. The efficacy assessments consisted of the Panic Disorder Severity Scale (PDSS) and the Quality-of-Life Scale (QOLS). The PDSS is a questionnaire developed for measuring the severity of PD and is considered a reliable tool for monitoring treatment outcome [24, 25]. The safety assessments included the Monitoring of Side Effects Scale (MOSES) and the Columbia-Suicide Severity Rating Scale (C-SSRS) [26, 27].

Statistical analysis

T tests were applied to compare the baseline scores for PDSS, QOLS, and MOSES to those for the same at the completion of the study for 18 patients (12 females and six males). Analyses and descriptive statistics were obtained using the R 3.1.1 statistical software (R foundation for Statistical Computing, Vienna, Austria).

Results

Patient population characteristics

From March to May 2016, 27 subjects were screened in the study, of which 20 were female. The median [IQR] age of the subjects was 39 (age range 23.5–49 years) (Fig. 2a). The median BMI of the patient population was 26.25 (range 23.58–29.2), and 59% were overweight (Fig. 2b). Major depressive disorder was the most frequent comorbidity in this patient population, followed by agoraphobia (Fig. 2c).

Significant decrease observed in overall PDSS scores and the frequency of panic attacks

PDSS score was used as a reliable method for measuring the severity of PD on each clinic visit. PDSS scores assess seven important criteria: panic frequency, distress during the panic attack, panic-focused anticipatory anxiety, phobic avoidance of situations, phobic avoidance of physical sensations, impairment in work functioning, and impairment in social functioning, and provide an overall score for PD severity. A total of 18 subjects, 12 females and six males, completed the study. A statistically significant decrease was observed between the baseline PDSS scores and final scores upon completing the study ($p < 0.05$), with a mean decrease of 8.89 (Fig. 3).

With respect to PDSS question one, regarding the frequency of panic attacks, a statistically significant improvement was observed between the baseline scores and those at the completion of the study ($p < 0.05$), with an observed decrease of 1.11 in the mean score.

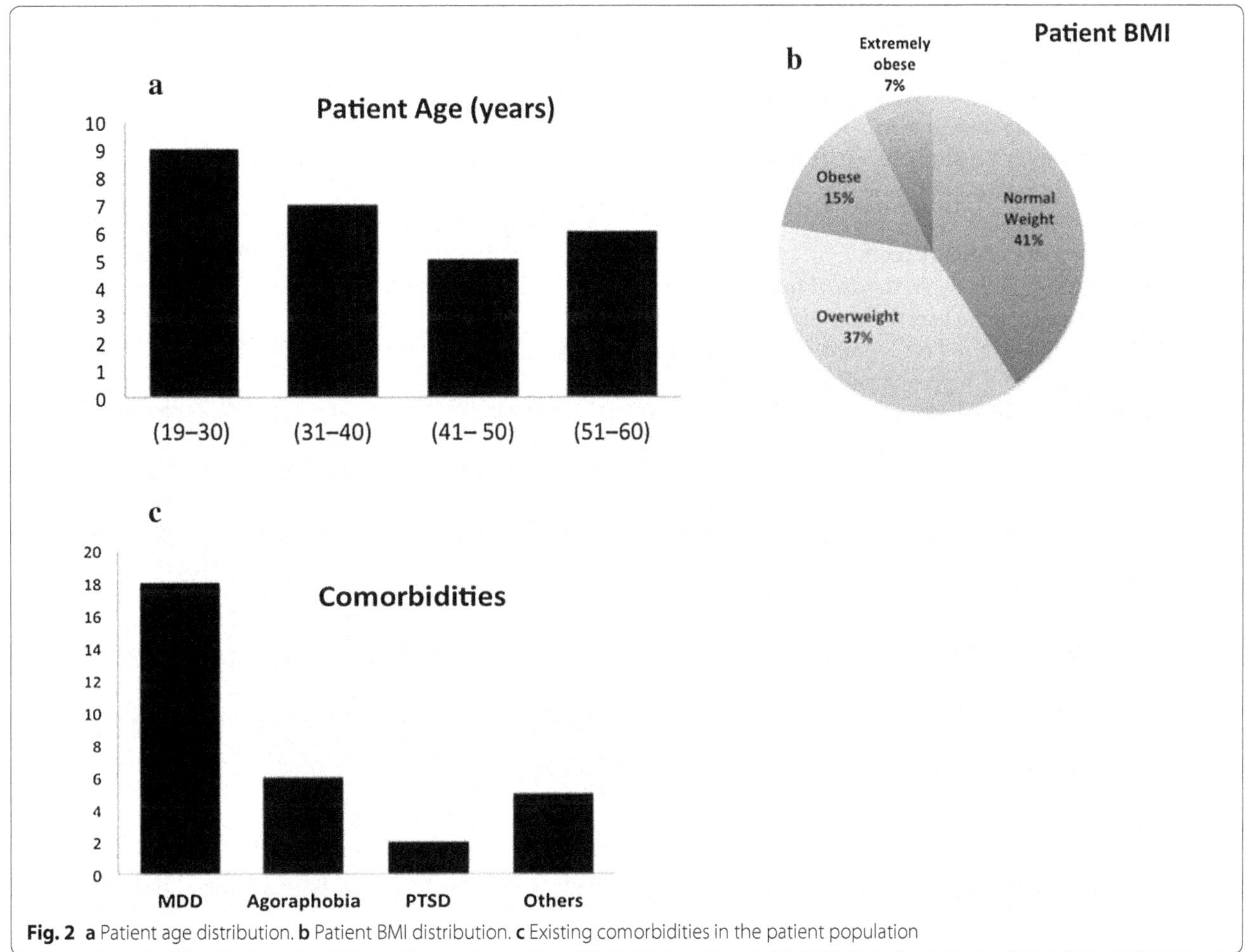

Fig. 2 **a** Patient age distribution. **b** Patient BMI distribution. **c** Existing comorbidities in the patient population

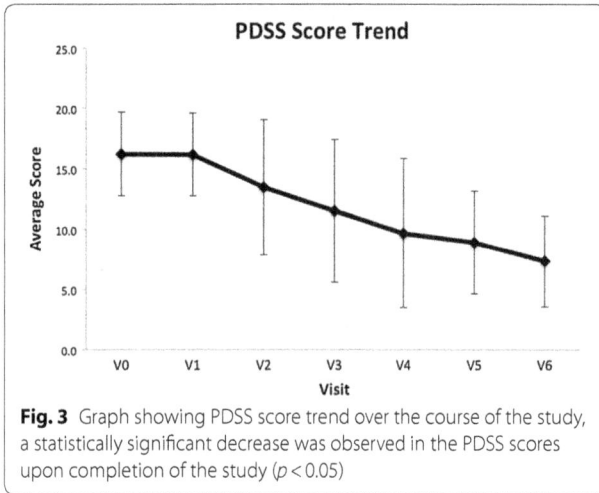

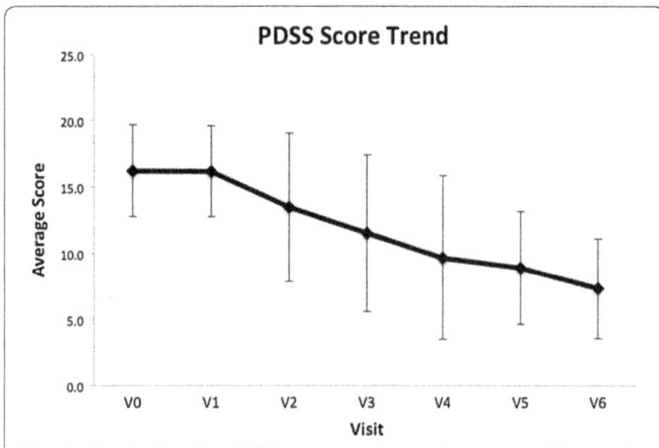

Fig. 3 Graph showing PDSS score trend over the course of the study, a statistically significant decrease was observed in the PDSS scores upon completion of the study ($p < 0.05$)

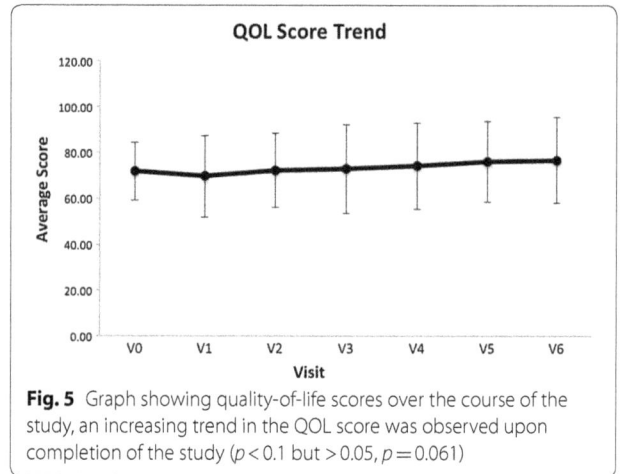

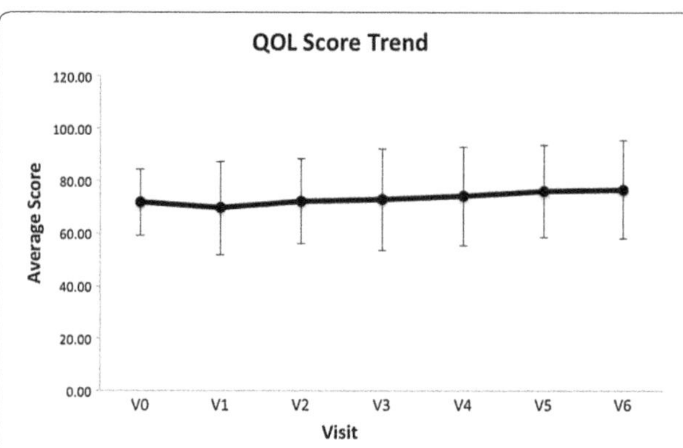

Fig. 5 Graph showing quality-of-life scores over the course of the study, an increasing trend in the QOL score was observed upon completion of the study ($p < 0.1$ but > 0.05, $p = 0.061$)

Statistically significant decrease observed in the MOSES score

The MOSES scale was used to document the safety and tolerability of vortioxetine. The MOSES has 73 items presented in layperson's language organized into nine body areas representing a typical physical examination. A statistically significant decrease (an improvement) was observed between the baseline MOSES score and the score upon completing the study ($p = 0.014$), with a mean decrease of 1.06 on the MOSES scale (Fig. 4).

An increase observed in the QOL score

The Quality-of-Life (QOL) scale is a valid instrument for measuring the quality of life across the patient groups [9]. The QOLS has 16 items rated on 7-point response scales. Higher scores indicate a higher quality of life. A trend towards an increase was observed in QOL score upon the completion of the study ($p = 0.061$), with a mean gain of 4.944 (Fig. 5).

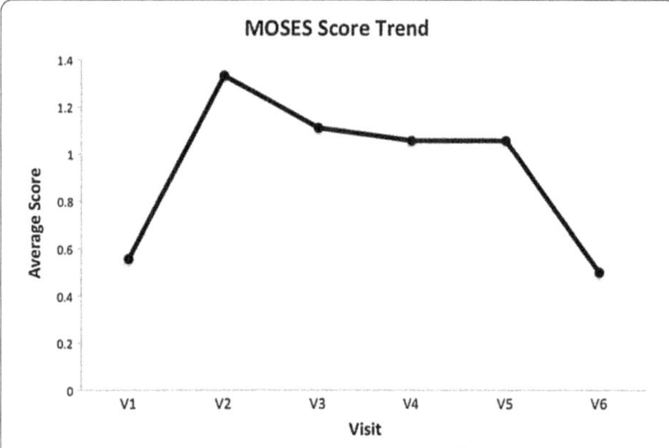

Fig. 4 Graph showing monitoring of the side effects over the course of the study, a significant decrease was observed in the MOSES score ($p = 0.014$)

Limitations

The sample size is small ($n = 22$) and mostly consisted of female subjects; with 18 subjects completing the study. There was neither a placebo or active control arm, nor randomization of subjects used for this study.

Discussion

Despite the current treatments available, as many as one-third of patients with PD have persistent and treatment-resistant panic attacks [28]. A previous meta-analysis study has shown that vortioxetine was efficacious in reducing depressive and anxiety symptoms in patients with MDD and high levels of anxiety [29]. We aimed to evaluate the effectiveness of vortioxetine in patients with panic disorder. Previous studies of vortioxetine efficacy have focused on different scoring measures, most notably the Hamilton Anxiety Rating Scale [30] and the personality diagnostic questionnaire (PDQ), which provides self-measurement of cognitive function [31]. We adopted the Panic Disorder Severity Scale which is a widely accepted clinical tool used for the measurement of panic disorder symptom severity. It has been shown to have acceptable internal consistency (Cronbach's $\alpha = 0.65$) and high inter-relater reliability with correlation coefficients ranging from 0.87 to 0.88 [32].

Using the PDSS, a statistically significant decrease in the occurrence of panic attacks was measured from baseline to study completion. The mean decrease in PDSS scores was 8.89 ($p < 0.05$), indicative of less severe PD. Regarding the frequency of panic attacks or question one on the scale, a statistically significant improvement was observed between baseline and study completion ($p < 0.05$), with an observed decrease of 1.11 in the mean frequency of attacks.

Administration of the MOSES scale provided an insight into the safety and tolerability of vortioxetine. The results of this monitoring showed a statistically significant decrease in the MOSES score upon study completion ($p = 0.014$), indicating a decrease in observed side effects. Likewise, the Quality-of-Life Scale (QOLS) showed an improvement in scores. This scale has been validated for measuring the quality of life across patient groups [8].

The prevalence of panic disorder remains high, with a large percentage of patients unable to remain gainfully employed and presenting with a higher rate of hospitalizations. Our results provide support for the use of vortioxetine in the management of panic disorder.

Conclusions

Our study provides support for the use of vortioxetine in the management of panic disorder.

Abbreviations

dPAG: dorsal periaqueductal gray; CRF: corticotrophic releasing factor; GABA: gamma-aminobutyric acid; MDD: major depressive disorder; MOSES: Monitoring of Side Effects Scale; PD: panic disorder; PDQ: personality diagnostic questionnaire; PDSS: Panic Disorder Severity Scale; QOLS: Quality-of-Life Scale; SNRI: serotonin and norepinephrine reuptake inhibitor; SSRI: selective serotonin reuptake inhibitor.

Authors' contributions

AS collected and analyzed patient data, and contributed to writing the manuscript. JN analyzed and interpreted patient data, and contributed to writing the manuscript. All authors read and approved the final manuscript.

Author details

[1] Siyan Clinical Corporation, 480 Tesconi Dr., Santa Rosa, CA 95401, USA.
[2] Northcutt Consulting, LLC, Orlando, USA.

Acknowledgements

None.

Competing interests

The authors declare that they have no competing interests.

Consent for publication

Not applicable.

Funding

This study was funded by Takeda Pharmaceuticals USA, Inc, but the Sponsor was not involved in study design, collection, analysis, and interpretation of data and in writing the manuscript.

References

1. Kessler RC, Chiu WT, Jin R, Ruscio AM, Shear K, Walters EE. The epidemiology of panic attacks, panic disorder, and agoraphobia in the national comorbidity survey replication. Arch Gen Psychiatry. 2006;63(4):415–24.
2. Roy-Byrne PP, Craske MG, Stein MB. Panic disorder. Lancet. 2006;368(9540):1023–32.
3. Moreno-Peral P, Conejo-Ceron S, Motrico E, Rodriguez-Morejon A, Fernandez A, Garcia-Campayo J, Roca M, Serrano-Blanco A, Rubio-Valera M, Bellon JA. Risk factors for the onset of panic and generalised anxiety disorders in the general adult population: a systematic review of cohort studies. J Affect Disord. 2014;168:337–48.
4. Taylor CB. Panic disorder. BMJ. 2006;332(7547):951–5.
5. Camuri G, Oldani L, Dell'Osso B, Benatti B, Lietti L, Palazzo C, Altamura AC. Prevalence and disability of comorbid social phobia and obsessive-compulsive disorder in patients with panic disorder and generalized anxiety disorder. Int J Psychiatry Clin Pract. 2014;18(4):248–54.
6. Zwanger P, Rupprecht R. Selective GABAergic treatment for panic? Investigations in experimental panic induction and panic disorder. J Psychiatry Neurosci. 2005;30(3):167–75.
7. Bandelow B, Reitt M, Röver C, et al. Efficacy of treatments for anxiety disorders: a meta-analysis. Int Clin Psychopharmacol. 2015;30(4):183–92. https://doi.org/10.1097/YIC0000000000000078.
8. Offidani E, Guidi J, Tomba E, Fava GA. Efficacy and tolerability of benzodiazepines versus antidepressants in anxiety disorders: a systematic review and meta-analysis. Psychother Psychosom. 2013;82(6):355–62.
9. Perna G, Alciati A, Riva A, Micieli W, Caldirola D. Long-term pharmacological treatments of anxiety disorders: an updated systematic review. Curr Psychiatry Rep. 2016;18(3):23.
10. Katzman MA, Jacobs L. Venlaxifine in the treatment of panic disorder. Neuropsychiatr Dis Treat. 2007;3(1):59–67.
11. Simon NM, Otto MW, Worthington LL, et al. Next-step strategies for panic disorder refractory to initial pharmacotherapy. J Clin Psychiatry. 2009;70(11):1563–70.
12. Fochtmann LJ, editor. Practice guideline for the treatment of patients with panic disorder. 2nd ed. Washington, D.C.: American Psychiatric Association; 2000.
13. Perna G, Dacco S, Menotti R, et al. Antianxiety medication for the treatment of complex agoraphobia: pharmacological interventions for a behavioral condition. Neuropsychiatr Dis Treat. 2011;7:621–37.
14. Pecknold JC, Luthe L, Iny L, et al. Fluoxetine in panic disorder: pharmacologic and tritiated platelet imipramine and paroxetine binding study. J Psychiatry Neurosci. 1995;20(3):193–8.
15. Bakker A, van Balkom AJLM, Stein DJ, et al. Evidence-based pharmacotherapy of panic disorder. Int J Neuropsychopharmcol. 2005;8:473–82.
16. Holt RL, Lydiard RB. Management of treatment-resistant panic disorder. Psychiatry. 2007;4(10):48–59.
17. Connolly KR, Thase ME. Vortioxetine: a new treatment for major depressive disorder. Expert Opin Pharmacother. 2016;17(3):421–31.
18. Katona CL, Katona CP. New generation multi-modal antidepressants: focus on vortioxetine for major depressive disorder. Neuropsychiatr Dis Treat. 2014;10:349–54.
19. Orsolini L, Tomasetti C, Valchera A, et al. New advances in the treatment of generalized anxiety disorder: the multimodal antidepressant vortioxetine. Expert Rev Neurother. 2016;16(5):483–95. https://doi.org/10.1586/14737175.2016.1173545.
20. Stahl SM. Modes and nodes explain the mechanism of action of vortioxetine, a multimodal agent (MMA): enhancing serotonin release by combining serotonin (5HT) transporter inhibition with actions at 5HT receptors (5HT1A, 5HT1B, 5HT1D, 5HT7 receptors). CNS Spectr. 2015;20(02):93–7.
21. Guilloux JP, Mendez-David I, Pehrson A, Guiard BP, Reperant C, Orvoen S, Gardier AM, Hen R, Ebert B, Miller S, et al. Antidepressant and anxiolytic potential of the multimodal antidepressant vortioxetine (Lu AA21004) assessed by behavioural and neurogenesis outcomes in mice. Neuropharmacology. 2013;73:147–59.
22. Boulenger JP, Loft H, Olsen CK. Efficacy and safety of vortioxetine (Lu AA21004), 15 and 20 mg/day: a randomized, double-blind, placebo-controlled, duloxetine-referenced study in the acute treatment of adult patients with major depressive disorder. Int Clin Psychopharmacol. 2014;29(3):138–49.
23. Areberg J, Søgaard B, Højer AM. The clinical pharmacokinetics of Lu AA21004 and its major metabolite in healthy young volunteers. Basic Clin Pharmacol Toxicol. 2012;111(3):198–205.
24. Shear MK, Brown TA, Barlow DH, Money R, Sholomskas DE, Woods SW, Gorman JM, Papp LA. Multicenter collaborative panic disorder severity scale. Am J Psychiatry. 1997;154(11):1571–5.
25. Shear MK, Rucci P, Williams J, Frank E, Grochocinski V, Vander Bilt J, Houck P, Wang T. Reliability and validity of the Panic Disorder Severity Scale: replication and extension. J Psychiatr Res. 2001;35(5):293–6.

26. Kalachnik JE. Measuring side effects of psychopharmacologic medication in individuals with mental retardation and developmental disabilities. Ment Retard Dev Disabil Res Rev. 1999;5(4):348–59.
27. Posner K, Melvin GA, Stanley B, Oquendo MA, Gould M. Factors in the assessment of suicidality in youth. CNS Spectr. 2007;12(2):156–62.
28. Friere RC, Zugliani MM, Garcia RF, et al. Treatment-resistant panic disorder: a systematic review. Expert Opin Pharmocother. 2016;17(2):159–68. https://doi.org/10.1517/14656566.2016.1109628.
29. Baldwin DS, et al. A meta-analysis of the efficacy of vortioxetine in patients with major depressive disorder (MDD) and high levels of anxiety. J Affect Disord. 2016;206:140–50. https://doi.org/10.1016/j.jad.2016.07.015.
30. Bidzan L, Mahableshwarkar AR, Jacobsen P, Yan M, Sheehan DV. Vortioxetine (Lu AA21004) in generalized anxiety disorder: results of an 8-week, multinational, randomized, double-blind, placebo-controlled clinical trial. Eur Neuropsychopharmacol. 2012;22(12):847–57.
31. Mahableshwarkar AR, Zajecka J, Jacobson W, Chen Y, Keefe RS. A randomized, placebo-controlled, active-reference, double-blind, flexible-dose study of the efficacy of vortioxetine on cognitive function in major depressive disorder. Neuropsychopharmacology. 2015;40(8):2025–37.
32. Keough ME, Porter E, Kredlow MA, Worthington JJ, Hoge EA, Pollack MH, Shear MK, Simon NM. Anchoring the panic disorder severity scale. Assessment. 2012;19(2):257–9.

25

Association of Schizoid and Schizotypal Personality disorder with violent crimes and homicides in Greek prisons

Athanasios Apostolopoulos[1*], Ioannis Michopoulos[1], Ioannis Zachos[3], Emmanouil Rizos[1], Georgios Tzeferakos[1], Vasiliki Manthou[3], Charalambos Papageorgiou[2] and Athanasios Douzenis[1]

Abstract

Background: Personality disorders (PDs) have been associated with both violent crimes and homicides in many studies. The proportion of PDs among prisoners reaches up to 80%. For male prisoners, the most common PD in the literature is antisocial PD. The aim of this study was to investigate the association between PDs and violent crimes/homicides of male prisoners in Greece.

Methods: A sample of 308 subjects was randomly selected from a population of 1300 male prisoners incarcerated in two Greek prisons, one urban and one rural. The presence of PDs was assessed using the Mini International Neuropsychiatric Interview (MINI) and the Personality Diagnostic Questionnaire-4 (PDQ-4). Using logistic regression models PD types and PD "Clusters" (independent variables) were associated with "violent/non-violent crimes" and "homicides/non homicides" (dependent variables).

Results: "Cluster A" PDs (Paranoid, Schizoid, and Schizotypal) were diagnosed in 16.2%, "Cluster B" (Antisocial, Borderline, Histrionic, Narcissistic) in 66.9% and "Cluster C" (Obsessive–Compulsive, Dependent, Avoidant) in 2.9% of the studied population. Violent crimes and homicides were found significantly associated with "Cluster A" PDs ($p=0.022$, $p=0.020$). The odds ratio of committing violent crimes was 2.86 times higher for patients with "Cluster A" PDs than the ones without PDs. In addition, the odds ratio of committing homicides was 4.25 times higher for patients with "Cluster A" PDs. In separate analyses, the commitment of violent crimes as well as homicides, was significantly associated with Schizoid ($p=0.043$, $p=0.020$) and Schizotypal PD ($p=0.017$, $p=0.030$).

Conclusions: The majority of prisoners was found to suffer from a PD, mainly the Antisocial "Cluster B", but the commitment of violent crimes and homicides was significantly associated only with "Cluster A" PDs and specifically with Schizoid and Schizotypal PD.

Keywords: Personality disorders, Prisoners, Cluster A, Schizotypal, Schizoid

Background

According to *DSM-IV, the proportion of Personality Disorder* (PD) types in the general population is: 5.7% for "Cluster A" (Paranoid, Schizoid, Schizotypal), 1.5% for "Cluster B" (Antisocial, Borderline, Histrionic, Narcissistic) and 6.0% for "Cluster C" (Obsessive–Compulsive, Dependent, Avoidant) [1]. Furthermore, in 9.1% of the cases, two or more PDs co-exist [1]. Fourteen studies examined the risk of antisocial and violent behavior in 10,007 individuals with PDs, compared with over 12 million general population controls [2]. The results showed a substantially increased risk of violent outcomes in all PD types. Meta-analysis revealed that Antisocial PD and male gender were associated with the higher risks [2].

"Cluster B" PDs are affecting behavior and lifestyle and cause significant problems not only to the disordered individual but to society as well [3]. Among criminal

*Correspondence: th.apostolopoulos@gmail.com
[1] 2nd Psychiatric Department of the University of Athens, Attikon Hospital, Athens, Greece
Full list of author information is available at the end of the article

offenders the proportion of Personality disorders is much higher [4] and can reach up to 80% in some studies [5]. Antisocial PD predominates among male offenders, while Borderline PD among female ones [6–8].

In a study by Riesco et al. [9] conducted in Spanish prisons, 91% of the prisoners had one or more PDs. Antisocial PD was diagnosed in 79% of the population while Paranoid PD and Borderline PD in 52% and 41%, respectively. Using the Mini International Neuropsychiatric Interview (MINI) and the Personality Diagnostic Questionnaire 4 (PDQ-4), Piselli et al. [10] found that the most frequent psychiatric disorder—in incarcerated offenders—was PD (51.9%). In a similar study by Coolidge et al. [11], 61% of prisoners had been diagnosed at least with one PD. Furthermore, Köhler et al. [12] found that the proportion of "Cluster B" PDs among incarcerated offenders was more than 62%. As mentioned before, Antisocial PD is found predominantly among male prisoners. This finding is supported by several studies: Kugu et al. reported a percentage of 48.6% [13], Naidoo and Mkize 46.1% [14] and Longato-Stadler et al. 56% [15]. In a systematic review of Fazel and Danesh [7]—23,000 incarcerated individuals with more than 9000 violent prisoners included—PDs were diagnosed in 42% of the sample, among which 21% was Antisocial PD. Among prisoners in Greece, Fotiadou et al. found that the percentage of Antisocial PD was 37.5% [16].

However, Antisocial PD is not the only PD related to violent crimes. According to Fountoulakis et al. [17], Paranoid, Antisocial, Narcissistic, Borderline and Schizoid PDs ("Clusters A and B") are all associated with violent crime. A significant association has been described, as well, between PDs of "Clusters A and B" and homicides. In case of homicide the most frequently encountered psychiatric diagnoses are PDs, drug addiction and alcohol abuse. More specifically, "Cluster B" PDs can be found in up to 60% of the cases. According to Crump et al. [18], people suffering from PDs and substance use disorders were more frequently convicted for homicide crimes. Richard-Devantoy et al. [8] claim, as well, that the association between comorbid Antisocial PD and alcoholism with murder is strong: Antisocial PD increased the risk of committing homicide 10 times compared to a Psychotic Disorder. In Finland, at least one diagnosis of PD was involved in 358 of the 593 homicides recorded from 1996 to 2004 [19].

As depicted, there is a much higher frequency of PDs in the prisons' population compared to the general population. These disorders are predominantly "Cluster B" (especially Antisocial PD), followed by "Cluster A" PDs. Despite the fact that in the recent years there seems to be an increased scientific interest in studying and understanding the link between PDs and typology of criminal behavior, there are many contradictory findings that need clarification. In Greece, there have been no studies addressing these questions in prisoners.

This study was an attempt to record PDs among male prisoners in Greece and investigate the possible association between these disorders and violent offences and homicides.

Method

Study design and population

This is a cross-sectional study conducted in two Greek prisons; one urban (Korydallos) and one rural (Domokos). Data were collected from March 2012 till August 2013. The sample comprised of 308 male individuals randomly sampled from a total of 1300 prisoners, aged between 18 and 77 years. The sample included Greek and foreign prisoners who either had the Greek citizenship or could read and speak in Greek. Every third name of the registry of the prison was chosen. In 88 cases of unavailability/difficulties in understanding the language or denial (57 cases), the next prisoner was asked to participate in the study.

Inmates who were found to be suffering from psychotic disorders during the interviews were excluded from the study.

Data collection

The psychiatric screening of prisoners was conducted with the Greek version 5.0.0 DSM-IV of Mini International Neuropsychiatric Interview (MINI) [20, 21] and the Greek version of Personality Diagnostic Questionnaire-4 (PDQ-4) [4, 22, 23]. The psychiatric examination was conducted by two psychiatrists. Initially demographics and other characteristics presented in Table 1 were recorded followed by a psychiatric assessment. The whole duration of the first interview was about 60 min. During the second interview, the PDQ-4 questionnaire was administered by the examiners, who were present till the end of the test (total duration about 60 min). Inmates who initially had shown mixed disorders or were not adequately assessed, were re-questioned (as suggested by the Personality Questionnaire manual) in order to conclude at one type of Personality Disorder. The third diagnostic interview's duration was about 45 min.

Regarding the criminal record of the individuals assessed, the total number of incarcerations as well as their index offence that led to their imprisonment at the time of the study, were recorded. The assessing psychiatrists had no knowledge of the index offence during the initial interview. The offences that led to imprisonment were divided and categorized, according to the Greek Penal Code into violent (crimes against life, personal injuries, crimes against personal freedom, crimes against

Table 1 Demographics and other characteristics of prisoners in Greece ($n = 308$)

	N (%)
Age (*M*, SD years)	38.3 (10.8)
Nationality	
Greek	270 (87.7)
Other	38 (12.3)
Educational status	
Primary school	162 (52.6)
Middle school	125 (40.6)
College	10 (3.2)
University	11 (3.6)
Family status	
Married	93 (30.4)
Single	160 (52.3)
Widowed	6 (2.0)
Divorced	39 (12.7)
Separated	8 (2.6)
Children	123 (39.9)
Violence between parents	152 (49.4)
Relationship with father	
Good	192 (62.3)
Bad	63 (20.5)
Casual	53 (17.2)
Relationship with mother	
Good	245 (80.1)
Bad	14 (4.6)
Casual	47 (15.4)
Tobacco use	295 (95.8)
Alcohol use	272 (88.3)
Cannabis use	208 (67.5)
Drug use	179 (58.5)
Pyromania during childhood/puberty	204 (66.2)
Gang member	151 (49.0)
Animal abuse	201 (65.3)
Psycho traumatic event	126 (41.0)
Living status prior to imprisonment	
Alone	78 (25.4)
With family	98 (31.9)
With parents	65 (21.2)
Other	66 (21.5)
Soldiering	
Fulfilled	201 (65.3)
Dispensation	107 (34.7)
First imprisonment	158 (51.3)
Type of crime	
Violent	95 (30.8)
Non-violent	213 (69.2)

M mean value, *SD* standard deviation

sexuality freedom, common danger crimes) and non-violent (crimes against ownership, debts to state, crimes related to drugs, crimes against property rights, crimes against honor, crimes related to marriage, crimes related to service, crimes related to currency). The crimes of homicide/attempted homicide were recorded separately from the other violent crimes and regardless the number of victims. Also for individuals that had multiple convictions, their most serious crime was recorded for the purpose of this study; e.g. for a conviction for both attempted murder and robbery, the individual was recorded under the category of "attempted murder".

Statistical analyses

Quantitative variables were expressed as mean values (*M*) and standard deviations (SD), while qualitative variables were expressed as absolute frequencies (*N*) and relative frequencies (%). For the comparison of proportions, Chi square and Fisher's exact tests were used. Multiple logistic regression models with a stepwise method (p for entry 0.05, p for removal 0.10) were used in order to test whether PD types and PD "Clusters" were independently associated with violent crimes and homicides. PD types and PD "Clusters" were used as independent variables, whereas "violent/non-violent crimes" and "homicides–attempted homicides/non homicides" as dependent variables. Variables that regarded social, economic, demographic or clinical characteristics were not included in the analysis due to sample size. More statistical tests could have led to a lower study power. Adjusted odds ratios (OR) and the respective 95% confidence intervals (CI) were computed. Statistical significance was set at $p \leq 0.05$. All reported p values are two-tailed and analyses were conducted using SPSS statistical software (version 19.0).

Results

The study population consisted of 308 participants from a total of 1300 prisoners. Their mean age was 38.3 years (SD = 10.8). Almost half of the participants (51.3%) were imprisoned for the first time. For 30.8% of the participants conviction was a result of a violent crime. Homicide was recorded for 38 of the cases (12.3%). Homicides along with attempted homicides were recorded for 46 cases (14.9%). Demographics and other characteristics are presented in Table 1.

PDs were diagnosed in 89% ($N = 275$) of the population. The types of PDs diagnosed are shown in Fig. 1. The most common PD was Antisocial (42.5%), followed by Borderline (15.9%), Narcissistic (7.8%), Schizoid (7.1%) and

Paranoid (7.1%). For 10.7% ($N=33$) of the participants no PD was diagnosed. "Cluster A" PDs were found in 16.2% of the participants, while "Clusters B and C" were found in 66.9% and 2.9% of the participants, respectively.

As extracted from Table 2, among prisoners with Antisocial, Borderline and Narcissistic Disorder, 77.1%, 65.3% and 58.3%, respectively, had been imprisoned for non-violent crimes. Nevertheless, most of the violent crimes ($N=30$) as well as homicides/attempted homicides ($N=12$) had been committed by individuals with Antisocial Disorder. Of those cases with Schizoid, Schizotypal and Paranoid disorder, 50.0%, 66.7% and 45.5%, respectively, had been incarcerated for violent crimes. On the other hand, 24.2% of violent crimes were committed by inmates with no diagnosis of a PD. Subjects of "Cluster A" PDs, in total, had committed 17 of the 46 homicides/attempted homicides.

Compared with prisoners without PD, the percentages of violent crimes and homicides/attempted homicides were significantly higher in those belonging to "Cluster A" and in those with Schizoid or Schizotypal PD alone (Table 2).

Multiple logistic regression analysis with "violent crimes/no violent crimes" as the dependent variable showed that the likelihood to commit a violence crime was significantly higher in "Cluster A" PDs ($p=0.022$, OR = 2.86). When all the PD types were included in the model instead of PDs "Clusters", it was found that Schizoid ($p=0.043$, OR = 3.49) and Schizotypal ($p=0.017$, OR = 10.5) PDs were significantly associated with a higher likelihood of violence crimes. Multiple logistic regression analysis with "homicides–attempted homicides/no homicides", as dependent variable, had similar results. Prisoners of "Cluster A" ($p=0.020$, OR = 4.25) and those with Schizoid ($p=0.020$, OR = 5.26) or Schizotypal ($p=0.030$, OR = 8.80) PDs had significantly increased likelihood for committing or attempting a homicide (Table 3).

Discussion

Personality disorders

The assessment of PDs, based on the DSM-IV classification and structured diagnostic instruments, is conflicting. It is possible individuals who meet the criteria for a particular Personality disorder meet as well the criteria for other Personality disorders. The new diagnostic approach in DSM-5 describes the Personality disorders as qualitatively distinct clinical syndromes. Nevertheless, in this study, diagnoses were based on MINI Interview and PDQ-4 Questionnaire because the use of the same instruments with other similar studies makes the results comparable and helps the scientific discussion on the association between violent crimes and psychiatric disorders.

PDs were diagnosed in the vast majority (89%) of the prisoners' sample. The most common PD was Antisocial

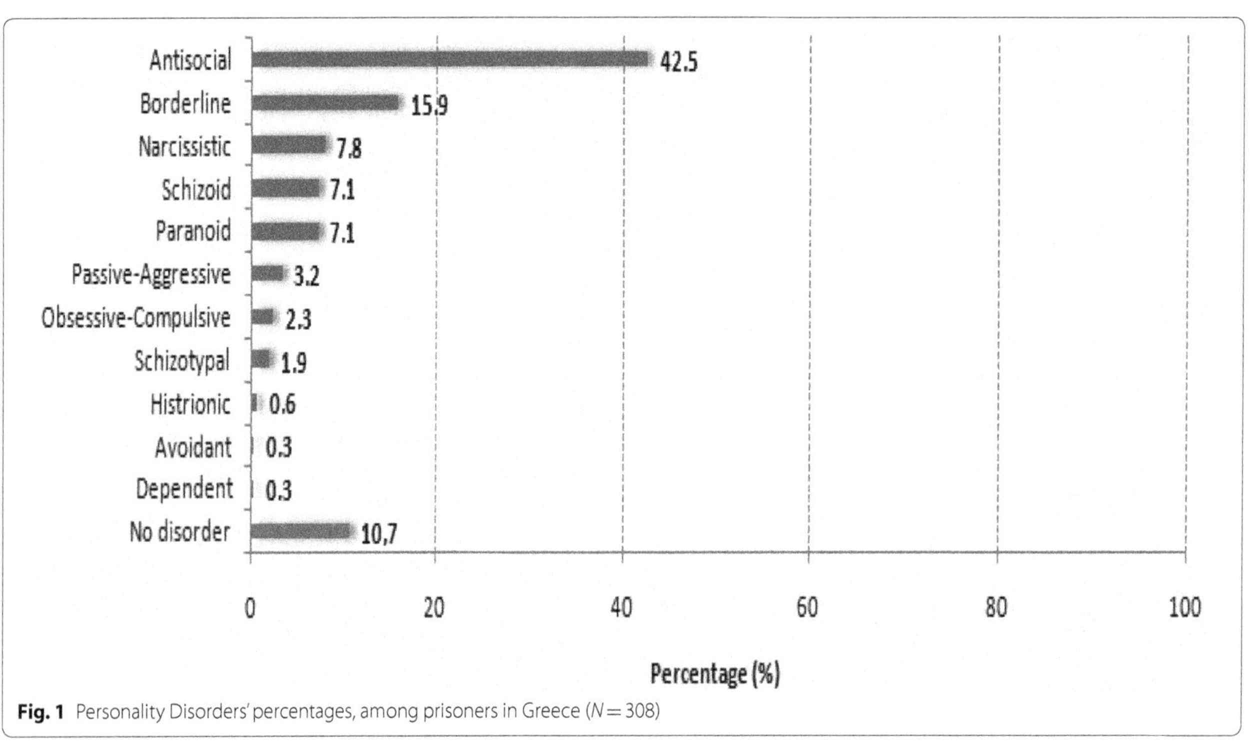

Fig. 1 Personality Disorders' percentages, among prisoners in Greece ($N=308$)

Table 2 Differences in Personality disorder percentages among prisoners in Greece with violent crimes and homicides–attempted homicides ($N = 308$)

	Violent crimes *N* (%)	*p**	Homicides/attempted homicides *N* (%)	*p**
PD diagnosis				
Antisocial	30 (22.9)	0.870	12 (9.2)	0.608
Borderline	17 (34.7)	0.313	10 (20.4)	0.328
Narcissistic	10 (41.7)	0.162	1 (4.2)	0.385**
Paranoid	10 (45.5)	0.100	6 (27.3)	0.175**
Histrionic	1 (50.0)	0.454**	0 (0.0)	1.000**
Schizoid	11 (50.0)	0.049	8 (36.4)	0.047**
Schizotypal	4 (66.7)	0. 050**	3 (50.0)	0.026**
Obsessive–Compulsive	0 (0.0)	0. 309**	0 (0.0)	1.000**
Dependent	0 (0.0)	1.000**	0 (0.0)	1.000**
Avoidant	0 (0.0)	1.000**	0 (0.0)	1.000**
Passive–aggressive	4 (40.0)	0.330	2 (20.0)	0.611**
No PD	8 (24.2)		4 (12.1)	
PD Cluster				
A	25 (50.0)	0.019	17 (34.0)	0.025
B	58 (28.2)	0.641	23 (11.2)	0.774**
C	0 (0.0)	0.168	0 (0.0)	0.561**

PD Personal Disorder, *Cluster A PD* Paranoid/Schizoid/Schizotypal PD, *Cluster B PD* Antisocial/Borderline/Histrionic/Narcissistic PD, *Cluster C PD* Obsessive/Compulsive/Dependent/Avoidant PD

* Chi square test for the comparison with those without PD, ** Fisher's exact test

(42.5%). The likelihood of committing a violent crime or homicide–attempt homicide,was significantly greater among those with Schizoid or Schizotypal PD.

The high prevalence of psychopathology in the population of incarcerated offenders is well documented in the literature and also reflected in this study. PDs were the most common disorders among prison inmates in Italy [10]. At least one type of PD was diagnosed in 61% of a prison population sample according to Coolidge et al. [11]. Langeveld and Melhus reported that PDs were found in 80% of the prisoners. In the same study, antisocial PD was present in more than 60% of the study population [24]. Results from a systematic review of 62 studies with a total sample of 23,000 prisoners reported that 65% of the population had PDs, and 47% had Antisocial PD [7]. Similar results were reported in Greek populations by Fountoulakis et al. [17] and Fotiadou et al. [16].

In this study Antisocial PD was diagnosed in 42.5% of the participants, Borderline PD in 15.9% and Narcissistic PD in 7.8%. Histrionic PD was diagnosed only in 0.6% of the individuals. A definite dominance of "Cluster B" PDs was obvious which is in concordance with the literature. Köhler et al. found that the prevalence of "Cluster B" PDs in a sample of male incarcerated juvenile offenders in Germany was up to 62%. Findings from this study were very similar to our results: the proportion of "Cluster B" PDs was 66.9%, whilst "Cluster A" was 16.2% and "Cluster C" 2.9%.

Personality disorders in relation to violent crimes

Of those diagnosed with Antisocial, Borderline and Narcissistic disorder in this study, 77.1%, 65.3% and 58.3%, respectively, had been imprisoned for non-violent crimes. Nevertheless, in absolute numbers, most of the violent offenses had been committed by inmates presenting Antisocial Disorder. However, a significant association of violent crimes and "Cluster B" PDs has not been established. According to Palmstierna, Antisocial PD and antisocial personality traits are connected with violence [25]. Similarly Pondé et al. and González et al. suggest a strong association of Antisocial and Borderline PDs with violent crime [26, 27].

High incidence of "Cluster B" PDs is often seen in the literature, although higher rates of "Cluster A" disorders have also been reported in prison's populations, usually associated with a high prevalence of Paranoid PD [9]. In this study, 16.2% of prisoners had "Cluster A" PDs; 1.9% Schizotypal; 7.1% Schizoid, and 7.1% Paranoid PD. Diagnosis with "Cluster A" disorders had an association with the commitment of violent crimes. Of those diagnosed

Table 3 Multiple logistic regressions with "violent crimes" and "homicides–attempted homicides" as dependent variables in two Greek prisons ($N = 308$)

	OR (95% CI)	*p*
Violent crimes		
PD Clusters		
No PDs	1.00[a]	
A	2.86 (1.16–7.04)	0.022
B	1.91 (0.85–4.31)	0.118
C	–[b]	–
PD diagnosis		
No PDs	1.00[a]	
Antisocial	2.23 (0.83–6.05)	0.114
Borderline	1.91 (0.67–5.67)	0.229
Narcissistic	2.76 (0.85–8.97)	0.092
Paranoid	2.99 (0.91–9.81)	0.071
Histrionic	10.58 (0.53–210.99)	0.122
Schizoid	3.49 (1.04–11.73)	0.043
Schizotypal	10.50 (1.53–71.89)	0.017
Passive-aggressive	2.41 (0.51–11.49)	0.268
Homicides or attempted homicides		
PD Clusters		
No PDs	1.00[a]	
A	4.25 (1.26–14.31)	0.020
B	1.41 (0.42–4.70)	0.574
C	–[b]	–
PD diagnosis		
No PDs	1.00[a]	
Antisocial	1.35 (0.37–4.90)	0.645
Borderline	3.34 (0.87–12.79)	0.078
Narcissistic	0.36 (0.04–3.50)	0.379
Paranoid	2.96 (0.71–12.26)	0.135
Schizoid	5.26 (1.30–21.23)	0.020
Schizotypal	8.80 (1.23–62.78)	0.030
Passive-aggressive	2.00 (0.30–13.25)	0.474

OR adjusted odds ratio, *CI* confidence intervals, *PD* Personal Disorder, *Cluster A PD* Paranoid/Schizoid/Schizotypal PD, *Cluster B PD* Antisocial/Borderline/Histrionic/Narcissistic PD, *Cluster C PD* Obsessive/Compulsive/Dependent/Avoidant PD

[a] Indicates reference category, [b] could not be computed due to no distribution

with Schizoid, Schizotypal and Paranoid disorder 50.0%, 66.7% and 45.5%, respectively, have been incarcerated for violent crimes. These results are in concordance with Esbec and Echeburúa who reported that increased symptoms of DSM-IV "Cluster A" or "Cluster B" PDs, such as paranoid, narcissistic and antisocial symptoms are significantly associated with violence [28]. Accordingly, Mouilso and Calhoun reported a strong association of Narcissistic PD with sexual assault [29]. On the other hand, increased borderline personality tendencies have been reported in female sexual abusers [30]. Serial offenders as well are more likely to have Narcissistic, Schizoid and/or Obsessive–Compulsive traits. They are also more likely to engage in sexual masochism, partialism, homosexual paedophilia, exhibitionism and/or voyeurism, according to Chan et al. [31]. In addition, Pulay et al. reported an association between Schizoid, Paranoid and Obsessive–Compulsive PDs with violent behavior [32]. Another study by Haller also suggested a significant association of paranoid disturbance with violent crimes [33]. Schizoid PD is related as well with features of psychopathy and Antisocial personality according to Kosson et al. [34]. Loza and Hanna argue that an association exists between Schizoid PD and violent acts [35]. This study found a significant relation only of "Cluster A" disorders with violent offenses.

"Cluster C" disorders accounted for a minority of cases; individuals with Obsessive–Compulsive PD were only 2.3% of the study sample, whereas Dependent PD and Avoidant PD were few (~ 0.3%). This is in concordance with findings from Finland; "Cluster C" disorders comprised 3.5% of the entire sample of 593 offenders [19]. However, in contrast with the aforementioned studies, there were no violent crimes committed by offenders with "Cluster C" PD in this study, possibly due to the very small proportion of this PD "Cluster" in the studied population.

As presented in logistic regressions' results (Table 3), prisoners with any type of PD have greater likelihood (OR) of committing a violent crime. Nevertheless, violent crimes were associated significantly ($p \leq 0.05$) only with Schizotypal and Schizoid PD likely because the comparison group was composed by another type of criminals, instead of being composed by the general population.

Diagnosis with Personality disorders and association with homicides–attempted homicides

PDs have been found as principal or secondary diagnosis between homicides and attempted homicides offenders [37]. According to Pera and Dailliet, in a sample of 32 Belgian offenders 17 had an Antisocial PD, 8 a Borderline PD, 4 a Paranoid, and 2 a Schizoid PD [38]. Also, in a sample of 36 convicted Jamaican murderers 66% had an Antisocial PD [39]. Antisocial PD and substance use disorders were the most prevalent psychiatric diagnoses among prisoners that had committed or attempted homicide, as suggested by Kugu et al. [13].

Concerning sexual murderers, they are often diagnosed with a PD, especially with Schizoid PD [40]. Myers and Monaco and others also found an association of Sadistic PD (as described in DSM-IV) with sexual homicide [41, 42]. Concerning serial homicide offenders, they are more likely to have Narcissistic, Schizoid and/or

Obsessive–Compulsive traits according to Chan et al. [31]. Loza and Hanna reported, as well, an association between Schizoid PD and violent homicidal behavior [35]. Analysis of case reports by Jeffrey Dahmer and Dennis Nilsen underlined an association between schizoid personality traits with violent antisocial behavior [43].

In children, schizotypal features elicit victimization from other children, which in turn predisposes to reactive retaliatory aggression [44]. Lam et al. found that schizotypal personality traits (schizotypy) are associated with antisocial behavior [45]. This relation is replicated in the literature linking Schizotypal Disorder with antisocial behavior and violent crime [45].

Regarding homicide–attempted homicide in this study, the majority was committed by individuals suffering from Antisocial PD. Subjects of "Cluster A" PDs, in total, had committed 17 of the 46 crimes of this type. These results are in contrast to Keue and Borchard [36] and Laajalo et al. [19] studies that found no association between disorders of "Cluster A" and homicides. Prisoners of this study, with disorders of "Cluster A", were 4.25 times more likely to commit murder, while individuals with "Cluster B" disorders were 1.41 times more likely to commit the particular offense, compared with subjects without PD. Specifically for Antisocial PD odds ratio was 1.35, for Borderline PD was 3.34, for Narcissistic PD was 0.36, for Paranoid PD was 2.96, for Schizoid PD was 5.26 and for Schizotypal PD was 8.80, compared with subjects without PD. However, the committed homicide–attempted homicide was significantly associated with only Schizotypal and Schizoid PD.

Possibly, there is a neurobiological contribution to the association between Schizoid and Schizotypal PD and commitment of homicides or violence crimes. In literature, Schizotypal traits are associated with high hostility levels [46]. According to Raine et al. schizotypy was associated with total and reactive aggression but not with proactive aggression [44]. Sexual murderers are often diagnosed with a Schizoid PD [40]. Lam et al. [45] suggested that orbitofrontal cortex gray matter mediated the effect of schizotypy on antisocial behavior by 53.5%. On the other hand, this association was not significant for prefrontal cortex sub-regions. These findings highlight the specificity of the orbitofrontal cortex in understanding the schizotypy–antisocial behavior relationship. A link between Schizoid PD and Schizotypal PD was suggested by Via et al. [47]. According to them, persons with Schizoid PD–Schizotypal PD have greater bilateral white matter volume in the superior part of the corona radiata, close to motor/premotor regions, compared to healthy controls.

Schug et al. reported that reduced skin conductance orienting to neutral tones may reflect a neurocognitive risk factor, for both Antisocial and Schizotypal PDs that indirectly reflects a common neural substrate to these disorders [48]. Other researchers reported that individuals with Schizotypal PD display heightened activation in the neural circuitry, involved in reward and decision making when viewing biological motion stimuli in addition to a positive correlation between increased blood oxygenation level-dependent, signal responses related to biological motions and clinical symptoms [49]. These findings suggest that enhanced responses arise within the reward network for individuals with Schizotypal PD and are possibly related to the "peculiar" ways that individuals with Schizotypal disorder behave in social contexts. It might be the "unemotional and cold part" of individuals with Schizoid and Schizotypal PD that contributes to the increased occurrence of "lethal violence".

This study addresses certain limitations. Although the number of the participants is quite large, a bigger sample of individuals would have enhanced our results. For example, association of Paranoid ("Cluster A") and Narcissistic ("Cluster B") PDs with violent crimes was slightly not statistically significant (p values were 0.09 and 0.07, respectively). Another limitation is that issues of "free" psychopathology and counter-transference were not addressed in the initial protocol. It is also likely that Personality disorders have been overestimated in this study as well as in studies using structured diagnostic instruments. Much higher prevalence possibly has been reported compared to clinically based studies.

Conclusions

Most of the Greek prison inmates were diagnosed with a PD with a clear predominance of Antisocial PD. Nevertheless, significant associations of violent crimes and the offense of homicides–attempted homicides were found for the Schizoid and Schizotypal PD. No association of "Cluster B" or "Cluster C" PDs with violent crimes was elicited. This study—conducted for the first time in a Greek prisoners' population—provides evidence that murders and attempted murders are strongly associated with Schizoid and Schizotypal PDs. Further research is necessary to study in more depth the possible association of PDs—especially of the "Cluster A"—and the type of crime in Greece. Also, studies with larger samples and higher statistical power could investigate the role of other social, economic, demographic and clinical determinants in appearance of violent crimes and committed or attempted homicides.

Abbreviations

PDs: Personality disorders; MINI: Mini International Neuropsychiatric Interview; PDQ-4: Personality Diagnostic Questionnaire-4; M: mean; N: absolute frequencies; SD: standard deviation; OR: odds ratios; CI: confidence intervals.

Authors' contributions

AA, AD and VM contributed to conception and design and acquisition of data; AA, VM and IZ to analysis and interpretation of data; AA, IM, IZ, GT, VM and AD have been involved in drafting and revising the manuscript; AA, ER, CP and AD have given final approval of the version to be published. Each author has participated sufficiently and agreed that questions related to the accuracy and integrity of the work are appropriately investigated and resolved. All authors read and approved the final manuscript.

Author details

[1] 2nd Psychiatric Department of the University of Athens, Attikon Hospital, Athens, Greece. [2] 1st Psychiatric Department of the University of Athens, Aeginition Hospital, Athens, Greece. [3] Organization Against Drugs, Athens, Greece.

Acknowledgements

Not applicable.

Competing interests

The authors declare that they have no competing interests.

Consent for publication

Not applicable.

Funding

The authors declare that no sponsor played a role in funding the design, collection, and analysis, interpretation of data or in writing the manuscript.

References

1. American Psychiatric Association. Diagnostic and statistical manual of mental disorders, DSM-IV. Washington: American Psychiatric Press Inc; 1994.
2. Yu R, Geddes JR, Fazel S. Personality Disorders, violence, and antisocial behavior: a systematic review and meta-regression analysis. J Pers Disord. 2012;26(5):775–92.
3. Douzenis A, Tsopelas C, Tzeferakos G. Medical comorbidity of cluster B Personality Disorders. Curr Opin Psychiatry. 2012;25(5):398–404.
4. Alevizopoulos G, Igoumenou A. Psychiatric disorders and criminal history in male prisoners in Greece. Int J Law Psychiatry. 2016;47:171–5.
5. Coid JW. Personality Disorders in prisoners and their motivation for dangerous and disruptive behavior. Crim Behav Ment Health. 2002;12(3):209–26.
6. Black DW, Gunter T, Allen J, Blum N, Arndt S, Wenman G, Sieleni B. Borderline personality disorder in male and female offenders newly committed to prison. Compr Psychiatry. 2007;48(5):400–5.
7. Fazel S, Danesh J. Serious mental disorder in 23000 prisoners: a systematic review of 62 surveys. Lancet. 2002;359(9306):545–50.
8. Richard-Devantoy S, Olie JP, Gourevitch R. Risk of homicide and major mental disorders: a critical review. Encephale. 2009;35(6):521–30.
9. Riesco Y, Pérez Urdániz A, Rubio V, Izquierdo JA, Sánchez Iglesias S, Santos JM, Carrasco JL. The evaluation of Personality Disorders among inmates by IPDE and MMPI. Actas Luso Esp Neurol Psiquiatr Cienc Afines. 1998;26(3):151–4.
10. Piselli M, Attademo L, Garinella R, Rella A, Antinarelli S, Tamantini A, Quartesan R, Stracci F, Abram KM. Psychiatric needs of male prison inmates in Italy. Int J Law Psychiatry. 2015;41:82–8.
11. Coolidge FL, Segal DL, Klebe KJ, Cahill BS, Whitcomb JM. Psychometric properties of the Coolidge Correctional Inventory in a sample of 3,962 prison inmates. Behav Sci Law. 2009;27(5):713–26.
12. Köhler D, Heinzen H, Hinrichs G, Huchzermeier C. The prevalence of mental disorders in a German sample of male incarcerated juvenile offenders. Int J Offender Ther Comp Criminol. 2009;53(2):211–27.
13. Kugu N, Akyuz G, Dogan O. Psychiatric morbidity in murder and attempted murder crime convicts: a Turkey study. Forensic Sci Int. 2008;175(2–3):107–12.
14. Naidoo S, Mkize DL. Prevalence of mental disorders in a prison population in Durban, South Africa. Afr J Psychiatry. 2012;15(1):30–5.
15. Longato-Stadler E, von Knorring L, Hallman J. Mental and Personality Disorders as well as personality traits in a Swedish male criminal population. Nord J Psychiatry. 2002;56(2):137–44.
16. Fotiadou M, Livaditis M, Manou I, Kaniotou E, Xenitidis K. Prevalence of mental disorders and deliberate self-harm in Greek male prisoners. Int J Law Psychiatry. 2006;29(1):68–73.
17. Fountoulakis KN, Leucht S, Kaprinis GS. Personality Disorders and violence. Curr Opin Psychiatry. 2008;21(1):84–92.
18. Crump C, Sundquist K, Winkleby MA, Sundquist J. Mental disorders and vulnerability to homicidal death: Swedish nationwide cohort study. BMJ. 2013;346:f557.
19. Laajalo T, Ylipekka M, Häkkänen-Nyholm H. Homicidal behavior among people with avoidant, dependent and obsessive–compulsive (cluster C) personality disorder. Crim Behav Ment Health. 2013;23(1):18–29.
20. Papadimitriou GN, Berati S, Matsoukas TH, Soldatos KR. Mini International Neuropsychiatric Interview, Greek Version 5.0.0. DSM-IV, 2005.
21. Black DW, Arndt S, Hale N, Rogerson R. Use of the Mini International Neuropsychiatric Interview (MINI) as a screening tool in prisons: results of a preliminary study. J Am Acad Psychiatry Law. 2004;32(2):158–62.
22. Tasoulas S, Siousioura D. Personality Diagnostic Questionnaire (PDQ-4) in the Greek Language. Tetr Psychiatr. 2005;92:87–96.
23. Abdin E, Koh KG, Subramaniam M, Guo ME, Leo T, Teo C, Tan EE, Chong SA. Validity of the Personality Diagnostic Questionnaire-4 (PDQ-4+) among mentally ill prison inmates in Singapore. J Pers Disord. 2011;25(6):834–41.
24. Lanqeveld H, Mehlus H. Are psychiatric disorders identified and treated by in-prison health services? Tidss Nor Laeqeforen. 2004;124(16):2094–7.
25. Palmstierna T. Personality disorders, violence and criminal behavior. Lakartidningen. 2016;113:1–3
26. Pondé MP, Caron J, Mendonca MS, Freire AC, Moraeu N. The relationship between mental disorders and types of crime in inmates in Brazilian prison. J Forensic Sci. 2014;59(5):1307–14.
27. González RA, Igoumenou A, Kallis C, Coid JW. Borderline personality disorder and violence in the UK population: categorical and dimensional trait assessment. BMC Psychiatry. 2016;16:180.
28. Esbec E, Echeburúa E. Violence and Personality Disorders: clinical and forensic implications. Actas Esp Psiquiatr. 2010;38(5):249–61.
29. Mouilso ER, Calhoun KS. Personality and perpetration: narcissism among college sexual assault perpetrators. Violence Against Women. 2016;22(10):1228–42.
30. Tsopelas C, Tsetsou S, Ntounas P, Douzenis A. Female perpetrators of sexual abuse of minors: what are the consequences for the victims? Int J Law Psychiatry. 2012;35(4):305–10.
31. Chan HC, Beauregard E, Myers WC. Single-victim and serial sexual homicide offenders: differences in crime, paraphilias and personality traits. Crim Behav Ment Health. 2015;25(1):66–78.
32. Pulay AJ, Dawson DA, Hasin DS, Goldstein RB, Ruan WJ, Pickering RP, Huang B, Chou SP, Grant BF. Violent behavior and DSM-IV psychiatric disorders: results from the national epidemiologic survey on alcohol and related conditions. J Clin Psychiatry. 2008;69(1):12–22.
33. Haller R. What makes a mental ill violent? Psychiatr Danub. 2005;17(3–4):143–53.
34. Kosson DS, Blackburn R, Byrnes KA, Park S, Logan C, Donnelly JP. Assessing interpersonal aspects of schizoid Personality Disorder: preliminary validation studies. J Pers Assess. 2008;90(2):185–96.
35. Loza W, Hanna S. Is schizoid personality a forerunner of homicidal or suicidal behavior?: a case study. Int J Offender Ther Comp Criminol. 2006;50(3):338–43.
36. Keue A, Borchard B, Hoyer J. Mental disorders in a forensic sample of sexual offenders. Eur Psychiatry. 2004;19(3):123–30.
37. Fazel S, Grann M. Psychiatric morbidity among homicide offenders: a Swedish population study. Am J Psychiatry. 2004;161(11):2129–31.
38. Pera SB, Dailliet A. Homicide by mentally ill: clinical and criminological analysis. Encephale. 2005;31(5Pt1):539–49.
39. Hickling FW, Walcott G. Personality Disorder in convicted Jamaican murderers. West Indian Med J. 2013;62(5):453–7.
40. Koch J, Berner W, Hill A, Briken P. Sociodemographic and diagnostic characteristics of homicidal and nonhomicidal sexual offenders. J Forensic Sci. 2011;56(6):1626–31.

41. Myers WC, Monaco L. Anger experience, styles of anger expression, sadistic personality disorder, and psychopathy in juvenile sexual homicide offenders. J Forensic Sci. 2000;45(3):698–701.
42. Leach G, Meloy JR. Serial murder of six victims by an African-American male. J Forensic Sci. 1999;44(5):1073–8.
43. Martens WH, Palermo GB. Loneliness and associated violent antisocial behavior: analysis of the case reports of Jeffrey Dahmer and Dennis Nilsen. Int J Offender Ther Comp Criminol. 2005;49(3):298–307.
44. Raine A, Fung AL, Lam BY. Peer victimization partially mediates the schizotypy-aggression relationship in children and adolescents. Schizophr Bull. 2011;37(5):937–45.
45. Lam BY, Yang Y, Raine A, Lee TM. Neural mediator of the schizotypy-antisocial behavior relationship. Transl Psychiatry. 2015;5:e669.
46. Schaub M, Boesch L, Stohler R. Association between aggressiveness, schizotypal personality traits and cannabis use in Swiss psychology students. Psychiatry Res. 2006;143:299–301.
47. Via E, Orfila C, Pedreño C, Rovira A, Menchón JM, Cardoner N, Palao DJ, Soriano-Mas C, Obiols JE. Structural alterations of the pyramidal pathway in schizoid and schizotypal cluster A Personality Disorders. Int J Psychophysiol. 2016;110:163–70.
48. Schug RA, Raine A, Wilcox RR. Psychophysiological and behavioral characteristics of individuals comorbid for antisocial personality disorder and schizophrenia-spectrum personality disorder. Br J Psychiatry. 2007;191:408–14.
49. Hur JW, Blake R, Cho KI, Kim J, Kim SY, Choi SH, Kang DH, Kwon JS. Biological motion perception, brain responses, and schizotypal personality disorder. JAMA Psychiatry. 2016;73(3):260–7.

26

The long-term outcome of patients with heroin use disorder/dual disorder (chronic psychosis) after admission to enhanced methadone maintenance

Angelo G. I. Maremmani[1,2,3], Alessandro Pallucchini[4], Luca Rovai[5^], Silvia Bacciardi[4], Vincenza Spera[4], Marco Maiello[4], Giulio Perugi[6] and Icro Maremmani[2,3,7*]

Abstract

Background: Over-standard methadone doses are generally needed in the treatment of heroin use disorder (HUD) patients that display concomitant high-severity psychopathological symptomatology. A flexible dosing regimen may lead to higher retention rates in dual disorder (DD), as we demonstrated in bipolar 1 HUD patients, leading to outcomes that are as satisfactory as those of HUD patients without high-severity psychopathological symptomatology.

Objective: This study aimed to compare the long-term outcomes of treatment-resistant chronic psychosis HUD patients (PSY-HUD) with those of peers without dual disorder (HUD).

Methods: 85 HUD patients who also met the criteria for treatment resistance—25 of them affected by chronic psychosis and 60 without DD—were monitored prospectively for up to 8 years while continuing to receive enhanced methadone maintenance treatment.

Results: The rates of endurance in the treatment of PSY-HUD patients were 36%, compared with 34% for HUD patients ($p = 0.872$). After 3 years of treatment, these rates tended to become progressively more stable. PSY-HUD patients showed better outcome results than HUD patients regarding CGI severity ($p < 0.001$) and DSM-IV-GAF ($p < 0.001$). No differences were found regarding good toxicological outcomes or the methadone dosages used to achieve stabilization. The time required to stabilize PSY-HUD patients was shorter ($p = 0.034$).

Conclusions: An enhanced methadone maintenance treatment seems to be equally effective in patients with PSY-HUD and those with HUD.

Keywords: Methadone maintenance, Long-term outcome, High-threshold methadone maintenance programme, Dual disorder, Chronic psychosis

Introduction

Opioid Use Disorder patients show a high rate of psychiatric comorbidities (anxiety, depression, sleep disorders) during agonist opioid treatment (AOT) [1]. The presence of psychotic and affective symptoms is a common feature of psychiatric disorders, and their link with substance use disorder (SUD) has been widely demonstrated in the literature [2]. Regarding patients with heroin use disorder (HUD), according to our previous studies, the onset of psychosis generally occurs before substance use begins, whereas affective symptoms develop afterwards [3, 4]. The natural history of HUD differs between psychotic and bipolar HUD patients, so these two categories of patients often present different clinical pictures at the moment of admission to their first Agonist Opioid Treatment (AOT). In HUD patients with chronic psychosis

*Correspondence: icro.maremmani@med.unipi.it
^ Deceased
[7] Vincent P. Dole Dual Diagnosis Unit, Department of Specialty Medicine, Santa Chiara University Hospital, University of Pisa, Pisa, Italy
Full list of author information is available at the end of the article

(PSY-HUD), the progression of the addictive disease is limited, whereas bipolar 1 HUD patients show a more severe substance (i.e. heroin) use illness [5]. In patients with PSY-HUD, a therapeutic use of heroin cannot be excluded, at least, at the beginning of their clinical history. This kind of situation was not reported in the case of bipolar HUD patients [4].

During AOT treatment, especially during methadone treatment, our patients with and without the diagnosis of a dual disorder (DD), considering DD patients as patients displaying SUD together with another concomitant mental illness, show extreme variability of the dose needed to prevent a relapse during treatment [6, 7]. In our patients, above-standard methadone doses are usually needed in the presence of high-severity psychopathological symptomatology characterized by somatization, depression, paranoid ideation and psychoticism [8]. Above-standard doses are likewise needed for DD patients [9]. Good outcomes are also related to methadone dosage in our previously studied bipolar 1 HUD patients [10].

The present study has aimed to compare the long-term outcomes of treatment-resistant PSY-HUD with those of HUD patients without psychiatric comorbidity (HUD). We decided to evaluate whether chronic psychosis was able to influence methadone treatment outcomes in patients who had previously been non-responders in front-line, low-threshold treatment facilities when those patients were included in a high-threshold, maintenance-oriented, high-dose methadone programme.

The study hypothesized that a diagnosis of chronic psychosis would not affect treatment outcomes if PSY-HUD patients received individualized (above-standard) doses of methadone, and that a good outcome would be related to long-term ongoing treatment (retention).

To test this hypothesis, PSY-HUD and HUD patients were followed in a naturalistic approach applied for up to 8 years in the context of the maintenance high-threshold, high-dose Pisa Methadone Programme, using retention in treatment and rates of heroin use as the primary end-point parameters.

Methods

Design of the study

A prospective cohort study was designed to evaluate the treatment outcome (in terms of retention in treatment, substance use, clinical improvement and general social adjustment) of patients included in a methadone programme, with reference to its relationship with chronic psychosis comorbidity.

Setting

In Italy, low-threshold facilities for HUD patients are available in each territorial district. In those settings, when opioid agonists are employed, dosage and duration of treatment are usually limited, regardless of clinical indication [11], which suggests the value of increased dosage or treatment duration. Patients are allowed to negotiate the lowering of dosages, regardless of urinalyses, and to have their medication tapered earlier than advisable on the basis of the scientific literature.

All the patients participating in the study were treated in the setting of the Pisa Methadone Maintenance Treatment Programme (Pisa-MMTP) at Santa Chiara University Hospital, following the methodology proposed by Dole and Nyswander [12, 13].

Dole and Nyswander's methodology involves four broad stages: (1) Induction—under medical supervision, the patient is transferred from street heroin to the maintenance medication. The induction phase involves an initial low dose, followed by titration over subsequent days to achieve a stable dose (which includes reaching a steady-state plasma concentration). (2) Stabilization—dose increments to deliver a maintenance dose that allows opioid withdrawal signs and symptoms to be alleviated without producing significant euphoria. (3) Maintenance—maintaining the patient on a stable regular dose of the medication. Monitoring is essential during this phase to monitor treatment progress and to change the dose level if necessary. Psychosocial interventions are offered during this period. (4) Medically supervised withdrawal—while retention in the treatment programme is an important target (with at least 12-month retention necessary for enduring positive changes to behaviour to be achieved), patients should be helped to withdraw from opioids if that is their informed choice. Safe withdrawal from the medication can be accomplished by gradual reductions in the dose—this minimizes the likelihood of significant withdrawal and allows time for neuronal re-adaptation to take place. After-care strategies, such as counselling and support, are developed at this time to maximize the possibility of enduring abstinence.

The length of each treatment phase, notably the stabilization and maintenance stages, can vary substantially among patients, with some patients remaining in the maintenance phase for years, or even a lifetime. Conversely, due to the chronic, relapsing nature of opioid dependence, many patients will not complete an entire treatment episode and may drop out at some point during the process. These patients may, after a while, begin a new treatment episode. Patients who have remained abstinent from drugs also may be liable to relapse into drug use. Thus, many opioid-dependent patients will enter treatment numerous times.

After patients at the PISA-MMTP had been safely inducted into treatment with methadone, their doses are gradually increased until the point is reached where there is no more than one urine drug screen which is positive for illicit opiates, cocaine or benzodiazepines in the previous 60-day period. Once this requirement is fulfilled, the patient is defined as having been "stabilized", and the dose at which this goal has been accomplished is referred to as the 'stabilization dose'. We consider these patients as reaching a good outcome. For more information, see Maremmani et al. [14].

Participants

All PSY-HUD patients referred by low-threshold facilities for HUD patients to the Pisa-MMT programme during the January 1997–December 2006 period ($N=25$) were consecutively enrolled in the study.

PSY-HUD patients were characterized by

- a diagnosis of HUD-concomitant chronic psychosis according to DSM-IV criteria for schizophrenia or delusional disorders,
- "absence of additional psychiatric DSM-IV diagnoses" and
- resistance to previous front-line, low-threshold methadone treatment programmes attended at local addiction treatment units.

Schizoaffective disorder, or bipolar disorder with psychotic features, was excluded from the PSY-HUD group because the present study aimed to discuss differences between PSY-HUD and HUD patients with reference to what we found in our previously studied bipolar 1 HUD patients.

We did not use a specific screening process other than the patient's wish to be treated and wanting to participate. Criteria for treatment resistance included at least two unsuccessful treatments in the 2-year period before being referred to our programme. Patients had been treated with the standard protocols for HUD (methadone maintenance with dosages up to 100 mg/day) and were discharged because of persisting positivity for opioid metabolites at urinalyses.

Axis 2 diagnoses were excluded from the study, since a wide range of personality disorders was usually displayed by SUD patients, which makes it challenging to define Axis 2 diagnostic subgroups. Addictive behaviours may carry diagnostic implications, as in the case of borderline and antisocial personality disorders [15–19]. HUD patients co-affected by Borderline Personality Disorders and Antisocial Personality Disorder, during treatment or during detoxification programmes, maintain significantly higher levels of crime, injection-related health problems, heroin overdose, major depression and poorer global mental health [20–22].

As control group, we considered patients we had previously compared with our bipolar 1 HUD patients [10]. We excluded 3 patients because of a positive family history of psychiatric disorders and a diagnosis of affective temperament according to the criteria of Hagop Akiskal [23].

All patients gave their written informed consent to the study after the procedure had been fully explained. The consent form and the study protocol were both approved by the ethics committee of the University of Pisa, according to the WMA Declaration of Helsinki—Ethical Principles for Medical Research Involving Human Subjects.

Instruments

Drug Addiction History Questionnaire (DAH-Q)

The DAH-Q [24] is a questionnaire comprising the following categories: sociodemographic information, physical health, mental health, substance use, treatment history, social adjustment and environmental factors. The questionnaire checks 10 areas: physical problems, mental problems, employment status, family situation, sexual problems, socialization and leisure time, legal problems, substance use, previous treatment and associated treatments. Items have been constructed in such a way as to ensure dichotomous (yes/no) answers. For more details, see [25]. The DAH-Q was administered at the beginning of treatment.

Global assessment of functioning, DSM-IV-GAF and clinical global impression (CGI)

The GAF considers psychological, social and occupational functioning within the sphere of a hypothetical mental health-illness continuum, without including any impairment of functioning due to physical or environmental limitations. The point allocation follows a specific code, with a maximum of 100 and a minimum of 0, with the possibility of using intermediate codes if necessary [26].

The CGI considers the severity of the disorder, the degree of improvement or worsening following the intervention and any adverse reactions [27].

CGI and GAF were administered monthly by a researcher who was blind as to the diagnosis of the patients.

Psychiatric diagnostic evaluation. Structured clinical interview for DSM-IV Axis I disorders (SCID-I)

This instrument [28] will help clinicians make standardized, reliable and accurate diagnoses while avoiding the common problem of premature closure (a premature focusing on one diagnostic possibility).

Toxicological urine analyses

The enzyme-multiplied immune technique for opiates was used. Toxicological urine analyses for morphine metabolites were carried out randomly every week during the induction phase and, randomly, almost every month, during the stabilization phase.

Procedures

Patients were evaluated outside acute phases at the end of their first hospitalization at our clinic, so as to reduce the diagnostic ambiguity between intoxication-related symptoms and spontaneous (substance-unrelated) mental disorders. In cases where further information emerged on clinical grounds during the monitoring period, diagnoses were reviewed.

Patients who stayed in treatment were assessed at the end of treatment. Among patients with poor outcomes, those who left the treatment were assessed at the time of treatment interruption, this being the last regular assessment.

PSY-HUD patients were treated with low oral dosages of second-generation antipsychotics during the acute phase of a psychotic episode and until its resolution. Psychotropic medications were not systematically used for the HUD patients. In summary, no differences were detected either in anti-psychotic use or in psychosocial management in the PSY-HUD group when compared with their previous low-threshold treatment. Long-term treatment with antipsychotics was not our main choice, considering the negative impact of antipsychotics on the anti-reward syndrome of SUD patients [29, 30]. In any case, in our unit, top priority was given to methadone dosage adaptation [31].

In our programme, patients are required to attend the clinic according to scheduled appointments, to participate in the development of their treatment plan, to work towards treatment goals, to meet with medical and case management staff, and to attend groups whenever necessary.

Take-home doses, without limitations, at most for a 7-day period, are allowed, once patients have shown complete compliance with the rules of the programme. Every 7-day period, medication management visits were applied.

Data analysis

Heroin use disorder patients and PSY-HUD patients were compared at treatment entry for demographic and addiction history using the Chi-square test for categorical variables, and Student's t test (designed for Independent Samples) for continuous variables.

The association between differences in demographic data, addiction history and retention in treatment was tested using Cox regression. In our model, we included each difference at treatment entry between groups as an independent variable, and poor outcomes for individual patients as dependent variables.

Retention in treatment was analysed by means of the Kaplan–Meier survival analysis and Wilcoxon statistics for comparison between the survival curves. For the purpose of this analysis, the term 'censored observations' refers to patients who were still in treatment at the end of the study or were leaving treatment for reasons unrelated to the treatment itself (e.g. patients moving on to other therapeutic communities, due to imprisonment for old crimes). We considered it to be a poor outcome (terminal event) when a patient had not reached stabilization within a year or had relapsed into addictive behaviour after a period of stabilization, abandoned the treatment or been expelled from it.

The toxicological urinalyses were expressed using two indices: The TGO index (per cent Toxicological Good Outcome) and TGO ratio (per total specimens Toxicological Good Outcome). The TGO index expresses the percentage ratio between urinalyses proving negative for the presence of morphine and the total number of urinalyses carried out for each patient during the treatment period. It is the percentage ratio between the number of urinalyses testing negative for the presence of morphine and the number of urine analyses that the protocol has envisaged throughout the process. The TGO index tends to give preference to patients who remain 'opiate-free' but who terminate the study in advance for reasons not correlated with the study (for example, imprisonment). The TGO ratio further comprises how long the patient remains in the protocol, but gives less precedence to these patients. These two indices represent the two extremes, and the results tend to balance out. Concerning these parameters, the comparison between the two groups was made using ANOVA Two Factors (group and outcome).

Regarding global clinical impressions and social adjustment outcomes, we compared the two groups using ANOVA Two Factors (group and outcome) for cross-sectional evaluation and repeated analysis of variance for longitudinal evaluations.

Regarding stabilization methadone dose and the time required to reach the stabilization phase, we compared the two groups using ANOVA Two factors (group and outcome).

The statistical tests were considered significant at the level of $p < 0.05$.

Results

Baseline evaluation (at the beginning of the treatment)

Table 1 shows the demographic and clinical characteristics of participants. The discriminant characteristics of PSY-HUD patients were as follows. PSY-HUD patients more frequently had education lasting less than 8 years, presented a lower level of social adjustment with a lower frequency of legal problems, and self-reported a lower severity of drug addiction history. More specifically, PSY-HUD patients less frequently showed physical concerns and polysubstance use, talked about having experienced unsuccessful treatments or having received ongoing psychosocial treatments at local units, declared 'daily or more' heroin intake before requesting treatment and reached stage 3 of heroin addiction. Also, PSY-HUD patients were older when they first started using heroin and when they began their continuous use of heroin. Lastly, the duration of their dependence was shorter. Cox regression analysis using the variables reported above—showing differences between PSY-HUD and HUD patients—as predictors, and patients' poor outcome as a criterion, did not show significant correlations except for a low educational level (HR = 3.72; 95% CI 1.69–8.16; $p=0.001$), ($\chi^2=22.54$; $df=13$; $p=0.047$).

Retention in treatment

Regarding the outcome of patients, as related to chronic psychotic comorbidity, at the end of the observational period, 12 (20.0%) HUD patients and 8 (32.0%) PSY-HUD patients completed their rehabilitation programme and either left the treatment or were referred to another programme as a "stabilized patient". Thirty-two (53.3%) HUD patients and 15 (60.0%) PSY-HUD patients had not reached stabilization within a year or had relapsed into heroin use during the programme, so they were terminated and referred to their local treatment services. Sixteen (26.7%) HUD patients and 2 (8.0%) PSY-HUD

Table 1 Demographic characteristics and drug addiction history of 85 heroin-dependent patients, comprising 25 with chronic psychosis (PSY-HUD) and 60 without Axis I psychiatric comorbidity (HUD)

	HUD patients *N* = 60	PSY-HUD patients *N* = 25	*t*/chi	*P*
Age (M ± s)	30.08 ± 5.9	30.64 ± 7.4	−0.36	0.715
Gender: male [*N* (%)]	46 (76.2)	15 (60.0)	2.41	0.185
Marital status: single [*N* (%)]	47 (79.7)	16 (64.0)	2.29	0.169
Education: < 8 years [*N* (%)]	12 (21.1)	11 (44.0)	4.53	0.033
Work [*N* (%)]				
White collar	12 (20.7)	8 (32.0)		
Blue collar	18 (31.0)	10 (40.0)		
Unemployed	28 (48.3)	7 (28.0)	3.04	0.218
CGI severity of illness[a] (*M* ± *s*)	5.54 ± 0.6	5.52 ± 0.7	0.12	0.900
GAF index from DSM-IV (*M* ± *s*)	44.75 ± 7.2	40.64 ± 10.6	2.06	0.042
1-Presence of physical concerns [*N* (%)]	48 (80.0)	14 (56.0)	5.15	0.023
2-Presence of altered mental status [*N* (%)]	54 (90.0)	25 (100.0)	2.69	0.101
3-Work concerns [*N* (%)]	42 (70.0)	14 (56.0)	1.53	0.215
4-Household concerns [*N* (%)]	14 (23.3)	9 (36.0)	1.43	0.231
5-Romantic concerns [*N* (%)]	24 (40.0)	13 (52.0)	1.03	0.309
6-Social/leisure concerns [*N* (%)]	33 (55.0)	12 (48.0)	0.34	0.556
7-Legal concerns [*N* (%)]	29 (48.3)	2 (8.0)	12.39	< 0.001
8-Polyabuse (more than 3) [*N* (%)]	45 (75.0)	11 (44.0)	7.454	0.006
9-Past treated [*N* (%)]	50 (83.3)	7 (28.0)	24.46	< 0.001
10-Combined treated [*N* (%)]	60 (100.0)	15 (60.0)	27.20	< 0.001
'Daily or more' heroin intake [*N* (%)]	55 (91.7)	14 (73.7)	4.22	0.040
Stable modality of use [*N* (%)]	21 (35.0)	12 (57.1)	3.15	0.076
Stage 3 of heroin addiction [*N* (%)]	47 (78.3)	5 (26.3)	17.37	< 0.001
Age at first use of heroin (*M* ± *s*)	18.22 ± 3.0	21.21 ± 5.0	−3.16	0.002
HUD: age at onset (*M* ± *s*)	20.10 ± 3.9	24.75 ± 5.9	−4.19	< 0.001
Dependence duration (years) (*M* ± *s*)	9.51 ± 6.1	4.15 ± 3.8	3.79	< 0.001
Age at first treatment (*M* ± *s*)	28.47 ± 6.8	30.64 ± 7.4	−1.30	0.195

[a] Between 1 = normal and 7 = extremely ill

patients were considered "stabilized" and were still in treatment at the end of the period of observation. These differences were not statistically significant (χ^2 4.12, $df=2$, $p=0.127$). No patients left the treatment because of side effects. Four HUD patients (6.6%) and none of the PSY-HUD patients were dismissed for violence ($p=0.136$); none were imprisoned or rehospitalized because of a psychotic episode.

Numbers of HUD patients entering annual intervals, according to the presence of chronic psychosis, are shown in Fig. 1. Twenty-two HUD patients (37%) and 7 PSY-HUD patients (28%) had not reached the stabilization phase in 1 year. None of the PSY-HUD patients relapsed into addictive behaviour (reusing heroin) after 3 years of treatment. In summary, according to the Kaplan–Meier methodology, the HUD patients' Cumulative Proportion Retained (CPR) in treatment at the end of the observational period was 0.34. The proportion of PSY-HUD patients was 0.36. These differences were not statistically significant ($p=0.872$).

Males (CPR=0.36) and females (CPR=0.30) showed a similar retention rate (Wilcoxon statistics=0.50; $df=1$; $p=0.478$). PSY-HUD (CPR=0.33) and HUD (CPR=0.37) males did not show a significantly different retention rate from HUD females (Wilcoxon statistics=0.22; $df=1$; $p=0.635$). The same results were observed in comparing PSY-HUD females (CPR=0.40) and HUD ones (CPS=0.27) (Wilcoxon statistics=0.81; $df=1$; $p=0.367$).

Outcome

Urinalyses

When the toxicological examination performed at the time of enrolment into the programme (which was required to be positive) was eliminated from the analysis, 10,674 urine samples were analysed in all: 7963 for good-outcome patients, 2711 for poor-outcome patients. A total of 7885 samples from HUD patients were examined, with 2788 from PSY-HUD ones. On average, 74.54% of samples tested negative for morphine. No patient provided positive samples for the entire duration of treatment. No patient provided exclusively negative samples.

In good-outcome PSY-HUD patients, the TPO index was 91.60±4.2; in good-outcome HUD patients, it was

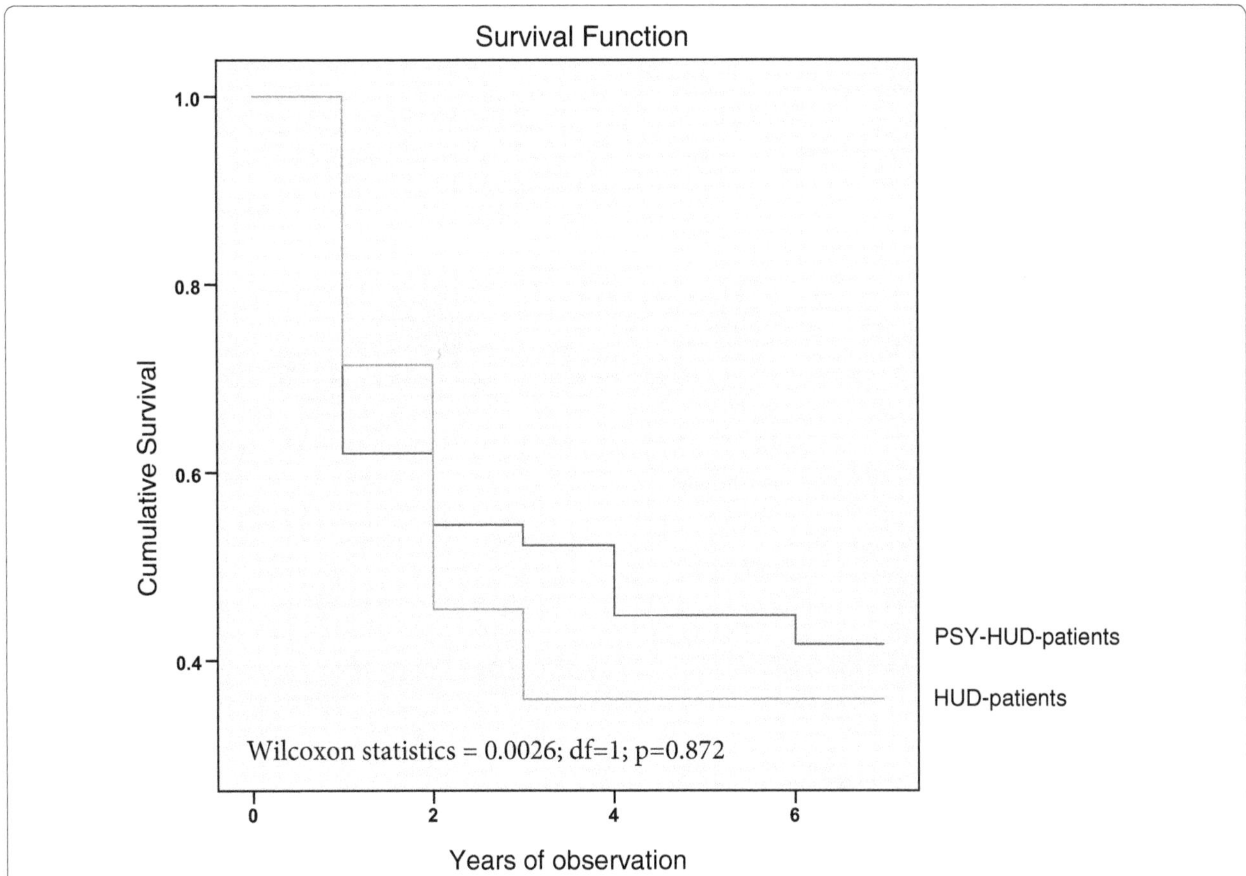

Fig. 1 Endurance in methadone maintenance of 25 treatment-resistant heroin-dependent patients with chronic psychosis (PSY-HUD) and of 60 without DSM-IV Axis 1 psychiatric comorbidity (HUD)

87.43±8.5 (Group effect: $F=1.13$; $df=1$; $p=0.290$; outcome effect: $F=146.78$, $p<0.001$; group-outcome effect: $F=0.74$, $p=0.391$). In good-outcome PSY-HUD patients, the TPO ratio was 0.47±0.2; in good-outcome HUD ones, it was 0.49±0.3 (Group effect: $F=0.09$; $df=1$; $p=0.758$; outcome effect: $F=46.32$, $p<0.001$; group-outcome effect: $F=0.00$, $p=0.978$). In summary, no differences were found regarding urinalyses for morphine between PSY-HUD and HUD patients during the observational period.

Global clinical impressions and social adjustment outcomes

The CGI severity of illness and the DSM-IV GAF (global assessment of functioning) showed the following significant trends in participants.

At the end-point evaluation, good-outcome PSY-HUD patients reported a lower severity of illness (1.90±0.9) than good-outcome HUD patients (2.46±0.7). Time effect ($F=3303.54$; $df=1$; $p<0.001$) and group-time effect ($F=48.38$; $df=1$; $p<0.001$) were significant. Interestingly, at baseline, the severity of illness was equal in the two groups. These differences were not related to the outcome ($F=0.55$; $df=1$; $p=0.458$).

At the end-point evaluation, good-outcome PSY-HUD patients reported a better level of social adjustment (78.30±8.1) than good-outcome HUD patients (74.39±9.8). Time effect ($F=376.01$; $df=1$; $p<0.001$) and group-time effect ($F=8.90$; $df=1$; $p=0.004$) were both significant. These differences were not related to the outcome ($F=0.05$; $df=1$; $p=0.824$).

Stabilization methadone dose and time to reach the stabilization phase

On average, PSY-HUD (115.20±41.2 mg/day; 60–190 ranged) and HUD patients (120.18±67.4 mg/day; 30–260 ranged) did not need statistically different methadone dosages in the stabilization phase ($F=0.28$; $p=0.597$). Differences between groups were not observed even when dosage was controlled by the outcome ($F=0.45$; $p=0.502$).

On average, PSY-HUD patients needed 2.76±0.9 months to reach the stabilization dosages; otherwise, HUD patients were stabilized in 6.35±9.3 months (Group effect: $F=4.65$, $p=0.034$; Outcome effect: $F=2.60$, $p=0.111$; Group-outcome effect: $F=4.15$, $p=0.045$).

Discussion

We have examined treatment retention and outcomes for PSY-HUD and HUD patients involved in an enhanced methadone treatment. We noted that:

- At baseline, PSY-HUD patients more frequently showed education lasting less than 8 years, a lower level of social adjustment and legal problems, and a lower severity of drug addiction history. These characteristics did not appear to be related to better retention or better outcome, the only exception being the low educational level.
- PSY-HUD and HUD patients were retained in treatment without differences. Males and females showed similar retention rates.
- Between groups, no differences were found regarding urinalyses for morphine or regarding methadone stabilization dosages.
- The time required to stabilize PSY-HUD patients was shorter.

It is not easy to correlate low educational level with poor outcome. It is known that, in SUD patients, successful treatment was associated with several baseline characteristics including older age, white race, having more than a high school education, lower level of care and not having a history of opioid use [32]. It is also true that, at first sight, control patients seem to be a more seriously ill control group. We assume, however, that only the drug-related history is less severe in PSY-HUD patients. The overall clinical judgment expressed by CGI stresses the same severity of disease in both groups. In addition, there is no doubt that from the psychopathological point of view, PSY-HUD patients are more seriously ill than their peers without DD.

In our study, the outcome and the retention rate in the therapy of treatment-resistant participants did not differ from that of long-term standard methadone programmes designed according to the methodology of Dole and Nyswander [33–35]. Participants were stabilized using middle-to-high dosages, but not with the above-standard dosages we used to stabilize bipolar 1 HUD patients [10].

Anecdotal evidence has been reported about the beneficial effects of opiates in reducing psychotic symptoms. In a 39-year-old man requesting treatment for positive psychotic symptoms, a low dose of quetiapine and 140 mg daily of methadone had controlled psychosis for years. After interrupting the use of anti-psychotic medication and methadone for complaints in the sexual area, he presented acute psychotic symptoms. After he started taking heroin regularly, treatment with methadone and quetiapine was resumed, and his symptoms subsided. A few months later, he again stopped using methadone, without relapsing into heroin use; his psychotic symptoms reappeared, even though he maintained the anti-psychotic medication [36]. The use of high methadone dosage has been confirmed in a series of psychotic HUD patients [37] and one patient responded to an increased dose of methadone [38]. Reports of the occurrence of a psychotic episode after methadone or buprenorphine discontinuation are, in the literature, a little bit more frequent [39–41].

Higher methadone doses have been used in Comorbid Psychiatric Disorder [42], as an anti-anxiety, anti-depressant and anti-psychotic treatment [43].

In our study, a possible explanation for the need for these relatively higher doses in patients who had previously been unresponsive to standard treatments may be related to a wide inter-individual variability in the methadone metabolism [44, 45], which may explain why a number of patients are under-medicated, if a standard (middle-to-low) dose of methadone is used. Unfortunately, we did not measure plasma methadone levels in studying participants during the stabilization phase, so we cannot resolve this doubt.

In study participants, only Axis I psychiatric disorders were taken into consideration, and the existence of a minor form of psychopathology in the other patients concealed under the main addictive symptoms cannot be excluded. We refer to the psychopathological symptoms of Axis II psychiatric disorders and/or psychopathological symptoms related to the HUD [46]. Participants were, however, followed up for a long time (up to 8 years), and diagnoses were subject to revision whenever further clinical evidence or retrospective information was gathered—a factor that reduces the likelihood of false HUD. Moreover, the duration of addiction was such as to make it improbable that participants rated as HUD had a silent psychiatric history. The availability of significant others was itself extremely helpful in increasing the level of diagnostic accuracy and grouping.

The high GAF score values recorded for PSY-HUD participants without hospitalizations throughout the treatment period showed that participants were simultaneously compliant both with MMT requirements and with the specific therapy adopted for their comorbid psychopathology. The use of new-generation antipsychotics for the treatment of psychiatric symptoms—medication not wholly changed by the need to treat addiction—may partly explain the positive outcomes obtained in psychotic participants. This effect cannot be attributed exclusively to the effects of pharmacotherapy. A lack whether of appropriately flexible methadone doses and/or of specific medications given in association with methadone treatment for PSY-HUD patients could have been responsible for the conflicting results obtained by other researchers, who reported that psychiatric disorders were linked to worse treatment outcomes (such as drug use and criminal activities) [47–49]. Also, the high therapeutic pressure associated with our programme could have been responsible for better results [50].

In the present study, methadone is potentially useful in treating psychosis, at least in HUD patients. This is in line with a series of observations about the correlation between opioid use and psychosis [51].

We are aware that it is very difficult to find published papers about the dosages of AO medications in dual-disorder patients, to corroborate the results of the present study. Our present results do, however, look stronger in the light of our previous studies, with all the limitations that this fact entails. The concern is that we may be over-interpreting our previous research despite the fact that it consisted of single site, small sample size, homogeneous population studies carried out in Europe (selected for patients who had failed to achieve results at lower levels of treatment). In the literature, there are still insufficient data to generalize the present results to cover all HUD patients with comorbid non-affective psychotic disorders. We wonder, of course, if our findings would apply to other HUD sub-populations (e.g. adolescents or psychiatric patients with HUD not seeking substance use disorder treatment). In any case, our previous studies do allow us to present some afterthoughts on the results of our present study.

In HUD patients admitted to hospital for an acute psychotic episode, we found that an increase in methadone dosage or the initiation of methadone treatment proved to be potentially effective in achieving control of psychotic symptoms by prescribing lower treatment dosages of antipsychotics and mood-stabilizing drugs, even when the period spent in hospital was the same [52].

We also found that the profile of psychotic HUD patients at their first treatment attempt displays a higher level of global symptom severity, even when coupled with less severe addictive symptoms and a shorter duration of addictive history than their non-psychotic peers [53].

Our psychotic HUD patients may be included among those who resort to street methadone as a regular practice before entering treatment, and this decision should be regarded as a self-harm-reducing behaviour rather than a pattern of use. Our patients may, in fact, have an independent motivation to look for treatment earlier and stay in treatment longer—an advantage that may overcome addictive ambivalence and improve compliance [54].

We also found that there is a distinction to be made between patients who had started heroin use after the onset of psychiatric disorders and those who had suffered from psychiatric disorders after the onset of their drug habit. Among the former, psychotic disorders and anxiety disorders were those best represented, and they were linked with a trend towards less severe addictive symptoms. The latter group mostly comprised patients with mood disorders, who had more severe addictive symptoms. This time sequence does not stand as a definite proof of self-medication dynamics, but it is broadly consistent with the idea that some disorders, rather than others, may lead to heroin use in a self-medication manner [3]. The same patients would then suffer from early impairment of their psychiatric disorders, due to acquired opiate imbalance, when the severity of their addictive disease is still lower, and they will benefit more directly from the opiate-balancing effect of agonist treatment [55].

Through the recent use of an exploratory factor analysis of the 90 items in the SCL-90, a five-factor solution was identified for HUD patients, namely "Worthlessness and Being Trapped", "Somatic Symptoms", "Sensitivity-Psychoticism", "Panic Anxiety" and "Violence-Suicide" [46]. Using this SCL-90, 5-factor solution, our HUD patients with prominently psychopathological "Sensitivity-Psychoticism" characteristics showed a better level of retention in treatment when treated with methadone [56].

According to our research group, methadone dosage would partly work as a psychotropic stabilizer, regardless of addictive symptoms, so that the eventual stabilization dosage is higher than in non-psychotic HUD patients. Once both psychopathological grounds (addictive and psychotic) have been neutralized, many HUD patients may achieve a positive outcome, reversing what might be expected in the absence of treatment [57, 58].

Lastly, in the present study, methadone should accelerate the stabilization process in psychotic HUD patients through the early normalizing of the opioid system.

Generally, patients requiring high-dose methadone are polydrug SUD patients or patients with psychiatric comorbidities [59]. That result was confirmed by us in HUD bipolar 1 patients [10], but not in psychotic ones, in which standard doses seem to be potentially effective, too. We should, in fact, keep in mind that an overall improvement in the psychiatric status of HUD patients has been reported, independently of the dosages used [60], and that a very high prevalence of psychiatric comorbidity is present in HUD patients receiving OAT [1].

Limitations

In any case, the validity of our study was limited by several factors—primarily, the observational nature of the protocol. Observational studies do, however, have the merit of capturing the most clinically significant data, such as data on the effectiveness and toxicity of therapies used by a heterogeneous population of patients in the 'real world.'

During the maintenance phase of the treatment, urine screening for cocaine and benzodiazepine was not performed systematically but randomly, every 6 months. All patients were evaluated almost at the same time, and patients with the presence of urine metabolites for cocaine and benzodiazepine were considered to be poor responders. Cannabinoid use was not assessed. The strength of the study was, however, the absence, in our patients, of cocaine or benzodiazepine comorbid diagnosis according to the DSM-IV-R criteria and the absence of cocaine and benzodiazepine use in all stabilized patients.

The sample size of this study was insufficient in number, and at the end of the observational period, only two participants were present in the DD group. In addition, it was not possible to have a follow-up evaluation in the case of the participants who dropped out. Of course, this small population and the fact that the majority of the patients have left the study before the end makes statistical analysis fairly tricky. This also makes it difficult to formulate any associations between population characteristics and treatment retention.

Lastly, one cannot fail to consider the multiple interferences caused by inter-individual variability (presence of mental disorder and personality traits and their neurobiological correlates), the possible selection biases, the clinical setting and the temporary use of adjunctive medications.

Conclusions

Opioid agonists deserve reconsideration, not only because of their anti-craving capability but also because of their helpfulness at the psychopathological level. They represent an adequate tool, even in the task of treating psychiatric symptomatology and psychiatric disorders, especially chronic psychosis, in HUD patients. In this case, a flexible dosing regimen that permits the administration of standard (middle-to-high) methadone doses may lead to satisfactory outcomes and to a retention rate very similar to that of HUD patients without other mental disorders while restraining psychotic symptoms and reducing the risk of rehospitalization. In conclusion, personalized methadone treatment seems to be capable of producing a good result in treatment-resistant HUD patients with or without chronic psychosis.

Authors' contributions

AGIM and IM conceived and designed the study, AP, LR, SB, VS and MM revised the literature and discussed data results, IM and AGIM analysed data, and GP participated with other authors in the interpretation of the data. AGIM drafted the manuscript and all authors revised it critically for important intellectual content. All authors gave final approval of the version to be published. All authors read and approved the final manuscript.

Author details

[1] Department of Psychiatry, North-Western Tuscany Local Health Unit, Versilian Zone, Viareggio, Italy. [2] AU-CNS, Association for the Application of Neuroscientific Knowledge to Social Aims, Pietrasanta, Lucca, Italy. [3] G. De Lisio Institute of Behavioural Sciences, Pisa, Italy. [4] School of Psychiatry, University of Pisa, Pisa, Italy. [5] Department of Psychiatry, North-Western Tuscany Local Health Unit, Apuan Zone, Massa, Italy. [6] Department of Clinical and Experimental

Medicine, University of Pisa, Pisa, Italy. [7] Vincent P. Dole Dual Diagnosis Unit, Department of Specialty Medicine, Santa Chiara University Hospital, University of Pisa, Pisa, Italy.

Acknowledgements
The authors acknowledge the decision of AU-CNS to offer open access fees.

Competing interests
The authors have no financial competing interests in relation to the publication of this manuscript. In addition, they have no political, personal, religious, ideological, academic or intellectual competing interests. IM served as Board Member for Molteni and Indivior.

Consent for publication
Not applicable.

Funding
No funding received for this work.

References

1. Roncero C, Barral C, Rodriguez-Cintas L, Perez-Pazos J, Martinez-Luna N, Casas M, Torrens M, Grau-Lopez L. Psychiatric comorbidities in opioid-dependent patients undergoing a replacement therapy programme in Spain: the PROTEUS study. Psychiatry Res. 2016;243:174–81.
2. Regier DA, Farmer ME, Rae DS, Locke BZ, Keith SJ, Judd LL, Goodwin FK. Comorbidity of mental disorders with alcohol and other drug abuse. JAMA. 1990;19(264):2511–8.
3. Maremmani AGI, Dell'Osso L, Pacini M, Popovic D, Rovai L, Torrens M, Perugi G, Maremmani I. Dual diagnosis and chronology of illness in 1090 treatment seeking Italian heroin dependent patients. J Addict Dis. 2011;30:123–35.
4. Maremmani AGI, Rovai L, Rugani F, Bacciardi S, Massimetti E, Gazzarrini D, Dell'Osso L, Fengyi T, Akiskal HS, Maremmani I. Chronology of illness in dual diagnosis heroin addicts. The role of mood disorders. J Affect Disord. 2015;179:156–60.
5. Maremmani AGI, Rugani F, Bacciardi S, Rovai L, Massimetti E, Gazzarrini D, Dell'Osso L, Maremmani I. Differentiating between the course of illness in bipolar 1 and chronic-psychotic heroin-dependent patients at their first Agonist Opioid Treatment. J Addict Dis. 2015;34:43–54.
6. Maremmani I, Pacini M. The issues of dosage. In: Maremmani I, editor. The principles and practice of methadone treatment. Pisa: Pacini Editore Medicina; 2009. p. 97–102.
7. Maremmani I, Pacini M, Canoniero S, Maremmani AGI, Tagliamonte A. Dose determination in dual diagnosed heroin addicts during [dovrebbe essere: during senza una maiuscola] methadone treatment. Heroin Addict Relat Clin Probl. 2010;12:17–24.
8. Maremmani I, Zolesi O, Agueci T, Castrogiovanni P. Methadone doses and psychopathological symptoms during methadone maintenance. J Psychoactive Drugs. 1993;25:253–6.
9. Maremmani I, Zolesi O, Aglietti M, Marini G, Tagliamonte A, Shinderman M, Maxwell S. Methadone dose and retention during treatment of heroin addicts with Axis I psychiatric comorbidity. J Addict Dis. 2000;19:29–41.
10. Maremmani AGI, Rovai L, Bacciardi S, Rugani F, Pacini M, Pani PP, Dell'Osso L, Akiskal HS, Maremmani I. The long-term outcomes of heroin-dependent treatment-resistant patients with bipolar 1 comorbidity after admission to enhanced methadone maintenance. J Affect Disord. 2013;151:582–9.
11. Schifano F, Bargagli AM, Belleudi V, Amato L, Davoli M, Diecidue R, Versino E, Vigna-Taglianti F, Faggiano F, Perucci CA. Methadone treatment in clinical practice in Italy: need for improvement. Eur Addict Res. 2006;12:121–7.
12. Dole VP, Nyswander ME. A medical treatment for diacetylmorphine (heroin) addiction: a clinical trial with methadone hydrochloride. JAMA. 1965;193:80–4.
13. Dole VP, Nyswander ME, Warner A. Successful treatment of 750 criminal addicts. JAMA. 1968;206:2708–11.
14. Maremmani I, Pacini M, Lubrano S, Perugi G, Tagliamonte A, Pani PP, Gerra G, Shinderman M. Long-term outcomes of treatment-resistant heroin addicts with and without DSM-IV axis I psychiatric comorbidity (dual diagnosis). Eur Addict Res. 2008;14:134–42.
15. Cerquetelli G. La clinica psichiatrica oggi: il sé e gli stati limite. Clinica Psichiatrica. 1980;16:9–110.
16. Glover E. On the etiology of drug addiction (1932). In: Glover E, editor. On the early development of the mind. New York: International Universities Press; 1956. p. 187–215.
17. Kernberg O. Sindromi marginali e narcisismo patologico. Torino: Boringhieri; 1978.
18. Kolb LC. Types and characteristics of drug addicts. Ment Hyg. 1925;9:300–13.
19. Reid WH. The psychopathology: a comprehensive study of antisocial disorders and behavior. New York: Wiley; 1978.
20. Gerra G, Ceresini S, Esposito A, Zaimovic A, Moi G, Bussandri M, Raggi MA, Molina E. Neuroendocrine and behavioural responses to opioid receptor-antagonist during heroin detoxification: relationship with personality traits. Int Clin Psychopharmacol. 2003;18:261–9.
21. Darke S, Ross J, Williamson A, Mills KL, Havard A, Teesson M. Borderline personality disorder and persistently elevated levels of risk in 36-month outcomes for the treatment of heroin dependence. Addiction. 2007;102:1140–6.
22. Darke S, Ross J, Williamson A, Teesson M. The impact of borderline personality disorder on 12-month outcomes for the treatment of heroin dependence. Addiction. 2005;100:1121–30.
23. Akiskal HS, Akiskal KK. TEMPS: Temperament Evaluation of Memphis, Pisa, Paris and San Diego. J Affect Disord. 2005;85(Special issue):1–242.
24. Maremmani I, Castrogiovanni P. Drug Addiction History Questionnaire (DAH-Q)—Heroin Version. Pisa: University Press; 1989.
25. Lovrecic B, Lovrecic M, Rovai L, Rugani F, Bacciardi S, Dell'Osso L, Maremmani AGI, Maremmani I. Ethnicity and drug addiction. A comparison between Italian and Slovenian heroin addicts. Heroin Addict Relat Clin Probl. 2012;14:5–18.
26. A.P.A. Diagnostic and statistical manual of mental disorders, DSM-IV. Washington: American Psychiatric Association; 1994.
27. Guy W. ECDEU Assessment Manual for Psychopharmacology. Clinical Global Impressions. Rockville: U.S. Department of Health, Education, and Welfare; 1976.
28. First MB, Spitzer RL, Gibbon M, Williams JBW. Structured clinical interview for DSM-IV Axis I disorders (SCID-I), clinician version. Arlington: American Psychiatric Publishing, Inc; 1997.
29. Karamatskos E, Mulert C, Lambert M, Naber D. Subjective well-being of patients with schizophrenia as a target of drug treatment. Curr Pharm Biotechnol. 2012;13:1490–9.
30. Blum K, Thanos PK, Oscar-Berman M, Febo M, Baron D, Badgaiyan RD, Gardner E, Demetrovics Z, Fahlke C, Haberstick BC, Dushaj K, Gold MS. Dopamine in the brain: hypothesizing surfeit or deficit links to reward and addiction. J Reward Defic Syndr. 2015;1:95–104.
31. Maremmani I, Perugi G, Pacini M, Akiskal HS. Toward a unitary perspective on the bipolar spectrum and substance abuse: opiate addiction as a paradigm. J Affect Disord. 2006;93:1–12.
32. Clark CB, Hendricks PS, Brown A, Cropsey KL. Anxiety and suicidal ideation predict successful completion of substance abuse treatment in a criminal justice sample. Subst Use Misuse. 2014;49:836–41.
33. Dole VP, Joseph H. Long term outcome of patients treated with methadone maintenance. Ann NY Acad Sci. 1978;311:181–9.
34. Strain EC, Stitzer ML, Liebson IA, Bigelow GE. Methadone dose and treatment outcome. Drug Alcohol Depend. 1993;33:105–17.
35. Fareed A, Casarella J, Roberts M, Sleboda M, Amar R, Vayalapalli S, Drexler K. High dose versus moderate dose methadone maintenance: is there a better outcome? J Addict Dis. 2009;28:399–405.
36. Ros-Cucurull E, Miquel L, Franco MQ, Casas M. Reduction of psychotic symptoms during the use of exogenous opiates. Heroin Addict Relat Clin Probl. 2012;14:57–8.
37. Walby FA, Borg P, Eikeseth PH, Neegaard E, Kjerpeseth K, Bruvik S, Waal H. Use of methadone in the treatment of psychotic patients with heroin dependence. Tidsskr Nor Laegeforen. 2000;120:195–8.

38. Feinberg DT, Hartman N. Methadone and schizophrenia. Am J Psychiatry. 1991;148:1750–1.
39. Cobo J, Ramos MM, Pelaez T, Garcia G, Marsal F. Psychosis related to methadone withdrawal. Acta Neuropsychiatrica. 2006;18:50–1.
40. Levinson I, Galynker II, Rosenthal RN. Methadone withdrawal psychosis. J Clin Psychiatry. 1995;56:73–6.
41. Karila L, Berlin I, Benyamina A, Reynaud M. Psychotic symptoms following buprenorphine withdrawal. Am J Psychiatry. 2008;165:400–1.
42. Parvaresh N, Masoudi A, Majidi S, Mazhari S. The correlation between methadone dosage and comorbid psychiatric disorders in patients on methadone maintenance treatment. Addict Health. 2012;4:1.
43. Deglon JJ, Wark E. Methadone: a fast and powerful anti-anxiety, anti-depressant and anti-psychotic treatment. Heroin Addict Relat Clin Probl. 2008;10:49–56.
44. Kharasch ED, Stubbert K. Role of cytochrome P4502B6 in methadone metabolism and clearance. J Clin Pharmacol. 2013;53:305–13.
45. Shinderman M, Maxwell S, Brawand-Amey M, Golay KP, Baumann P, Eap CB. Cytochrome P4503A4 metabolic activity, methadone blood concentrations, and methadone doses. Drug Alcohol Depend. 2003;69:205–11.
46. Maremmani I, Pani PP, Pacini M, Bizzarri JV, Trogu E, Maremmani AGI, Perugi G, Gerra G, Dell'Osso L. Subtyping patients with heroin addiction at treatment entry: factors derived from the SCL-90. Ann Gen Psychiatry. 2010;9:15.
47. Darke S, Mills K, Teesson M, Ross J, Williamson A, Havard A. Patterns of major depression and drug-related problems amongst heroin users across 36 months. Psychiatry Res. 2009;166:7–14.
48. Friedmann PD, Lemon SC, Anderson BJ, Stein MD. Predictors of follow-up health status in the drug abuse treatment outcome study (DATOS). Drug Alcohol Depend. 2003;69:243–51.
49. Fernandez Miranda J, Gonzalez Garcia-Portilla M, Saiz Martinez P, Gutierrez Cienfuegos E, Bobes Garcia J. Influence of psychiatric disorders in the effectiveness of a long-term methadone maintenance treatment. Actas Luso Esp Neurol Psiquiatr Cienc Afines. 2001;29:228–32.
50. Amato L, Minozzi S, Davoli M, Vecchi S. Psychosocial and pharmacological treatments versus pharmacological treatments for opioid detoxification. Cochrane Database Syst Rev. 2011;9:CD005031.
51. Maremmani AG, Rovai L, Rugani F, Bacciardi S, Dell'Osso L, Maremmani I. Substance abuse and psychosis. The strange case of opioids. Eur Rev Med Pharmacol Sci. 2014;18:287–302.
52. Pacini M, Maremmani I. Methadone reduces the need for antipsychotic and antimanic agents in heroin addicts hospitalized for manic and/or acute psychotic episodes. Heroin Addict Relat Clin Probl. 2005;7:43–8.
53. Maremmani AG, Rugani F, Bacciardi S, Rovai L, Massimetti E, Gazzarrini D, Dell'Osso L, Maremmani I. Differentiating between the course of illness in bipolar 1 and chronic-psychotic heroin-dependent patients at their first agonist opioid treatment. J Addict Dis. 2015;34:1–12.
54. Maremmani I, Pacini M, Pani PP, Popovic D, Romano A, Maremmani AG, Deltito J, Perugi G. Use of street methadone in Italian heroin addicts presenting for opioid agonist treatment. J Addict Dis. 2009;28:382–8.
55. Maremmani I, Canoniero S, Pacini M. Psycho(patho)logy of "addiction". Interpretative hypothesis. Ann Ist Super Sanita. 2002;38:241–57.
56. Maremmani AGI, Rovai L, Pani PP, Pacini M, Lamanna F, Rugani F, Schiavi E, Dell'Osso L, Maremmani I. Do methadone and buprenorphine have the same impact on psychopathological symptoms of heroin addicts? Ann Gen Psychiatry. 2011;10:17.
57. Maremmani AGI, Bacciardi S, Rovai L, Rugani F, Akiskal HS, Maremmani I. Do bipolar patients use street opioids to stabilize mood? Heroin Addict Relat Clin Probl. 2013;15:25–32.
58. Pani PP, Agus A, Gessa GL. Methadone as a mood stabilizer [Letter]. Heroin Addict Relat Clin Probl. 1999;1:43–4.
59. Eiden C, Leglise Y, Clarivet B, Blayac JP, Peyriere H. Psychiatric disorders associated with high-dose methadone (> 100 mg/d): a retrospective analysis of treated patients. Therapie. 2012;67:223–30.
60. Herrero MJ, Domingo-Salvany A, Brugal MT, Torrens M, Itinere I. Incidence of psychopathology in a cohort of young heroin and/or cocaine users. J Subst Abuse Treat. 2011;41:55–63.

Off-label prescription of psychiatric drugs by non-psychiatrist physicians in three general hospitals in Germany

Caroline Lücke[1], Jürgen M. Gschossmann[2], Teja W. Grömer[3], Sebastian Moeller[1], Charlotte E. Schneider[1], Aikaterini Zikidi[1], Alexandra Philipsen[1] and Helge H. O. Müller[1,3*]

Abstract

Background: Off-label prescribing of psychoactive drugs is a common practice in psychiatry. Here, we sought to investigate the frequency of off-label prescribing in a population of hospitalized patients with a somatic illness who were also suffering from a psychiatric pathology.

Methods: Using a prospective, observational design, we collected data from 982 hospitalized patients with a somatic illness for whom a psychiatric consultation was requested because of the presence of additional psychiatric symptoms. Data were collected at three hospitals in Germany. Demographic and clinical data, including the previous psychoactive medications and an assessment of the suitability of the previous medications, were recorded and analyzed.

Results: Data on the previous psychiatric medications were available for 972 patients. In 16.6% of patients, at least one psychoactive drug had been prescribed off-label, 20.2% had received on-label medication, and 63.2% had not received any psychiatric medication. Among all patients receiving psychiatric medication, 45.1% had received off-label medication. The logistic regression analysis showed a significant influence of age on the likelihood of receiving off-label medication ($p = 0.018$). Benzodiazepines were the most frequent off-label prescription (25.8% of off-label prescriptions), followed by atypical antipsychotics (18.2%) and low-potency antipsychotics (17.2%). Notably, 57.1% of off-label prescriptions were judged to be 'not indicated' by experienced psychiatrists.

Conclusions: Our data show a high frequency of the off-label prescription of psychoactive drugs by physicians treating patients with somatic illnesses in general hospitals. Because more than half of these cases were judged to be "not indicated", these prescriptions indicate a potential risk to patients. Furthermore, the classes of drugs that were most frequently prescribed off-label, benzodiazepines and antipsychotics, both show a substantial risk profile, particularly for elderly patients.

Keywords: Off-label prescription, Psychotropic medication, Risk profile

Background

Off-label prescribing, the prescription of drugs not licensed for the intended use in the country of conduct, is a common phenomenon. The term "off-label" not only refers to the use of a medication outside its licensed indication but also includes the use of dosages above the recommended range, a treatment duration for periods longer than recommended or the use in special patient groups, such as children, the elderly, or patients with contraindications. Moreover, the use of different routes of administration or a change in the formulation, i.e., when a tablet is crushed to be easier to swallow, may result in different pharmacokinetics and constitute an off-label use. Pediatrics is the subspecialty with the largest number of off-label prescriptions due to the special age group of the patients [1, 2], but clear evidence exists for

*Correspondence: helge.mueller1@uni-oldenburg.de
[1] Medical Campus University of Oldenburg, School of Medicine and Health Sciences, Psychiatry and Psychotherapy-University Hospital, Karl-Jaspers-Klinik, Hermann-Ehlers-Straße 7, 26160 Bad Zwischenahn, Germany
Full list of author information is available at the end of the article

extensive off-label use in psychiatry, as well [3]. According to a cross-sectional questionnaire-based survey from the United Kingdom (UK), 65% of respondents had been prescribed a medication for an off-label indication in the past month [4]. A subsequent UK study analyzing inpatient prescriptions in psychiatric wards reported an off-label prescription rate of 7.5% [5], whereas another study conducted in a German Psychiatric hospital found that 20% of prescriptions were clearly off-label and another 19% of prescriptions were classified as "probably off-label" [6]. However, these studies were conducted more than 15 years ago. More recently, 40% of drugs were prescribed off-label in a prospective study conducted at an Indian outpatient psychiatric department, with 79% of patients receiving at least one off-label drug [7]. Classes of drugs that are commonly prescribed off-label very in psychiatric practice are antipsychotics [5, 8] and benzodiazepines [7, 9], the latter of which is often being prescribed off-label for long-term use.

In some situations, off-label prescribing is a feasible or even necessary practice. Conditions for the use of off-label medications in accordance with professional organizations in most countries include the lack of an equally safe and effective licensed alternative, the existence of sufficient scientific evidence to support the use of the drug for the intended condition, and the presence of fully informed consent from the patient to be treated off-label [10].

However, in many cases, these requirements are not or are only partially fulfilled [10, 11]. Often, the level and quality of the scientific evidence supporting the intended off-label use of a drug is overestimated by physicians [12], and the possible risks of side effects are underestimated [13]. In particular, when drugs are used in off-licensed age groups, such as geriatric patients, the risk of side effects may increase considerably [14]. Although the bias due to the underreporting of adverse events is difficult to estimate, the rate of spontaneous reporting seems lower for unlicensed medicines compared to licensed medicines [13], which may be due to the fear of legal consequences by physicians. Furthermore, patients are often not informed about the unlicensed status of the drug that they receive [15, 16].

In the present analysis, we specifically examined the number of off-label prescriptions of psychotropic drugs for patients who were hospitalized due to a somatic illness and showed additional psychiatric pathology. Psychopharmacological prescriptions were administered to this population prior to specific psychiatric consultations in nearly all cases by the physician treating the somatic illness. Since physicians in a somatic setting typically do not have extensive psychiatric training, the off-label prescription of psychiatric drugs in this setting might constitute a particular risk of the non-optimal or even hazardous treatment of patients.

Methods

In a prospective, observational design, data from 982 hospitalized patients with a somatic illness were collected and evaluated. Only patients who showed psychiatric symptoms and thus required a psychiatric consultation were included. Patient data were collected from three different hospitals in Germany; 345 cases were from a large university clinic (University Clinic Erlangen) and 636 cases were from two medium-sized general hospitals (545 from Klinikum Forchheim and 91 from Evangelisches Krankenhaus Oldenburg).

Data were collected by the consultation-liaison psychiatrist who conducted the psychiatric consultation and comprised the demographical and clinical psychiatric data, including current psychopathology, previous treatments, psychiatric diagnosis (current and pre-known), and recommended treatment. For patients who previously received a psychiatric treatment, the psychiatrist also evaluated and recorded whether this treatment was medically justified in the given situation. Furthermore, the psychiatric diagnosis suspected by the somatically treating physician prior to the psychiatric consultation was recorded in addition to a judgement by the psychiatrist regarding whether this diagnosis was correct.

All patients received information about the study design from the psychiatrist and provided informed consent to participate. All data were assessed as part of the routine psychiatric consultation, and participating patients did not undergo any additional study-related procedures.

Study results on psychiatric pathology, diagnoses, and further treatment have already been published elsewhere [17]. The current psychoactive medications used by the patients prior to treatment recommendations by the psychiatrist were recorded and classified into groups in the database. Drug prescriptions were then classified as on- or off-label according to the drug's license in Germany at the time of use.

Data were collected from September 2011 to April 2012 at the University Clinic Erlangen, from March 2014 to September 2015 at Klinikum Forchheim and from January 2016 to September 2017 at Evangelisches Krankenhaus Oldenburg. All psychiatric consultations performed at these clinics during the specified periods were included in the study, unless the patients did not consent to data collection. The physicians treating the somatic illness usually made the decision to request a psychiatric consultation for patients, based on the current psychopathology shown by the patients. Over 90% of consultations were conducted by the same three psychiatrists. The majority of the patients (85.3%) came from the department of internal medicine.

Data were processed and analyzed using SPSS Statistics 23 (IBM, Armonk, NY, USA). Since the design of this analysis was exploratory and based on a large database with several study endpoints, data were primarily analyzed using descriptive statistics. In addition, influences of co-factors such as gender and age were tested using multi- or binomial regression analyses.

This study was approved by the ethics committee of the Friedrich-Alexander-University of Erlangen-Nuremberg.

Results

Nine hundred and eighty-two patients participated in this study, and information on the previous psychiatric medications was available for 975 patients. Of these patients, 60.3% were female and 39.7% were male. The mean age was 64.3 years.

The rate of off-label prescriptions for psychoactive medications in our patient population was 16.6%. On-label psychiatric medications were prescribed to 20.2% of patients, whereas 63.2% of patients had not received any previous psychiatric medication. When restricting the analysis to patients who had received psychoactive medications, the rate of off-label prescriptions was 45.1%.

A logistic regression analysis was performed to examine the influence of the factors age and gender on the likelihood of off-label prescriptions in patients. The models showed a statistically significant influence of age on the comparison of "on-label use" versus "off-label use" ($p = 0.018$) and the comparison of "no psychiatric medication" versus "off-label use ($p = 0.047$); patients who received off-label prescriptions were slightly older than the other two groups (Table 1). The ratio of male-to-female patients was nearly equal in all groups, and the logistic regression analysis did not show a statistically significant influence of gender (Table 1).

Among all the previous off-label prescriptions, 57.1% were judged as 'not indicated' by the liaison psychiatrist and additional 37.5% were judged as 'partially indicated'. Only 3.4% of off-label prescriptions were judged to be 'indicated'.

The distribution of drug classes that were prescribed off-label is shown in Table 2. Benzodiazepines were the class of drugs that were most frequently prescribed off-label, with 25.8% of off-label prescriptions, followed by atypical antipsychotics (18.2%) and low-potency antipsychotics (17.2%). Selective serotonin reuptake inhibitors constituted 12.0% of off-label prescriptions. Taking together all antipsychotics of any generation and potency, antipsychotics were the most frequently prescribed off-label drug class, with 38.3% of off-label prescriptions.

Table 2 Off-label prescriptions of psychiatric drugs

Class of drug	Responses	
	N	Percent (%)
Low-potency antipsychotics	36	17.2
Atypical antipsychotics	38	18.2
Typical antipsychotics	6	2.9
Benzodiazepines	54	25.8
Other hypnotics	6	2.9
SSRI	25	12.0
Mirtazapine	9	4.3
Tricyclic antidepressants	7	3.3
Lithium	2	1.0
Pregabalin	6	2.9
Others	20	9.6
Total	209	100.0

Table 1 Demographics and psychiatric medication

	On-label use	Off-label use	No psychiatric medication	Total
Gender				
Male				
Count	76	62	249	387
Percent within psych. medication (%)	38.8	38.3	40.6	39.9
Female				
Count	120	100	364	584
% within psych. mediation (%)	61.2	61.7	59.4	60.1
Mean age (years)	62.9*	67.5*,+	64.2+	64.3
Total				
Count	196	162	613	971
Percent within psych. medication (%)	100.0	100.0	100.0	100.0

* $p = 0.018$, + $p = 0.047$

Psychiatric disorders with high rates of off-label prescriptions were somatoform disorders (28.0%), organic mental disorders (21.9%), and anxiety disorders (22.1%). Sleep disorders and drug-related disorders had high rates of off-label prescriptions as well, but too few patients were included in these categories to provide a valid result. In the single case of a patient with the diagnosis of sleep disorder who had received psychiatric medication, an atypical antipsychotic had been prescribed off-label. Table 3 shows the rates of off-label prescriptions in the different psychiatric diagnoses as determined by the psychiatrist as a result of the consultation.

To investigate whether the high percentage of unjustified off-label prescriptions was related to a high amount of incorrect diagnoses, we also analyzed the suspected psychiatric diagnoses made by the non-psychiatrist physicians prior to the psychiatric consultation. Among all cases of off-label prescription for which these data were available ($n = 104$), 48.1% of diagnoses were classified by the psychiatrists as "correct", 35.6% were "partially correct" (e.g., depressive episode versus adjustment disorder), and 16.3% were "incorrect".

Furthermore, we performed an exploratory analysis of the distribution of off-label prescribing in the different medical specialties. The vast majority of participants were seen in the internal medicine department, and 74.5% of off-label prescriptions were written by physicians in internal medicine. However, compared to other specialties, internal medicine was slightly below average, with 14.5% of patients receiving off-label medications. The specialty with the highest rate of off-label prescriptions was the emergency department (62.5%), followed by trauma surgery (27.8%), neurology (26.3%), and intensive care (20.0%). Patients from other departments were very rarely prescribed off-label medications; thus, the numbers were too small for interpretation.

Table 3 Off-label prescriptions in different psychiatric diagnoses

	Psychiatric medication		
	On-label use	Off-label use	No psych. medication
Organic mental disorders			
N	37	41	109
%	19.8	21.9	58.3
Alcohol-related disorders			
N	11	17	72
%	11.0	17.0	72.0
Other drugs			
N	4	5	14
%	17.4	21.7	60.9
Psychosis			
N	13	3	26
%	31.0	7.1	61.9
Affective disorders			
N	71	51	223
%	20.6	14.8	64.6
Anxiety disorders			
N	16	15	37
%	23.5	22.1	54.4
Reaction to severe stress/adjustment disorder			
N	8	14	70
%	8.7	15.2	76.1
Dissociative and conversion disorders			
N	0	1	7
%	0.0	12.5	87.5
Somatoform disorders			
N	11	14	25
%	22.0	28.0	50.0
Eating disorders			
N	1	1	4
%	16.7	16.7	66.7
Sleep disorders			
N	0	1	2
%	0.0	33.3	66.7
Other diagnoses			
N	1	4	17
%	4.5	18.2	77.3
No psychiatric disorder			
N	4	4	40
%	6.4	8.5	85.1

Discussion

To our knowledge, this study represents the first large and systematic analysis that specifically examines the off-label prescribing of psychiatric drugs by non-psychiatrists in a naturalistic clinical hospital environment. We observed a surprisingly high rate of off-label prescriptions in this population, with 16.6% of patients receiving off-label psychoactive medications. Among the patients who received any psychopharmacological medication, 45.1% received at least one off-label drug. Compared to the literature, this rate is clearly higher than the rates of off-label prescriptions reported in British and German psychiatric wards in the previous studies [5, 6]. Several possibilities may explain this discrepancy. The difference may be partially due to a general increase in the number of off-label prescriptions since the early 2000s. Unfortunately, more recent data from Western populations are not available for comparison, which is a surprising finding of the lack of (needed) systematic examinations in the field of in-house off-label prescribing.

Second, differences between the populations studied (psychiatric wards versus medical wards) could account for the discrepancy, since the distribution of psychiatric diagnoses in our population differed from the distribution typically found in psychiatric wards, particularly for organic mental disorders. However, an additional reason for the high rates of off-label prescriptions observed in our population may be because prescribers in our population were mostly physicians from specialties other than psychiatry. These physicians may either have a generally more uncritical view of off-label prescribing or are simply less informed about the licensed indications and the recommended use of the drugs prescribed. If the latter is true, it implies a potential risk for patients, since a responsible off-label prescribing practice requires good knowledge of the scientific evidence supporting the off-label use of the drug in question for a specific condition. Those facts also highlight the need for the systematic education of non-psychiatric prescribers in the field of psychopharmacological treatment options. In some cases, an "unjustified" off-label prescription may have simply been the result of an incorrect psychiatric diagnosis by the prescriber prior to the psychiatric consultation. Our data show that the rate of "incorrect" diagnoses among cases of off-label prescription was 16.3%, whereas a further 35.6% were only "partially correct". Thus, a prescription may have been on-label based on the physician's diagnosis at the time of prescription, but off-label based on the correct diagnosis made by the psychiatrist. This effect may have further contributed to the high rate of off-label prescriptions in our patient population. Since the distribution of correct versus incorrect diagnoses was similar in cases of on-label prescription and in cases of no psychiatric medication, we do not believe that this is the primary explanation for our main results regarding off-label prescribing. Nevertheless, the high amount of incorrect or partially correct diagnoses further highlights the necessity of a qualified psychiatric diagnosis prior to prescription of psychopharmacological medication in hospitals.

Our results on the evaluation of previous off-label treatments by specialists support the hypothesis that the frequent off-label prescribing practice in hospitals is very often not in the patients' interest. More than half of off-label cases were judged to be 'not indicated' by psychiatrists, and the off-label prescription was only clearly advisable for 3.4% of patients. These results are consistent with the previous studies, showing that the majority of off-label prescriptions, particularly for psychiatric indications, are not supported by solid scientific evidence [12, 15, 18]. The fact that the justification of off-label prescribed medications was based on the psychiatrists' assessment and not controlled by standardized rules or a literature search may constitute a certain limitation of our study; however, all psychiatrists performing the consultations were experienced specialists with fundamental scientific knowledge in the area of psychopharmacology.

Consistent with the literature, the classes of drugs that were most frequently prescribed off-label were antipsychotics and benzodiazepines. The off-label prescription of antipsychotics is very common in psychiatry [11, 19–21] and has significantly increased over the years [22, 23]. With some exceptions, atypical antipsychotics are often only licensed for use in patients with schizophrenia and often bipolar disorder, but they are frequently prescribed for other indications as well, particularly anxiety, affective disorders, and organic mental disorders [19, 24, 25], due to their stabilizing effects on agitation. Since the development of atypical antipsychotics with reduced risks of extrapyramidal symptoms (EPS), the reputation of antipsychotics has significantly improved; however, the second-generation antipsychotics may also have significant side effects, particularly regarding metabolic changes. These changes may be negligible in relation to the immediate dangers of acute psychosis or manic phases, but the uncritical use of antipsychotics in other, less threatening conditions may not always be justified. Furthermore, extrapyramidal side effects may still occur with atypical antipsychotics [14], and tardive dyskinesia is of particular concern because of its potential irreversibility. In a 2006 prospective cohort study of patients receiving maintenance antipsychotic treatment, the risk of tardive dyskinesia following treatment with quetiapine was as high as 13% [26]. The study also confirmed previously known risk factors for the development of EPS, including an older age and duration of treatment [26–28]. Other potentially serious risks of antipsychotics are cardiac side effects [29–31] which may be of particular concern in patients with preexisting heart disease. Thus, uncritical off-label use of antipsychotics seems especially problematic in elderly populations, such as our study population [32].

Long-term benzodiazepine use causes tolerance, addiction, and potential abuse; thus, licenses and national guidelines usually recommend the prescription of benzodiazepines for only a very limited amount of time. In addition to addiction, including the danger of potentially severe withdrawal symptoms, long-term benzodiazepine use is associated with side effects such as psychomotor retardation, cognitive impairment, affective symptoms, paradoxical inhibition, and drug interactions [33]. Again, elderly patients are at an increased risk for the occurrence of these side effects [33–35]; however, the prescription of benzodiazepines to patients simultaneously increases with increasing age [32, 36]. CNS effects, such as cognitive impairment and sedation, as well as drug interactions play a significant role in elderly patients [33,

35, 37]. Of particular concern is the increased risk of falls in elderly patients receiving benzodiazepine treatment [38, 39], with potentially life-threatening consequences.

The medical departments with the highest amounts of off-label use were departments with a focus on the treatment of acute cases and emergencies (emergency unit, trauma surgery, intensive care, and neurology/stroke unit). Psychiatric drugs in these situations were mostly given for acute sedation with protection from the stress and anxiety of the situation or/and prophylaxis of delirium. In emergency situations, there is usually no time for a medical clinician to consult a psychiatrist about the choice of drugs; thus, acute treatment decisions need to be made by physicians based on their previous knowledge. We recommend the establishment of treatment standards in departments according to the respective national guidelines, since recommendations may differ according to the status of licenses for different drugs in different countries. In example, the guidelines for "Analgesia, sedation and management of delirium" published by an interdisciplinary consortium of 12 German medical societies, including the German society of Psychiatry and Psychotherapy, Psychosomatics and Neurology (DGPPN) [40], recommends the carefully monitored use of benzodiazepines for symptom-oriented treatment of agitation and anxiety as well as sedation (alternatives in intensive care settings: Propofol and Clonidine). Neuroleptics are recommended for the treatment of psychotic symptoms only, for example, in delirium and are not to be regularly used as sedatives. A pharmacological prophylaxis of delirium is recommended for at-risk patients only using low-dose Haloperidol (as licensed). However, these recommendations can only provide very general guidelines, since treatment of individual patients in a given situation often requires acknowledgement of diverse factors, and the establishment of one standard treatment for all patients is difficult. Therefore, a regular review of cases with the consultation-liaison psychiatrist could improve patient care in the time following an acute situation and could help to train physicians on treatment decisions in future cases.

A limitation of our study is the lack of information on the exact causes of a prescription being off-label, since these data were not recorded at the time of data collection. Although information on factors such as dose, length of treatment, patient's age, and means of administration were available to the psychiatrists and included in their assessment of off-label use at the time of data collection, the distribution of causes for prescriptions being off-label cannot be retrospectively analyzed from our database. Future studies of off-label medication use should include the detailed recording of this information to obtain a more differentiated picture of common, potentially problematic prescribing situations in different drug categories.

Conclusions

In summary, the off-label prescription of psychotropic drugs, particularly antipsychotics and benzodiazepines, is a very common phenomenon in German hospital wards of non-psychiatric specialties, at least in the investigated hospitals. Furthermore, most of these prescriptions are not supported by solid clinical and scientific knowledge and may thus constitute a potential risk for patients, particularly when patients are administered multiple off-label medications. Better training on psychiatric pharmacology for physicians from other specialties is necessary, as is a policy for the timely consultation of a specialized psychiatric colleague in hospitalized patients presenting with a psychiatric pathology.

Abbreviations

UK: United Kingdom; EPS: extrapyramidal symptoms.

Author's contributions

HHOM and JGM collected the data. CL and HHOM wrote the final draft of the manuscript. TWG, SM, CS, AZ, and AP critically reviewed and improved the manuscript. All authors read and approved the final manuscript.

Author details

[1] Medical Campus University of Oldenburg, School of Medicine and Health Sciences, Psychiatry and Psychotherapy-University Hospital, Karl-Jaspers-Klinik, Hermann-Ehlers-Straße 7, 26160 Bad Zwischenahn, Germany. [2] Department of Internal Medicine, Klinikum Forchheim, Forchheim, Germany. [3] Department of Psychiatry and Psychotherapy, Friedrich-Alexander-University Erlangen-Nuremberg, Erlangen, Germany.

Acknowledgements

None.

Competing interests

The authors declare that they have no competing interests.

Consent for publication

Not applicable.

Funding

This research did not receive any specific grants from funding agencies in the public, commercial, or not-for-profit sectors.

References

1. Ekins-Daukes S, Helms PJ, Taylor MW, McLay JS. Off-label prescribing to children: attitudes and experience of general practitioners. Br J Clin Pharmacol. 2005;60(2):145–9.
2. Wertheimer A. Off-label prescribing of drugs for children. Curr Drug Saf. 2011;6(1):46–8.
3. Baldwin DK, Kosky N. Off-label prescribing in psychiatric practice. Adv Psychiatr Treat. 2007;13:414–22.
4. Lowe-Ponsford FL, Baldwin DS. Off-label prescribing by psychiatrists. Psychol Bull. 2000;24:415–7.
5. Douglas-Hall P, Fuller A, Gill-Banham S. An analysis of off-licence prescribing in psychiatric medicine. Pharmaceut J. 2001;267:890–1.

6. Assion HJ, Jungck C. Off-label prescribing in a German psychiatric hospital. Pharmacopsychiatry. 2007;40(1):30–6.
7. Kharadi D, Patel K, Rana D, Patel V. Off-label drug use in psychiatry outpatient Department: a prospective study at a Tertiary Care Teaching Hospital. J Basic Clin Pharm. 2015;6(2):45–9.
8. Haw C, Stubbs J. Off-label use of antipsychotics: are we mad? Expert Opin Drug Saf. 2007;6(5):533–45.
9. Haw C, Stubbs J. Benzodiazepines–a necessary evil? A survey of prescribing at a specialist UK psychiatric hospital. J Psychopharmacol. 2007;21(6):645–9.
10. Sutherland A, Waldek S. It is time to review how unlicensed medicines are used. Eur J Clin Pharmacol. 2015;71(9):1029–35.
11. Hickie IB. Reducing off-label prescribing in psychiatry. Med J Aust. 2014;200(2):65–6.
12. Haw C, Stubbs J. Off-label psychotropic prescribing for young persons in medium security. J Psychopharmacol. 2010;24(10):1491–8.
13. Evidence of harm from offlabel and unlicensed medicine in children. EMEA. [http://www.ema.europa.eu/docs/en_GB/document_library/Other/2009/10/WC500004021.pdf]. Accessed Oct 2004.
14. Remington G, Hahn M. Off-label antipsychotic use and tardive dyskinesia in at-risk populations: new drugs with old side effects. J Psychiatry Neurosci. 2014;39(1):E1–2.
15. Brauner JV, Johansen LM, Roesbjerg T, Pagsberg AK. Off-label prescription of psychopharmacological drugs in child and adolescent psychiatry. J Clin Psychopharmacol. 2016;36(5):500–7.
16. Culshaw J, Kendall D, Wilcock A. Off-label prescribing in palliative care: a survey of independent prescribers. Palliat Med. 2013;27(4):314–9.
17. Lucke C, Gschossmann JM, Schmidt A, Gschossmann J, Lam AP, Schneider CE, Philipsen A, Muller HH. A comparison of two psychiatric service approaches: findings from the Consultation vs Liaison Psychiatry-Study. BMC Psychiatry. 2017;17(1):8.
18. Radley DC, Finkelstein SN, Stafford RS. Off-label prescribing among office-based physicians. Arch Intern Med. 2006;166(9):1021–6.
19. Hodgson R, Belgamwar R. Off-label prescribing by psychiatrists. Psychiatr Bull. 2006;30(2):55–7.
20. Leslie DL, Mohamed S, Rosenheck RA. Off-label use of antipsychotic medications in the department of Veterans Affairs health care system. Psychiatr Serv. 2009;60(9):1175–81.
21. Hoff R, Braam AW. Off-label prescriptions in acute psychiatry: a practice-based evaluation. Tijdschr Psychiatr. 2013;55(4):233–45.
22. McKean A, Monasterio E. Off-label use of atypical antipsychotics: cause for concern? CNS Drugs. 2012;26(5):383–90.
23. Alexander GC, Gallagher SA, Mascola A, Moloney RM, Stafford RS. Increasing off-label use of antipsychotic medications in the United States, 1995–2008. Pharmacoepidemiol Drug Saf. 2011;20(2):177–84.
24. Sridharan K, Arora K, Chaudhary S. Off-label drug use in psychiatry: a retrospective audit in a tertiary care hospital. Asian J Psychiatr. 2016;24:124.
25. Weih M, Thurauf N, Bleich S, Kornhuber J. Off-label use in psychiatry. Fortschr Neurol Psychiatr. 2008;76(1):7–13.
26. Casey DE. Implications of the CATIE trial on treatment: extrapyramidal symptoms. CNS Spectr. 2006;11(7 Suppl 7):25–31.
27. Carton L, Cottencin O, Lapeyre-Mestre M, Geoffroy PA, Favre J, Simon N, Bordet R, Rolland B. Off-label prescribing of antipsychotics in adults, children and elderly individuals: a systematic review of recent prescription trends. Curr Pharm Des. 2015;21(23):3280–97.
28. Kane JM, Smith JM. Tardive dyskinesia: prevalence and risk factors, 1959–1979. Arch Gen Psychiatry. 1982;39(4):473–81.
29. Gupta S, Masand PS, Gupta S. Cardiovascular side effects of novel antipsychotics. CNS Spectr. 2001;6(11):912–8.
30. Howland RH. Atypical antipsychotics are not all alike: side effects and risk assessment. J Psychosoc Nurs Ment Health Serv. 2014;52(9):13–5.
31. Ikeno T, Okumura Y, Kugiyama K, Ito H. Analysis of the cardiac side effects of antipsychotics: Japanese adverse drug event report database (JADER). Nihon Shinkei Seishin Yakurigaku Zasshi. 2013;33(4):179–82.
32. Kamble P, Sherer J, Chen H, Aparasu R. Off-label use of second-generation antipsychotic agents among elderly nursing home residents. Psychiatr Serv. 2010;61(2):130–6.
33. Longo LP, Johnson B. Addiction: Part I. Benzodiazepines-side effects, abuse risk and alternatives. Am Fam Physician. 2000;61(7):2121–8.
34. Kruse WH. Problems and pitfalls in the use of benzodiazepines in the elderly. Drug Saf. 1990;5(5):328–44.
35. Madhusoodanan S, Bogunovic OJ. Safety of benzodiazepines in the geriatric population. Expert Opin Drug Saf. 2004;3(5):485–93.
36. Olfson M, King M, Schoenbaum M. Benzodiazepine use in the United States. JAMA Psychiatry. 2015;72(2):136–42.
37. Dautzenberg PL, van der Zande JA, Conemans JM, Rikkert MG. Off-label drug use on a Dutch geriatric ward. Int J Geriatr Psychiatry. 2009;24(10):1173–4.
38. Softic A, Beganlic A, Pranjic N, Sulejmanovic S. The influence of the use of benzodiazepines in the frequency falls in the elderly. Med Arch. 2013;67(4):256–9.
39. Pariente A, Dartigues JF, Benichou J, Letenneur L, Moore N, Fourrier-Reglat A. Benzodiazepines and injurious falls in community dwelling elders. Drugs Aging. 2008;25(1):61–70.
40. Association of the Scientific Medical Societies in Germany (AWMF): S3-Leitlinie, Analgesie, Sedierung und Delirmanagement in der Intensivmedizin (DAS-Leitlinie 2015). http://www.awmf.org/. Accessed Aug 2015.

28

Psychometric properties of the Chinese version of the empathy quotient among Chinese minority college students

Yanjun Zhang[1], JiuYu Xiang[2], Jianlin Wen[3*], Wei Bian[4], Liangbin Sun[5] and Ziran Bai[5]

Abstract

Background: When the minority college students from the ethnic minority communities come to study in Chinese Han region, they encounter adapting difficulties of culture and socio-psychology, in which empathy plays a crucial role. Current instruments used to measure empathy have many limited effectiveness. The empathy quotient (EQ) scale which has been validated in many countries was explicitly designed for clinical applications and was intended to be sensitive to a lack of empathy. This study is to develop a complete Chinese version of the EQ scale and to assess its reliability and validity among Chinese minority college students in the Han Chinese region.

Methods: A total of 1638 Chinese minority college students in the Han region were selected and were randomly divided into two groups. One group of 818 students took part in the implementation of the exploratory factor analysis while the other group of 820 students participated in the confirmatory factor analysis.

Results: Twenty-nine items of the EQ were retained based on the factor analysis and four factors were extracted: self-awareness, cognitive empathy, social skills, and emotional reactivity, which can explain 51.793% of the total variance. The factors of the EQ scale were significantly correlated with each other, with the correlation coefficient ranging from 0.316 to 0.563. The coefficient of internal consistency (Cronbach's α) was 0.824 for the total scale and ranged from 0.640 to 0.818 for the subscales. Confirmatory factor analysis proved that the measured data fitted well with the hypothesized four-factor model. All of the items in the scale fitted the model well, and the point-measure correlation coefficient had acceptable consistency.

Conclusions: The refined 29-item Chinese version of the EQ possesses good reliability and validity, and can be applied in assessing empathy among Chinese minority college students.

Keywords: Empathy, Empathy quotient, Reliability, Validity, Chinese minority nationality college students

Introduction

As an important ability for social communication, empathy in the broadest sense refers to the reactions of one individual to the observed experiences of another [1]. For its clinical implication, empathy helps to accurately represent others' psychological states and, therefore, enables self-control and adequate behavior in social contexts [2]. Researchers pointed out that the impairment of empathy may cause some mental psychiatric conditions including antisocial personality disorders and psychopathy [3, 4]. When the minority college students come to study in the Chinese Han region, they will inevitably find themselves immersed in a brand-new environment in which their interpersonal relationships and efforts to assimilate with the students of the Han nationality require an adapting process of psychology. For these minority college students, these 4 years of college life can also be viewed as a form of immigration. Language obstacles and a diverse culture make it difficult for them to understand what are taught in the class. Some of the minority students can successfully assimilate themselves into the new groups,

*Correspondence: 634798780@qq.com
[3] School of Marxism, Chongqing University, No. 174 Shazhengjie, Shapingba, Chongqing 400044, People's Republic of China
Full list of author information is available at the end of the article

but quite a number of them exhibit an abortive adaptation. During their adaptation, stressors like having trouble in understanding what teachers say, fearing about passing examinations, and the feeling of being excluded from groups will finally lead to psychological disorders such as anxiety, depression, and autism. In this study, we chose Uyghur and Hui nationalities as our study samples because Uyghur and Hui nationalities are typically representative with big population and widely distributed people among China's 55 ethnic minorities. Accounting for a large proportion of the minority college students in China, the two nationalities share the Islamic faith and their cultures are noticeably different from Han culture.

In the multicultural adaptation of Chinese minority college students, empathy helps to abate the cultural anxiety that emerges from the course of interpersonal communication because it could be viewed as the "glue" of the social world, drawing us to help others and stopping us from hurting others [5].

Although empathy without question plays a crucial role in interpersonal relationships, it is difficult for researchers to agree on a consistent definition and use of the term empathy [6]. Traditionally, researchers in this area have fallen into two camps: those who conceptualized empathy as more cognitive and those who conceptualized it as more affective [7]. However, a consensus has recently been reached in that both approaches have been essential to conceptualizing empathy and recognizing its multidimensional nature: the cognitive and affective approaches cannot be easily separated. Due to the historical divergence of recognizing the nature of empathy, instruments of various kinds have been developed to measure empathy. Among them, self-report questionnaires are one of the most widely used instruments because they are easy to use and can access multiple dimensions more straightforwardly than can other methods [8]. Some questionnaires for measuring empathy were developed, but it is doubtful that many of them are suitable instruments for measuring empathy. Here, we illustrate three typical types of questionnaires for measuring empathy: the empathy scale [9], the Questionnaire Measure of Emotional Empathy (QMEE) [10], and the Interpersonal Reactivity Index (IRI) [11].

The empathy scale was intended to measure empathy in a cognitive sense, but it later was found to have four independent factors: social self-confidence, even-temperedness, sensitivity, and nonconformity [12]. Of these four factors, only sensitivity is thought to be directly relevant to empathy; so, the empathy scale was not considered a pure measure of empathy but sort of a measure of social skills [13]. The Questionnaire Measure of Emotional Empathy (QMEE) was designed to assess an individual's tendency to react strongly to another's experience [10]. The authors of the QMEE suggest that the split-half reliability is high (0.84), which indicates the items are likely to tap a single construct, but this single construct may be emotional arousability to the environment in general, rather than to people's emotions in particular [14]. The IRI comprises four subscales: perspective-taking, empathic concern, personal distress, and fantasy. Because three of the four factors are directly relevant to empathy, the IRI was once thought to be the best way to measure empathy. But items of the fantasy subscale that state, "I daydream and fantasize, with some regularity, about things that might happen to me" and items of the personal distress subscale saying, "In emergency situations, I feel apprehensive and ill at ease" indicate that the IRI may measure processes broader than empathy and that these factors are not empathy itself [5].

To address the deficiencies of the existing questionnaires, Baron-Cohen and Wheelwright [5] developed a new self-report measure of empathy: the empathy quotient (EQ). The EQ was explicitly designed for clinical applications and was intended to be sensitive to a lack of empathy as a feature of psychopathology. The original, the Japanese [15], the French [2], the Korean [8], the Italian [16], and the Chinese [17] versions of the EQ have been validated in samples of university students and of the general population, in adults with high-functioning autism or Asperger's disorder, and with depersonalization disorder [18]. The aim of our study was to develop a Chinese version of the EQ and to establish its psychometric properties based on Chinese minority college students, a potentially useful assessment in working with Chinese minority college students who may suffer from mental disorders during the process of this typical immigrant adaptation.

Methods

Objects

A convenience sampling of 1650 Uyghur and Hui nationality college students (freshmen to seniors) from two Chinese universities (Chongqing University and Zhejiang Normal University) were recruited in May 2016. Approval for this study was obtained from the office of social science of the two universities. Inclusion criteria were as follows: (1) from Xinjiang Autonomous Region; (2) aged 17 years or older; (3) can read and understand Mandarin; (4) were not taking any anti-anxiety or antidepressant medication; and (5) did not have any other systematic diseases. The medical records of the students had been collected from the students file.

All questionnaires were returned, and there were no students refusing to participate. But twelve were incorrectly completed, leaving a total sample of 1638 subjects. 818 participants were randomly selected for the implementation of the exploratory factor analysis (EFA). The remaining 820 participants were arranged to participate in the confirmatory factor analysis (CFA).

A demographic data sheet including the age, gender, grade, and geographic area was also collected in the beginning of the study.

Instruments

Empathy quotient (EQ)

The empathy quotient (EQ), prepared by Professor Baron-Cohen and Professor Wheelwright [5] in 2004, is a scale specifically used to test the status of empathy among adults. It was organized into the three subscales of cognitive empathy, emotional reactivity, and social skill subscales. The original scale consists of 60 items, including 40 scoring items and 20 filler items. All the items were measured on a 4-point Likert-type scale ranging from complete agreement and half agreement to half disagreement and total disagreement. The final score was the total of all scoring items. The highest score was 80 (best EQ), while the lowest was 0 (worst EQ).

Translation and adaptation

We developed the Chinese version of the empathy quotient scale after obtaining the permission from Professor Baron-Cohen and his team, followed by a standard forward and backward translation procedure [19]. Firstly, two professional translators were employed to translate the EQ into Chinese, and panelists (including two psychologists and three education experts) were invited to conduct language and culture adjustments, perform content evaluation of the preliminary scale, and determine the first draft of the scale. The back-translation was conducted by two bilingual experts to translate the first draft into English, make comparisons with the original scale, find the differences, make corresponding amendments to the translated first draft, and ultimately reach a consistent opinion. The whole process was conducted rigorously to ensure semantic, idiomatic, experiential and conceptual equivalence to respect cultural considerations.

Fifty Uyghur college students were then selected to participate in the pretest, after which further amendments were made according to the results, and the final Chinese (language) version of the EQ was developed.

Data collection

The investigators directly distributed the scale to the participants of study, informed them of the purpose and process of this research, and had them sign the informed consent. Next, the objects of study carefully filled out the form item by item. At the time of collecting questionnaire, investigators immediately checked whether the questionnaire was entirely filled in. In case of any missing items, it was required to have them refilled at once and the questionnaire was collected only after proper checks and verifications were finalized. One week after the first round of investigation, 50 participants were randomly selected from the 818 participants to conduct the second round of filling out the questionnaire, for the purpose of testing the test–retest reliability of the questionnaire.

Data analysis

Data analysis was carried out by the SPSS 17.0 software package and checked by two researchers to ensure consistency. AMOS 21.0 was applied to test the confirmatory factor analysis. Descriptive statistics were used to summarize sample characteristics and the Kolmogorov–Smirnov test was used to examine the normal distribution of the data. Construct validity was statistically tested by means of principal component factor analysis with varimax rotation.

The reliability analysis of the EQ was tested by calculating the Cronbach's α and test–retest reliability by intraclass correlation coefficient. A Cronbach's $\alpha \geq 0.70$ was considered adequate [20].

Construct validity was evaluated by factor analysis. Regarding factor analysis, the principal components method was used to extract common factors based on the eigenvalues > 1 criterion and also scree plots, and the varimax rotation method to reveal relations (factor loadings) between common factors and items [21].

A content validity index (CVI) was used to describe the content validity. The expert panel was asked to score each item regarding the relevance to the total questionnaire on a 4-point scale of 4 = very relevant, 3 = quite relevant, 2 = somewhat relevant, and 1 = not relevant. The CVI was calculated by the percentage of items receiving a rating of 3 or 4, and a CVI value exceeding 0.80 indicated good content validity [20].

Convergent validity was evaluated by the correlation coefficient between the scores of every subscale and the total score.

A confirmatory factor analysis was conducted to examine the EQ structure to see if the factor structure reflected the proposed theoretical model. Statistical methods were used to test the fit of the model: χ^2/df, the goodness of fit index (GFI), adjusted goodness of fit index (AGFI), incremental fit index (IFI) value, comparative fit index (CFI), and Tucker–Lewis Index (TLI), and root mean square error of approximation (RMSEA). A χ^2 test with $P > 0.05$ shows a good model fit. Also, A model with $1 < \chi^2/df < 5$, IFI > 0.9, GFI > 0.9, AGFI > 0.9, CFI > 0.9, TLI > 0.9, RMSEA < 0.05 suggested a good model fit. Additionally, average variance extracted (AVE) was calculated from model estimates using the AVE formula given by, and the AVE for all exceeded the recommended level of 0.50. The maximum shared squared variance (MSV), and average shared squared variance (ASV) was less than AVE.

Results

Demographic data of the participants

Of all the 1638 participants who returned valid questionnaires, 941 students are with Uyghur nationality, 697 students are with Hui nationality. 884 (54.0%) of the participants are males, with an age range of 17–24, and 936 (57.1%) are from urban areas; 909 (55.5%) of the participants are only child.

A total of 818 participants were randomly selected for the implementation of exploratory factor analysis (EFA) while the remaining 820 participants participated in confirmatory factor analysis (CFA). Among the EFA group, there were 431 males and 387 females, with an average age of (20.69 ± 2.12). Among the CFA group, 453 were males and 367 were females, with an average age of (21.73 ± 3.24). There was no statistical significance between the two groups with regard to the demographic data.

Construct validity

The Kaiser–Meyer–Olkin (KMO) score for the Chinese version of the EQ scale was 0.888 and the Bartlett's test for sphericity was significant ($P < 0.001$), suggesting that the EQ scale was suitable for principal component analysis (PCA). As for the factor extraction, the factors with their extraction characteristic values of PCA greater than 1 are selected. Regarding the factor rotation method, the method combining both orthogonal rotation and oblique rotation is adopted. During the process of exploratory factor analysis, by grounding the factor analysis on the entry deletion criteria, those entries with factor loading smaller than 0.4, multiplicity factor loading, and unexplained dimensionality of belonging were deleted or retained after the panel discussion. Moreover, the factor analysis was conducted a second time for each deleted entry. As a result, four factors were extracted and 29 items ultimately retained. The scree plot suggested generating a four-factor model (Fig. 1).

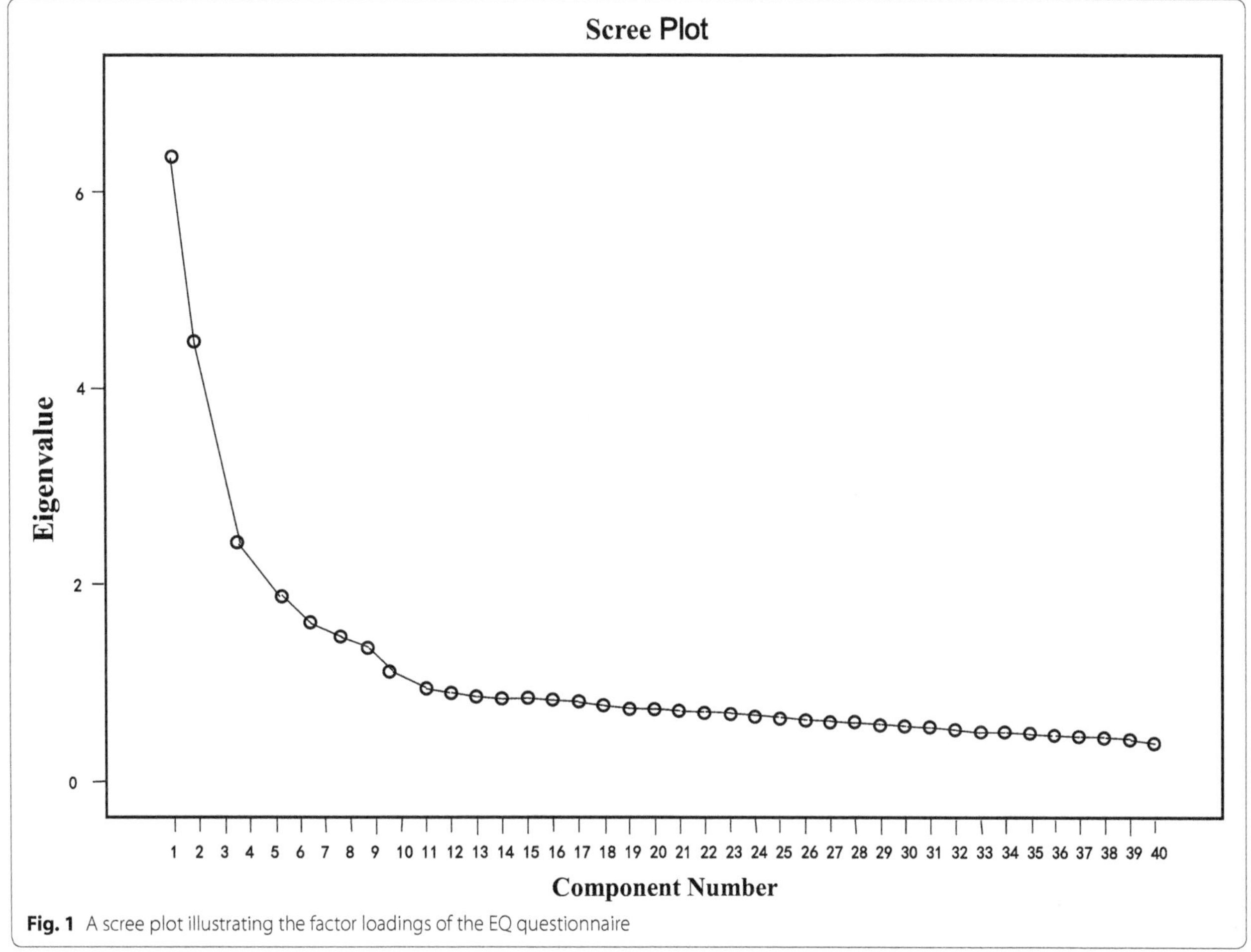

Fig. 1 A scree plot illustrating the factor loadings of the EQ questionnaire

The first factor, "cognitive empathy," which refers to the process of investigation in terms of recognizing and understanding the emotional feelings of others, accounted for 18.994% of the total variance. The second factor, "self-consciousness," referring to the process of investigation in terms of understanding the self-competence from individuals, accounted for 15.260% of the total variance. The third factor, "emotional empathy," the common experience of the emotional feelings of others, accounted for 13.386% of the total variance. Finally, the fourth factor, "social skills," or the skills and abilities manifested during the interactions between individuals and others, accounted for 13.073% of the total variance. See Table 1.

Reliability

The result showed that Cronbach's α of the EQ total scale was 0.824, and Cronbach's α of every subscale ranged between 0.714 and 0.818. The test–retest reliability of total scale was 0.896, and the test–retest reliabilities of every subscale ranged between 0.718 and 0.943 (see Table 2).

Content validity

The expert panel was invited to review the contents of the scale, and to make language and culture adjustments to entries so as to make them relevant to the expression of Chinese people. All the experts agreed that the Chinese version of the EQ scale was suitable for the determination of empathy status among Uyghur college students and the representativeness of entries was fine. And the CVI was 0.928, indicating adequate content validity.

Convergent validity

The correlation coefficient between each subscale of the EQ was significant, ranging between 0.316 and 0.563 and indicating moderate correlation. The correlation coefficient between each subscale and the total score ranged between 0.525 and 0.827, indicating high correlation (see Table 2).

Confirmatory factor analysis (CFA)

As indicated in the result, $\chi^2/df = 2.51 < 5$, and the goodness of fit index (GFI), adjusted goodness of fit index (AGFI), incremental fit index (IFI) value, comparative fit index (CFI), and Tucker–Lewis Index (TLI) were 0.942, 0.928, 0.920, 0.919, 0.909, respectively. All of them were greater than 0.9, and the root mean square error of approximation (RMSEA) was $0.043 < 0.06$. The results showed that the EQ scale fitted well into a four-factor model and all items were found to contribute significantly to their respective latent constructs. The four-factor model path diagram with standardized parameter estimates and factor inter-correlations is shown in Fig. 2.

The calculation of AVE and MSV showed that the AVE for all exceeded the recommended level of 0.50 and the MSV was less than AVE (shown in Table 3).

Comparison of EQ scale scores between different genders

A *T* test with independent samples was conducted among all the scores of the participants. The result showed that the median scores for the total EQ as well as "self-consciousness," "social skills," and "emotional empathy" subscales were significant higher in female college students compared with male college students ($P < 0.001$; see Table 4).

Comparison of different EQ models

The original EQ (60 items) has 40 items that measure empathy as a single construct and another 20 filler items. In the new Chinese EQ, 29 entries and 4 factors were ultimately retained which include three of the previous factors F1 (10 items): cognitive empathy, F3 (6 items): emotional empathy, and F4 (5 items): social skills, and one more added factor F2 (8 items): self-consciousness. The differences between the items available for the English version and the Chinese version are as the following Table 5.

In Table 5, seven structural models have been reported for the EQ, and the model description and CFA results for each model are provided. Cronbach's α values for the scores on the EQ − 40 and EQ − 15 were both 0.86. The Cronbach's α of every subscale of this study ranged between 0.714 and 0.818. Cronbach's α values for the scores on the other EQ models are provided in Table 5. The final modified model of this study showed a good fit to the data (see Table 5).

In this modified study, the approximate values of six other structural models were gotten in a rounded way with data citations from "validation of the empathy quotient in Mainland China" [22].

Discussion

A Chinese version of the EQ (29 items) was validated in this study with the samples of Uyghur and Hui Minority College Students in Mainland China. This study, in line with three other studies which based on Chinese populations [23–25], provides evidence to support the notion that the cognitive and emotional empathy may coexist, rather than be clearly differentiated, which was originally put forward by Baron-Cohen and Wheelwright [5].

Compared to other validations worldwide, this study also showed similarities and statistically significant gender differences in findings. Through a *T* test with

Table 1 Factor loading, eigenvalues, and percent of variance for EQ scale items emerging from the principal components analysis ($n = 818$)

Items	Factors			
	Cognitive empathy	Self-consciousness	Emotional empathy	Social skills
1. EQ36				
Good at understanding others	0.787			
2. EQ26				
Quick to feel others are uncomfort	0.760			
3. EQ41				
Sensitive to others' feelings	0.756			
4. EQ19				
Insightful to others' talk	0.743			
5. EQ54				
Sensitive to others' talk intention	0.693			
6. EQ52				
Tune into how someone feels	0.588			
7. EQ58				
Good at prediction	0.579			
8. EQ55				
Sensitive to others' talk intention	0.568			
9. EQ44				
I can sense if I am intruding	0.567			
10. EQ01				
Sensitive to others' intention	0.536			
11. EQ15				
Focus on my own thoughts in talk		0.711		
12. EQ34				
Regard my bluntness as rudeness		0.682		
13. EQ27				
Say offendence		0.668		
14. EQ28				
Reply someone truthfully		0.676		
15. EQ30				
Being often told unpredictable		0.668		
16. EQ31				
Enjoy being the center		0.642		
17. EQ24				
Like impulsion		0.555		
18. EQ29				
Can't always see offendence cause		0.527		
19. EQ06				
Enjoy caring for other people			0.779	
20. EQ50				
Emotionally detached with a film			0.727	
21. EQ38				
Feel upsets to see animals in pain			0.683	
22. EQ42				
Get upset if see sufferings			0.632	
23. EQ21				
Hard to find upset			0.597	

Table 1 (continued)

Items	Factors			
	Cognitive empathy	Self-consciousness	Emotional empathy	Social skills
24. EQ59				
Involved with a friend's problems			0.519	
25. EQ08				
Hard to know what to do				0.750
26. EQ35				
Don't tend to find confusion				0.641
27. EQ04				
Difficult to explain to others				0.627
28. EQ48				
People say I am insensitive				0.583
29. EQ33				
Enjoy discussing about politics				0.548
Eigenvalues	4.679	2.213	2.159	1.857
Variance explained	18.994%	15.260%	13.386%	13.073%

Only factor loading values over 0.4 was listed here

Table 2 Correlation between scores for each EQ scale and the total EQ scale score

	Self-consciousness	Cognitive empathy	Social skills	Emotional empathy
Self-consciousness	1			
Cognitive empathy	0.316[a]	1		
Social skills	0.563[a]	0.383[a]	1	
Emotional empathy	0.494[a]	0.474[a]	0.375[a]	1
Total	0.827[a]	0.544[a]	0.646[a]	0.525[a]

[a] $P<0.01$

independent samples, this research showed that the median scores for the total EQ as well as "self-consciousness," "social skills," and "emotional empathy" subscales were significantly higher in female college students compared with male college students ($P<0.001$); however, there was no distinct difference in the scores of cognitive empathy between male and female participants. It is consistent with the findings in the majority of studies [2, 18, 26], which proved the findings of the emotion study: men are more likely to suppress their emotions while women are more inclined to express them [18]. However, it is not only completely inconsistent with Bailey's (1996) findings and Guan's (2012) findings [24], in which "no statistically significant gender differences were found", but also absolutely inconsistent with Preti and Vellante's (2011) findings, "cognitive empathy factor scores were consistently higher among females than males; there were no differences by gender on the social skills, or the emotional reactivity factor" [27]. Meanwhile, it is also different with Baron-Cohen and Wheelwright's [5] findings, in which "sex differences (female superiority) were also found on both cognitive empathy and emotional reactivity but not on the 'social skills'". It might be that the participants were college students from either Hui or Uyghur nationality which were Chinese ethnic minorities in a cross-culture environment.

Dutch cultural anthropologist Hofstede described the multicultural conflicts as having four stages: curiosity, cultural disturbance, acculturation, and stabilizing [28]. The less time one spends in the stage of cultural disturbance and acculturation, the faster he or she will adapt into the new cultural environment. But the truth is that so many minority college students in Chinese Han region failed to convert this conflict due to their long time span in the stages of cultural disturbance and acculturation. Researches showed that, confronted with the dual-cultural environment, namely Han culture and their own national culture, minority college students in Chinese Han region have a sense of cultural alienation because of the friction between their mother culture and the mainstream culture of the Han nationality [29]. They have to accept the influence of Han culture on the one hand and inherit the culture of their own nationality on the other. This adapting process inevitably incurs conflicts between their native cultural position and the extraneous ones. Therefore, their scores of compulsion, depression and paranoid ideation of Xinjiang ethnic minority students in colleges of Han region were significantly higher than those of other students [30]. As a result, negative emotions such as inferiority, autism, and anxiety show up

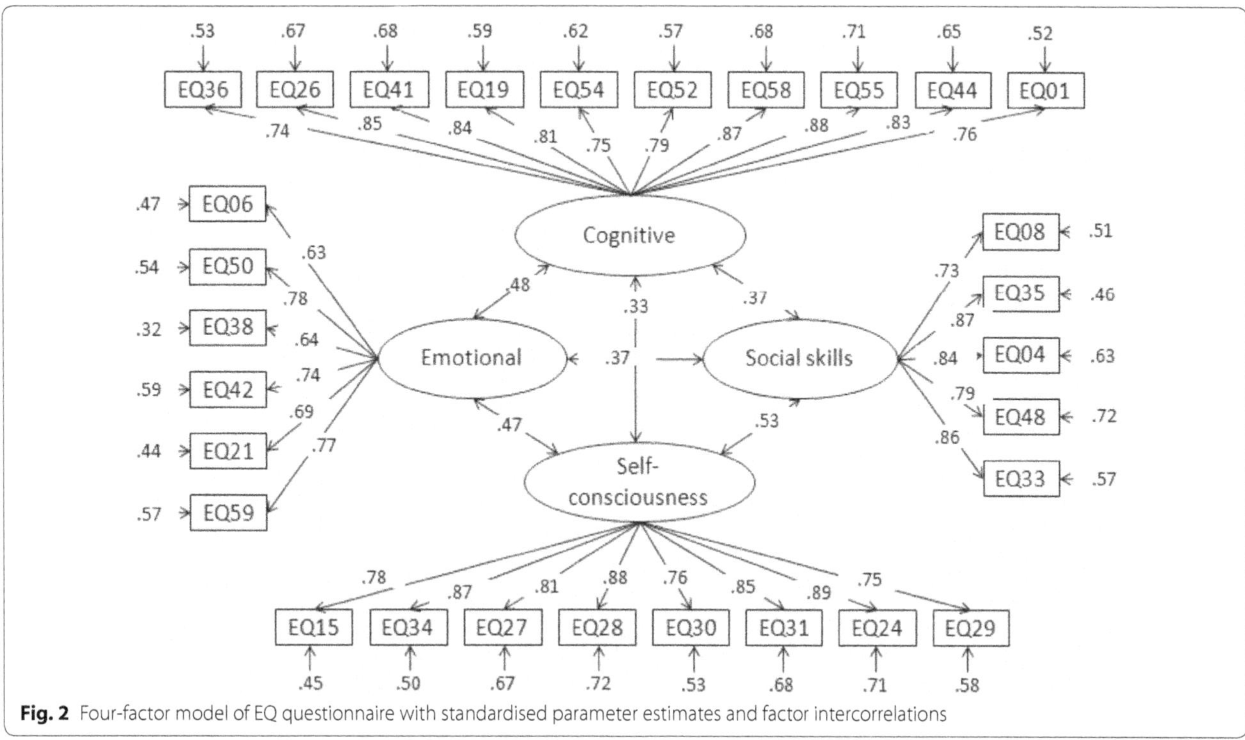

Fig. 2 Four-factor model of EQ questionnaire with standardised parameter estimates and factor intercorrelations

and their academic performance starts to decline, which inevitably endangers their physical and mental health. Obviously, the cultivation of empathy skills can help to shorten the time span of the cultural disturbance and acculturation stages and finally improve the ability for cross-cultural communication.

By this means, their negative emotions can be decreased progressively and their positive emotions can increase correspondingly which help individuals to become adapted to the main cultural environment in a short time. The EQ scale has first been implemented in the population of minority college students, and the cross validation for the EQ scale has been made by exploratory factor analysis and confirmatory factor analysis. Firstly, according to the exploratory factor analysis and taking into account the original structure of the EQ scale, we deleted some items, finally obtaining 29 items and four factors which have the same nomenclature as the original EQ scale. We named the four factors as cognitive empathy, self-awareness, emotional empathy, and social skills. Secondly, confirmatory factor analysis was used to verify the structural model and the results show that the model fitting is preferable. All the indicators of reliability and validity analysis showed that this version of EQ scale had a good validation.

In this study, we ranked the contribution ability of four factors in order from high to low: cognitive empathy, self-awareness, emotional empathy, and social skills. The cumulative percent of the four factors was 60.713%. This result was different from Lawrence and Baron-Cohen's study of a British population. In their study, three factors were obtained with the contribution ability ranked in the following order (high to low): cognitive empathy, emotional empathy, and social skills. By comparison, the cumulative percent of our four factors improved upon that found in the study by Lawrence and his colleagues on the British population by 19.313%, suggesting that the EQ scale in the Chinese version is quite fit for measuring empathy in the population of Chinese Uyghur and Hui Nationality College students. Further analysis showed that in both Western and Eastern culture, cognition plays a vital role in the process of the dynamically social and psychological phenomenon of empathy. When individuals confront one or more definite emotional situations, empathy occurs according to the following steps: firstly, the emotions and feelings were shared; then, on the premise of recognizing the difference between oneself and others, cognitive assessments on the whole situation were made; consequently, the response to the emotions and feelings with appropriate actions came into being [31].

In this study, we detached a new factor, self-awareness, which plays a vital role in the empathy skills of minority college students. Compared with Han students in mainland Chinese cities, minority students' way of thought and action on the value of orientation normally stem

Table 3 Results for the measurement model

Construct	Items	Factor loading	ASV	MSV	AVE	CR
Self-consciousness	EQ15	0.711	0.220	0.317	0.508	0.891
	EQ34	0.682				
	EQ27	0.668				
	EQ28	0.676				
	EQ30	0.668				
	EQ31	0.642				
	EQ24	0.555				
	EQ29	0.527				
Cognitive empathy	EQ36	0.787	0.157	0.225	0.502	0.909
	EQ26	0.760				
	EQ41	0.756				
	EQ19	0.743				
	EQ54	0.693				
	EQ52	0.588				
	EQ58	0.579				
	EQ55	0.568				
	EQ44	0.567				
	EQ01	0.536				
Emotional empathy	EQ06	0.779	0.201	0.317	0.517	0.810
	EQ50	0.727				
	EQ38	0.683				
	EQ42	0.632				
	EQ21	0.597				
	EQ59	0.519				
Social skills	EQ08	0.750	0.203	0.244	0.570	0.797
	EQ35	0.641				
	EQ04	0.627				
	EQ48	0.583				
	EQ33	0.548				

Table 4 Score comparison of the Chinese version of the empathy quotient (EQ) scale for male and female college students ($\overline{X} \pm s$)

Subscales	Total ($n=1638$)	Male ($n=884$)	Female ($n=754$)	t	P
Self-consciousness	10.0±0.4	9.1±0.4	11.0±0.4	−6.24	<0.001
Cognitive empathy	6.3±0.7	6.1±0.7	6.4±0.7	−1.68	0.092
Social skills	3.3±0.6	2.9±0.9	3.7±0.5	−5.26	<0.001
Emotional empathy	4.3±0.9	4.0±0.8	4.6±0.9	−4.66	<0.001
Total	23.9±0.6	22.2±0.4	25.7±0.5	−6.89	<0.001

from their inherent cultural habits and customs, while the former have more opportunities to be well informed and to enrich social communication. The manners of thought and action of minority college students represent an unconscious status of "always being right" while never thinking "must always be right?" Consequently, this cultural and psychological structure formed the distinct psychological characteristics featured by self-centeredness, strong independence, self-respect, and sensitivity.

In addition, gender difference was scored in this revised Chinese version of the EQ scale. The results showed that there was no distinct difference in the scores of cognitive empathy between male and female participants, but the total score and scores of self-awareness, social skills, and emotional empathy were higher for females than for males. The difference of the EQ index for different genders in our study is consistent with the research results of Lawrence and Baron-Cohen [18], which proved the findings of the emotion study: men are more likely to suppress their emotions while women are more inclined to express them [32].

There are some limitations in our study. Firstly, we used the convenience sample to recruit the college students

Table 5 Differences of EQ structural models and CFA results

EQ model	Factors (item number) Cronbach's α				CFA results			
	F1	F2	F3	F4	χ^2/df	CFI	TLI	RMSEA
Baron-Cohen and Wheelwright [5]	EM (40) 0.86	–	–	–	4.383	0.73	0.71	0.076
Lawrence et al. [18]	CE (11) 0.87	ER (11) 0.69	SS (6) 0.57	–	4.577	0.84	0.83	0.078
Wakabayashi et al. [33]	EM (22) 0.86	–	–	–	5.744	0.86	0.84	0.090
Muncer and Ling [34]	CE (5) 0.78	ER (5) 0.55	SS (5) 0.56	–	4.138	0.90	0.88	0.073
Allison et al. [35]	AG (13) 0.80	DI (13) 0.74	–	–	2.459	0.91	0.90	0.050
Guan et al. [24]	EM (15) 0.86	–	–	–	4.690	0.94	0.93	0.079
Zhao et al. [17, 22, 25, 26]	EM (15) 0.86	–	–	–	4.036	0.95	0.95	0.072
This study	CE (10) 0.818	SC (8) 0.793	EE (6) 0.714	SS (5) 0.746	2.51	0.919	0.909	0.043

CFI comparative fit index, *TLI* Tucker–Lewis Index, *RMSEA* root mean square error of approximation, *EQ* empathy quotient, *EM* empathy, *CE* cognitive empathy, *ER* emotional reactivity, *SS* social skills, *AG* agreement, *DI* disagreement, *SC* self-consciousness, *EE* emotional empathy

from only two universities as our research targets, so there was a sample selection bias in this study. Thus, our results may not be representative of the wider minority College Students in China. Additionally, this study used classical test theory to assess the psychometric properties of the EQ. Modern psychometric theory such as Rasch analysis was not used.

Conclusion

In summary,this study developed a complete Chinese version of the EQ scale and found that it had a good reliability and validity among Chinese Uyghur and Hui nationality college students in the Han Chinese region. Also, the related research findings with this Chinese version EQ scale could be the reference of offering suggestions for various related educators and policy-makers to help a large quantity of minority students to improve their empathy ability and to adapt to a new learning environment much easier. A much larger number of samples will be collected, various analyzing methods such as Rasch analysis have to be used in future to verify the EQ scale structure, and an examination of factors that influence the EQ skills will be made.

Abbreviations

EQ: empathy quotient scale; EFA: exploratory factor analysis; CFA: confirmatory factor analysis; QMEE: Questionnaire Measure of Emotional Empathy; IRI: Interpersonal Reactivity Index; PANAS: positive and negative affect scale; SSRS: social support review survey; SCSQ: simplified coping style questionnaire; CVI: content validity index; GFI: goodness of fit index; AGFI: adjusted goodness of fit index; IFI: incremental fit index value; CFI: comparative fit index; TLI: Tucker–Lewis Index; RMSEA: root mean square error of approximation.

Authors' contributions

YZ, JX, JW and WB together contributed to the conception, conducted the design, performed the data analyses, YZ and JW prepared the manuscript draft, and conducted the project management. JX contributed to calculate the AVE and MSV. WB contributed to the study design, data analyses, clinical consultation, and manuscript revision. LS contributed to study design, data collection, manuscript writing and revision. ZB provided advice and assistance with statistical operations. JW supervised the study. All authors read and approved the final manuscript.

Author details

[1] College of Teacher Education, Zhejiang Normal University, Jinhua, zhejiang Province, People's Republic of China. [2] School of Marxism, Wuhan University, Wuhan, Hubei Province, People's Republic of China. [3] School of Marxism, Chongqing University, No. 174 Shazhengjie, Shapingba, Chongqing 400044, People's Republic of China. [4] Southwest Eye Hospital, Third Military Medical University, Chongqing, People's Republic of China. [5] School of Journalism and Communication, Chongqing University, Chongqing, People's Republic of China.

Acknowledgements

Thanks to Dr. Simon Baron-Cohen and his team for providing the EQ scale and for his assistance in the amendment of the Chinese version of the EQ scale.

Competing interests

The authors declare that they have no competing interests.

Consent to publication

Not applicable.

Funding

This study was funded by National Social Science Foundation of China (15XKS042) and Ministry of Education Subordinate University (CQDXWL-2012-157) and project of the Internet Plus Educational Research of Ideology and Policy of Chongqing University (2017CDJSK01PT30) to Jianlin Wen.

References

1. Davis Mark H. Measuring individual differences in empathy evidence for multidimensional approach. J Pers Soc Psychol. 1983;44(1):113–26.
2. Berthoz S, Wessa M, Kedia G, Wicker B, Grèzes J. Cross-cultural validation of the empathy quotient in a French-speaking sample. Can J Psychiatry. 2008;53(7):469–77.
3. Jolliffe D, Farrington DP. Empathy and offending: a systematic review and meta-analysis. Aggress Violent Behav. 2004;9(5):441–76.
4. Blair RJR. Responding to the emotions of others: dissociating forms of empathy through the study of typical and psychiatric populations. Conscious Cogn. 2005;14(4):698–718.
5. Baron-Cohen S, Wheelwright S. The empathy quotient: an investigation of adults with Asperger syndrome or high functioning autism and normal sex differences. J Autism Dev Disord.2004;34(2):163–175. https://doi.org/10.1023/B:JADD.0000022607.19833.00
6. de Vignemont F, Singer T. The empathic brain: how, when and why? Trends Cogn Sci. 2006;10(10):435–41.
7. Chakrabarti B, Baron-Cohen S. Empathizing: neurocognitive developmental mechanisms and individual differences. Progr Brain Res. 2006;156:403–17.
8. Kim J, Lee SJ. Reliability and validity of the Korean version of the empathy quotient scale. Psychiatry Invest. 2010;7(1):24–30.
9. Hogan R. Development of an empathy scale. J Consult Clin Psychol. 1969;33(3):307–16.
10. Mehrabian A, Epstein N. A measure of emotional empathy. J Pers. 1972;40(4):525–43.
11. Davis MH. A multidimensional approach to individual differences in empathy. JSAS Catalog Sel Doc Psychol. 1980;10:85.
12. Johnson JA, Cheek JM, Smither R. The structure of empathy. J Pers Soc Psychol. 1983;45(1):1299–312.
13. Davis MH. Empathy: a social psychological approach. Boulder: Westview Press USA; 1996.
14. Mehrabian A, Young AL, Sato S. Emotional empathy and associated individual differences. Curr Psychol Res Rev. 1988;7(3):221–40.
15. Wakabayashi A, Baron-Cohen S, Uchiyama T, Yoshida Y, Kuroda M, Wheelwright S. Empathizing and systemizing in adults with and without autism spectrum conditions: cross-cultural stability. J Autism Dev Disord. 2007;37(10):1823–32.
16. Preti A, Vellante M, Baron-Cohen S, Zucca G, Petretto DR, Masala C. The Empathy quotient: a cross-cultural comparison of the Italian version. Cogn Neuropsychiatry. 2011;16(1):50–70.
17. Zhao Q, Neumann DL, Cao X, Baron-Cohen S, Sun X, Cao Y, Yan C, Wang Y, Shao L, Shum DHK. Validation of the empathy quotient in Mainland China. J Pers Assess. 2017. https://doi.org/10.1080/00223891.2017.1324458.
18. Lawrence EJ, Shaw P, Baker D, Baron-Cohen S, David AS. Measuring empathy: reliability and validity of the empathy quotient. Psychol Med. 2004;34(5):911–9.
19. Garyfallos G, Karastergiou A, Adamopoulou A, Moutzoukis C, Alagiozidou E, Mala D, et al. Greek version of the general health questionnaire: accuracy of translation and validity. Acta Psychiatr Scand. 1991;84:371–8.
20. Polit D, Beck C. Nursing research: principles and methods. Philadelphia: Lippincott Williams & Wilkins, cop.; 2004.
21. Fabrigar L, MacCallum R, Wegener DT, Strahan EJ. Evaluating the use of exploratory factor analysis in psychological research. Psychol Methods. 1999;4:272–99.
22. Zhao Q, Neumann DL, Cao X. Validation of the empathy quotient in Mainland China. J Pers Assess. 2017. https://doi.org/10.1080/00223891.2017.1324458.
23. Siu AM, Shek DT. Validation of the interpersonal reactivity index in a Chinese context. Res Soc Work Pract. 2005;15:118–26. https://doi.org/10.1177/1049731504270384.
24. Guan R, Jin L, Qian M. Validation of the empathy quotient-short form among Chinese healthcare professionals. Soc Behav Pers. 2012;40:75–84. https://doi.org/10.2224/sbp.2012.40.1.75.
25. Zhao Q, Neumann DL, Cao X. Validation of the empathy quotient in Mainland China. J Pers Assess. 2017. https://doi.org/10.1080/00223891.2017.1324458.
26. Zhao Q, Neumann DL, Cao X. Validation of the empathy quotient in Mainland China. J Pers Assess. 2017. https://doi.org/10.1080/00223891.2017.1324458.
27. Preti A, Vellante M, Baron-Cohen S, Zucca G, Petretto DR, Masala C. The empathy quotient: a cross-cultural comparison of the Italian version. Cogn Neuropsychiatry. 2011;16:50–70. https://doi.org/10.1080/13546801003790982.
28. Hofstede GJ. Cultures and organizations: software of the mind. 2nd ed. New York: McGraw-Hill; 2005.
29. Yudi C, Baojuan Y. The effect of cultural alienation on well-being of minority students in Han District colleges: the moderating effect of emotion regulation strategies. Chin J Clin Psychol. 2016;24(01):49–52.
30. Li M, Long Y. Research of factors influencing mental health of Xinjiang minority college students in the Hinterland. J Res Educ Ethnic Minor. 2018;29(01):76–82. https://doi.org/10.15946/j.cnki.1001-7178.2018.01.011.
31. Liu C, Wang Y, Yu G, Wang Y. Related theories and exploration on dynamic model of empathy. Adv Psychol Sci. 2009;17(5):964–72.
32. Huang S, Liu P, Zhang W, Liang S. Reliability and validity of Chinese version of the regulatory emotional self-efficacy scale in junior middle school students. Chin J Clin Psychol. 2012;20(2):158–61.
33. Wakabayashi A, Baron-Cohen S, Wheelwright S, Goldenfeld N, Delaney J, Fine D, Weil L. Development of short forms of the Empathy Quotient (EQ–Short) and the Systemizing Quotient (SQ–Short). Personal Individ Differ. 2006;41:929–40.
34. Muncer SJ, Ling J. Psychometric analysis of the Empathy Quotient (EQ) scale. Personal Individ Differ. 2006;40:1111–9.
35. Allison C, Baron-Cohen S, Wheelwright S, Stone MH, Muncer SJ. Psychometric analysis of the Empathy Quotient (EQ). Personal Individ Differ. 2011;51:829–35.

29

The association between parental depression and adolescent's Internet addiction in South Korea

Dong-Woo Choi[1,2], Sung-Youn Chun[1,2], Sang Ah Lee[1,2], Kyu-Tae Han[3] and Eun-Cheol Park[2,4*]

Abstract

Background: A number of risk factors for Internet addiction among adolescents have been identified to be associated with their behavior, familial, and parental factors. However, few studies have focused on the relationship between parental mental health and Internet addiction among adolescents. Therefore, we investigated the association between parental mental health and children's Internet addiction by controlling for several risk factors.

Methods: This study used panel data collected by the Korea Welfare Panel Study in 2012 and 2015. We focused primarily on the association between Internet addiction which was assessed by the Internet Addiction Scale (IAS) and parental depression which was measured with the 11-item version of the Center for Epidemiologic Studies Depression Scale. To analyze the association between parental depression and log-transformed IAS, we conducted multiple regression analysis after adjusting for covariates.

Results: Among 587 children, depressed mothers and fathers comprised 4.75 and 4.19%, respectively. The mean IAS score of the adolescents was 23.62 ± 4.38. Only maternal depression ($\beta = 0.0960$, $p = 0.0033$) showed higher IAS among children compared to nonmaternal depression. Strongly positive associations between parental depression and children's Internet addiction were observed for high maternal education level, adolescents' gender, and adolescent's academic performance.

Conclusions: Maternal depression is related to children's Internet addiction; particularly, mothers who had graduated from the university level or above, male children, and children's normal or better academic performance show the strongest relationship with children's Internet addiction.

Keywords: Maternal depression, Internet addiction, Mental health, Adolescent, CESD-11, Internet Addiction Scale

Introduction

The Internet has become an integral part of our daily lives. We have come to depend so much on the Internet that we are unable to imagine a world without it. However, this dependence causes Internet addiction. Although Internet addiction is not yet recognized as an established disorder, it is considered an emerging behavioral problem, particularly among adolescents [1].

While more than 80% of the population in the United Kingdom, United States, and Asia have access to the Internet, a smaller proportion of the population in South America (45–55%) have Internet access, and the proportion of young Internet users in Africa and the Middle East has increased by about 3000% over the past decade [2]. According to international research, over 30% of children under the age of 2 used tablets or smartphones, while 80% of teenagers owned similar devices [3].

A number of risk factors for Internet addiction among adolescents have been identified to be associated with their behavior, familial, and parental factors such as family relationships, dysfunction families, parental attitudes, and parenting styles [4–8]. However, few studies

*Correspondence: ecpark@yuhs.ac
[4] Department of Preventive Medicine, Yonsei University College of Medicine, 50 Yonsei-ro, Seodaemun-gu, Seoul 03722, Republic of Korea
Full list of author information is available at the end of the article

have focused on the relationship between parental mental health and Internet addiction among adolescents [9]. Parental depression has extensive consequences on family life and children's social adjustment and mental health, and these results induce major psychiatric problems such as depression and anxiety among these children [10, 11]. Therefore, parental mental health problems need to be managed for their own good as well as that of their children.

In this study, we focused on Internet addiction among adolescents in relation to parental depression, considering other risk factors. We hypothesized that parental mental health problems are associated with a negative impact on Internet addiction among children, and that particularly, the mother's role is more important in curbing this addiction compared to the father.

Methods

Study population

This study used panel data collected by the Korea Welfare Panel Study (KOWEPS) between 2012 and 2015 from nationally representative samples of Korean households with two-stage-stratified cluster sampling. The KOWEPS included information of 18,856 participants from 7072 households, regarding socioeconomic status, health status, and insurance and welfare status. Moreover, it included an additional survey of students aged 11–19 years, regarding health status, education status, and school life triennially. Among 775 children who participated in this study, 188 provided no answer for survey questionnaires about variables including school type, school record, stress and academic performance, mental health score indexes, parental depression, and socioeconomic status, and were excluded. Accordingly, 587 children were included in this study.

Variables

Internet addiction was assessed by the Internet Addiction Scale (IAS) for children, which was developed by the National Information Society Agency. This scale was a self-assessment tool developed as a short form of the *K*-scale considering it was too long for children to fill out and hardly reflected the characteristics appropriately in Korea [12]. It consisted of 20 questions for each of the four categories assessing Internet addiction from 'never true' to 'always true.' Therefore, the IAS score was obtained by summing the individual values of the answers to the 20 questions. This standard scale was validated to screen and evaluate Internet addiction by previous studies [13, 14].

We focused primarily on parental depression. Parental depression was measured with the 11-item version of the Center for Epidemiologic Studies Depression Scale (CESD-11). The CESD-11 is a shorter version of the 20-item CESD and is a self-reported screening tool which is well validated [15]. The CESD-11 consisted of 11 questions for each of the four categories measuring depression symptoms and the total score was calculated by adding the scores for all questions and multiplying this value by 20/11. Depression was diagnosed by obtaining a CESD-11 score of above 16.

Covariates were used such as sex, parental economic status ('salary employee,' 'employer or self-employed,' and 'not employed or unemployed'), parental education level ('high school or below' and 'university or above'), household income ('low,' 'mid-low,' 'mid-high,' 'high'), school type ('elementary school' and 'high school'), academic performance ('poor or very poor,' 'normal,' and 'good or very good'), academic achievement stress and score on the Korean version of the Child Behavior Checklist (K-CBCL) [16, 17]. The Academic Achievement Stress Scale was measured by four items measuring students' perceived stress from score 1 to 4 (performance, homework, concern of College entrance exams, and burn-out for study). Total score is the sum of each item that indicates a level of adolescent's perceived stress. The K-CBCL consists of five items, including depression and anxiety, attention problems, social problems, delinquency, and aggression. Each question has The K-CBCL scale was the modified Korean version of Achenbach's CBCL and has three answer categories ranging from 'never felt,' 'sometimes felt,' and 'strongly felt,' and each category score is valued as 0, 1, or 2, and the total score is obtained by summing the scores of all items.

Statistical analysis

For all statistical analyses, we used weights to improve the representativeness of the samples provided by the KOWEPS. First, the frequencies and percentages of the study population and weighted mean of IAS score for each variable were determined by t test and analysis of variance. Thereafter, we performed a log-transformation of the IAS score to improve normality. To analyze the association between parental depression and log-transformed IAS, we performed multiple regression analysis after controlling for covariates such as parental economic status, parental education level, household income, adolescent's sex, school type, academic performance, academic achievement stress score, and K-CBCL score. Finally, we performed subgroup analyses for the association between adolescents' IAS score and different factors according to parental depression after adjusting for covariates. All statistical analyses were performed using SAS 9.4 (SAS Institute Inc., Cary, NC, USA), and p-values less than 0.05 were considered statistically significant.

Table 1 The general characteristics of the study population in this study

Variables	N/mean	% (weighted)/SD	IAS		
			Mean	SD	p-value
Parents					
Mother's depression					0.0049
Yes	36	4.75	25.61	±5.08	
No	551	95.26	23.53	±4.33	
Father's depression					0.9898
Yes	30	4.19	24.38	±4.55	
No	557	95.81	23.59	±4.38	
Mother's economic status					0.0016
Salary employee	287	48.76	24.17	±4.54	
Employer or self-employed	91	15.32	23.19	±4.65	
Not employed or unemployed	209	35.92	23.08	±3.99	
Father's economic status					0.2665
Salary employee	400	71.19	23.75	±4.66	
Employer or self-employed	157	24.32	23.20	±3.55	
Not employed or unemployed	30	4.50	23.93	±4.70	
Mother's education level					0.1000
High school or under	347	56.53	23.90	±4.62	
University or above	240	43.47	23.27	±4.01	
Father's education level					0.0003
High school or under	318	48.81	24.32	±4.72	
University or above	269	51.19	22.97	±3.86	
Household income					0.5061
Low	147	19.78	23.82	±4.16	
Mid-low	149	22.97	23.37	±4.08	
Mid-high	148	25.63	24.04	±4.59	
High	143	31.62	23.36	±4.72	
Adolescents					
Gender					< 0.0001
Male	293	52.28	24.44	±4.62	
Female	294	47.72	22.73	±3.98	
School type					
Elementary school	303	41.70	23.24	±3.90	
High school	284	58.30	23.90	±4.84	
Academic performance					< 0.0001
Bad or very bad	105	19.44	25.28	±5.61	
Normal	199	36.50	23.70	±4.72	
Good or very good	283	44.07	22.83	±3.34	
Academic achievement stress score[a]	8.74	±2.92			
Depression and anxiety score[a]	4.14	±4.38			
Attention problems score[a]	3.45	±3.79			
Social problem score[a]	2.35	±2.84			
Delinquency score[a]	0.73	±1.45			
Aggression score[a]	2.79	±3.69			
Total	587	100.00	23.64	±4.38	

[a] Mean and standard deviation (SD) of the continuous independent variables in this study

Results

Table 1 shows the general characteristics of the study population. The prevalence rates of maternal and paternal depression were 4.75 and 4.19%, respectively. Regarding education level, 56.53 and 43.47% of mothers and fathers had graduated from high school or below, respectively, and 43.47 and 51.19% of mothers and fathers had graduated from university or above, respectively. Of the children surveyed, 52.28% were males and 47.72% were females. The average IAS score for the adolescents was 23.62 ± 4.38.

Table 2 shows the results of the multiple regression analysis performed to investigate the relationship between factors and the Internet addiction among adolescents. As shown in Table 2, maternal depression ($\beta = 0.0960$, $p = 0.0033$) yielded higher IAS compared to nonmaternal depression, unlike paternal depression which did not show significantly different findings between groups ($p = 0.7555$). Maternal education at the high school level or below ($\beta = 0.0380$, $p = 0.0173$) yielded higher IAS than those with education at the university level or above. On the other hand, paternal education level did not show statistically significant findings ($p = 0.2132$). Male children showed higher IAS ($\beta = 0.0815$, $p < 0.0001$) compared to that of female children. Moreover, children who performed poorly academically had higher IAS ($\beta = 0.0480$, $p = 0.0286$) compared to those with good or very good academic performance.

Figure 1 shows the results of the subgroup analysis for the association between parental depression and IAS according to the children's maternal education level, adolescents' gender, and academic performance. Adolescents' mothers with depression who graduated from high school or below had higher IAS ($\beta = 0.0770$, $p = 0.0187$) compared to those who did not have depression. Likewise, among adolescents' mothers who graduated from university or above, children with maternal depression ($\beta = 0.2291$, $p < 0.0001$) had higher IAS compared to those whose mothers did not have depression. However, there were not significant results in paternal depression ($p > 0.05$). Male children whose mothers had depression showed higher IAS ($\beta = 0.1138$, $p = 0.0383$) than those who had no depression. Female adolescents whose mothers had depression also had higher IAS ($\beta = 0.0724$, $p = 0.0300$) compared to those whose mothers had no depression. However, there was no statistically significant association for children of fathers with depression (male: p = 0.6209, female: $p = 0.4951$).

Table 2 The results of multiple regression analysis performed to investigate the relationship between factors and adolescent's Internet addiction

Variables	Log-transformed IAS		
	β	SE	*p*-value
Parents			
Mother's depression			
Yes	0.0960	0.0325	0.0033
No	Ref	–	–
Father's depression			
Yes	−0.0107	0.0343	0.7555
No	Ref	–	–
Mother's economic status			
Salary employee	0.0296	0.0156	0.0575
Employer or self-employed	−0.0090	0.0237	0.7054
Not employed or unemployed	Ref	–	–
Father's economic status			
Salary employee	0.0041	0.0289	0.8865
Employer or self-employed	−0.0244	0.0303	0.4210
Not employed or unemployed	Ref	–	–
Mother's education level			
High school or under	0.0380	0.0159	0.0173
University or above	Ref	–	–
Father's education level			
High school or under	−0.0203	0.0162	0.2132
University or above	Ref	–	–
Household income			
Low	−0.0033	0.0213	0.8777
Mid-low	−0.0183	0.0190	0.3338
Mid-high	−0.0173	0.0180	0.3368
High	Ref	–	–
Adolescents			
Gender			
Male	0.0815	0.0143	< 0.0001
Female	Ref	–	–
School type			
Elementary school	0.0178	0.0174	0.3046
High school	Ref	–	–
Academic performance			
Bad or very bad	0.0480	0.0219	0.0286
Normal	0.0175	0.0159	0.2715
Good or very good	Ref	–	–
Academic achievement stress score	0.0053	0.0028	0.0624
Depression and anxiety score	−0.0002	0.0026	0.9341
Attention problems score	0.0088	0.0030	0.0029
Social problem score	0.0022	0.0041	0.5997
Delinquency score	−0.0072	0.0077	0.3484
Aggression score	0.0127	0.0033	0.0001

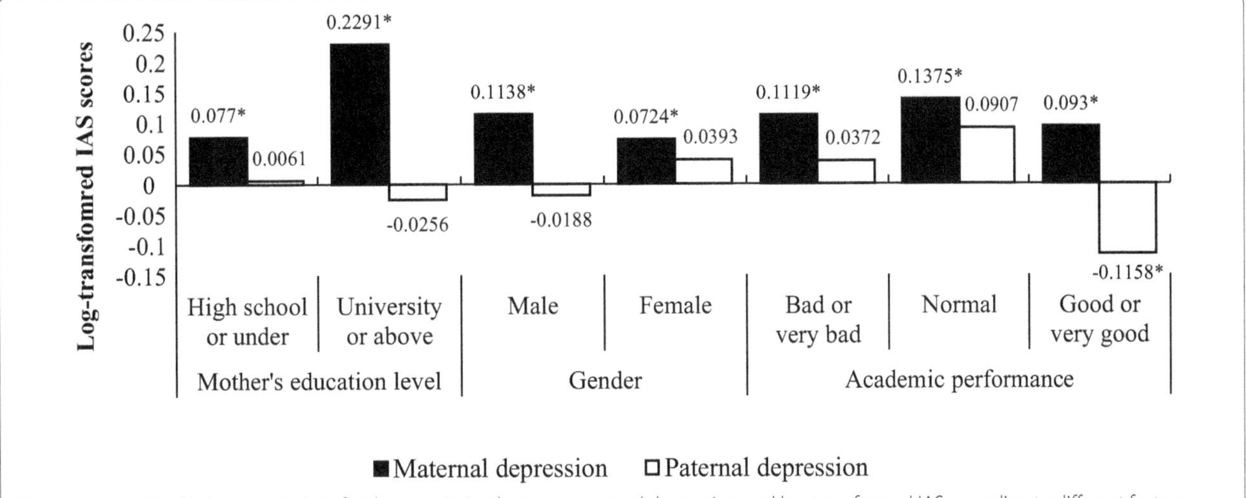

Fig. 1 The results of subgroup analysis for the association between parental depression and log-transformed IAS according to different factors. *Statistically significant results ($p < 0.05$). [§]Analyses were adjusted for the following covariates: economic status, father's education level, household income, gender, school type, academic performance, academic achievement stress score, depression and anxiety score, attention problems score, social problem score, delinquency score, and aggression score

Discussion

The association between parental depression and adolescent Internet addiction was the main finding of this study. As shown above, the most important finding was that maternal depression could result in Internet addiction among children. On the other hand, paternal depression was not significantly associated with the development of Internet addiction among children. Moreover, this result was also consistently maintained in the subgroup analysis according to high maternal education levels such as university or above, male children, and normal or better academic performance.

Previous studies have found an association between Internet addiction among children and family factors such as adolescent–parent conflict, parental monitoring, and parental attitude [4, 5]. Particularly, parental depression has been known as one of the major risk factors for adverse behavioral and emotional functioning among children by numerous studies and reviews [18–20]. Unfortunately, we could find just a few studies about the association between parental depression and Internet addiction among children. Lam found that the association between parental depression and Internet addiction among adolescents might reflect the relationship of the children's depression status and their parents' depression [9]. In addition, parental mental health also plays a significant role in the development of Internet addiction among children. Interestingly, our study found that only maternal depression adversely was associated with Internet addiction among children. It could be guessed that depression might adversely affect mothers' parenting attitudes [21, 22]. South Koreans have a strong tendency of mother's parenting responsibility [23]. Mothers take care of all for their children such as their schedule of school, private academy, and a college entrance examination [24]. In other words, children are more affected by mother's care for children than father's. Moreover, the association between maternal depression and parenting behavior was manifest most strongly for negative effect including increased hostility, high rates of negative interactions, being fewer responsive to child behavior, to communicate less effectively and to have fewer interactions with their children [25]. Therefore, mothers with depression could take less care of their children's behaviors and mental development, and the quality of the relationship between this mother and her children might be worse compared to others who are not depressed [20, 26]. As a result, these factors might strongly be associated with the development of Internet addiction among children.

In particular, this finding showed a stronger correlation when the mother's educational level was at the university level or above. The results of our study were contradictory to those of other studies. Lam's study indicated that mother's education level was not associated with Internet addiction among children, and another study also showed that parental educational attainment was only associated with male children's addictive Internet use [9]. However, our study showed a correlation between maternal high education level and Internet addiction among children. Moreover, children's Internet addiction showed a strong correlation with mother's high education level when their mother had depression. Previous study found that mothers who had high education level provide better home environment for their children by educating musical instruments, special lessons, and books [27]. When high educated mother got depressed, it would be difficult to support their children compared to those who did not get depressed. Thus, we could guess that high educated mother was more strongly associated with the development of children's Internet addiction.

Male adolescents had high potential Internet addiction compared to female adolescents. This finding is supported by the difference in Internet addiction between genders found in several studies, and male gender was one of the risk factors identified by Young and Greenfield [28–30]. They demonstrated that male adolescents tended to use the Internet mainly for purposes related to entertainment and leisure, whereas women use it primarily for interpersonal communication and educational assistance.

Below normal academic performance groups showed strong associations between mother's depression and Internet addiction of their children. A previous study showed that poor academic performance was a risk factor for Internet addiction [31]. Moreover, children who had poor performance were likely to have strong mother's care, because their mother would be worried about their children's future [32]. Therefore, when their mother was depressed it might happen that children with below normal academic performance had a high potential Internet addiction because there was no mother's care.

Although many studies and literature have focused on the association between mental health of children and maternal depression, it has not yet been clearly discovered that maternal mental health is directly associated with Internet addiction among their children. Therefore, this study may suggest that Internet addiction among children may not only be affected by their behavior and mental problems, but may also be affected by the mental health of the mother.

This study has several limitations that should be considered when interpreting our results. First, this study is a cross-sectional study; thus, caution should be exercised in interpreting causality between parental depression and children's Internet addiction. Second, there are not enough previous studies which could support to the results of the relationship between parental depression and children's Internet addiction. However, it is likely to be one of evidence for a possibility of the relationship between parental mental health and children's Internet addiction. Third, there is a risk of recall bias because the data were collected via self-reported surveys and interviews to assess parental depression, children's Internet addiction, and children's mental health. Finally, although we included several lifestyle covariates as potential confounders, it is likely that we have not included all independent variables related to children's Internet addiction.

Despite these limitations, this study has several strengths. First, we used data from a nationwide survey with randomly sampled data, increasing the representativeness of the data for the general Korean population. Compared with previous studies, this study focuses on the parental depression. Therefore, it suggests that children's Internet addiction is not only association with their behaviors and mental health, but also by parental mental health. Moreover, it might serve as a new perspective on the causes of Internet addiction among children.

In conclusion, maternal depression is related to children's Internet addiction; particularly, mothers who graduated from the university or higher, male children, and normal or better academic performance show the strongest relationship with children's Internet addiction. To prevent children's Internet addiction, parents' mental health, as well as children's behavior, needs to be managed. Especially, maternal care might be one of the important roles for alleviating their children's Internet addiction. Therefore, mothers who have children need to manage their children to use Internet appropriately. The results of this study could provide other researchers with additional inspiration to study the impact of parental mental health and children's Internet addiction. In addition, since there is a lack of research on parental depression and children's Internet addiction, we hope that further research will be uncovered to clarify the association between them.

Authors' contributions

DWC participated in designing of the study and interpretation of data, and writing the initial manuscript. SAL and SYC participated in analyzing the data. KTH reviewed the manuscript. ECP is the guarantor of this work and, as such, had full access to all the data in the study and takes responsibility for the integrity of the data and the accuracy of the data analysis. All authors read and approved the final manuscript.

Author details

[1] Department of Public Health, Graduate School, Yonsei University, Seoul, Republic of Korea. [2] Institute of Health Services Research, Yonsei University, Seoul, Republic of Korea. [3] Department of Policy Research Affairs, National Health Insurance Service Ilsan Hospital, Koyang, Republic of Korea. [4] Department of Preventive Medicine, Yonsei University College of Medicine, 50 Yonsei-ro, Seodaemun-gu, Seoul 03722, Republic of Korea.

Acknowledgements

Not applicable.

Competing interests

The authors declare that they have no competing interests.

Consent for publication

Not applicable.

Funding
This study was not supported by any financial supports.

References

1. Young KS. Internet addiction: the emergence of a new clinical disorder. Cyberpsychol Behav. 1998;1:237–44.
2. World Internet Users Statistics and World Population Stats. http://www.internetworldstats.com/stats.htm. Accessed 11 Nov 2017.
3. Health Online. 2013. http://www.pewinternet.org/files/old-media//Files/Reports/PIP_HealthOnline.pdf. Accessed 11 Nov 2017.
4. Park SK, Kim JY, Cho CB. Prevalence of internet addiction and correlations with family factors among South Korean adolescents. Adolescence. 2008;43:895–909.
5. Yen J-Y, Yen C-F, Chen C-C, Chen S-H, Ko C-H. Family factors of internet addiction and substance use experience in Taiwanese adolescents. CyberPsychol Behav. 2007;10:323–9.
6. Li W, Garland EL, Howard MO. Family factors in internet addiction among Chinese youth: a review of English- and Chinese-language studies. Comput Hum Behav. 2014;31:393–411.
7. Ko CH, Wang PW, Liu TL, Yen CF, Chen CS, Yen JY. Bidirectional associations between family factors and internet addiction among adolescents in a prospective investigation. Psychiatry Clin Neurosci. 2015;69:192–200.
8. Xiuqin H, Huimin Z, Mengchen L, Jinan W, Ying Z, Ran T. Mental health, personality, and parental rearing styles of adolescents with internet addiction disorder. Cyberpsychol Behav Soc Netw. 2010;13:401–6.
9. Lam LT. Parental mental health and internet addiction in adolescents. Addict Behav. 2015;42:20–3.
10. Lieb R, Isensee B, Höfler M, Pfister H, Wittchen H. Parental major depression and the risk of depression and other mental disorders in offspring: a prospective-longitudinal community study. Arch Gen Psychiatry. 2002;59:365–74.
11. Nomura Y, Wickramaratne PJ, Warner V, Mufson L, Weissman MM. Family discord, parental depression, and psychopathology in offspring: ten-year follow-up. J Am Acad Child Adolesc Psychiatry. 2002;41:402–9.
12. Kim DI, Chung YJ, Lee EA, Kim DM, Cho YM. Development of internet addiction proneness scale-short form (KS scale). Korean Counsel Assoc. 2008;9:1703–22.
13. Jang KW, Lee JH. Development and validation of the Korean version of the game addiction/engagement scale (KGAES). Korean J Health Psychol. 2007;12:517–27.
14. Kang M, Oh I. Development of internet addiction scale for Korean adolescent. Korean J Educ Psychol. 2002;16:247–74.
15. Kohout FJ, Berkman LF, Evans DA, Cornoni-Huntley J. Two shorter forms of the CES-D (Center for Epidemiological Studies Depression) depression symptoms index. J Aging Health. 1993;5:179–93.
16. Oh K, Lee H, Hong K, Ha E. K-CBCL. Seoul: Chung Ang Aptitude Publishing Co; 1997.
17. Achenbach TM, Edelbrock C. Manual for the child behavior checklist/4–18 and 1991 profile. Burlington: Department of Psychiatry, University of Vermont; 1991.
18. Downey G, Coyne JC. Children of depressed parents: an integrative review. Psychol Bull. 1990;108:50.
19. Goodman SH, Gotlib IH. Children of depressed parents: mechanisms of risk and implications for treatment. Worcester: American Psychological Association; 2002.
20. Olsson MB, Hwang C. Depression in mothers and fathers of children with intellectual disability. J Intellect Disabil Res. 2001;45:535–43.
21. Cox JE, Buman M, Valenzuela J, Joseph NP, Mitchell A, Woods ER. Depression, parenting attributes, and social support among adolescent mothers attending a teen tot program. J Pediatr Adolesc Gynecol. 2008;21:275–81.
22. Hoffman C, Crnic KA, Baker JK. Maternal depression and parenting: implications for children's emergent emotion regulation and behavioral functioning. Parenting. 2006;6:271–95.
23. Jahng KE, Lim HJ. A study on the predictors of parenting responsibility of mothers with infants. Korean J Early Childhood Educ. 2015;35:49–71.
24. Kim H-O, Hoppe-Graff S. Mothers roles in traditional and modern korean families: the consequences for parental practices and adolescent socialization. Asia Pac Educ Rev. 2001;2:85–93.
25. Lovejoy MC, Graczyk PA, O'Hare E, Neuman G. Maternal depression and parenting behavior: a meta-analytic review. Clin Psychol Rev. 2000;20:561–92.
26. Burke L. The impact of maternal depression on familial relationships. Int Rev Psychiatry. 2003;15:243–55.
27. Carneiro P, Meghir C, Parey M. Maternal education, home environments, and the development of children and adolescents. J Eur Econ Assoc. 2013;11:123–60.
28. Ko C-H, Yen J-Y, Yen C-F, Chen C-S, Wang S-Y. The association between internet addiction and belief of frustration intolerance: the gender difference. Cyberpsychol Behav. 2008;11:273–8.
29. Greenfield DN. Psychological characteristics of compulsive internet use: a preliminary analysis. Cyberpsychol Behav. 1999;2:403–12.
30. Bakken IJ, Wenzel HG, Götestam KG, Johansson A, Øren A. Internet addiction among Norwegian adults: a stratified probability sample study. Scand J Psychol. 2009;50:121–7.
31. Chen Y-L, Chen S-H, Gau SS-F. ADHD and autistic traits, family function, parenting style, and social adjustment for internet addiction among children and adolescents in Taiwan: a longitudinal study. Res Dev Disabil. 2015;39:20–31.
32. Baker DP, Stevenson DL. Mothers' strategies for children's school achievement: managing the transition to high school. Sociol Educ. 1986;59:156–66.

30

Compassion fatigue and substance use among nurses

Reem Jarrad[1*], Sawsan Hammad[2], Tagreed Shawashi[1] and Naser Mahmoud[3]

Abstract

Aim: This study aimed to detect if there were differences in compassion fatigue (CF) among nurses based on substance use and demographic variables of gender, marital status, type of health institution and income.

Background: Compassion fatigue is considered an outcome of poorly handled stressful situations in which nurses may respond with self-harming behaviours like substance use. Evidence in this area is critically lacking.

Methods: This study used a descriptive design to survey differences in CF of 282 nurses. The participants completed a demographic survey and indicated whether they consume any of the following substances on a frequent basis: cigarettes, sleeping pills, power drinks, anti-depressant drugs, anti-anxiety drugs, coffee, analgesics, amphetamines and alcohol. Compassion Fatigue scores were surveyed using CF self-test 66 items developed by Stamm and Figely (Compassion satisfaction and fatigue test. http://www.isu.edu/~bhstamm/tests.htm, 1996).

Results: There were significant differences in CF scores in favour of nurses who used cigarettes, sleeping pills, power drinks, anti-depressants and anti-anxiety drugs. While no significant differences in CF were found between nurses who used coffee, analgesics, amphetamines and alcohol, significant differences in nurses' CF were found in relation to type of institution, gender and marital status. But nurses' income did not bring differences to CF scores.

Conclusion: Nurses who might be lacking resilience cope negatively with CF using maladaptive negative behaviours such as substance use.

Implications for nursing management: Nursing management should be aware of the substance use drive among nurses and build organizational solutions to overcome compassion fatigue and potential substance use problems.

Keywords: Compassion fatigue, Substance use, Nurses, Demographic variables

Introduction

Compassion fatigue (CF) is a recent concept that refers to the emotional and physical exhaustion that affects helping professionals and caregivers over time. It is associated with a gradual desensitization to patient stories, a decrease in quality of care, an increase in clinical errors, higher rates of depression and anxiety disorders and rising rates of stress leave and a sense of humiliation in workplace climate [1].

Compassion fatigue in nurses can be explained as a cumulative and progressive absorption process of patient's pain and suffering formed from the caring interactions with patients and their families. The physical, emotional, spiritual, social and organizational consequences of CF are so extensive that they threaten the existential integrity of the nurse [2]. Such consequences include, but not limited to, decreased level of job satisfaction, decreased productivity, increased rates of absenteeism, burnout, turnover, stress, insomnia, nightmares, headaches, gastrointestinal complaints, anxiety and depression [3].

Compassion fatigue can happen to any nurse, at any time during the job course, though some nurses may be at greater risk to develop CF than other nurses. For example, those who work in oncology, emergency, intensive care units, paediatric units and hospice care are at a greater risk of developing CF because of the frequent

*Correspondence: r.jarrad@ju.edu.jo; rawshehcoffee2009@gmail.com
[1] Clinical Nursing Department-School of Nursing, The University of Jordan, Amman 11942, Jordan
Full list of author information is available at the end of the article

encounters with patient/family tragedies and deaths [4].When close, caring relationships are formed with patients, the risk of CF is increased. Sometimes a particular patient may remind the nurse of someone important in his or her life. If that patient dies, the nurse may be triggered emotionally in the most debilitating ways [5]. One of the greatest risks for compassion fatigue comes when nurses forgo their own self-care while immersing themselves intensely in their patients' traumatization, suffering, grief and pain [6].

Theoretical framework

Nurses are particularly vulnerable to traumatic experiences and resultant CF because they usually enter the lives of patients at very critical health junctures and become directly and deeply involved in providing multidimensional care as well as end-of-life care [7]. The negative effects of providing care are aggravated by the severity of the traumatic experiences to which nurses are exposed. Those traumatic experiences may bring to life a group of unpleasant feelings such as exhaustion, anger, irritability, diminished sense of enjoyment and impaired ability to make decisions and care for patients. Subsequently, some nurses develop negative coping behaviours including alcohol and drug use or abuse [8, 9].

There are several styles with which a care giver respond to CF poorly handled stressful situations. For example, the Coping Inventory for Stressful Situations, by Endler and Parker [10] identified three coping styles: task-oriented coping (i.e. taking actions to solve the situation), emotion-oriented coping (e.g. self-blame and anxiety), and avoidance-oriented coping (replacement behaviours to substitute the problem); the last two coping styles may result in care giver self-harm and self-destructive behaviours that include, but are not limited to, substance use. In support of this explanative framework Adriaenssens et al. [11] asserted that what matters is how individuals respond to stressors not the stressors themselves. The response could be in an action oriented and problem solving manner (adaptive coping response) or resort to ineffective coping responses and defensive mechanisms like substance use and withdrawal.

An understanding of the coping responses of nurses can help develop resilience-promoting interventions tailored to ease the resolution of CF issues and maximize retention rates in work places [12]. Those outcomes are directly supported by the concept of resilience which implies the ability to effectively cope and adapt when faced with loss or hardship and minimize the negative results of exposure to adverse situations [13].

Zander et al. [14] aimed to develop strategies that can be implemented at an organizational level to support the development of resilience in nurses and hence counteract the wide spectrum of negative consequences of compassion fatigue. Ginzburg [15] stated that resilience is a survival skill that is often manifested as the difference between individuals' conceptualizing themselves as survivors versus victims and individuals who can take care of themselves and others, versus those who become unable to care for themselves or others when subjected to significant stressors; which is definitely an unwanted outcome in health care facilities.

Hereby, this study hypothesized that nurses with the highest level of compassion fatigue may turn to maladaptive, less resilient, negative coping behaviours to manage their feelings. Such behaviours may include surrendering to some forms of substance use or abuse.

Research questions

This study aimed to detect if there were differences in CF scores, the dependent variable, among Jordanian nurses based on substance use. The independent variables were: cigarette smoking, sleeping pills, power drinks, antidepressant drugs, anti-anxiety drugs, coffee, analgesics, amphetamines and alcohol. The second objective was to evaluate if there were differences in CF scores among Jordanian nurses based on demographic variables of: gender, type of health institution, marital status and income.

Methods

Sample and design

This study used a descriptive cross-sectional convenient sampling design to survey CF and some associated demographic and drug use related variables among Jordanian nurses. The sample included 282 nurses selected from three types of major and high occupancy rate hospitals covering psychiatric, governmental and educational sectors. The sample included nurses who had spent at least 3 months in the current unit.

The areas selected from within the governmental and educational hospitals included several types of intensive care units (ICUs), emergency departments, medical and surgical floors which received some oncology cases that clinically ranged from early diagnosis to terminal illness conditions. The specialized psychiatric hospital had clients with a variety of mental illnesses such as schizophrenia, depression and bipolar disorders in variable levels of acuity.

Measures

The participants were asked to complete a single page demographic form which had two sections. Section one included questions regarding: age, income, duration of experience, gender, unit, hospital type, marital status and income, while section two requested a yes/no response to statements about frequent use of cigarettes, sleeping pills, power drinks, anti-depressant drugs, anti-anxiety drugs, coffee, analgesics, amphetamines and alcohol.

The Compassion Fatigue scores were surveyed using a face and content validated translation to Arabic version of the CF self-test which was adapted with permission of Dr. Charles Figely [17]. This survey measures three concepts which are: compassion fatigue, compassion satisfaction and burn out. The survey has been used by many researchers in variable target groups such as: educators, clinicians, social workers, nurses, therapists, chaplains, counsellors, etc. The compassion fatigue section of the test showed a strong alpha value of 0.87; the analysis of variance did not provide evidence of differences based on country of origin, type of work or sex when age was used as a control variable [16].

The CF self-test has 66 items (Appendix 1). Each item is evaluated by the care provider on a Likert scale out of five. Zero means never; one means rarely, two means a few times, three means somewhat often, four means often and five means very often. The CF score is the sum of the following 23 test items: 4, 6, 7, 8, 12, 13, 15, 16, 18, 20–22, 28, 29, 31–34, 36, 38–40 and 44. If the calculated score is 26 or less there would be an extremely low risk for CF. When the score is 27–30 there would be low risk of CF. Score a 31–35 refers to moderate CF risk. Whereas a score of 36–40 is considered a high CF risk and a score of 41 or above indicates an extremely high risk for CF [17].

Results and statistical analysis

Sample characteristics

The sample of this study consisted of 64% ($n=181$) females and 36% ($n=101$) males. Their mean age was 32.3 years (SD = 6.6). Half the sample were working in governmental hospitals ($n=141$), the minority were in educational (training) hospitals 17% ($n=48$) and almost a third were from a specialized psychiatric institution ($n=93$). The majority of the participants were married 68% ($n=98$) and 74% ($n=209$) have a monthly individual income of 600 JD or less. The participants had mean of 9.9 years of experience as nurses and 6.3 years of experience in the current unit or ward. This is quite enough range of time to measure certain nurses' emotional outcomes such as compassion fatigue (Table 1).

Table 1 Description of the personal demographics, *N* = 282

Variable	*n* (%)	*M* (SD)
Type of hospital		
Psychiatric hospital	93 (33)	
Governmental hospital	141 (50)	
Educational (training) hospital	48 (17)	
Gender		
Male	101 (36)	
Female	181 (64)	
Age		32.3 (6.6)
Marital status		
Married	192 (68)	
Not married	90 (32)	
Experience as a nurse		9.9 (6.5)
Experience in the current unit/ward		6.3 (5.4)
Income		
Less or equal 600	209 (74)	
More than 600	73 (26)	

Substance use among Jordanian nurses

Table 2 displays the frequency of substance use among the nurses participating in the study. The highest frequencies were for coffee 69% ($n=194$), analgesic drugs 41% ($n=115$), cigarette smoking 29% ($n=81$), and power drinks 52 (18%). The lowest frequencies were for alcohol 8% ($n=23$), amphetamines 12% ($n=33$), antidepressants 15% ($n=41$), sleeping pills 16% (46), and anti-anxiety drugs 17% ($n=48$).

Table 2 Description of the substance use among nurses, *N* = 282

Variable	Yes *n* (%)	No *n* (%)
Smoking	81 (29)	201 (71)
Alcohol	23 (8)	259 (92)
Sleeping pills	46 (16)	236 (84)
Power drinks	52 (18.0)	230 (82)
Coffee	194 (69)	88 (31)
Antidepressants	41 (15)	241 (86)
Anti-anxiety drugs	48 (17)	234 (83)
Stimulants (amphetamines)	33 (12)	249 (88)
Analgesic drugs	115 (41)	167 (59)

Differences in compassion fatigue level in relation to socio-demographic and substance use variables

In this study, the mean as well as the median scores of CF among all nurses was 41 (SD = 17.7). This aligns with the category of "extremely high risk for CF", regardless of any contributing variables. To test the differences in CF level among nurses in the three health sectors (three different groups), analysis of variance (ANOVA) test was carried out and the result revealed statistically significant differences (F (279, 2) = 8.92, $p=.000$). Based on Scheffe post hoc criterion for multiple group comparison, nurses working in the psychiatric hospital scored significantly higher CF than nurses in governmental hospitals ($P=.004$). Nurses working in educational (training) hospitals scored significantly higher CF than nurses in governmental hospitals ($P=.003$). There was no significant difference in CF between nurses working in psychiatric hospitals compared to educational hospitals ($P=.764$) (Table 3).

Table 3 Differences in compassion fatigue level in relation to socio-demographic and substance use

Variable	*M* (SD)	Test value	*P* value
Type of hospital			
Psychiatric hospital	44.4 (19.2)	8.92	.000
Governmental hospital	36.7 (16.5)		
Educational (training) hospital	46.7 (15.1)		
Gender			
Male	44.3 (19.3)	2.43	.015
Female	39.0 (16.4)		
Marital status			
Married	42.8 (17.2)	2.66	.008
Not married	36.9 (18.0)		
Income			
Less or equal 600	40.3 (18.3)	.959	.34
More than 600	42.6 (15.7)		
Smoking			
Yes	44.5 (17.4)	2.19	.029
No	39.4 (17.6)		
Alcohol			
Yes	44.1(21.8)	.912	.363
No	40.6 (17.3)		
Sleeping pills			
Yes	50.5 (19.4)	4.13	.000
No	39.0 (16.7)		
Power drinks			
Yes	47.6 (19.3)	3.10	.002
No	39.4 (16.9)		
Coffee			
Yes	41.3 (18.6)	.493	.62
No	40.1 (15.5)		
Antidepressants			
Yes	48.0 (16.9)	2.82	.005
No	39.7 (17.6)		
Anti-anxiety drugs			
Yes	45.9 (16.9)	2.17	.031
No	39.9 (17.7)		
Amphetamines			
Yes	45.5 (15.3)	1.60	.10
No	40.3 (17.9)		
Analgesic drugs			
Yes	41.2 (20.5)	.257	.797
No	40.7 (15.6)		

Based on socio-demographic variables, and using a Student's *t* test for comparison for each two independent groups, a significant difference was found in regard to gender ($t\ (280)=2.43$, $p=.015$). Male nurses scored higher CF (M=44.3, SD=19.3) than female nurses ($M=39.0$, SD=16.4). In addition, a statistically significant difference was found among nurses based on marital status ($t\ (280)=2.66$, $p=.008$) in which married nurses scored higher CF ($M=42.8$, SD=17.2) than the unmarried nurses ($M=36.9$, SD=18.0). Compassion fatigue level did not differ significantly ($t\ (280)=.959$, $p=.34$) in relation to income (Table 3).

In regard to substance use, there was a significant difference in smoking ($t\ (280)=2.19$, $p=.29$) as nurses who smoked cigarettes scored higher CF ($M=44.5$, SD=17.4) than nurses who did not smoke ($M=39.4$, SD=17.6). In regard to sleeping pills, results revealed a significant difference ($t\ (280)=4.13$, $p<.001$). Nurses who used sleeping pills scored higher CF ($M=50.5$, SD=19.4) than nurses who did not ($M=39.0$, SD=16.7). Nurses who used power drinks scored higher CF ($M=47.6$, SD=19.3) than nurses who did not ($M=39.4$, SD=16.9, $t\ (280)=3.10$, $p=.002$). Other significant differences were found in nurses who took antidepressants ($t\ (280)=2.82$, $p=.005$) with a mean of ($M=48.0$, SD=16.9) compared to nurses who did not ($M=39.7$, SD=17.6). Similarly, nurses who took anti-anxiety drugs scored higher CF ($M=45.9$, SD=16.9) than nurses who did not ($M=39.9$, SD=17.7) with a significant difference ($t\ (280)=2.17$, $p=.031$). Finally, results revealed no significant difference in CF scores in regard to coffee use, amphetamines, alcohol or analgesic use (Table 3).

Discussion

Compassion fatigue and type of health institution

Work environment and prevailing work conditions, demands, burdens and stressors along with patient's problems and stories add to the nurses' potential for CF. Examples of work stressors are paperwork, the electronic medical records, changes in leadership or staffing, accreditation requirements and expectations of best practices [18]. Moreover, nurses often spend considerable time with people who live outside the regular norms of society such as individuals who are extremely poor, victims of abuse or neglect, people with mental illnesses or others who are demented, debilitated, paralytic, comatose or abandoned. Such people with special scenarios absorb the nurses' physical, intellectual and emotional power; in a way that is adding to the CF provoking effects of work environment which is often stressful, understaffed and overwhelmed with negativity [8, 19].

Those factors indeed play a major role in making some hospitals more CF predisposing environments than others. Hence, our study found that psychiatric health care nurses are more prone to CF than nurses working in non-psychiatric settings. Training-based hospital nurses are more prone to CF than their partners in governmental hospitals, who may be holding less responsibilities and simpler job descriptions. It should not be disregarded here that the mean and the median scores of our sample were within the extremely high risk for CF category, regardless of the hospital type. It is worth noting that that literature comparing CF between different health settings or units are limited in Jordan as well as elsewhere.

Compassion fatigue and gender

Compassion fatigue differs by some nurse-related socio-demographic variables. In regard to gender, Mooney et al. [20] reported that ICU and oncology male nurses exhibited significantly lower CF ($p=.014$) than female nurses. Those findings were not noted in our study. The variation could be attributed to differences in sample size (86–282), different measurement scales of CF (The Professional Quality of Life (ProQOL) scale to CF self-test 66 items) and different sample characteristics (ICU and oncology nurses in a community hospital versus a more variable mix of different nursing specialities from different types of health settings).

Compassion fatigue and nurses' marital status and income level

Nurses' marital status scored significant differences in relation to CF. Married nurses were more prone to CF than the unmarried. When compared to a research done by Hee and Kyung [21], our finding was inconsistent with theirs. This could be attributed, at least partially, to cultural and economic differences of surveyed populations. Here, in Jordan, the life demands of married people are significantly higher than those who are unmarried; additionally the cost of living is high when compared to personal income [22]. The combination of the escalating burdens of married life, the absence of governmental financial support to families, and the accelerating prices and taxes that touches even the most basic goods, adds extra stress on Jordanian nurses which increase their CF level [23]. It is evident that 74% of the study sample individual income was below 600 Jordanian dinars, and this applies to most Jordanian nurses and regular citizens which is considered low when compared to other Arab countries like Qatar and Kuwait [24].

Compassion fatigue and substance use

There were significant differences in nurses' CF scores based on their substance use; namely, cigarette smoking, sleeping pills, power drinks, anti-depressants and anti-anxiety drugs. Nurses who consumed these substances on a frequent basis reported significantly higher CF scores than those who did not; supporting the initial hypothesis. It is recommended that the resiliency characteristics and the coping styles of the participants of similar studies be surveyed in the future.

The term substance use includes prescribed or non-prescribed use, misuse and/or abuse of legal substances such as caffeine, nicotine, alcohol, over-the-counter drugs, prescribed drugs, alcohol concoctions, indigenous plants, solvents, inhalants and illicit drugs. Simply, substance use refers to any substance that, when taken by a person, modifies perception, mood, cognition, behaviour or motor functions, and could be considered a maladaptive behavioural pattern [25].

Substance use among health workers such as nurses is a dangerous behaviour that may lead to negative personal, social and organizational consequences and should be carefully investigated and properly managed [26]. Nurses, like most people with substance use disorders, abuse drugs, tobacco or alcohol to relieve stress and emotional or physical pain. In many cases, the abuse initially helps boost performance; for example when drinking stimulants such as coffee, power drinks or amphetamines, nurses stay wake and energetic during night shifts. This behaviour, if not controlled, will gradually turn into dependence which is an unwanted outcome [27]. The nurses that become abusers sadly become victims, and burdens on the health care system and will eventually require massive interventional rehabilitation programmes to maintain their career lives [28].

When combating stressful feelings of compassion fatigue at work, nurses may turn to negative styles of coping. Maladaptive, non-resilient behaviours of using substances (nicotine, high concentrations of caffeine in the form of power drinks, sleeping pills, antidepressants and anti-anxiety drugs) may be enhanced by the presence of certain negative elements in the work environment. Examples of those elements would be high work demands, low job satisfaction, long duty hours, irregular shifts, fatigue/exhaustion, repetitious duties, periods of inactivity or boredom, irregular supervision and easy access to substances [29].

Nurses working in most health care sectors in Jordan are challenged by multiple negative work environment elements. For example, the ever present nursing shortage, the feminized image of a nurse thereby causing a male-nurse stigma, lower wages when compared to international nursing salaries and poor communication among healthcare team. In addition, Jordanian nurses suffer from a lack of autonomy, non-supportive leadership and/or co-workers, autocratic managers and frequent "floating" of nurses between different units and floors. Besides, nurses often tend to recall the non-supportive or troubled personal relationships, low self-esteem among colleagues, ambiguous nursing roles and the high patient acuities [30–34]. These factors may play a role in pushing nurses toward variable forms of substance use or abuse. Subsequently, it is recommended to study those elements adequately to intervene timely on the behalf of nurses.

Implications for nursing management

This research strongly indicates that there is a serious nursing compassion fatigue problem which is sometimes accompanied with some sort of substance use behaviour. The fact that the mean and the median scores of CF among nurses was falling within the category of "extremely high risk for CF", ascertains the need to identify the most risky target groups, like male nurses, married nurses and nurses working in either psychiatric care facilities or overloaded work environments like large training hospitals. There is a need to establish saving managerial strategic interventional plans to rescue those target groups before further personal and organizational damage is inflicted. With regard to the compassion fatigue substance use related behaviour, the health authorities are obliged to follow up this problem comprehensively, specify its prevalence, motives, correlations, outcomes and possible practical solutions. After all healthy nurses will always be vital to an efficient and sustainable Jordanian as well as global healthcare systems.

Limitations

The sample from this study only included governmental and semi-governmental hospitals, so future studies in Jordan are encouraged to involve both military health services and the private sector and to adopt randomization when picking the included health institutions, type of units and participating subjects in order to enhance the generalizability of the findings. Researchers from other countries and different cultural, social and economic backgrounds are highly recommended to replicate our study to see if the conclusions drawn about nurses' CF, substance use and the other variables will be the same. Also, comparative studies between different types of health institutions and nursing specialities are required both locally and internationally to set a solid literature data for the phenomena. Besides, future studies are to survey the variables that our study did not cover especially the environmental and personal stressors that lead to compassion fatigue and resultant substance use among nurses as well as the nurses dominating resiliency characteristics and coping styles used when facing diversity and hardship at work.

Conclusion

This is a pioneer study in Jordan as well as in the region that holds a great value in exploring nurses' compassion fatigue, associated feelings, characteristics and behaviours. It is necessary to conduct a survey that determines the factors that drive nurses the most towards maladaptive less resilient coping behaviours of substance use; and to further investigate the correlation between CF and such use behaviours.

Authors' contributions

JR contributed to the major building of the manuscript. HS contributed to the "Results and statistical analysis" section. ST supervised quality of data collection processes and helped in the manuscript editing, while MN contributed to the data collection, piloting, SPSS coding and analysis. All authors read and approved the final manuscript.

Author details

[1] Clinical Nursing Department-School of Nursing, The University of Jordan, Amman 11942, Jordan. [2] Community Health Department-School of Nursing, The University of Jordan, Amman, Jordan. [3] Jordan Ministry of Health-Fuheis Psychiatric Hospital, Amman, Jordan.

Acknowledgements

Hereby, we acknowledge the great help, efforts and facilitation received from the following parties: The University of Jordan, The Ministry of Health, AL Hussein Cancer Centre, AL Fuheis Psychiatric Hospital and its nursing management, The University of Jordan Hospital and Full brighter Brenda Moore PHD, RN.

Competing interests

This statement asserts that none of the authors have any competing interests of any kind.

Consent for publication

This item is not applicable.

Funding

This statement declares that is research is funded by the Deanship of Scientific and Academic Research in The University of Jordan.

Appendix 1: compassion fatigue self-test 66 items

Helping others puts you in direct contact with other people's lives. As you probably have experienced, your compassion for those you help has both positive and negative aspects. This self -test helps you estimate your compassion status: how much at risk you are of burnout and compassion fatigue and also the degree of satisfaction with you helping others. Consider each of the following characteristics about you and your current situation. Write in the number that honestly reflects how frequently you experienced these characteristics in the last week. Then follow the scoring directions at the end of the self-test.

0 = Never 1 = Rarely 2 = A few times 3 = Somewhat often 4 = Often 5 = Very often

Items about you

1. I am happy
2. I find my life satisfying
3. I have beliefs that sustain me
4. I feel estranged from others
5. I find that I learn new things from those I care for
6. I force myself to avoid certain thoughts or feelings that remind me of a frightening experience
7. I find myself avoiding certain activities or situations because they remind me of a frightening experience
8. I have gaps in my memory about frightening events
9. I feel connected to others
10. I feel calm
11. I believe that I have a good balance between my work and my free time
12. I have difficulty falling or staying asleep
13. I have outburst of anger or irritability with little provocation
14. I am the person I always wanted to be
15. I startle easily
16. While working with a victim, I thought about violence against the perpetrator
17. I am a sensitive person
18. I have flashbacks connected to those I help
19. I have good peer support when I need to work through a highly stressful experience
20. I have had first-hand experience with traumatic events in my adult life
21. I have had first-hand experience with traumatic events in my childhood
22. I think that I need to "work through" a traumatic experience in my life
23. I think that I need more close friends
24. I think that there is no one to talk with about highly stressful experiences
25. I have concluded that I work too hard for my own good
26. Working with those I help brings me a great deal of satisfaction
27. I feel invigorated after working with those I help
28. I am frightened of things a person I helped has said or done to me
29. I experience troubling dreams similar to those I help
30. I have happy thoughts about those I help and how I could help them
31. I have experienced intrusive thoughts of times with especially difficult people I helped
32. I have suddenly and involuntarily recalled a frightening experience while working with a person I helped
33. I am pre-occupied with more than one person I help
34. I am losing sleep over a person I help's traumatic experiences
35. I have joyful feelings about how I can help the victims I work with
36. I think that I might have been "infected" by the traumatic stress of those I help
37. I think that I might be positively "inoculated" by the traumatic stress of those I help
38. I remind myself to be less concerned about the wellbeing of those I help
39. I have felt trapped by my work as a helper
40. I have a sense of hopelessness associated with working with those I help
41. I have felt "on edge" about various things and I attribute this to working with certain people I help
42. I wish that I could avoid working with some people I help
43. Some people I help are particularly enjoyable to work with
44. I have been in danger working with people I help
45. I feel that some people I help dislike me personally

Items about being a helper and your helping environment

46. I like my work as a helper
47. I feel like I have the tools and resources that I need to do my work as a helper
48. I have felt weak, tired, run down as a result of my work as helper
49. I have felt depressed as a result of my work as a helper
50. I have thoughts that I am a "success" as a helper
51. I am unsuccessful at separating helping from personal life
52. I enjoy my co-workers
53. I depend on my co-workers to help me when I need it
54. My co-workers can depend on me for help when they need it
55. I trust my co-workers
56. I feel little compassion toward most of my co-workers
57. I am pleased with how I am able to keep up with helping technology
58. I feel I am working more for the money/prestige than for personal fulfillment
59. Although I have to do paperwork that I don't like, I still have time to work with those I help
60. I find it difficult separating my personal life from my helper life
61. I am pleased with how I am able to keep up with helping techniques and protocols
62. I have a sense of worthlessness/disillusionment/resentment associated with my role as a helper
63. I have thoughts that I am a "failure" as a helper
64. I have thoughts that I am not succeeding at achieving my life goals
65. I have to deal with bureaucratic, unimportant tasks in my work as a helper
66. I plan to be a helper for a long time

References

1. Bride B. Secondary traumatic stress. In: Figley CR, editor. Encyclopedia of trauma. Thousand Oaks: Sage Publications; 2012.
2. Saberya M, Hosseinib M, Tafreshib M, Mohtashamib J, Ebadic A. Concept development of "compassion fatigue" in clinical nurses: application of Schwartz-Barcott and Kim's Hybrid Model. Asian Pac Isl Nurs J. 2017;2(1):37–47.
3. Kelly L, Runge J, Spencer C. Predictors of compassion fatigue and compassion satisfaction in acute care nurses. J Nurs Scholarsh. 2015;47:522–8. https://doi.org/10.1111/jnu.12162.
4. Sheppard K. Compassion fatigue: are you at risk? J Am Nurse Today. 2016;11(1):53–5.

5. Cetrano G, Tedeschi F, Rabbi L ,Gosetti G, Lora A , Lamonaca D , Manthorpe J, Amaddeo F (2017). How are compassion fatigue, burnout, and compassion satisfaction affected by quality of working life? Findings from a survey of mental health staff in Italy. BMC Health Serv Res. 17:755. https://doi.org/10.1186/s12913-017-2726-x. https://bmchealthservres.biomedcentral.com/articles/10.1186/s12913-017-2726-x. Accessed 9 Mar 2018.
6. Cocker F, Joss N. Compassion fatigue among healthcare, emergency and community service workers: a systematic review. Int J Environ Res Public Health. 2016;13(6):618. https://doi.org/10.3390/ijerph13060618.
7. Boyle D. Countering compassion fatigue: a requisite nursing agenda. Online J Issues Nurs. 2011;16(1):Man02. https://doi.org/10.3912/OJIN.Vol16No01Man02.
8. Mathieu F. Running on empty: compassion fatigue in health professionals. Rehab Community Care Med. 2007, 4:1–7. http://www.compassionfatigue.org/pages/RunningOnEmpty.pdf. Accessed 9 Mar 2018.
9. Drury V, Craigie M, Francis K, Aoun S, Hegney DG. Compassion satisfaction, compassion fatigue, anxiety, depression and stress in registered nurses in Australia: phase 2 results. J Nurs Manag. 2014;22:519–31. https://doi.org/10.1111/jonm.12168.
10. Endler NS, Parker JDA. Multidimensional assessment of coping: a critical evaluation. J Pers Soc Psychol. 1990;58(5):844–54.
11. Adriaenssens J, de Gucht V, Maes S. The impact of traumatic events on emergency room nurses: findings from a questionnaire survey. Int J Nurs Stud. 2012;49:1411–22.
12. Delgado C, Upton D, Ranse K, Furness T, Foster K. Nurses' resilience and the emotional labour of nursing work: An integrative review of empirical literature. Int J Nurs Stud. 2017, 70:71–88. https://doi.org/10.1016/j.ijnurstu.2017.02.008. https://www.sciencedirect.com/science/article/pii/S0020748917300421. Accessed 2 Feb 2018.
13. Zimmerman MA. Resiliency theory: strengths-based approach to research and practice for adolescent health. Health Educ Behav. 2013;40(4):381–3. https://doi.org/10.1177/1090198113493782.
14. Zander M, Hutton A, King L. Exploring resilience in paediatric oncology nursing staff. Collegian. 2013;20(1):17–25.
15. Ginzburg H. Resilience. In: Figley CR, editor. Encyclopedia of Trauma. Thousand Oaks: Sage Publications; 2012.
16. Stamm BH, Figely CR. Compassion satisfaction and fatigue test. 1996. http://www.isu.edu/~bhstamm/tests.htm.
17. Figely CR. Compassion fatigue, New York: Brunner/Mazel. B. Hudnall Stamm, traumatic stress research group; 1995–1998. 1995. http://www.dartmouth.edu/~bhstamm/index.htm. Accessed 9 Mar 2018.
18. Nolte A, Downing C, Temane A, Hastings-Tolsma M. Compassion fatigue in nurses: a meta-synthesis. J Clin Nurs. 2017, 26(23–24):4364–4378. https://doi.org/10.1111/jocn.13766. http://onlinelibrary.wiley.com/doi/10.1111/jocn.13766/full. Accessed 1 Feb 2018.
19. Portnoy D. Burnout and compassion fatigue watch for the signs. J Cathol Health Assoc US. 2011, 47–50. http://www.compassionfatigue.org/pages/healthprogress.pdf. Accessed 9 Mar 2018.
20. Mooney C, Fetter K, Gross B, Rinehart C, Lynch C, Rogers F. Abstract: a preliminary analysis of compassion satisfaction and compassion fatigue with considerations for nursing unit specialization and demographic factors. J Trauma Nurs. 2017, 24(3): 158–163. http://journals.lww.com/journaloftraumanursing/Abstract/2017/05000/A_Preliminary_Analysis_of_Compassion_Satisfaction.5.aspx. Accessed 9 Mar 2018.
21. Hee YY, Kyung KJ. A literature review of compassion fatigue in nursing. Korean J Adult Nurs. 2012;24(1):38–51.
22. Numbeo database. Cost of living in Amman. 2018. https://www.numbeo.com/cost-of-living/in/Amman. Accessed 1 Feb 2018.
23. AL Arabiya English. Will 2018 be the year of high prices in Jordan?. 2017. http://english.alarabiya.net/en/business/economy/2017/11/21/Will-2018-be-the-year-of-high-prices-in-Jordan-.html. Accessed 30 Jan 2018.
24. Eastern Amman Investors Industrial association. Economic report about Jordanian income. 2017. http://www.eaiia.org/industry-news-in-jordan/news-activities-and-developments/10208-11-19/ Accessed 9 Sep 2017.
25. American Psychiatric Association (APA). Diagnostic and statistical manual of mental disorders. 4th text. Revision ed. Washington, DC: American Psychiatric Association; 2000.
26. Mokaya AG, Mutiso V, Musau A, Tele A, Kombe Y, Ng'ang'a Z, Frank E, Ndetei DM, Clair V. Substance use among a sample of healthcare workers in Kenya: a cross-sectional study. J Psychoactive Drugs. 2016;48(4):310–9. https://doi.org/10.1080/02791072.2016.1211352.
27. Arria A, Caldeira K, Bugbee B, Vincent K, O'Grady K. Trajectories of energy drink consumption and subsequent drug use during young adulthood, J Drug Alcohol Depend. 2017, 179, 424–432. http://dx.doi.org/10.1016/j.drugalcdep.2017.06.008. http://www.drugandalcoholdependence.com/article/S0376-8716(17)30332-0/fulltext. Accessed 1 Feb 2018.
28. Snyder R. Drug abuse among health professionals. 2016. http://c.ymcdn.com/sites/papharmacists.site-ym.com/resource/resmgr/CE_Home_Studies/HP_Drug_Abuse_CE_Article.pdf. Accessed 9 Sep 2017.
29. Canadian Centre for occupational Health and Safety (CCOHS). Substance abuse in the workplace. 2008. https://www.ccohs.ca/oshanswers/psychosocial/substance.html. Accessed 9 Mar 2018.
30. Mrayyan MT. Nursing practice problems in private hospitals in Jordan: students' perspectives. Nurse Educ Prac. 2007;7:82–7.
31. Al-khasawneh AL, Futa SM. The relationship between job stress and nurses performance in the Jordanian hospitals: a case study in King Abdullah the Founder Hospital. Asian J Bus Manag. 2013;5(2):267–75.
32. Ahmed AS. Verbal and physical abuse against Jordanian nurses in the work environment. East Mediterr Health J (EMHJ). 2012;18(4):318–24.
33. Subih M, Alamer R, Al Hadid L, Alsatari M. Stressors amongst Jordanian nurses working in different types of hospitals and the effect of selected demographic factors: a descriptive—explorative study. Jordan Med J. 2011;45(4):331–40.
34. Mrayyan MT. Job stressors and social support behaviours: comparing intensive care units to wards in Jordan. Contemp Nurse. 2009;31:163–75.

Permissions

All chapters in this book were first published in AGP, by BioMed Central; hereby published with permission under the Creative Commons Attribution License or equivalent. Every chapter published in this book has been scrutinized by our experts. Their significance has been extensively debated. The topics covered herein carry significant findings which will fuel the growth of the discipline. They may even be implemented as practical applications or may be referred to as a beginning point for another development.

The contributors of this book come from diverse backgrounds, making this book a truly international effort. This book will bring forth new frontiers with its revolutionizing research information and detailed analysis of the nascent developments around the world.

We would like to thank all the contributing authors for lending their expertise to make the book truly unique. They have played a crucial role in the development of this book. Without their invaluable contributions this book wouldn't have been possible. They have made vital efforts to compile up to date information on the varied aspects of this subject to make this book a valuable addition to the collection of many professionals and students.

This book was conceptualized with the vision of imparting up-to-date information and advanced data in this field. To ensure the same, a matchless editorial board was set up. Every individual on the board went through rigorous rounds of assessment to prove their worth. After which they invested a large part of their time researching and compiling the most relevant data for our readers.

The editorial board has been involved in producing this book since its inception. They have spent rigorous hours researching and exploring the diverse topics which have resulted in the successful publishing of this book. They have passed on their knowledge of decades through this book. To expedite this challenging task, the publisher supported the team at every step. A small team of assistant editors was also appointed to further simplify the editing procedure and attain best results for the readers.

Apart from the editorial board, the designing team has also invested a significant amount of their time in understanding the subject and creating the most relevant covers. They scrutinized every image to scout for the most suitable representation of the subject and create an appropriate cover for the book.

The publishing team has been an ardent support to the editorial, designing and production team. Their endless efforts to recruit the best for this project, has resulted in the accomplishment of this book. They are a veteran in the field of academics and their pool of knowledge is as vast as their experience in printing. Their expertise and guidance has proved useful at every step. Their uncompromising quality standards have made this book an exceptional effort. Their encouragement from time to time has been an inspiration for everyone.

The publisher and the editorial board hope that this book will prove to be a valuable piece of knowledge for researchers, students, practitioners and scholars across the globe.

List of Contributors

Jacek Kurpisz, Monika Mak and Jerzy Samochowiec
Department of Psychiatry, Pomeranian Medical University, Szczecin, Poland

Michał Lew-Starowicz
Institute of Psychiatry and Neurology, 3rd Psychiatric Clinic, Warsaw, Poland.

Krzysztof Nowosielski
Department of Sexology and Family Planning, Medical College in Sosnowiec, Sosnowiec, Poland
Department of Obstetrics and Gynaecology, Specialistic Teaching Hospital, Tychy, Poland

Przemysław Bieńkowski
Institute of Psychiatry and Neurology, Warsaw, Poland

Robert Kowalczyk
Department of Sexology, Andrzej Frycz Modrzewski Cracow University, Kraków, Poland

Błażej Misiak
Department of Genetics, Wroclaw Medical University, Wrocław, Poland

Dorota Frydecka
Department of Psychiatry, Wroclaw Medical University, Wrocław, Poland

Wen-Lin Chu and Kuo-Sheng Cheng
Department of Biomedical Engineering, National Cheng Kung University, Tainan 701, Taiwan

Min-Wei Huang
Department of Biomedical Engineering, National Cheng Kung University, Tainan 701, Taiwan
Department of Psychiatry, Chiayi Branch, Taichung Veterans General Hospital, Chia-Yi 600, Taiwan

Bo-Lin Jian
Department of Aeronautics and Astronautics, National Cheng Kung University, Tainan 701, Taiwan

I. S. Haussleiter, B. Emons, C. Armgart and A. Schramm
Dept. of Psychiatry, LWL Institute of Mental Health, LWL University Hospital, Ruhr-University Bochum, Alexandrinenstr.1, 44791 Bochum, Germany

Knut Hoffmann, F. Illes, J. Jendreyschak and G. Juckel
Dept. of Psychiatry, LWL Institute of Mental Health, LWL University Hospital,
Ruhr-University Bochum, Alexandrinenstr.1, 44791 Bochum, Germany
Department of Psychiatry, LWL-University Hospital Bochum, Alexandrinenstr. 1, 44791 Bochum, Germany

A. Diehl
NRW Center for Health, Gesundheitscampus 9, 44801 Bochum, Germany

Kingsley Afeti and Samuel Harrenson Nyarko
Department of Population and Behavioural Sciences, School of Public
Health, University of Health and Allied Sciences, Hohoe, Ghana

Hsiu-Hung Wang
College of Nursing, Kaohsiung Medical University, Kaohsiung, Taiwan

Shu-Ching Ma
College of Nursing, Kaohsiung Medical University, Kaohsiung, Taiwan.
Nursing Department, Chi-Mei Medical Center, Tainan, Taiwan

Tsair-Wei Chien
Research Department, Chi-Mei Medical Center, 901 Chung Hwa Road, Yung Kung Dist., Tainan 710, Taiwan
Department of Hospital and Health Care Administration, Chia-Nan University of Pharmacy and Science, Tainan, Taiwan

Sevinc Kutluturkan and Elif Sozeri
Department of Nursing, Gazi University Faculty of Health Sciences, Besevler, 06500 Ankara, Turkey

Nese Uysal
Yıldırım Beyazıt Üniversity Faculty of Health Science, Ankara, Turkey

Figen Bay
Gazi University Health Research and Application Center, Gazi Hospital, Ankara, Turkey

Eiji Kirino
Department of Psychiatry, Juntendo University Shizuoka Hospital, 1129
Nagaoka, Izunokunishi, Shizuoka 4102211, Japan.
Department of Psychiatry, Juntendo University School of Medicine, 2-1-1 Hongo, Bunkyoku, Tokyo 1138421, Japan.
Juntendo Institute of Mental Health, 700-1 Fukuroyama, Koshigayashi, Saitama 3430032, Japan

Elena Dragioti, Britt Larsson and Björn Gerdle
Pain and Rehabilitation Centre, Department of Medical and Health Sciences
(IMH), Linköping University, 581 85 Linköping, Sweden

Lars-Åke Levin and Lars Bernfort
Division of Health Care Analysis, Department of Medical and Health Sciences, Linköping University, 581 85 Linköping, Sweden

Berihun Assefa Dachew
Department of Epidemiology and Biostatistics, Institute of Public Health, College
of Medicine and Health Sciences, University of Gondar, Gondar, Ethiopia

Berhanu Boru Bifftu, Bewket Tadesse Tiruneh and Degefaye Zelalem Anlay
School of Nursing, College of Medicine and Health Sciences, University of Gondar, Gondar, Ethiopia

Meseret Adugna Wassie
Department of Health Informatics, Teda Health Science College, Gondar, Ethiopia

Shinichi Honda, Tomohiro Nakao, Hiroshi Mitsuyasu, Kayo Okada, Hirokuni Sanematsu, Keitaro Murayama, Keisuke Ikari, Masumi Kuwano and Shigenobu Kanba
Department of Neuropsychiatry, Graduate School of Medical Sciences, Kyushu University, 3-1-1 Maidashi Higashi-ku, Fukuoka, Japan

Hiroaki Kawasaki
Department of Neuropsychiatry, Graduate School of Medical Sciences, Kyushu University, 3-1-1 Maidashi Higashi-ku, Fukuoka, Japan
Department of Psychiatry, Faculty of Medicine, Fukuoka University, Fukuoka, Japan

Leo Gotoh
Department of Mental Retardation and Birth Defect Research, National Institute of Neuroscience, National Center of Neurology and Psychiatry, Tokyo, Japan

Mayumi Tomita
Kurume University Graduate School of Psychology, Fukuoka, Japan

Takashi Yoshiura
Department of Radiology, Graduate School of Medical and Dental Sciences, Kagoshima University, Kagoshima, Japan

Yasunori Oda, Masatomo Ishikawa, Satoshi and Masaomi Iyo
Department of Psychiatry, Graduate School of Medicine, Chiba University, 1-8-1 Inohana, Chuo-ku, Chiba 260-8670, Japan

Tomihisa Niitsu
Department of Psychiatry, Graduate School of Medicine, Chiba University, 1-8-1 Inohana, Chuo-ku, Chiba 260-8670, Japan Fujita Hospital, 3292-Ho Yokaichiba, Sosa-shi, Chi-ba 289-2146, Japan

Hiroshi Kimura
Department of Psychiatry, Graduate School of Medicine, Chiba University, 1-8-1 Inohana, Chuo-ku, Chiba 260-8670, Japan

Kokoronokaze Funabashi Clinic, 1-26-2 Motomachi, Funabashi-shi, Chiba 273-0005, Japan

Tasuku Hashimoto
Present Address: Department of Psychiatry, Graduate School of Medicine, Chiba University, 1-8-1 Inohana, Chuo-ku, Chiba 260-8670, Japan
Sodegaura Satsukidai Hospital, 5-21 Nagauraeki-mae, Sodegaura-shi 299-0246, Japan

Akihiro Shiina Tadashi Hasegawa
Department of Psychiatry, Chiba University Hospital, 1-8-1 Inohana, Chuo-ku, Chiba 260-0856, Japan.
Kokoronokenko Tsudanuma Clinic, 2-13-13 Maebaranishi, Funabashi-shi, Chiba 274-0825, Japan.

Matsuki
Research Center for Child Mental Development, Graduate School of Medicine, Chiba University, 1-8-1 Inohana, Chuo-ku, Chiba 260-8670, Japan
Kisarazu Hospital, 2-3-1 Iwane, Kisarazu-shi, Chiba 292-0061, Japan

Michiko Nakazato
Research Center for Child Mental Development, Graduate School of Medicine, Chiba University, 1-8-1 Inohana, Chuo-ku, Chiba 260-8670, Japan
Kokoronokaze Funabashi Clinic, 1-26-2 Motomachi, Funabashi-shi, Chiba 273-0005, Japan

Masumi Tachibana
Fujita Hospital, 3292-Ho Yokaichiba, Sosa-shi, Chiba 289-2146, Japan

Katsumasa Muneoka
Kimura Hospital, 6-19 Higashihoncho, Chuo-ku, Chiba 260-0004, Japan

Kelelemua Haile and Getinet Ayano
Department of Psychiatry, Amanuel Mental Specialized Hospital, Addis Ababa, Ethiopia

Tadesse Awoke
Department of Epidemiology and Biostatistics, University of Gondar, Gondar, Ethiopia.

Minale Tareke and Andargie Abate
College of Medicine and Health Science, Bahir Dar University, Bahir Dar, Ethiopia

Mulugeta Nega
College of Medicine and Health Science, Haramaya University, Harer, Ethiopia

Christoph U. Correll
Hofstra North Shore LIJ School of Medicine, Manhasset, NY, USA
The Zucker Hillside Hospital, Glen Oaks, NY, USA

Daisy S. Ng-Mak and Krithika Rajagopalan
Sunovion Pharmaceuticals Inc., 84 Waterford Dr., Marlborough, MA 01752, USA

Dana Stafkey-Mailey and Eileen Farrelly
Xcenda, Palm Harbor, FL, USA

Antony Loebel
Sunovion Pharmaceuticals Inc., Fort Lee, NJ, USA

Jae Ho Chung and Yong Won Lee
Department of Internal Medicine, International St. Mary's Hospital, Catholic Kwandong University College of Medicine, Incheon, Republic of Korea

Sun- Hyun Kim
Department of Family Medicine, International St. Mary's Hospital, Catholic Kwandong University College of Medicine, Simgokro 100 Gil 25 Seo-gu, Incheon 22711, Republic of Korea

Lidija Injac Stevovic
Clinical Department of Psychiatry, Clinical Centre of Montenegro, Podgorica, Montenegro.
Department of Psychiatry, School of Medicine, University of Montenegro, Dzona Dzeksona bb, Podgorica, Montenegro

Sanja Vodopic
Clinical Department of Neurology, Clinical Centre of Montenegro, Dzona Dzeksona bb, Podgorica, Montenegro

Marc-Andreas Edel, Brian Blackwell, Tanja Fox and Patrik Roser
Department of Psychiatry, Psychotherapy and Preventive Medicine, LWL University Hospital, Ruhr University Bochum, Alexandrinenstr. 1-3, 44791 Bochum, Germany

Ida Sibylle Haussleiter and Georg Juckel
Department of Psychiatry, Psychotherapy and Preventive Medicine, LWL University Hospital, Ruhr University Bochum, Alexandrinenstr. 1-3, 44791 Bochum, Germany
Institute of Mental Health, LWL University Hospital Bochum, Bochum, Germany

Markus Schaub Barbara Emons and Friederike Tornau
Institute of Mental Health, LWL University Hospital Bochum, Bochum, Germany

Bernward Vieten
LWL Hospital Paderborn, Paderborn, Germany

Hiroko Kashiwagi, Mayuko Koyama, Daisuke Saito and Naotsugu Hirabayashi
Department of Forensic Psychiatry, National Center Hospital of Neurology and Psychiatry, 4-1-1, Ogawahigashicho, Kodaira, Tokyo 187-8553, Japan

Akiko Kikuchi
Department of Forensic Psychiatry, National Institute of Mental Health, National Center of Neurology and Psychiatry, Kodaira, Tokyo, Japan

Bereket Duko
Faculty of Health Sciences, College of Medicine and Health Sciences, Hawassa University, Ethiopia

Getinet Ayano
Research and Training Directorate, Amanuel Mental Specialized Hospital, Addis Ababa, Ethiopia.

Claudia Carmassi, Camilla Gesi, Martina Corsi, Ivan M. Cremone, Carlo A. Bertelloni, Enrico Massimetti, Ciro Conversano and Liliana Dell'Osso
Section of Psychiatry, Department of Clinical and Experimental Medicine, University of Pisa, Via Roma 67, 56100 Pisa, Italy

Maria Cristina Olivieri and Massimo Santini
Emergency Medicine and Emergency Room Unit, AOUP, Pisa, Italy

Reindolf Anokye, Enoch Acheampong and Adjei Gyimah Akwasi
Centre for Disability and Rehabilitation Studies, Department of Community Health, Kwame Nkrumah University of Science and Technology, Kumasi, Ghana

Amy Budu-Ainooson
School of Public Health, Department of Health Education and Promotion, Kwame Nkrumah University of Science and Technology, Kumasi, Ghana

Edmund Isaac Obeng
Methodist University College, Accra, Ghana

Hiba Alblooshi
School of Human Sciences, The University of Western Australia, Crawley, WA, Australia.
School of Psychiatry and Clinical Neurosciences, The University of Western Australia, Crawley, WA, Australia

Gary Hulse
School of Psychiatry and Clinical Neurosciences, The University of Western Australia, Crawley, WA, Australia
School of Medical and Health Sciences, Edith Cowan University, Perth, WA, Australia

Guan K. Tay
School of Psychiatry and Clinical Neurosciences, The University of Western Australia, Crawley, WA, Australia
School of Medical and Health Sciences, Edith Cowan University, Perth, WA, Australia
Center of Biotechnology, Khalifa University of Science, Technology and Research, Abu Dhabi, United Arab Emirates
Faculty of Biomedical Engineering, Khalifa University of Science, Technology and Research, Abu Dhabi, United Arab Emirates

Wael Osman
Center of Biotechnology, Khalifa University of Science, Technology and Research, Abu Dhabi, United Arab Emirates

Habiba Al Safar
Center of Biotechnology, Khalifa University of Science, Technology and Research, Abu Dhabi, United Arab Emirates
Faculty of Biomedical Engineering, Khalifa University of Science, Technology and Research, Abu Dhabi, United Arab Emirates

Ahmed El Kashef, Mansour Shawky and Hamad Al Ghaferi
United Arab Emirates National Rehabilitation Center, Abu Dhabi, United Arab Emirates

Frank Kruisdijk
Department Innova, GGz Centraal Innova, Amersfoort, The Netherlands
Body@Work, TNO-VU University Medical Center, Amsterdam, The Netherlands

Ingrid Hendriksen and Erwin Tak
Body@Work, TNO-VU University Medical Center, Amsterdam, The Netherlands

The Netherlands Organisation for Applied Scientific Research TNO, Leiden, The Netherlands

Marijke Hopman-Rock
Body@Work, TNO-VU University Medical Center, Amsterdam, The Netherlands
The Netherlands Organisation for Applied Scientific Research TNO, Leiden, The Netherlands
Department of Public and Occupational Health, EMGO Institute for Health and Care Research, VU University Medical Center, Amsterdam, The Netherlands

Aart-Jan Beekman
Department of Psychiatry, VU University Medical Center, Amsterdam, The Netherlands

Angela J. Pereira-Morales and Diego A. Forero
Laboratory of Neuropsychiatric Genetics, Biomedical Sciences Research Group, School of Medicine, Universidad Antonio Nariño, Bogotá 110231, Colombia

Ana Adan
Department of Clinical Psychology and Psychobiology, School of Psychology, University of Barcelona, Barcelona, Spain.
Institute of Neurosciences, University of Barcelona, Barcelona, Spain

Sandra Lopez-Leon
Novartis Pharmaceuticals Corporation, One Health Plaza, East Hanover, NJ 07936-1080, USA

Anish Shah
Siyan Clinical Corporation, 480 Tesconi Dr., Santa Rosa, CA 95401, USA

Joanne Northcutt
Northcutt Consulting, LLC, Orlando, USA

Athanasios Apostolopoulos, Ioannis Michopoulos, Emmanouil Rizos, Georgios Tzeferakos, and Athanasios Douzenis
2nd Psychiatric Department of the University of Athens, Attikon Hospital, Athens, Greece

Charalambos Papageorgiou
1st Psychiatric Department of the University of Athens, Aeginition Hospital, Athens, Greece

Ioannis Zachos and Vasiliki Manthou
Organization Against Drugs, Athens, Greece

Angelo G. I. Maremmani
Department of Psychiatry, North-Western Tuscany Local Health Unit, Versilian
Zone, Viareggio, Italy
AU-CNS, Association for the Application of Neuroscientific Knowledge to Social Aims, Pietrasanta, Lucca, Italy
G. De Lisio Institute of Behavioural Sciences, Pisa, Italy

Icro Maremmani
AU-CNS, Association for the Application of Neuroscientific Knowledge to Social Aims, Pietrasanta, Lucca, Italy
G. De Lisio Institute of Behavioural Sciences, Pisa, Italy
Vincent P. Dole Dual Diagnosis Unit, Department of Specialty Medicine, Santa Chiara University Hospital, University of Pisa, Pisa, Italy
Alessandro Pallucchini4, Silvia Bacciardi4, Vincenza Spera, Marco Maiello, School of Psychiatry, University of Pisa, Pisa, Italy

Luca Rovai
Department of Psychiatry, North-Western Tuscany Local Health Unit, Apuan Zone, Massa, Italy

Giulio Perugi
Department of Clinical and Experimental Medicine, University of Pisa, Pisa, Italy

Caroline Lücke, Sebastian Moeller, Charlotte E. Schneider, Aikaterini Zikidi and Alexandra Philipsen
Medical Campus University of Oldenburg, School of Medicine and Health Sciences, Psychiatry and Psychotherapy-University Hospital, Karl-Jaspers-Klinik, Hermann-Ehlers-Straße 7, 26160 Bad Zwischenahn, Germany

Helge H. O. Müller
Medical Campus University of Oldenburg, School of Medicine and Health Sciences, Psychiatry and Psychotherapy-University Hospital, Karl-Jaspers-Klinik, Hermann-Ehlers-Straße 7, 26160 Bad Zwischenahn, Germany
Department of Psychiatry and Psychotherapy, Friedrich-Alexander-University Erlangen-Nuremberg, Erlangen, Germany

Jürgen M. Gschossmann
Department of Internal Medicine, Klinikum Forchheim, Forchheim, Germany

Teja W. Grömer
Department of Psychiatry and Psychotherapy, Friedrich-Alexander-University Erlangen-Nuremberg, Erlangen, Germany

Yanjun Zhang
College of Teacher Education, Zhejiang Normal University, Jinhua, Zhejiang Province, People's Republic of China

JiuYu Xiang
School of Marxism, Wuhan University, Wuhan, Hubei Province, People's Republic of China

Jianlin Wen
School of Marxism, Chongqing University, No. 174 Shazhengjie, Shapingba, Chongqing 400044, People's Republic of China

Wei Bian
Southwest Eye Hospital, Third Military Medical University, Chongqing, People's Republic of China

Liangbin Sun and Ziran Bai
School of Journalism and Communication, Chongqing University, Chongqing, People's Republic of China

Dong-Woo Choi, Sung-Youn Chun and Sang Ah Lee
Department of Public Health, Graduate School, Yonsei University, Seoul, Republic of Korea
Institute of Health Services Research, Yonsei University, Seoul, Republic of Korea

Eun-Cheol Park
Institute of Health Services Research, Yonsei University, Seoul, Republic of Korea
Department of Preventive Medicine, Yonsei University College of Medicine, 50 Yonsei-ro, Seodaemun-gu, Seoul 03722, Republic of Korea

Kyu-Tae Han
Department of Policy Research Affairs, National Health Insurance Service Ilsan Hospital, Koyang, Republic of Korea

Reem Jarrad and Tagreed Shawashi
Clinical Nursing Department-School of Nursing, The University of Jordan, Amman 11942, Jordan

Sawsan Hammad
Community Health Department-School of Nursing, The University of Jordan, Amman, Jordan

Naser Mahmoud
Jordan Ministry of Health-Fuheis Psychiatric Hospital, Amman, Jordan

Index

www.ingramcontent.com/pod-product-compliance
Lightning Source LLC
Chambersburg PA
CBHW061311190326
41458CB00011B/3780

* 9 7 8 1 6 3 2 4 2 7 8 6 1 *